中国食物成分表 2004

China Food Composition 2004

（第二册／Book 2）

中国疾病预防控制中心营养与食品安全所　编著

Institute of Nutrition and Food Safety, China CDC

编　委　Edited by

主　编　杨月欣　Yang Yuexin

副主编　何　梅　He Mei

　　　　潘兴昌　Pan Xingchang

编校人员　（按姓氏笔画排序）

门建华　王　竹　王光亚　王国栋　王红伟

王惠君　石　磊　边立华　刘　兰　李　东

李建文　沈　湘　何宇纳　杨晶明　杨晓光

杨晓莉　涂晓明　周瑞华　郑玉梅　徐　筠

郭　军　唐华澄　韩军花　薛　颖　翟凤英

北京大学医学出版社

Peking University Medical Press

ZHONGGUO SHIWU CHENGFENBIAO

图书在版编目（CIP）数据

中国食物成分表2004/杨月欣主编. —北京：北京大学医学出版社，2005（2018.3重印）
ISBN 978-7-81071-678-9

Ⅰ. 中…　Ⅱ. 杨…　Ⅲ. 食物营养－营养成分－数据－中国－2004　Ⅳ. R151. 3

中国版本图书馆 CIP 数据核字（2004）第 136238 号

中国食物成分表 2004

主　　编：杨月欣
出版发行：北京大学医学出版社
地　　址：（100191）北京市海淀区学院路 38 号 北京大学医学部院内
电　　话：发行部 010-82802230；图书邮购 010-82802495
网　　址：http://www.pumpress.com.cn
E-mail：booksale@bjmu.edu.cn
印　　刷：北京圣彩虹制版印刷技术有限公司
经　　销：新华书店
责任编辑：赵　莳　**责任校对**：何士茹　**责任印制**：罗德刚
开　　本：889mm × 1194mm　1/16　**印张**：23　**彩插**：6　**字数**：579 千字
版　　次：2005 年 5 月第 1 版　2018 年 3 月第 10 次印刷
书　　号：ISBN 978-7-81071-678-9
定　　价：148.00 元

人人讲营养
全民都健康

于若木

序 FOREWORD

食物成分数据是一个国家必需的科学数据，也是公共卫生体系基础建设的重要组成部分。我国食物资源丰富，种类繁多，研究和了解各种食物的组成和营养学特性，不仅是医学、营养学、食品科学必不可少的基础性资料，也是国家制定食物发展纲要、实施有关营养政策和健康教育的基础。众多流行病学调查和营养学研究已经证实：膳食构成不仅影响着人体的生长发育、体质强弱、工作效率等，同时与心脑血管病、糖尿病、癌症等各种慢性病的发生、发展以及人群的亚健康状态有着密切的联系。随着我国经济的发展，国民生活水平的不断提高，人们对食物的要求不再仅为安全卫生的概念，“营养健康”、“膳食平衡”已开始成为一个普遍追求的生活理念。因此，正确认识食物，加强营养指导，科学引导消费，预防营养缺乏病和营养相关性慢性病，提高整个中华民族的身体素质，乃是营养和食品卫生工作者的重要任务。

一些国际组织，如联合国粮农组织(FAO)、世界卫生组织(WHO)和国际科技数据委员会(CODATA)等，近年来积极倡导科技数据的建设和共享，并认为科技数据的建设和共享是发展国民经济和提高社会效益的极为重要的环节。最近几年食物成分数据作为我国国家科学数据的重要组成部分，受到科技界的普遍重视。国家科技部加大了对研究机构获得此类数据的投入和支持的力度，从而促进了公共卫生体系内涵建设的发展。在中国疾病预防控制中心的学者们的努力下，《中国食物成分表2004》即将出版。这是对我国食物成分数据的又一次丰富和发展，将更有利于促进我国居民的营养健康状况和防病治病工作；对预防医学领域的研究和全国营养调查工作的开展也将会有较大的支持和推动。值此书出版之际，欣然作序，以示祝贺，并希望广大营养工作者今后更好地服务于我国公共卫生体系建设。

王陇德　副部长

中华人民共和国卫生部

2004年10月

FOREWORD

National food composition data is an important asset for a country of the world, which is also the integral part of any public health system of a country. China holds abundance and variety of food resources. Studying and understanding Chinese foods and establishing a Chinese food composition database will not only provide essential information to health professionals working in medicine, nutrition, dietetics and food sciences but also contribute to the formulation of national food development programs, food and nutrition-related policies, and health education strategies. Numerous researches of epidemiological and nutritional studies have found that food and nutrients intake not only contributes to the building blocks of human body and working efficiency but also links to the risk of developing diet-related chronic diseases such as cardiovascular diseases, cerebrovascular diseases, diabetes and cancers, as well as the sub-healthy status of a population, etc. In recent decades, a remarkable economic growth and a steady improvement in living standards of people has taken place in China. Nowadays, the Chinese people are more concerned with the health significance of foods and dietary balance rather than only with food sanitation and safety. Hence, the responsibility of health professionals is to provide updated scientific information on food nutrition and dietary guidelines to the general publics in order to help them prevent malnutrition, diet-related chronic diseases, and to continuously improve the health status of whole people in the nation.

FAO, WHO and CODATA have advocated developing a scientific and uniformed food composition database in recent years, for which the data can be shared with each other in all countries. They believe that this is the best approach to benefit the economic growth of a nation and the common interest of international societies.

The development of the Chinese food composition data, as a major part of the nation's scientific database, has drawn a great deal of attention in many scientific communities in China. The Ministry of Science and Technology of the People's Republic of China has increased investment and financial supports on this project, which will expedite the public health system of our nation. I would like to express my appreciation to the scientists and experts from the China CDC who provided tremendous inputs on this project. The studies on food composition data have further enriched and consolidated the existing food composition database in China. The publication of the Food Composition 2004 will make a further great stride for improving the health and nutritional status of Chinese people, promote disease prevention and control, and support the works on preventive medicine and nutrition surveys. On this special occasion of publishing this book, it would be my great pleasure to write a preface with my heartfelt congratulations, and it is also my sincere hope that our efforts on the public health in China will make a better serve for Chinese people.

Vice Minister: Wang Longde
Ministry of Health of the People's Republic of China
Oct. 2004

前言

PREFACE

21世纪，人类进入信息时代。作为重要的信息资源，众多科学数据兼具学术、经济、社会等多种价值，成为产生经济和社会效益的重要环节，成为知识创新工程、社会发展和进步的极为重要的资源。

在国家有关部委的支持下，中国食物成分数据研究工作近年来得到较大发展。自2000年以来，中国CDC营养与食品安全所在食物成分数据的研究方面先后完成了四个项目。这些工作不仅是对我国食物成分数据的有力补充，更是对营养学和食物科学研究、疾病预防等公共卫生体系建设的重要支持。

2004年版的食物成分数据仍力求在食物分类及编码、营养成分的数据表达等方面与国际组织INFOODS的规范和国内现有标准相一致。除此之外，本版与2002年的修订版相比还有几个突出的特点：首先是所有的食物数据都是新分析的数据，而且有较多的加工食品和消费量大的基本食物如大米、蔬菜等。某些食物虽然过去有数据，但同20世纪80年代相比，由于种植条件和加工方法早已发生变化，所以重新分析这些基本食物是有重要意义的。其次是补充了食物样品描述信息，便于使用者了解食物的具体信息和寻找对应的食物。第三是增加了总膳食纤维、可溶性膳食纤维、不溶性膳食纤维、维生素B_6、维生素B_{12}、维生素K_1、生物素、泛酸、胆碱、叶酸等对健康有益成分的数据。我们相信这些改进必将有力地支持营养学方面的研究，并有助于推进食品工业的发展。

鉴于国家居民营养调查和研究的需要，本书中收录了一些常见包装食品。这些食品的营养成分数据多是征得生产者同意后摘抄其营养标签，仅有少量是分析的数据。因为我国多数包装食品配方还不能长久固定，使用时仅供参考。

本书是一本以专业人员为主要读者的科学参考书，包括了757条食物的近5万个数据。这些数据既是营养学研究的基础，也是营养学发展进步的成果，又是推动农作物更新、食品营养强化、新资源食品、保健食品以及食品工业不断发展进步的关键。我们高兴地将此书献给在营养学、流行病学、医学、食品工业等各相关领域工作的每一位科技工作者，并希望它能够与您的工作构成良性的互馈，成为您工作的助手和成就的阶石。

本书的数据整理、核对和编辑花费了大量的人力、物力和时间，由于其数据较多、涉及专业面广以及我们水平有限，可能存在这样或那样的失误或错误。我们衷心盼望广大读者能函告我们，并提出宝贵意见和建议。来函请寄：nutri@163.com；或北京市宣武区南纬路29号，中国疾病预防控制中心营养与食品安全所，邮编：100050。

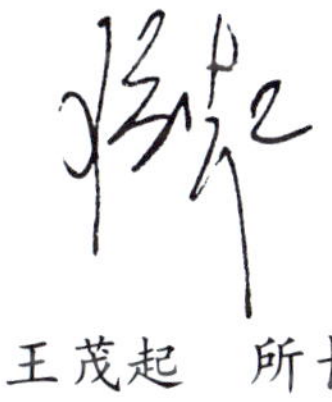

王茂起　所长

中国 CDC 营养与食品安全所

2004 年 10 月　北京

PREFACE

The 21st century is an era of information. Enormous scientific information bearing academic, economic and social significance has made big contribution to the economic growth and social development, which also provide fundamental resources for knowledge-based innovation programs.

With the strong support from the national ministries and commissions, the research on Chinese food composition data has made rapid progress in recent years. Since 2000, the Institute of Nutrition and Food Safety, China CDC has accomplished four projects related to the development of food composition data. Furthermore, the expanded data in 2004 edition has made a complementation to the existing food composition database and has provided the most updated information to the researchers in the areas of nutrition and food sciences.

During the development of the 2004 edition, we had complied strictly to the standards at national and international level. In terms of food classification, coding and expression of nutrient contents, etc. we made an effort to meet the requirement of FAO INFOODS and national standards. Several remarkable features in the 2004 edition could be found when compared with the 2002 edition. Firstly, many new processed food items are added, and many core foods commony consumed by people, such as rice and vegetables are reanalyzed. Although some previous data are still in place, the reanalysis on these 'core foods' still makes a sense, because a substantial changes on the mode of cultivation and food processing taken place since 1980s. Secondly, the descriptions of food items are given, so as to facilitate the readers to search for a right food item. The last but not the least, the number of food nutrients is expanded and some non-nutrient components that are beneficial to human health were added, namely, total dietary fiber, soluble dietary fiber, insoluble dietary fiber, vitamin $B_{6,}$ vitamin $B_{12,}$ vitamin K_1, biotin, pantothenic acid and folate, etc. We are sure that these new features in 2004 edition will definitely facilitate for the development of nutritional science and food industry.

In response to the demands in nutrition research and dietary survey, the data for some popular packaged foods are included in this edition; most of the data for these packaged foods were supplied by the manufacturers while only a few data was based on analytical results. Because the food components of packaged foods available in China may be changed from time to time, the information on the food labeling is only for reference.

There are about fifty thousand food composition data on 757 food items in the 2004 edition of Chinese Food Composition Table. This book is served as a professional reference book for scientists working in nutrition and dietetics, epidemiology, medical science and for food industries. These data are not only the ground work of nutritional sciences but also the result of a substantial progress in nutrition field. Furthermore, these data can be worked as key reference materials for crop renovation, food enrichment with nutrients and developing novel foods and functional foods. We hope that this edition will assist you and become a cornerstone in your success.

A great deal of time, manpower and resources has been taken to carry out the analysis on food components, data evaluation and data compilation. Some inaccuracies and errors might exist in this book, because the volume of data is so large, the range of specialized fields is so wide, and the limitation of our knowledge is existed to some extent. We sincerely hope that the readers would let us know if any error or inaccuracy spotted in this book. Your comments and suggestions would be the precious gifts for us. Please email us at nutri@163.com or send letters to the Institute of Nutrition and Food Safety, China CDC, #29, Nanwei Road, Xuanwu District, Beijing, 100050, China.

Director: Wang Maoqi
Institute of Nutrition and Food Safety, China CDC
Oct. 2004, Beijing

致谢

ACKNOWLEDGEMENTS

本书所包含的近5万个食物成分数据，从筹划到立项、从研究到今天出版，历经了四年有余的时间，今天终于可以面对广大的使用者了。在本书完成之际，我代表项目执行单位衷心感谢所有给予中国食物成分数据工作关心、支持和指导的国内外专家学者和科研基金机构。

本书所包含的所有数据是在政府的重视下完成的，没有国家科技部、北京市自然科学基金委、中国CDC达能营养中心等基金的支持，没有参加这些项目的百余名科技工作者的努力，我们无论如何也不能把过去50年才完成的数据，在这短短的四年内完成！这里首先要感谢国家科技部、北京市自然科学基金委和中国CDC达能营养中心对国家食物数据的重视和鼎力支持；同时也感谢与我共同奋斗了四年的项目组全体成员，特别是合作单位北京市疾病预防控制中心、北京市营养源研究所等单位的学者们。我知道从第一次讨论立项到最后的项目总结，从食物的采集到逐个食物的营养成分分析，从一个个记录的核对到全书出版，处处都有大家的辛勤和努力，更渗透着项目组全体成员的知识和智慧！

我们还特别感谢香港中文大学的Warren TK Lee博士、FAO INFOODS的Barbara Burlingame博士和本所的闻芝梅教授。在本项目的执行和本书的编辑出版过程中，他们不但给予了友好跟踪关注、帮助和建议，而且还多次修改了英文版本，在保障本书的食物成分概念、定义、分析方法以及英文译文的正确性、准确性等方面给予了无私的帮助。正是有了他们的帮助，才使我们不断减少错误，逐步接近国际先进水平，并与世界食物成分数据研究同路前进。

本书首次收集了居民日常膳食消费量较大的一些包装食品的数据，我们衷心感谢这些食品生产企业在产品营养成分数据方面给予的全面支持。

特别值得说明的是，书中的21大类757条食物的近5万个数据，基本上是经本书的编者和校核者之手在1200多天的时间里分析出来的，而且也是经他们之手反复核实、对比和核定的结果。在本书出版之际，向所有参与或给予中国食物成分数据关心、支持和指导的专家学者、提供科学基金的组织表示衷心的感谢！

杨月欣

中国CDC营养与食品安全所

2004年10月 北京

ACKNOWLEDGEMENTS

On behalf of the working group of the Chinese Food Composition Data Program, I would like to extend my heartfelt appreciation to all scientists and experts, research institutes and foundations for their concerns, supports and guidance on the development of the Chinese food composition data.

There is total about fifty thousand food composition data comprised in this book. The preparation and implementation of these programs, from grant application and laboratory analysis to data publication, have spent more than four years. The accomplishment of these projects represent the result of collective research efforts of all project team members, without the cooperative efforts of more than one hundred scientists, the achievement is impossible. I would like to express my heartfelt thanks to all project team members working with us for four years, especially those experts from the collaborating institutions, including Beijing Center for Disease Control and Prevention, Beijing Institute of Nutrient Source Research, and also other colleagues from our institute. The efforts from discussing the study design, collecting and analyzing food samples, checking records one-by-one, summarizing to publishing data, etc., reflected the collective knowledge and intelligence of all team members.

The funding agencies in China are very supportive for these projects. We are grateful to the Ministry of Science and Technology, Beijing Natural Science Foundation and the Danone Institute affiliated to the China CDC. We wish to give thanks particularly to Dr. Warren TK Lee from the Chinese University of Hong Kang, Dr. Barbara Burlingame, Dr. Ruth from INFOODS of FAO, and Prof. ZhimeiWen from our institute, who gave advices on the definition, concept and description of foods in English version of this book. Their precious comments and advices made us to minimize the error, inaccuracy and misinterpretation on data, and help us to comply with the international codes and standards.

Special thanks are also due to those food enterprises that provided us with package food samples and food data. This is the first time for us to include the data of common packaged foods in the Chinese Food Composition Table. We wholeheartedly thank those food manufacturers who have made considerable progress in nutrient analysis and offered supports. With these achievements and supports, we firmly believe that a continuous improvement on China's food composition database to meet the public demands is possible.

It is worth mentioning that more than 1200 days and nights have been taken for the editors and collators to analyze, verify, compare and review hardly for about fifty thousand data on 21 food categories. On this special occasion, it would be a great pleasure for me to express my devout appreciation to all scientists and experts rendering concerns, supports and guidance to the production of Chinese food composition data and those organizations providing funds to support this scientific project.

Yang Yuexin
Institute of Nutrition and Food Safety, China CDC
Oct. 2004, Beijing

目录

CONTENTS

使用说明

1 概述

《中国食物成分表2004》内容包括五个部分：使用说明、食物描述、食物成分表、附录和食物图片。

本书共包含757条食物，其中一部分是1992年全国营养调查中居民消费量较高的前100种基本食物，一部分是1999～2000年间食物消费频率调查中消费量较高的前20类加工食品。另外，还涉及一些新品种食物、工业产品及珍稀食品。

食物成分表中的营养成分包括了能量、水分、灰分、膳食纤维和宏量营养素共10种，维生素15种，矿物质11种，氨基酸20种，脂肪酸38种。

为提高对数据理解和应用的准确性，本书还给出了较为详细的食物描述，并附有部分食物图片，以供参考。

2 数据来源

《中国食物成分表2004》中包括的数据主要是国家科技部2001年公益基金项目、国家科技部基础项目、北京自然科学基金项目(3002010)以及达能营养基金项目(2001)的研究结果。少数数据引用国内外食物成分表和科学文献中发表的数据以及食品标签中的营养成分数据。对于借鉴和引用的数据，在“食物描述”部分中的“数据来源”一栏中予以注明。具体说明如下：

“UK-FCT” ——英国食物成分表(2002)
“USA-FCT” ——美国食物成分数据库(SR16)
“Japan-FCT” ——日本食物成分表(2000)
“Korea-FCT” ——韩国食物成分表(2001)
“ShH-FCT” ——上海食物成分表(1990)
“FJ-FCT” ——福建食物成分表(1991)
“YN-FCT” ——云南食物成分表(2003)
“FNL” ——食品营养标签

3 食物的名称、分类与编码

3.1 食物名称

食物名称由中文学名和别名组成，均在食物名称中列出。附录中还给出了全部食物的英文名称、部分食物的拉丁文名称和图片。

为了便于使用者对食物信息的了解，食物描述表中对食物的颜色、形状、质地、生产加工方式、地区来源以及配方等做了较为详细的说明，对食物的分析部位和样品前处理的方法等也有介绍。

3.2 食物分类

《中国食物成分表2004》中的食物分类方法与2002版基本相同，共分为21大类。每一大类中根据食物的属性和加工方法又分为不同的亚类，并将那些难以分配到某一具体亚类的食物归入到相应食物类中的名为“其它”的亚类中。

我国标准化管理委员会于2002年制定的食品工业标准体系分类标准，将食品工业制品分为19大类，其中各大类又分为若干门类。本书食物分类中亚类的设置也参照了此标准。具体的食物分类及食物数量见表 1。

表 1　食物分类及食物数量一览表

食物类编码	食物类名称	食物条数	亚类编码	亚类名称	食物条数
01	谷类及制品	29			
			1	小麦	11
			2	稻米	9
			3	玉米	4
			4	大麦	1
			5	小米	1
			9	其它	3
02	薯类、淀粉及制品	11			
			1	薯类	6
			2	淀粉类	5
03	干豆类及制品	17			
			1	大豆	11
			2	绿豆	0
			3	赤豆	2
			4	芸豆	0
			5	蚕豆	1
			9	其它	3
04	蔬菜类及制品	82			
			1	根菜类	8
			2	鲜豆菜和豆苗类	9
			3	茄果、瓜菜类	20
			4	葱蒜类	3
			5	嫩茎、叶、花菜类	35
			6	水生蔬菜类	1
			7	薯芋类	2
			8	野生蔬菜类	4
05	菌藻类	31			
			1	菌类	28
			2	藻类	3
06	水果类及制品	24			
			1	仁果类	1
			2	核果类	6
			3	浆果类	2
			4	柑橘类	2
			5	热带、亚热带水果	12
			6	瓜果类	1
07	坚果、种子类	22			
			1	树坚果	15
			2	种子	7

续表

食物类编码	食物类名称	食物条数	亚类编码	亚类名称	食物条数
08	畜肉类及制品	59			
			1	猪	35
			2	牛	15
			3	羊	7
			4	驴	1
			5	马	0
			9	其它	1
09	禽肉类及制品	15			
			1	鸡	8
			2	鸭	3
			3	鹅	1
			4	火鸡	1
			9	其它	2
10	乳类及制品	47			
			1	液态乳	17
			2	奶粉	20
			3	酸奶	2
			4	奶酪	4
			5	奶油	1
			9	其它	3
11	蛋类及制品	10			
			1	鸡蛋	7
			2	鸭蛋	2
			3	鹅蛋	1
			4	鹌鹑蛋	0
12	鱼虾蟹贝类	44			
			1	鱼	34
			2	虾	3
			3	蟹	2
			4	贝	2
			9	其它	3
13	婴幼儿食品	58			
			1	婴幼儿配方粉	43
			2	婴幼儿断奶期辅助食品	3
			3	婴幼儿补充食品	12
14	小吃、甜饼	13			
			1	小吃	5
			2	蛋糕、甜点	8
15	速食食品	115			
			1	快餐食品	24
			2	方便食品	62

续表

食物类编码	食物类名称	食物条数	亚类编码	亚类名称	食物条数
			3	休闲食品	29
16	饮料类	63			
			1	碳酸饮料	1
			2	果汁及果汁饮料	17
			3	蔬菜汁饮料	1
			4	含乳饮料	5
			5	植物蛋白饮料	5
			6	茶叶及茶饮料	2
			7	固体饮料	8
			8	冰激凌、棒冰类	12
			9	其它	12
17	含酒精饮料	32			
			1	发酵酒	12
			2	蒸馏酒	13
			3	露酒(配制酒)	7
18	糖、果脯和蜜饯、蜂蜜	31			
			1	糖	0
			2	糖果	12
			3	果脯和蜜饯	14
			4	蜂蜜	5
19	油脂类	9			
			1	动物油脂	0
			2	植物油	9
20	调味品类	33			
			1	酱油	3
			2	醋	0
			3	酱	10
			4	腐乳	3
			5	咸菜类	13
			6	香辛料	1
			7	盐、味精及其它	3
21	其它	12			

3.3 食物编码

食物编码主要根据食物分类的规则进行。一条食物的编码共有6位数字，前2位是食物的类别编码，第3位是食物的亚类编码，最后3位是食物在亚类中的排列序号。食物类别编码、食物亚类编码见表1。

任一食物的编码在食物成分表中具有唯一性，即同一条食物在食物一般营养成分表、食物氨基酸含量表、食物脂肪酸含量表以及食物胆碱、生物素、泛酸、维生素K、维生素D含量表中采用同一编码。

4 食物的可食部

所有营养素的含量均以100g可食部食物来表达。很多食物具有不可食部分，对于从市场上采集来的食物（称为“样品”），分析工作者按照居民通常的加工、烹调和饮食习惯，去掉其中不可食用的部分后，剩余的即为食物的可食部。如香蕉要去掉皮，猪排要去掉骨头等。“可食部”栏中的数值表示某一食物中可食用部分占食物样品的百分比，用于计算食物可食部分的重量。计算 1000g 食物中营养成分的含量，可用下面的公式：

$$X = A \times 10 \times (EP / 100)$$

其中 X：1000g 市售食物中某营养素的含量；

A：食物成分表中每 100g 可食部中该种营养素的含量；

EP：食物成分表中可食部比例。

食物的可食部比例不是固定不变的，它会因运输、贮藏和加工处理等方面的不同而有所差异。因此，当认为食物实际的可食部比例与表中的数值有较大出入时，可以采用自己实际测定的食物可食部的比例来计算营养素含量。

5 食物成分的定义

5.1 能量

能量为计算值，采用各供能营养素（蛋白质、脂肪、碳水化合物、酒精）含量乘以相应的能量折算系数（表 2），再求和而得。能量的单位采用千卡 (kilocalorie, kcal) 和千焦耳 (kilojoule, kJ)，彼此间的换算为 1 卡能量相当于 4.184 焦耳。

表 2　能量折算系数 *

营养素名称	kcal/g	kJ/g
蛋白质	4	17
脂肪	9	37
碳水化合物	4	17
酒精（乙醇）	7	29

* Royal Society (1972)

最近，世界粮农组织 (FAO) 推荐使用 2 kcal/g 为膳食纤维的能量值。基于与 2002 版食物成分数据的一致性，本书暂仍采用 2002 年食物成分表的原则，即食物成分表中膳食纤维的能量值为 0。

另外，当使用“( )”或“Tr”表示供能营养素如蛋白质、脂肪或碳水化合物的数值时，由此所计算的能量数值也可能存在着一定程度的偏差。借鉴、引用的食物成分数据，其能量值为原文引用数值。当借鉴、引用的食物能量数据仅给出千卡或千焦耳的数值时，本书中以4.184作为换算系数进行计算，并以字母“c”加以标注。当某些食物的能量值不能由其成分计算时，用“un”加以标注。某些婴幼儿食品的能量值为厂家提供的数据，没有采用表中的折算系数。

5.2 宏量营养素

蛋白质和氨基酸　食物蛋白质是用凯氏微量定氮法 (Kjeldahl法) 测定食物的总氮量，再乘以相应的蛋白质折算系数换算而得。在多数食物中总氮占蛋白质的 16%，所以由总氮计算蛋白质含量的折算系数一般用 6.25 (100/16)。但是有些食物中非蛋白质来源的氮含量较高，因此折算系数也不同。本书采用了联合国粮农组织和世界卫生组织 (FAO/WHO) 1973 年推荐使用的食物蛋白质折算系数（表 3）。

表3 蛋白质折算系数*

食 物	折算系数	食 物	折算系数
小麦		蛋类	
全麦	5.83	全蛋	6.25
麦糠麸皮	6.31	蛋白	6.32
胚芽	5.80	蛋黄	6.12
胚乳	5.70	肉类和鱼类	6.25
燕麦	5.83	动物明胶	5.55
大麦及大麦粉	5.83	乳及乳制品	6.38
黑麦及黑麦粉	5.83	酪蛋白	6.40
小米	6.31	人乳	6.37
玉米	6.25	豆类	
稻米及米粉	5.95	大豆	5.71
坚果		其它豆类	6.25
杏仁	5.18	其它食物	6.25
巴西果	5.46		
花生	5.46		
其它	5.30		

* FAO/WHO (1973)

通常，食物蛋白质含量应相当于或高于其各种氨基酸含量之和。但是，利用折算系数计算的食物蛋白质含量与实际分析的氨基酸总和可能不能较好地吻合。为保持数据的准确性，本书食物中各种氨基酸的总和与蛋白质数值正负相差不超过 5%。

碳水化合物 本书中使用减差法计算食物中的总碳水化合物含量，其中包括了膳食纤维部分。计算公式为：

$$碳水化合物 = 100 - (水分 + 蛋白质 + 脂肪 + 灰分)$$

利用上述公式计算的食物中碳水化合物的值一般应大于或等于0。由于用减差法计算的碳水化合物的数值包含了水分、蛋白质、脂肪、灰分等成分在实际分析测定过程中的误差，因此该数值可能存在一定的偏差。本书中规定，每 100g 食物中水分、蛋白质、脂肪、灰分、碳水化合物各部分总和应≤ 105g。1998 年，FAO/WHO 强调在食物成分数据库（FCD）的研究中应该弃用这个方法，但由于各国对碳水化合物分析技术的不同及受分析条件的限制，现在 FCD 研究中大多数国家仍然使用减差法。

膳食纤维 本书数据中食物的膳食纤维检测方法主要有两种：中性洗涤剂法和 AOAC 的酶重量法。中性洗涤剂法是用中性洗涤剂来溶解除去样品中的糖、淀粉、脂肪、蛋白质、果胶等成分，剩余的残渣用淀粉酶酶解，洗净后干燥称重，即为不溶性膳食纤维部分，也可能包括少许不溶性灰分。酶重量法可以测定总膳食纤维、可溶性和不可溶性膳食纤维。可溶性膳食纤维包括果胶、寡糖等成分，不溶性膳食纤维包括纤维素、半纤维素、木质素、角质、二氧化硅等。实际上，在蔬菜和谷类等食物中，由于可溶性部分较少，不溶性膳食纤维与总膳食纤维的含量差别不大。

在本书中，用中性洗涤剂法测得的不溶性纤维数据用字母“a”加以标示；另外一些借鉴和引用的数据是用粗纤维测定法获得的，用字母“b”加以标示；未作任何标示的数据均为用酶重量法测定。

脂肪和脂肪酸 食物脂肪的测定数值实际代表粗脂肪，因其中除脂肪外，尚有游离脂肪酸、蜡、磷脂、固醇、松脂及色素等脂溶性物质。

脂肪酸数据中包含了两种表达形式：一种是各单体脂肪酸占总脂肪酸的百分比；另一种是先通过脂肪酸折算系数乘以粗脂肪含量计算出食物中总脂肪酸的含量，再利用饱和脂肪酸、单不饱和脂肪酸和多不饱和脂肪酸占总脂肪酸的百分比计算三类脂肪酸的含量。本书中所采用的“脂肪酸折算系数” 见表 4。

表 4　脂肪酸折算系数 *

食物名称	折算系数	食物名称	折算系数
小麦、大麦和黑麦		牛肉（瘦）	0.916
全麦	0.720	牛肉（肥）	0.953
面粉	0.670	羊肉（瘦）	0.916
麦麸	0.820	羊肉（肥）	0.953
燕麦	0.940	猪肉（瘦）	0.910
大米	0.850	猪肉（肥）	0.953
豆类		家禽	0.945
大豆及制品▲	0.930	脑	0.561
其它豆类▲	0.775	心	0.789
蔬菜和水果	0.800	肾	0.747
鳄梨	0.956	肝	0.741
菌藻类▲	0.562	乳及乳制品	0.945
坚果	0.956	蛋类	0.830
花生▲	0.951	鱼	
莲子▲	0.930	鱼肉 (含油多)	0.900
油脂类		鱼肉	0.700
油脂类 (椰子油除外)	0.956	虾、蟹类▲	0.723
椰子油	0.942	果酱、蜜饯类▲	0.686

* FAO (2002)

▲ USDA nutrition database (SR16)

5.3　维生素

维生素 A (Vitamin A)　维生素 A 有多种化学形式，每种有不同的生物活性。为了计算总维生素 A 生物活性，常常需要测定食物中不同形式的维生素 A，包括视黄醇、β-胡萝卜素和其它类型的胡萝卜素。维生素 A 的生物活性通常用视黄醇当量 (retinol equivalent, RE) 来表示。计算总的维生素 A 生物活性使用下述公式。

$$维生素A\ (\mu gRE) = 视黄醇\ (\mu g) + \beta\text{-}胡萝卜素\ (\mu g) / 6 + 其它类型的胡萝卜素\ (\mu g) / 12$$

在植物性食物中只有胡萝卜素，没有视黄醇。而绝大多数动物体内仅有视黄醇。植物性来源的胡萝卜素测定采用层析法，未能分型，计算中均按 β-胡萝卜素计算，即乘以系数 1 / 6。因此，视黄醇、胡萝卜素的国际单位与视黄醇当量间的转换关系如下：

$$\begin{aligned} 1\ \mu g\ RE\ Vit\ A &= 1\ \mu g\ 视黄醇 \\ &= 3.33\ IU\ 维生素A \\ &= 6\ \mu g\ \beta\text{-}胡萝卜素 \\ &= 10\ IU\ \beta\text{-}胡萝卜素 \end{aligned}$$

维生素 D (Vitamin D)　维生素 D 有两种具有生物活性的形式：维生素 D_2(麦角固醇 ergocalciferol 或钙化醇 calciferol) 和维生素 D_3(胆钙化醇 cholecalciferol)。维生素 D_2 主要由人工合成。维生素 D_3 是由表皮下 7-脱氢胆固醇 (7-dehydrocholesterol) 经紫外线光照射而形成的。现在常用的单位为重量单位微克 (μg)，而国际单位 (IU) 逐步被替代。以 0.025μg 维生素 D 作为一个活性单位，即 1 IU 维生素 D = 0.025μg 维生素 D。本书中所登载的食物中维生素 D 的数据仍用国际单位 (IU) 表示。

维生素 E (Vitamin E)　维生素 E 同维生素 A 一样，在食物中有多种存在形式，如 α、β、γ、δ-生育酚，α、β、γ、δ-二烯生育酚等，其中 α-生育酚生物活性最高。膳食中的天然维生素 E 为 d-α型生育酚，其活性以

α-生育酚当量 (α-tocopherol equivalent，α-TE) 表示，1mg α-TE 相当于 1mg α-生育酚的活性。合成的维生素 E 为 dl-α-生育酚，其活性大大低于食物中天然存在的生育酚。不同形式的维生素 E 在体内利用率不同，因此当考虑生物利用率时，计算食物中α-生育酚当量使用以下公式：

$$\alpha\text{-TE (mg)} = \alpha\text{-生育酚 (mg)} + 0.5 \times \beta\text{-生育酚 (mg)} + 0.1 \times \gamma\text{-生育酚 (mg)} + 0.3 \times \text{三烯生育酚 (mg)}$$

维生素 E 的生物活性单位还可用国际单位 (IU) 表达，与α-生育酚当量间的转换关系为：

$$1\ \text{mg}\ \alpha\text{-TE} = 1.49\ \text{IU 维生素 E}$$

各种形式维生素 E 的总和是指简单的加和。即

$$\text{维生素 E (mg)} = \alpha\text{-生育酚 (mg)} + \beta\text{-生育酚 (mg)} + \gamma\text{-生育酚 (mg)} + \delta\text{-生育酚 (mg)}$$

为与以往食物成分数据保持一致，本书同时给出食物中各种形式维生素 E 的总和、α-TE。当只有其中一个数据而又无法转换时，另一数据以“un”标示。

维生素 K (Vitamin K)　维生素 K 包括维生素 K_1 和维生素 K_2。维生素 K_1 存在于植物中，其化学名称为叶绿醌，是人类食物中维生素 K 的主要来源。维生素 K_2 存在于肠道细菌中，化学名称为甲萘醌，动物组织中含维生素 K_1 和维生素 K_2。本书中所登载的维生素 K 的数据未进行分型。

维生素 C (Vitamin C)　维生素 C 的化学结构是含有 6 个碳的 α-酮基内酯的弱酸，其天然形式为 L-型 α-异构体，膳食补充剂中的维生素 C 也是 L-抗坏血酸。L-抗坏血酸可以被氧化而成为脱氧抗坏血酸，也具有相同的生理活性，而 D-型异构体的生理活性仅为 L-型的 10%。维生素 C 存在于植物性食物中，动物性食品中含量极少，但动物血液中含有少量的维生素 C。

维生素 B_1 和 B_2 (Vitamin B_1 & B_2)　维生素 B_1 又称硫胺素 (thiamin)，因为能够预防和治疗脚气病 (beriberi)，又称为抗神经炎素。硫胺素富含于谷粒的外皮如麦麸和米糠中，动植物性食物中也含有硫胺素。维生素 B_2 又称核黄素 (Riboflavin)，存在于动植物食物中。硫胺素和核黄素是体内多种酶的辅酶，具有生理活性，并在代谢中起重要作用。

烟酸 (Niacin)　又称尼克酸。早期的名称为抗癞皮病因子 (preventive pellagra, pp)，因此又称维生素 pp，亦曾被排名为维生素 B_4 或维生素 B_5，终未成名。烟酰胺是烟酸的衍生物，是烟酸的生理活性形式。在动物性食物如肉及内脏中烟酸含量较多，植物性食物如谷类食物中的含量也不少，但植物性食物所含烟酸大部分 (约50%～70%) 为结合型，不能被人体利用。食物中的色氨酸可在人体内转变成烟酸，因此在估计其摄入量时还应考虑食物中所含色氨酸的量。一般采用 60：1 来计算色氨酸转换成烟酸的量。

维生素B_6 (Vitamin B_6)　又名吡哆素。有三种形式：吡哆醇 (PN)，吡哆醛 (PL) 和吡哆胺 (PM)，这三种形式的化合物均具有生理活性。其磷酸酯是转氨酶的辅酶，广泛存在于自然界中。本书中所给出的维生素 B_6 的数据是应用微生物法检测，检测结果为三种形式含量的总和。

维生素 B_{12} (Vitamin B_{12})　维生素 B_{12} 是一组含钴的类咕啉化合物，由 4 个还原型吡咯环相连接，中心为钴元素，该大环称为咕啉 (corrin) 环，是维生素 B_{12} 结构的核心。维生素 B_{12} 的化学名为 α-5,6-二甲苯并咪唑—氰钴胺，其分子结构中心的氰基 (CN) 可由其它基团替代，成为不同类的钴胺素。维生素 B_{12} 在食物中存在形式多样，但一般含量较少，主要存在于动物性食物及发酵食品中如动物肝脏、腐乳等。本书中列出的维生素 B_{12} 的数据为使用微生物法检测的结果。

叶酸 (Folate)　叶酸属于B族维生素，是由蝶酰和谷氨酸组成的化合物。天然食物中的叶酸含有一个或多个谷氨酸，膳食中的叶酸 3 / 4 是以蝶酰多谷氨酸的形式存在。叶酸结构中的谷氨酸分子越多则吸收率越低。本书中叶酸检测方法为微生物法。

胆碱 (Choline)　胆碱是磷脂和乙酰胆碱的重要组成部分。胆碱具强吸湿性，在空气中很快吸水，胆碱易与酸反应生成稳定的结晶。氯化胆碱在碱性条件下也不稳定，但对热稳定。胆碱广泛存在于各类动植物性食物中，尤其是蛋黄和内脏及植物胚芽中。本书胆碱数据采用柱层析－比色法检测。

生物素 (Biotin) 已知生物素有8种异构体，但仅α-生物素是天然存在的，具有生理活性。富含生物素的食物有酵母、动物的肝和其它内脏。本书中数据为微生物法检测结果。

泛酸 (Pantothnic acid) 根据译音又称之为遍多酸，也是 B 族维生素中的一种。泛酸的化学结构为 α，γ-二羟基，β，β-二甲基丁基-β-丙氨酸 (dihydroxy-β，β-dimethyl-butyl-β-alanine)。泛酸的人工合成物为泛酸钙。泛酸的主要生理功能是以乙酰辅酶 A(CoA)的形式参与二碳单位的代谢，即起传递乙酰基的作用。本书中的数据是微生物法的检测结果。

5.4 矿物质

矿物质中每日膳食需要量在100mg以上的称为常量元素，如钙、磷、镁、钾、钠、氯等。人体必需微量元素指人体需要量甚微，自身不能合成，但却有重要的生理功能，这一类微量元素必须靠食物和水供给。1990年FAO / WHO / IAEA 三个国际组织的专家委员会认定人体必需微量元素共8种，即碘、锌、硒、铜、钼、铬、钴及铁。

本书数据仅就11种矿物质 (即钙、磷、 钾、 钠、镁、铁、锌、硒、铜、锰和碘) 进行分析归纳。分析方法为火焰原子吸收法和比色法等。

6 食物成分的表达和描述

本书食物成分表中对营养成分的表达仍然沿用了 2002 版的原则。营养素名称采用《中国居民膳食营养素参考摄入量》一书中的学名或通用名称，同时还 列出英文名称。

表 5 ～ 7 列出了各个成分的具体表达方式， INFOODS 推荐的各营养素的 Tagname 暂未在一般营养成分表中使用。

表5 食物一般营养成分的表达

营养成分		计量单位	INFOODS Tagname	分析或计算方法
能量	Energy	kcal / kJ	ENERC	各供能营养素×相应的能量折算系数，并求和 *本书中能量值未包括膳食纤维提供的能量
水分	Water	g	WATER	重量法
蛋白质	Protein	g	PROCNT	凯氏定氮法 蛋白质 = 总氮×蛋白质折算系数
脂肪	Fat	g	FAT	索氏提取法、酸水解法、罗高氏法
碳水化合物	Carbohydrate (CHO)	g	CHOCDF	碳水化合物＝100－(水分＋蛋白质＋脂肪＋灰分)
总膳食纤维	Total dietary fiber	g	FIBTG	酶重量法
可溶性膳食纤维	Soluble dietary fiber	g	FIBSOL	酶重量法
不溶性膳食纤维	Insoluble dietary fiber	g	FIBINS	酶重量法
灰分	Ash	g	ASH	重量法
胆固醇	Cholesterol	mg	CHOLE	比色法
维生素 A	Vitamin A (Vit A)	μg RE	VITA	维生素 A (μg RE)＝视黄醇 (μg)＋胡萝卜素 (μg)/6
胡萝卜素	Total carotene	μg	CAROT	纸层析测定法
β-胡萝卜素	β-Carotene	μg	CARTB	
硫胺素	Thiamin (Vit B_1)	mg	THIA	荧光测定法
核黄素	Riboflavin (Vit B_2)	mg	RIBF	荧光测定法
烟酸	Niacin	mg	NIA	微生物测定法
维生素 C	Vitamin C (Vit C)	mg	VITC	荧光测定法
维生素 D	Vitamin D (Vit D)	IU	VITD	高效液相色谱法

续表

营养成分		计量单位	INFOODS Tagname	分析或计算方法
维生素 E	Vitamin E (Vit E)	mg		高效液相色谱法 维生素 E＝α-生育酚＋β-生育酚＋γ-生育酚＋δ-生育酚
α-生育酚当量	α-Tocopherol equivalent (α-TE)	mg	VITE	高效液相色谱法 α-TE＝α-生育酚＋0.5×β-生育酚＋0.1×γ-生育酚＋0.3×三烯生育酚
叶酸	Folate	μg	FOL	微生物测定法
生物素	Biotin	μg	BIOT	微生物测定法
泛酸	Pantothenic acid	mg	PANTAC	微生物测定法
胆碱	Choline	mg	CHOLN	柱层析-比色法
维生素 B_6	Pyridoxine (Vit B_6)	mg	VITB6A	微生物测定法
维生素 B_{12}	Cobalamin (Vit B_{12})	μg	VITB12	微生物测定法
维生素 K	Vitamin K (Vit K)	μg	VITK	高效液相色谱法
钙	Calcium (Ca)	mg	CA	原子吸收分光光度法
磷	Phosphorus (P)	mg	P	比色法
钾	Potassium (K)	mg	K	原子吸收分光光度法
钠	Sodium (Na)	mg	NA	原子吸收分光光度法
镁	Magnesium (Mg)	mg	MG	原子吸收分光光度法
铁	Iron (Fe)	mg	FE	原子吸收分光光度法
锌	Zinc (Zn)	mg	ZN	原子吸收分光光度法
硒	Selenium (Se)	μg	SE	荧光法
铜	Copper (Cu)	mg	CU	原子吸收分光光度法
锰	Manganese (Mn)	mg	MN	原子吸收分光光度法
碘	Iodine (I)	μg	ID	碱灰化砷铈接触比色法

表 6　食物氨基酸的表达

氨基酸		计量单位	INFOODS Tagname	分析或计算方法
异亮氨酸	Isoleucine (Ile)	mg	ILE	氨基酸自动分析仪法
亮氨酸	Leucine (Leu)	mg	LEU	氨基酸自动分析仪法
赖氨酸	Lysine (Lys)	mg	LYS	氨基酸自动分析仪法
含硫氨基酸	Sulfur-containing ami-no acids (SAA)	mg	AAS	含硫氨基酸 = 蛋氨酸 + 胱氨酸
蛋氨酸	Methionine (Met)	mg	MET	氨基酸自动分析仪法
胱氨酸	Cysteine (Cys)	mg	CYS	过甲酸氧化，氨基酸自动分析仪法
芳香族氨基酸	Aromatic amino acids (AAA)	mg	AAA	芳香族氨基酸 = 苯丙氨酸 + 酪氨酸
苯丙氨酸	Phenylalanine (Phe)	mg	PHE	氨基酸自动分析仪法
酪氨酸	Tyrosine (Tyr)	mg	TYR	氨基酸自动分析仪法
苏氨酸	Threonine (Thr)	mg	THR	氨基酸自动分析仪法
色氨酸	Tryptophan (Try)	mg	TRP	荧光法

续表

氨基酸		计量单位	INFOODS Tagname	分析或计算方法
缬氨酸	Valine (Val)	mg	VAL	氨基酸自动分析仪法
精氨酸	Arginine (Arg)	mg	ARG	氨基酸自动分析仪法
组氨酸	Histidine (His)	mg	HIS	氨基酸自动分析仪法
丙氨酸	Alanine (Ala)	mg	ALA	氨基酸自动分析仪法
天冬氨酸	Aspartic acid (Asp)	mg	ASP	氨基酸自动分析仪法
谷氨酸	Glutamic acid (Glu)	mg	GLU	氨基酸自动分析仪法
甘氨酸	Glycine (Gly)	mg	GLY	氨基酸自动分析仪法
脯氨酸	Proline (Pro)	mg	PRO	氨基酸自动分析仪法
丝氨酸	Serine (Ser)	mg	SER	氨基酸自动分析仪法

表 7　食物脂肪酸的表达

脂肪酸		计量单位	INFOODS Tagname	分析或计算方法
单体脂肪酸	Individual fatty acid	%*	▲	气相色谱分析法
总脂肪酸	Total fatty acid	g	FACID	脂肪 × 脂肪酸折算系数
饱和脂肪酸	Saturated fatty acid	g	FASAT	总脂肪酸 × 全部饱和脂肪酸所占百分比
单不饱和脂肪酸	Monounsaturated fatty acid	g	FAMS	总脂肪酸 × 全部单不饱和脂肪酸所占百分比
多不饱和脂肪酸	Polyunsaturated fatty acid	g	FAPU	总脂肪酸 × 全部多不饱和脂肪酸所占百分比

* % 指单体脂肪酸占总脂肪酸的百分比

▲ 单体脂肪酸 INFOODS Tagname 命名基本规则："F" + 脂肪酸中的碳原子数 + "D" + 不饱和键数 + "F"。如脂肪酸 C8 : 0 表示为 F8D0F，脂肪酸 C15 : 1 表示为 F15D1F。由于本次使用百分比表示单体脂肪酸的含量，没有相对应的 Tagname

7　食物成分分析方法

各种食物成分分析所使用的方法如表 5 ～ 7 所述。关于方法的详细说明和操作规程，详见由杨月欣、王光亚主编中国轻工业出版社出版的《实用食物营养成分分析手册》一书。

8　符号及缩写说明

数据表达中所涉及的符号、标注及其意义说明如下：

符　号	意　义
—	未检测：理论上食物中应该存在一定量的该种成分，但未实际检测
Tr	微量：低于目前应用的检测方法的检出限或未检出
(0)	估计零值：理论上估计不存在该营养素，未实际检测
( )	估计数值：参照相同或相似食物的给出值，未实际检测
un	不能计算
a*	中性洗涤剂法
b*	粗纤维测定法
c*	无原始数据，通过换算系数 4.184 进行能量值换算而得

* 为上标

本书所用计量单位符号如下：

缩写	单位名称
g	克
mg	毫克
μg	微克
kcal	千卡
kJ	千焦

Introduction

1 General introduction

The *China Food Composition 2004* consists of five parts, introduction, food description, food composition, appendices and food pictures.

There are 757 food items in this edition. The selection of food items were based on two parts：100 kinds of core foods frequently consumed during the National Nutrition Survey in 1992; the top 20 processed food products best sold in 1999-2000, as well as some novel foods.

The food components included in this book are 10 kinds of macronutrients, 15 kinds of vitamins, 11 kinds of minerals, 20 kinds of amino acids and 38 kinds of fatty acids.

2 Data source

Most data in *China Food Composition 2004* are the results from four research programs sponsored by the National Ministry of Science and Technology, Beijing Natural Science Foundation and Danone Nutrition Institute affiliated to the China CDC. A small portion of data was quoted from other food composition tables (FCT) published in China and other countries. The source of data was shown in the remark columns as follows:

"UK-FCT" —— *McCance and Widdowson's The Composition of Foods (6th, 2002)*
"USA-FCT" —— *USDA Nutrition Database for Standard Reference—Release 16*
"Japan-FCT" —— *Standard Tables of Food Composition in Japan (5th, 2000)*
"Korea-FCT" —— *Korea Food Composition Table (6th, 2001)*
"ShH-FCT" —— *Shanghai Food Composition, China (1990)*
"FJ-FCT" —— *Fujian Food Composition, China (1991)*
"YN-FCT" —— *Yunnan Food Composition, China (2003)*
"FNL" —— Food Nutrition Labeling

3 Food description and classification

3.1 Food description

The name of a food is composed of the scientific name and its alias in Chinese. In order to facilitate the user to obtain detailed information, the description provides the characteristics of a food, such as color, shape, texture, ingredient, manufacturing or processing methods, the treatment of samples and the parts selected for analysis.

The English and Latin food names are listed in the appendices. For better understanding, the photocopies of foods are provided too.

3.2 Food Classification

The classification of foods used in the edition 2004 follows the same rule in the edition 2002. There are 21 groups of foods; each group was subdivided into several sub-groups according to one of their specific attributes or processing methods. Moreover, all those foods considered difficult to be classed into a specific sub-group will come to a sub-group marked as

"Others" under the corresponding food group.

The processed foods were classified according to the food classification criteria of the China Food Industry Standardization Management Committee. The detailed food classification and the number of food items in this book are listed in Table 1.

Table 1 Food groups and sub-groups in the food composition tables

Code	Group	N	Sub-code	Sub-group	N
01	Cereals and cereal products	29			
			1	Wheat	11
			2	Rice	9
			3	Corn	4
			4	Barley	1
			5	Millet	1
			9	Others	3
02	Tubers, starches and products	11			
			1	Tubers	6
			2	Starches	5
03	Dried legumes and legume products	17			
			1	Soybean	11
			2	Mung bean	0
			3	Adzuki bean	2
			4	Kidney bean	0
			5	Broad bean	1
			9	Others	3
04	Vegetables and vegetable products	82			
			1	Root vegetables	8
			2	Leguminous vegetables, sprouts and seedings	9
			3	Cucurbitaceous and solanaceous vegetables	20
			4	Allium vegetables	3
			5	Stem, leafy and flowering vegetables	35
			6	Aquatic vegetables	1
			7	Tubers	2
			8	Wild vegetables	4
05	Fungi and algae	31			
			1	Fungi	28
			2	Algae	3
06	Fruits and fruit products	24			
			1	Kernel fruits	1
			2	Drupe fruits	6
			3	Berries	2
			4	Citrus fruits	2
			5	Tropical fruits	12
			6	Melons	1

Code	Group	N	Sub-code	Sub-group	N
07	Nuts and seeds	22			
			1	Nuts	15
			2	Seeds	7
08	Meat and meat products	59			
			1	Pig	35
			2	Cattle	15
			3	Mutton	7
			4	Ass	1
			5	Horse	0
			9	Others	1
09	Poultry and poultry products	15			
			1	Chicken	8
			2	Duck	3
			3	Goose	1
			4	Turkey	1
			9	Others	2
10	Milk and milk products	47			
			1	Liquid cow's milk	17
			2	Cow's milk powder	20
			3	Yogurt	2
			4	Cheese	4
			5	Butter and cream	1
			9	Others	3
11	Eggs and egg products	10			
			1	Hen egg	7
			2	Duck egg	2
			3	Goose egg	1
			4	Quail egg	0
12	Fish, shellfish and mollusc	44			
			1	Fish	34
			2	Prawn and shrimp	3
			3	Crab	2
			4	Shellfish	2
			9	Others	3
13	Infant foods	58			
			1	Infant formulas	43
			2	Formulated weaning foods	3
			3	Supplementary foods	12
14	Ethnic foods and cakes	13			
			1	Ethnic foods	5
			2	Cakes	8

Code	Group	N	Sub-code	Sub-group	N
15	Fast foods	115			
			1	Handy foods	24
			2	Convenience foods	62
			3	Snacks	29
16	Beverages	63			
			1	Carbonated drinks	1
			2	Fruit juices and fruit flavoured drinks	17
			3	Vegetable juices and drinks	1
			4	Milk drinks	5
			5	Vegetable protein drinks	5
			6	Teas and tea beverages	2
			7	Powdered beverages	8
			8	Ice creams and popsicles	12
			9	Others	12
17	Liquor and alcoholic beverages	32			
			1	Fermented alcoholic beverages	12
			2	Liquor (distilled spirits)	13
			3	Cordial (integrated alcoholic beverages)	7
18	Sugars, preserves and honeys	31			
			1	Sugars	0
			2	Confectionery	12
			3	Preserves	14
			4	Honeys	5
19	Fats and oils	9			
			1	Animal fats	0
			2	Plant oils	9
20	Condiments	33			
			1	Sauces	3
			2	Vinegar	0
			3	Sauces and pastes	10
			4	Fermented soybean curd	3
			5	Pickles	13
			6	Spices	1
			7	Salt and others	3
21	Others	12			

3.3 Food code

A six-digit code was used for coding foods. The first two digits refer to the group of a food, the third digit refers to the sub-group of a food, and the last three digits refer to the sequence number of a food. The detailed information can be found from Table 1. Each food item has a unique code in different nutrient tables, which means that the code of a food item is the same in the general nutrients content table, amino acid content table, fatty acid content table, and cholin, biotin, pantothenic acid, vitamin K and vitamin D content table.

4 Edible portion

The data in the tables are the nutrient content per 100 g edible portion (EP) of a food. Many foods purchased from markets have some inedible parts that need to be removed before cooking and processing, such as the peel of banana and the bone of pork chop. Only the nutrient content in the edible portion of a food sample was analyzed. The data showed in the EP column are the percentage of edible portion to the whole sample. The calculation for the nutrient contents in 1kg of the sampled food is shown as follows.

$$X = A \times 10 \times (EP / 100)$$

X is the nutrient content in 1kg food sample.

A is the nutrient content in 100 g edible portion of the food sample.

EP is the percentage of edible portion to whole food sample.

The edible portion of a food item tends to be varied depending on the transportation, storage and processing methods used. Therefore, it is appropriate to measure the actual proportion of edible parts instead of the data shown in the table to calculate the nutrient content of a food when you consider a difference existed.

5 Definition of nutrients and expression

5.1 Energy

The energy value of a food is the sum of all energy-producing nutrients (e.g., protein, fat, carbohydrate and alcohol) multiplied with corresponding energy conversion factor (see Table 2). The energy value in the table is expressed as both in kilocalorie (kcal) and kilojoule (kJ). The exchange factor for the unit of energy is that 1 kilocalorie equals to 4.184 kilojoule.

Table 2 Energy conversion factor*

Energy-producing nutrients	Energy	
	kcal/g	kJ/g
Protein	4	17
Fat	9	37
Carbohydrate	4	17
Alcohol	7	29

* Royal Society (1972)

Recently, FAO recommends 2 kcal/g as the energy value for dietary fiber. In consideration of the consistency with China Food Composition 2002, we still follow the rules as previous edition; which means that the carbohydrate values given in the food composition table include the dietary fiber contents, but the energy value of dietary fiber is assumed zero in the calculation of encrgy.

In addition, when the mark '( )' or 'Tr' is used to express the content of protein, fat or carbohydrate, the energy value may exist some deviation. The mark 'c' is used to express the energy value of a quoted data that had only kcal or kJ, the conversion factor of 4.184 is used for the calculation. When the energy value of a food can not be calculated from its components it is marked with 'un'.

5.2 *Macro nutrients*

Protein and amino acid

Protein content of a food is calculated by the total nitrogen determined by Kjeldahl method and multiplied with a corresponding protein conversion factor. The average nitrogen content of most protein in foods is 16% by weight; therefore, the protein content of a food can be calculated by multiplying the total nitrogen with 6.25 (100/16). The non-protein nitrogen content were varied slightly by food; therefore, the protein content in different food categories can be adjusted by calculating the total nitrogen content with different conversion factors recommended by FAO/WHO in 1973, which are shown in table 3.

Table 3 Factors for the conversion of nitrogen values to protein (per g N)*

Food	Conversion factor	Food	Conversion factor
Wheat		Eggs	
whole	5.83	Whole	6.25
bran	6.31	albumin	6.32
embryo	5.80	vitellin	6.12
endosperm	5.70	Meat and fish	6.25
Oats	5.83	Gelatin	5.55
Barley and barley flour	5.83	Milk and milk products	6.38
Rye and rye flour	5.83	Casein	6.40
Millet	6.31	Human milk	6.37
maize	6.25	Beans	
Rice and rice flour	5.95	soybean	5.71
Nuts		other beans	6.25
almond	5.18	All other foods	6.25
brazil	5.46		
peanut	5.46		
others	5.30		

* FAO/WHO (1973)

Theoretically, the protein content is equivalent to or higher than the sum of various amino acids. However, it was likely that the protein content derived from the conversion factor was matched not very well with the sum of various amino acids measured directly. To avoid notable misinformation, the difference between the sum of amino acids and protein content was controlled within $\pm 5\%$. Otherwise, the data would be reanalyzed.

Carbohydrate

A difference subtracting method was used herein to calculate the total carbohydrate content in food, therefore, in which the dietary fiber is included. The calculation is as follow:

$$\text{carbohydrate} = 100 - (\text{protein} + \text{fat} + \text{water} + \text{ash})$$

Due to the fact that the carbohydrate content is not determined directly, any error occurred during the determination of water, protein, fat and ash might has some effects on the result of carbohydrate, the actual deviation is more likely to be higher than the theoretical one. In 1998, FAO/WHO emphasized that the difference subtracting method should be rejected from the research on food composition database. However, because of the limitation in analytical coudition, the difference subtracting method is still used by many countries.

Dietary fiber

Two methods are adopted for dietary fiber here, i.e. neutral detergent method and enzyme gravimetric method from AOAC. Some data borrowed from other FCTs, determined by crude fiber method. The neutral detergent method is used to determine the insoluble fiber. In this method, sugar, starch, protein and pectin are removed by dissolving the sample in a neutral detergent, and the remains are then decomposed with amylase, then the insoluble part is dried and weighted as the insoluble fiber which might contain some insoluble ash. The enzyme gravimetric method from AOAC is used to determine the total dietary fiber including soluble and insoluble dietary fiber; the soluble fiber includes pectin and oligosaccharide etc. and the insoluble fiber includes cellulose, hemicellulose, lignin and silicon dioxide.

These data are expressed by total, insoluble and soluble dietary fiber in the book. The insoluble dietary fiber data are differentiated by ‘a’ as neutral detergent method, and by ‘b’ as crude fiber method.

Total fat and fatty acid

The total fat measured is virtually the total content of crude fat, because many soluble substances other than neutral fat, such as free fatty acid, wax, phospholipids, sterol, turpentine and pigment existed.

Fatty acid expressed in this book both as the percentage of individual fatty acid to the total fatty acid and the content of saturated fatty acid, monounsaturated fatty acid and polyunsaturated fatty acid in 100 grams of food. The content of fatty acids is calculated by multiplying the fat content with fatty acid conversion factors shown in Table 4.

Table 4 Conversion factors to give values for total fatty acid in fat*

Food	Conversion factor	Food	Conversion factor
Wheat, barley and rye		Beef lean	0.916
whole grain	0.720	Beef fat	0.953
flour	0.670	Lamb, take as beef	
bran	0.820	Pork lean	0.910
Oat, whole	0.940	Pork fat	0.953
Rice, milled	0.850	Poultry	0.945
Beans		Brain	0.561
soybean and its products ▲	0.930	Heart	0.789
Other beans ▲	0.775	Kidney	0.747
Vegetables and fruit	0.800	Liver	0.741
Avocado pears	0.956	Milk and milk products	0.945
Fungi and algea ▲	0.562	Eggs	0.830
Nuts	0.956	Fish	
Peanut ▲	0.951	fatty	0.900
Lotus seed ▲	0.930	white	0.700
Fats and oils		Shrimp and crab ▲	0.723
all except coconut oil	0.956	Jam and preserved foods ▲	0.686
coconut oil	0.942		

* FAO (2003)

▲ USDA Nutrition Database, SR16

5.3 Vitamins

Vitamin A

Vitamin A refers to a variety of chemical forms with different biological activity, including retinol, β carotene and other carotenoids. The biological activity of vitamin A is usually expressed as retinal equivalent (RE) calculated by the following formula:

$$\text{Vitamin A } (\mu\text{gRE}) = \text{Retinol } (\mu\text{g}) + 1/6\ \beta\text{-Carotene } (\mu\text{g}) + 1/12 \text{ Other Carotenoids } (\mu\text{g})$$

Retinol is present only in animal foods, where as β-carotene and other carotenoids existed in plant foods. Total carotenoids were determined by the chromatographic method without further separating. Therefore, in calculating the RE of carotenoids in vegetable food with a coefficient 1/6, the result tends to be higher than it should be.

The international unit (IU) of retinol and β-carotene can be converted into retinol equivalent (RE) as follows:

$$\begin{aligned} 1\ \mu\text{g RE Vitamin A} &= 1\ \mu\text{g retinol} \\ &= 3.33 \text{ IU Vitamin A} \\ &= 6\ \mu\text{g } \beta\text{-carotene} \\ &= 10 \text{ IU } \beta\text{-carotene} \end{aligned}$$

Vitamin D

There are two forms of vitamin D, i.e., vitamin D_2 (ergocalciferol or calciferol) and vitamin D_3 (cholecalciferol). Vitamin D_2 is rare in natural environment and is produced largely from the irradiated ergosterol for medical use. Vitamin D_3 is formed from the 7-dehydrocholesterol beneath the epidermis by sunlight or ultraviolet ray irradiation. Currently, the unit of vitamin D is expressed as μg instead of international unit (IU), and 0.025μg Vitamin D is recognized as one active unit, which means that Vitamin D_3 1 IU=0.025μg.

Vitamin E

Vitamin E of food exists as α-, β-, γ-and δ-tocopherol, as well as α-, β-, γ-and δ-triene tocopherol. Vitamin E in most natural foods is d-α-tocopherol, which has the highest biological activity. The activity of vitamin E is expressed as α-tocopherol equivalent (α-TE). The bioavailability for different forms of vitamin E is different, therefore, the total α-TE of a food is calculated as follows:

$$\alpha\text{-TE (mg)} = \alpha\text{-tocopherol (mg)} + 0.5 \times \beta\text{-tocopherol (mg)} + 0.1 \times \gamma\text{-tocopherol (mg)} + 0.3 \times \text{triene tocopherol (mg)}$$

The biologically active unit of vitamin E can also be expressed as international unit (IU):

$$1\ \alpha\text{-TE (mg)} = 1.49 \text{ IU vitamin E}$$

The total vitamin E expressed in the tables is the sum of various forms of vitamin E by weight without considering its bioavailability.

The data of vitamin E are listed both as α-TE and total vitamin E in this book. When a mark "un" is used, it means that only α-TE or total vitamin E is available, no transformation could be done from each other.

Vitamin K

Vitamin K is the generic name for vitamin K_1 (phylloquinone) and vitamin K_2 (menaquinone). Phylloquinone is formed in plants and vegetables which is the major source of vitamin K in human food. Menaquinone is formed in bacteria. Both forms of vitamin K could be found in animal tissue. The data acquired herein were not typed.

Vitamin C

Vitamin C is a weak acid with a chemical structure of α-keto-lactone containing six carbon atoms. The natural form of vitamin C is the L-α-isomer, the biological activity of which is nine times more than the D-type isomer. L-Ascorbic acid is used for dietary supplements, which can be oxidized to dehydroascorbic acid with the same activity. Vitamin C is mostly present in plant foods and rare in animal foods. Nonetheless, there is a slight quantity of vitamin C in animal blood.

Vitamin B_1 & B_2

Vitamin B_1 is called as thiamine or aneurin because of its capability to treat and prevent beriberi. Vitamin B_1 is rich in cereal bran, and is present both in animal and plant foods. Vitamin B_2 is also called as riboflavin, which is present in animal and plant foods. The derivatives of thiamine and riboflavin serve as the coenzyme of enzyme in human body and play important roles in metabolism.

Niacin

Niacin is also known as vitamin PP (preventive pellagra). Nicotinic acid amide (nicotinamide) is the biological active form. Niacin is distributed widely in animal and plant foods; meat (including liver and other viscera), yeast, cereals and legumes are the good sources of niacin. Milk, fish and green leafy vegetables also contain appreciable amount of niacin. Most niacin in plant foods (50% ~ 70%) may bond with some macromolecules and cannot be available in mammals. Since niacin can be synthesized in the liver of human body from the amino acid tryptophan, the content of tryptophan in foods is also considered in a factor of 60 : 1 for the conversion of tryptophan to niacin.

Vitamin B_6

Vitamin B_6 is also known as pyridoxol. There are three forms, namely, pyridoxine (PN), pyridoxal (PL) and pyridoxamine (PM), all of which are biologically active. The phosphoric acid ester of pyridoxal (PLP) is the coenzyme for aminotransferase. The data of vitamin B_6 is determined by microbiological method, representing the total of these three forms.

Vitamin B_{12}

Vitamin B_{12} is a group of corrinoid compounds. In vitamin B_{12}, cobalt is the center of the big corrin ring interlinked with four reductive pyrrole rings. The chemical name is called α-5.6 xylene imidazole 1-berubigen. There is a small amount of vitamin B_{12} in animal foods and fermented foods such as liver and preserved bean curd. The data on vitamin B_{12} herein is acquired by using microbiological method.

Folate

Folate falls in the category of B vitamins and its chemical structure is in the pteroylglutamic acid family. It is a chemical compound comprised of pteroyl and glutamic acid. In natural foods, there are one or more glutamic acids in the folic acid, and three out of four folic acids existed in the form of pteroyl polyglutamine. The more glutamic acid molecules in the folic acid, the lower absorbance is in the body. The data on folate herein is acquired by using a microbiological method.

Choline

Choline is the methyl donor for phospholipids and acetylcholine. Choline is highly moisture retentive in open air and is more readily reacted with acid to generate stably thermostatic crystal. Choline is present extensively in various foods, especially in animal foods, such as egg yolk and entails, as well as in vegetable foods, such as egg embryo buds. The data on choline herein is acquired by using the colorimetric method.

Biotin

Eight isomers of biotin have been found so far, of which only the α-biotin is natural and biological active. It is largely present in yeast, liver and other animal entails. The data on biotin herein is acquired by the colorimetric method.

Pantothenic acid

Pantothenic acid is also one kind of B vitamins with a chemical structure of dihydroxy-β, β-dimethyl-butyl-β-alanine. Calcium pantothenate is more stable than the pure pantothenic acid. The major physiological function of pantothenic acid lies in the synthesis of CoA in the body for the transmission of acetyl group. The data on pantothenic acid herein were acquired by the microbiological method.

5.4 Minerals

The minerals that can not be synthesized in human body and have to be got from foods and water are known as essential minerals. The essential minerals can be divided into macro-elements and microelements, based on the quantity of daily needs. Macro-elements are defined as the needs being more than 100 mg per day, such as calcium, phosphorus, magnesium, sodium and chlorine. Micro-elements play very important physiological roles in human body but the daily needs being very slight. In 1990, the Expert Committee of FAO, WHO and IAEA jointly defined that there are 8 kinds of essential microelements so far, namely, iodine, zinc, selenium, copper, molybdenum, chromium, cobalt and iron.

Eleven minerals were analyzed and included in this edition, i.e., calcium, phosphorus, magnesium, sodium, potassium, iron, zinc, selenium, copper, manganese and iodine, by means of flame atomic absorption method and colorimetric method.

6 Expression and description of food components

The expression of nutrients in this edition is the same as that in *the China Food Composition 2002*. The detailed expression is shown in Table 5 to 7. Total dietary fiber, insoluble dietary fiber, soluble dietary fiber, vitamin E in α-TE, vitamin B_6, vitamin B_{12}, choline, biotin and folic acid are the nutrients newly added in this edition.

Table 5 The expressions of main food components

Food components		Unit	INFOODS Tagname	Analytical or computing method
能量	Energy	kcal / kJ	ENERC	The sum of individual energy-producing nutrients multiplied with correspouding energy conversion factors. *The energy from dietary fiber is not included
水分	Water	g	WATER	Gravimetric method
蛋白质	Protein	g	PROCNT	Kjeldahl Method Total nitrogen × protein conversion factor
脂肪	Fat	g	FAT	Soxhlet extraction method, acid hydrolysis
碳水化合物	Carbohydrate (CHO)	g	CHOCDF	100−(water + protein + fat + ash)
总膳食纤维	Total dietary fiber	g	FIBTG	Enzyme gravimetric method
可溶性膳食纤维	Soluble dietary fiber	g	FIBSOL	Enzyme gravimetric method
不溶性膳食纤维	Insoluble dietary fiber	g	FIBINS	Enzyme gravimetric method
灰分	Ash	g	ASH	Gravimetric method
胆固醇	Cholesterol	mg	CHOLE	Colorimetric method
维生素 A	Vitamin A (Vit A)	μgRE	VITA	Vit A (μg RE) = Retinol (μg) + Carotene (μg) / 6
胡萝卜素	Total carotene	μg	CAROT	Paper chromatography
β-胡萝卜素	β-Carotene	μg	CARTB	Paper chromatography
视黄醇	Retinol	μg	RETOL	HPLC*
硫胺素	Thiamin (Vit B_1)	mg	THIA	Fluorimetry
核黄素	Riboflavin (Vit B_2)	mg	RIBF	Fluorimetry
烟酸	Niacin	mg	NIA	Microbiological assay
维生素 C	Vitamin C (Vit C)	mg	VITC	Fluorimetry
维生素 D	Vitamin D (Vit D)	IU	VITD	HPLC
维生素 E	Vitamin E (Vit E)	mg		HPLC The sum of α-, β-, γ-, and δ-tocopherol
α-生育酚当量	α-Tocopherol equivalent (α-TE)	mg	VITE	HPLC α-TE = (α-tocopherol) + 0.5 × (β-tocopherol) + 0.1 × (γ-tocopherol) + 0.3 × (triene tocopherol)
叶酸	Folate	μg	FOL	Microbiological assay
生物素	Biotin	μg	BIOT	Microbiological assay
泛酸	Pantothenic acid	mg	PANTAC	Microbiological assay
胆碱	Choline	mg	CHOLN	Column chromatography-colorimetric method

Food components		Unit	INFOODS Tagname	Analytical or computing method
维生素 B_6	Pyridoxine (Vit B_6)	mg	VITB6A	Microbiological assay
维生素 B_{12}	Cobalamin (Vit B_{12})	μg	VITB12	Microbiological assay
维生素 K	Vitamin K (Vit K)	μg	VITK	HPLC
钙	Calcium (Ca)	mg	CA	AAS ▲
磷	Phosphorus (P)	mg	P	Colorimetric method
钾	Potassium (K)	mg	K	AAS
钠	Sodium (Na)	mg	NA	AAS
镁	Magnesium (Mg)	mg	MG	AAS
铁	Iron (Fe)	mg	FE	AAS
锌	Zinc (Zn)	mg	ZN	AAS
硒	Selenium (Se)	μg	SE	Fluorescence method
铜	Copper (Cu)	mg	CU	AAS
锰	Manganese (Mn)	mg	MN	AAS
碘	Iodine (I)	μg	ID	Alkaline ashing arsenic and cerium contact colorimetric method

* HPLC: high performance liquid chromatography

▲ AAS: atomic absorption spectrophotometry

Table 6 The expression of amino acid

Amino acid		Unit	INFOODS Tagname	Analytical or computing method
异亮氨酸	Isoleucine (Ile)	mg	ILE	Automatic amino acid analyzer
亮氨酸	Leucine (Leu)	mg	LEU	Automatic amino acid analyzer
赖氨酸	Lysine (Lys)	mg	LYS	Automatic amino acid analyzer
含硫氨基酸	Sulfur-containing am -ino acids (SAA)	mg	AAS	The sum of methionine and cysteine
蛋氨酸	Methionine (Met)	mg	MET	Automatic amino acid analyzer
胱氨酸	Cysteine (Cys)	mg	CYS	Automatic amino acid analyzer, after oxidation with peroxyformic acid
芳香族氨基酸	Aromatic amino acids (AAA)	mg	AAA	The sum of phenylalanine and tyrosine
苯丙氨酸	Phenylalanine (Phe)	mg	PHE	Automatic amino acid analyzer
酪氨酸	Tyrosine (Tyr)	mg	TYR	Automatic amino acid analyzer
苏氨酸	Threonine (Thr)	mg	THR	Automatic amino acid analyzer
色氨酸	Tryptophan (Try)	mg	TRP	Fluorescence method
缬氨酸	Valine (Val)	mg	VAL	Automatic amino acid analyzer
精氨酸	Argininc (Arg)	mg	ARG	Automatic amino acid analyzer
组氨酸	Histidine (His)	mg	HIS	Automatic amino acid analyzer
丙氨酸	Alanine (Ala)	mg	ALA	Automatic amino acid analyzer
天冬氨酸	Aspartic acid (Asp)	mg	ASP	Automatic amino acid analyzer
谷氨酸	Glutamic acid (Glu)	mg	GLU	Automatic amino acid analyzer

续表

脂肪酸	Fatty acids	Unit	INFOODS Tag name	Analytical or computing method
甘氨酸	Glycine (Gly)	mg	GLY	Automatic amino acid analyzer
脯氨酸	Proline (Pro)	mg	PRO	Automatic amino acid analyzer
丝氨酸	Serine (Ser)	mg	SER	Automatic amino acid analyzer

Table 7 Expression of fatty acid

脂肪酸	Fatty acids	Unit	INFOODS Tag name	Analytical or computing method
单体脂肪酸	Individual fatty acid	%*	▲	Gas chromatography
总脂肪酸	Total fatty acid	g	FACID	Fat × fatty acid conversion factor
饱和脂肪酸	Saturated fatty acid	g	FASAT	Total fatty acid × the percentage of total saturated fatty acid
单不饱和脂肪酸	Monounsaturated fatty acid	g	FAMS	Total fatty acid × the percentage of total monounsaturated fatty acid
多不饱和脂肪酸	Polyunsaturated fatty acid	g	FAPU	Total fatty acid × the percentage of total polyunsaturated fatty acid

* The "%" refers to the percentage of individual fatty acid to the total fatty acid

▲The basic rule for the designation of individual fatty acid in INFOODS Tagname is as follows: 'F' + the number of carbon atoms in fatty acid + 'D' + the number of unsaturated bonds + 'F'. For example, fatty acid C8:0 stands for F8D0F and C15:1 for F15D1F. Since the individual fatty acid is expressed as the percentage of total fatty acid herein, no corresponding Tagname is available for individual fatty acid calculated from the percentage of total fatty acids.

7 Analytic methods

The analytic methods for food components are shown in table 5 to 7. For the detailed description and operating instructions of these methods, please refer to a *Practical Handbook of Food Composition Analysis*, China Light Industry Press, edited by Yang Yuexin and Wang Guangya.

8 Mark and abbreviation

The symbols and their meanings referred to the data expression are shown as follows:

Symbols	Meaning
—	Untested: Theoretically, there may exist a certain quantity or trace amount of such nutrient in the food, with little possibility of nonexistence
Tr	Trace amount: The result is lower than the detection line or not detected based on current test methods
(0)	Estimated zero value: Theoretically, there is no such nutrient existed although not tested
( )	Estimated value: Derived from reference data for the same or similar food
un	Cannot calculate
a*	Insoluble fiber tested by neutral detergent method
b*	Insoluble fiber tested by crude fiber method
c*	No original data, the value of dietary fiber is converted with a energy conversion factor of 4.184

* superscript

The measuring units used herein include:

Abbreviation	Full name
g	gram
mg	milligram
μg	microgram
kcal	kilocalorie
kJ	kilojoule

Notes

食物描述

Description of Foods

Notes

食物描述 Description of foods

编码	食物类别和名称	食物描述	样品处理	数据来源	采样日期	采样地点	产地
	谷类及制品						
小麦							
01-1-206	小麦面粉 (标准粉)	散装	数份等量混合均匀		2002.7	北京市宣武区太平街粮店	
01-1-207	小麦面粉 (富强粉、特一粉)	散装	数份等量混合均匀		2002.7	北京市宣武区太平街粮店	
01-1-208	小麦面粉 (特制)	袋装。商品名：特制家庭面粉。铁人牌	数袋等量混合均匀		2001.6	送检	天津
01-1-313	挂面 (富强粉)	主要原料：小麦面粉、食盐等。生	数包等量混合均匀磨碎		2002.7	北京市宣武区太平街粮店	
01-1-314	龙须面 (素)	主要原料：小麦面粉、食盐等。生。味都牌	数包等量混合均匀磨碎		2001.10	送检	上海
01-1-315	龙须面 (鸡蛋)	主要原料：小麦面粉、鸡蛋粉、食盐等。生。康师傅牌	数包等量混合均匀磨碎		2001.11	送检	天津
01-1-316	面条 (富强粉, 切面)	生, 散装	混合打匀		2002.7	北京市宣武区太平街粮店	北京
01-1-317	面条 (富强粉, 煮)	生切面 314g, 开水煮 15 分钟, 沥去水后重 559g	混合打匀		2002.7	北京市宣武区太平街粮店采集原料, 实验室煮制	
01-1-410	花卷 (加牛奶)	主要原料：小麦面粉、牛奶、白砂糖、水等。熟, 冷冻。商品名：奶油香花卷。康乐牌	数袋中取数个混合均匀磨碎		2001.11	送检	广东
01-1-411	馒头 (富强粉)	主要原料：富强粉、水等	数个等量混合均匀磨碎		2002.7	北京市宣武区太平街粮店	北京
01-1-503	面筋 (肉馅)	主要原料：面筋、猪肉、盐、糖、酱油、味精等。熟。三梅牌	数袋混合打匀		2001.11	送检	江苏
稻米							
01-2-106	粳米 (极品精米)	生, 袋装。大荒地牌	数袋等量混合均匀磨碎		2001.7	送检	吉林
01-2-107	粳米 (西域王米)	生, 袋装	数袋等量混合均匀磨碎		2001.6	送检	新疆
01-2-108	粳米 (小站稻米)	生, 袋装。盛传牌	数袋等量混合均匀磨碎		2001.7	送检	天津
01-2-214	籼米	生, 散装	混合均匀磨碎		2002.7	北京市宣武区太平街粮店	
01-2-215	香米	生, 袋装。商品名：泰香米	数袋等量混合均匀磨碎		2001.7	送检	泰国
01-2-408	籼米饭 (蒸)	籼米 300g、水 800ml, 电饭煲蒸 30 分钟, 米饭重 856g	混合打匀		2002.7	北京市宣武区太平街粮店采集原料, 实验室蒸制	

食物描述 Description of foods

编码	食物类别和名称	食物描述	样品处理	数据来源	采样日期	采样地点	产地
01-2-409	籼米粥	籼米 170g、水 1000ml, 煮 36 分钟	混合打匀		2002.7	北京市宣武区太平街粮店 采集原料, 实验室煮制	
01-2-410	米粉	主要原料：大米、淀粉、水等。细粉条状。商品名：张师傅米粉。振兴牌	数包等量混合均匀打碎		2001.10	送检	广东
01-2-411	河粉	主要原料：大米、水等。粗粉条状。商品名：张师傅沙河粉。振兴牌	数包等量混合均匀打碎		2001.10	送检	广东
玉米							
01-3-108	玉米粒 (黄, 干)	生, 散装	混合均匀磨碎		2002.7	北京市宣武区太平街粮店	
01-3-109	玉米面 (黄)	散装	混合均匀磨碎		2002.7	北京市宣武区太平街粮店	
01-3-110	玉米糁 (黄)	散装	混合均匀磨碎		2002.7	北京市宣武区太平街粮店	
01-3-202	玉米面面条	主要原料：玉米面、小麦面粉等。生	数包混合均匀磨碎			送检	北京
大麦							
01-4-102	黑大麦	生。奥比牌	混合均匀磨碎			送检	江苏
小米							
01-5-104	小米 (黄)	生。太后香牌	数包等量混合均匀磨碎		2001.11	送检	山西
其它							
01-9-010	荞麦面	太后香牌	数包等量混合均匀磨碎		2001.11	送检	山西
01-9-011	莜麦面	太后香牌	数包等量混合均匀磨碎		2001.11	送检	山西
01-9-201	高粱面面条	主要原料：高粱面、小麦面粉等。生	数包等量混合均匀磨碎			送检	北京
	薯类、淀粉及制品						
薯类							
02-1-104	马铃薯 [土豆、洋芋]	生、鲜	数十个各取 1/4, 去皮, 混合打匀		2002.8	北京市崇文门菜市场	
02-1-105	马铃薯 (烤)	烤熟, 去皮		Korea-FCT			

编码	食物类别和名称	食物描述	样品处理	数据来源	采样日期	采样地点	产地
02-1-106	马铃薯(蒸)	蒸熟,去皮		Korea-FCT			
02-1-107	马铃薯(煮)	煮熟,去皮		Korea-FCT			
02-1-108	马铃薯全粉		数袋混合均匀			送检	内蒙古
02-1-205	甘薯(红心)[山芋、红薯]		十余个各取1/4,去皮,混合打匀		2002.8	北京市崇文门菜市场	
淀粉类							
02-2-108	淀粉(小麦)			Japan-FCT			
02-2-109	淀粉(大米)			Japan-FCT			
02-2-110	淀粉(马铃薯)			Korea-FCT			
02-2-111	淀粉(甘薯)			Korea-FCT			
02-2-112	煎炸粉	以马铃薯淀粉为原料,煎炸食品时用		Korea-FCT			
	干豆类及制品						
大豆							
03-1-104	黄豆		数斤混匀磨碎			送检	
03-1-206	豆奶粉(维维牌)	主要原料：大豆、牛奶、白砂糖、奶粉等。商品名：维维豆奶粉	数包混合均匀			送检	江苏
03-1-207	豆奶粉(多力牌)	主要原料：大豆、白砂糖、全脂乳粉、全鸡蛋粉等。强化钙。商品名：新一代钙强化豆奶粉	数包混合均匀		2001.7	送检	江苏
03-1-208	豆奶粉(大磨牌)	主要原料：大豆粉、鲜牛奶、脱盐乳精粉等。强化钙、铁,无糖。商品名：中老年钙+铁无糖豆奶粉	数包混合均匀		2001.6	送检	黑龙江
03-1-306	豆腐(北豆腐)	主要原料：黄豆、水等。黄豆浸泡后磨浆，卤水点制	数份数斤混合打匀		2002.7	北京市宣武区永安路菜市场	北京
03-1-307	豆腐(南豆腐)	主要原料：黄豆、水等。黄豆浸泡后磨浆，石膏点制	数份数斤混合打匀		2002.7	北京市宣武区永安路菜市场	北京
03-1-405	豆浆	主要原料：黄豆、水等。新南洋牌	数包混合均匀		2001.8	送检	北京
03-1-406	豆浆(甜)	主要原料：黄豆、水、糖等。新南洋牌	数包混合均匀			送检	北京

食物描述 Description of foods

编码	食物类别和名称	食物描述	样品处理	数据来源	采样日期	采样地点	产地
03-1-527	豆腐皮	主要原料：黄豆等。禾宝牌	数包混合均匀磨碎		2002.3	送检	辽宁
03-1-528	腐竹	主要原料：黄豆等。象山牌	数包混合均匀磨碎		2001.8	送检	广西
03-1-529	豆腐干	主要原料：黄豆等。老爸牌	数包混合均匀磨碎		2001.7	送检	浙江
赤豆							
03-3-204	红豆沙	主要原料：白砂糖、红小豆(去皮)、软化水等	数袋等量混合均匀磨碎			送检	北京
03-3-205	红豆馅	主要原料：白砂糖、红小豆、软化水等	数袋等量混合均匀磨碎			送检	北京
蚕豆							
03-5-203	蚕豆(煮)			USA-FCT			
其它							
03-9-204	豇豆(煮)			Korea-FCT			
03-9-303	豌豆(煮)			Korea-FCT			
03-9-401	鹰嘴豆[桃豆]	干。见附图	数袋等量混合均匀磨碎			送检	北京
	蔬菜类及制品						
根菜类							
04-1-111	白萝卜[莱菔]	生、鲜，大白萝卜、白皮、白心。见附图	去蒂，数个等量混合均		2002.8	北京市崇文门菜市场	
04-1-112	白萝卜(圆)	生、鲜，小圆球形、白皮、白心。见附图	去蒂，数十个混合打匀		2002.9	北京市朝阳区潘家园农贸市场	
04-1-113	青萝卜	生、鲜，青绿色皮、绿心。见附图	去蒂，数个混合打匀		2002.8	北京市崇文门菜市场	
04-1-114	变萝卜[红皮萝卜]	生、鲜，圆形、红皮、白心。见附图	去蒂，数个等量混合打匀		2002.9	北京市朝阳区潘家园农贸市场	
04-1-115	樱桃萝卜	生、鲜，小球形、紫红色皮、白心。见附图	去蒂，数十个混合打匀		2002.8	北京市蔬菜研究中心	北京
04-1-204	胡萝卜	生、鲜，黄色。见附图	去蒂，数个混合打匀		2002.8	北京市崇文门菜市场	
04-1-402	根芹[根洋芹、球根塘蒿]	生、鲜，土色皮，不规则球形根。见附图	去蒂、去皮，数个混合打匀		2002.8	北京市蔬菜研究中心	北京

编码	食物类别和名称	食物描述	样品处理	数据来源	采样日期	采样地点	产地
04-1-403	紫菜头	生、鲜，紫皮、紫心。见附图	去蒂，数个混合打匀		2002.9	北京市崇文门菜市场	
鲜豆菜和豆苗类							
04-2-118	扁豆	生、鲜。见附图	去蒂、去筋，数斤混合打匀		2002.8	北京市崇文门菜市场	
04-2-119	豇豆	生、鲜。见附图	去蒂、去筋，数斤混合打匀		2002.7	北京市崇文门菜市场	
04-2-120	四季豆 [菜豆、芸豆]	生、鲜。见附图	去蒂、去筋，数斤混合打匀		2002.8	北京市崇文门菜市场	
04-2-121	四棱豆 [杨桃豆、翅豆]	生、鲜。见附图	去蒂、去筋，数斤混合打匀		2002.7	北京市崇文门菜市场	
04-2-122	甜脆荷兰豆 [甜豆]	生、鲜。见附图	去蒂、去筋，数斤混合打匀		2002.9	北京市崇文门菜市场	
04-2-205	黄豆芽	生、鲜。见附图	去根，数斤混合打匀		2002.8	北京市崇文门菜市场	
04-2-206	绿豆芽	生、鲜。见附图	去根，数斤混合打匀		2002.7	北京市崇文门菜市场	
04-2-207	黑豆苗	生、鲜	去根，数斤混合打匀		2002.9	北京市家乐福超市	
04-2-208	豌豆苗	生、鲜。见附图	去根，数斤混合打匀		2002.8	北京市崇文门菜市场	
茄果、瓜菜类							
04-3-115	茄子 (白皮，长)	生、鲜。见附图	去蒂、去皮，数个混合打匀		2002.7	北京市崇文门菜市场	
04-3-116	茄子 (紫皮，长)	生、鲜。见附图	去蒂、去皮，数个混合打匀		2002.7	北京市崇文门菜市场	
04-3-117	茄子 (紫皮，圆)	生、鲜。见附图	去蒂、去皮，数个混合打匀		2002.7	北京市崇文门菜市场	
04-3-118	香瓜茄	生、鲜。见附图	去蒂、去皮，数个混合打匀		2002.9	北京市蔬菜研究中心	北京
04-3-119	番茄 [西红柿]	生、鲜。见附图	去蒂，数个混合打匀		2002.8	北京市崇文门菜市场	
04-3-120	樱桃番茄 [小西红柿]	生、鲜。见附图	去蒂，紫樱柿、春桃圣女、圣女果三个品种等量混合打匀		2002.8	北京市崇文门菜市场	
04-3-121	辣椒 (小红尖辣椒)	生、鲜	去蒂，数斤混合打匀		2002.9	北京市崇文门菜市场	
04-3-122	辣椒 (小红尖辣椒，干)	生、鲜	去蒂，数斤混合打匀		2002.8	北京市崇文门菜市场	
04-3-123	辣椒 (青，尖)	生、鲜。见附图	去蒂、去籽，数十个混合打匀		2002.8	北京市崇文门菜市场	
04-3-124	甜椒 [灯笼椒、柿子椒]	生、鲜，绿色。见附图	去蒂、去籽，数十个混合打匀		2002.8	北京市崇文门菜市场	
04-3-125	彩椒	生、鲜，红、黄、紫、白数种颜色的甜椒。见附图	去蒂、去籽，红、黄、紫、白等多种颜色样品等量混合打匀		2002.8	北京市蔬菜研究中心	北京

食物描述 Description of foods

编码	食物类别和名称	食物描述	样品处理	数据来源	采样日期	采样地点	产地
04-3-126	秋葵 [黄秋葵、羊角豆]	生、鲜。见附图	去蒂，数十个混合打匀		2002.9	北京市蔬菜研究中心	北京
04-3-221	冬瓜	生、鲜。见附图	去皮、去瓤，数个等量混合打匀		2002.8	北京市崇文门菜市场	
04-3-222	飞碟瓜	生、鲜。见附图	去蒂，数个等量混合打匀		2002.9	北京市蔬菜研究中心	北京
04-3-223	黄金西葫芦	生、鲜。见附图	去蒂，数个等量混合打匀		2002.9	北京市蔬菜研究中心	北京
04-3-224	黄茎瓜	生、鲜	去蒂，数个混合打匀			送检	四川
04-3-225	迷你黄瓜 [荷兰乳黄瓜]	生、鲜。见附图	去蒂，十余个混合打匀		2002.7	北京市崇文门菜市场	
04-3-226	秋黄瓜 [旱黄瓜]	生、鲜。见附图	去蒂，十余个混合打匀		2002.7	北京市崇文门菜市场	
04-3-227	南瓜 (栗面)	生、鲜。见附图	去皮、去瓤，数个等量混合打匀		2002.8	北京市蔬菜研究中心	北京
04-3-228	丝瓜	生、鲜。见附图	去蒂、去皮，数个混合打匀		2002.8	北京市崇文门菜市场	
葱蒜类							
04-4-206	大葱	生、鲜。见附图	去根、粗叶和外皮，十余根混合打匀		2002.8	北京市崇文门菜市场	
04-4-207	细香葱 [香葱、四季葱]	生、鲜。见附图	去根须、老叶和外皮，数斤混合打匀		2002.8	北京市崇文门菜市场	
04-4-404	韭菜	生、鲜。见附图	去老叶，数斤混合打匀		2002.8	北京市崇文门菜市场	
嫩茎、叶、花菜类							
04-5-117	大白菜 (白口)	生、鲜。见附图	去粗根、老帮儿，数棵各取1/4、混合打匀		2002.8	北京市崇文门菜市场	
04-5-118	大白菜 (青口)	生、鲜。见附图	去粗根、老帮儿，数棵各取1/4、混合打匀		2002.8	北京市崇文门菜市场	
04-5-119	酸白菜 [酸菜]	生，大白菜用开水渍后冷却、发酵	晾干表面水分，数斤混合打匀		2002.7	北京市崇文门菜市场	
04-5-120	小白菜 [青菜]	生、鲜。见附图	去根，数份取数斤混合打匀		2002.7	北京市崇文门菜市场	
04-5-121	奶白菜	生、鲜。见附图	数份取数斤混合打匀		2002.9	北京市家乐福超市	北京
04-5-122	鸡毛菜	生、鲜。见附图	数份数斤混合打匀		2002.8	北京市崇文门菜市场	

编码	食物类别和名称	食物描述	样品处理	数据来源	采样日期	采样地点	产地
04-5-123	娃娃菜	生、鲜。见附图	去根，数棵各取1/4、混合打匀		2002.8	北京市蔬菜研究中心	北京
04-5-124	乌塌菜 [塌菜、塌棵菜]	生、鲜。见附图	去根，数份数斤混合打匀		2002.9	北京市家乐福超市	北京
04-5-125	油菜	生、鲜。见附图	去根，数份取数斤混合打匀		2002.7	北京市崇文门菜市场	
04-5-126	油菜心	生、鲜。见附图	数份取数斤混合打匀		2002.8	北京市崇文门菜市场	
04-5-210	结球甘蓝（绿）[圆白菜]	生、鲜。见附图	去粗根，数个各取1/4，混合打匀		2002.7	北京市崇文门菜市场	
04-5-211	结球甘蓝（紫）	生、鲜。见附图	去粗根，数个各取1/4，混合打匀		2002.8	北京市崇文门菜市场	
04-5-212	抱子甘蓝	生、鲜。见附图	去蒂、数斤混合打匀		2002.8	北京市蔬菜研究中心	北京
04-5-213	羽衣甘蓝	生、鲜。见附图	数斤混合打匀		2002.8	北京市蔬菜研究中心	北京
04-5-214	盖菜	生、鲜。见附图	去根，数份数斤混合打匀		2002.8	北京市崇文门菜市场	
04-5-215	芥蓝 [甘蓝菜、盖蓝菜]	生、鲜。见附图	去老茎，数斤混合打匀		2002.8	北京市崇文门菜市场	
04-5-216	菜花 [花椰菜]	生、鲜。见附图	去粗茎，数个各取1/4、混合打匀		2002.8	北京市崇文门菜市场	
04-5-217	西兰花 [绿菜花]	生、鲜。见附图	去粗茎，数个各取1/4、混合打匀		2002.8	北京市崇文门菜市场	
04-5-327	番杏 [新西兰菠菜、夏菠菜]	生、鲜。见附图	数份数斤混合打匀		2002.8	北京市崇文门菜市场	
04-5-328	樱桃萝卜缨	生、鲜	数份数斤混合打匀		2002.8	北京市蔬菜研究中心	北京
04-5-329	白凤菜	生、鲜。见附图	数份数斤混合打匀		2002.8	北京市蔬菜研究中心	北京
04-5-330	紫背天葵 [红凤菜、血皮菜]	生、鲜。见附图	数斤混合打匀		2002.8	北京市蔬菜研究中心	北京
04-5-331	芹菜（茎）	生、鲜。见附图	去根、去叶，十余棵混合打匀		2002.8	北京市崇文门菜市场	
04-5-332	西芹 [西洋芹菜、美芹]	生、鲜。见附图	去根、去叶，十余棵混合打匀		2002.9	北京市崇文门菜市场	
04-5-333	生菜	生、鲜，圆球形叶菜。见附图	去粗根，数斤混合打匀		2002.8	北京市崇文门菜市场	

食物描述 Description of foods

编码	食物类别和名称	食物描述	样品处理	数据来源	采样日期	采样地点	产地
04-5-334	油麦菜	生、鲜。见附图	去根，数斤混合打匀		2002.8	北京市崇文门菜市场	
04-5-335	叶甜菜 (白梗)	生、鲜。见附图	数斤混合打匀		2002.9	北京市蔬菜研究中心	北京
04-5-336	莴笋叶 [莴苣菜]	生、鲜。见附图	数份数斤混合打匀		2002.8	北京市崇文门菜市场	
04-5-337	蕹菜 [空心菜、藤藤菜]	生、鲜。见附图	数份数斤混合打匀		2002.7	北京市崇文门菜市场	
04-5-338	观达菜 [根达菜、牛皮菜]	生、鲜。见附图	数份混合打匀			送检	北京
04-5-339	球茎茴香 [甜茴香、意大利茴香]	生、鲜，叶鞘膨大形成的球形茎。见附图	去根、外皮，十余个混合打匀		2002.9	北京市蔬菜研究中心	北京
04-5-415	芦笋 (绿) [石刁柏、龙须菜]	生、鲜，绿色、细长杆状。见附图	去老茎，数斤混合打匀		2002.8	北京市崇文门菜市场	
04-5-416	芦笋 (紫)	生、鲜，紫色、细长杆状。见附图	去老茎，数斤混合打匀		2002.9	北京市蔬菜研究中心	北京
04-5-417	结球菊苣	生、鲜，红色。见附图	去根，数个各取1/4、混合打匀		2002.8	北京市蔬菜研究中心	北京
04-5-418	软化白菊苣	生、鲜，黄白色。见附图	去根，数个混合打匀		2002.8	北京市蔬菜研究中心	北京
水生蔬菜类							
04-6-010	藕 [莲藕]	生、鲜。见附图	去节，数个混合打匀		2002.8	北京市崇文门菜市场	
薯芋类							
04-7-203	芋头 [芋艿、毛芋]	生、鲜。见附图	去皮，数斤混合打匀		2002.9	北京市朝阳区潘家园农贸市场	
04-7-204	芋头 (煮)			Korea-FCT			
野生蔬菜类							
04-8-081	苦苣菜 [苦菜、天精菜]	生、鲜。见附图	数斤混合打匀			送检	
04-8-082	苜蓿 [草头、金花菜]	生、鲜		ShH-FCT			上海
04-8-083	鱼腥草 (叶) [蕺菜、臭菜]	生、鲜。见附图	数斤混合打匀		2002.8	北京市蔬菜研究中心	北京
04-8-084	鱼腥草 (根)	生、鲜。见附图	去根须、数斤混合打匀		2002.8	北京市蔬菜研究中心	北京

编码	食物类别和名称	食物描述	样品处理	数据来源	采样日期	采样地点	产地
	菌藻类						
菌类							
05-1-028	白蘑菇 [双孢蘑菇、洋蘑菇]	见附图		TW-FCT			台湾
05-1-029	北风菌 [荷叶离褶伞、一窝羊]	见附图		YN-FCT			云南
05-1-030	草菇 [大黑头细花草、稻菇]	主要原料：鲜草菇、水、盐等。罐装。特供牌	数罐混合打匀		2001.11	送检	北京
05-1-031	茶树菇(干) [柱状田头菇、茶薪菇]	见附图	数包等量混合磨碎		2001.7	送检	江西
05-1-032	干巴菌	见附图		YN-FCT			云南
05-1-033	红奶浆菌 [多汁乳菇、谷熟菌]	见附图		YN-FCT			云南
05-1-034	黄蘑(干)	野生。丹华牌	数包等量混合磨碎		2001.7	送检	吉林
05-1-035	黄伞菇(干) [多脂鳞伞、黄丝菌]	见附图	数包等量混合磨碎		2001.9	送检	北京
05-1-036	鸡腿菇(干) [毛头鬼伞]	十爹牌	数包等量混合磨碎		2001.8	送检	广东
05-1-037	鸡油菌 [黄丝菌、杏菌]			YN-FCT			云南
05-1-038	鸡纵 [蚁纵、伞把菇、鸡纵菌]	见附图		YN-FCT			云南
05-1-039	鸡纵(干)	野生。野香牌	数包等量混合磨碎		2001.7	送检	四川
05-1-040	鸡纵(油炸) [油鸡纵]	油浸，加盐		YN-FCT			云南
05-1-041	鸡纵花			YN-FCT			云南
05-1-042	白牛肝菌 [美味牛肝菌]	见附图		YN-FCT			云南
05-1-043	白牛肝菌(干) [美味牛肝菌]	野香牌	数包等量混合磨碎		2001.7	送检	四川
05-1-044	黑牛肝菌 [铜色牛肝菌]	见附图		YN-FCT			云南

食物描述 Description of foods

编码	食物类别和名称	食物描述	样品处理	数据来源	采样日期	采样地点	产地
05-1-045	黄皮牛肝菌 [黄皮疣柄牛肝菌、黄癞头]	见附图		YN-FCT			云南
05-1-046	乳牛肝菌(干) [粘盖牛肝菌、松树菌]	野香牌	数包等量混合磨碎		2001.7	送检	四川
05-1-047	牛眼睛菌 [马勃菌]			YN-FCT			云南
05-1-048	平菇 [糙皮侧耳、青蘑]		数份数斤混合打匀		2002.8	北京市崇文门菜市场	
05-1-049	青头菌 [变绿红菇、绿菇]	见附图		YN-FCT			云南
05-1-050	松蘑(干) [松茸、松口蘑]	野香牌。见附图	数包等量混合磨碎		2001.7	送检	四川
05-1-051	杏鲍菇	见附图	数份数斤混合打匀			送检	河南
05-1-052	血红菇(干)	见附图	数包等量混合磨碎		2001.9	送检	北京
05-1-053	元蘑(干) [亚侧耳、冬蘑、黄蘑]	野生。丹华牌。见附图	数包等量混合磨碎		2001.7	送检	吉林
05-1-054	竹荪(干) [竹笙、竹参]			YN-FCT			云南
05-1-055	榛蘑(干) [小蜜环菌]	野生。丹华牌。见附图	数包等量混合磨碎		2001.7	送检	吉林
藻类							
05-2-009	螺旋藻(干)			YN-FCT			云南
05-2-010	裙带菜(干) [海芥菜、海木耳]	海王星牌	数罐等量混合磨碎		2003.7	北京市崇文门菜市场	辽宁
05-2-011	海带菜	主要原料：鲜海带、白糖、芝麻、碘盐等。姑香牌	数袋混合打匀		2002.3	送检	山东
	水果类及制品						
仁果类							
06-1-907	蛇果	见附图	去皮、去果芯，数斤混合打匀		2002.9	北京市崇文门菜市场	

食物描述 Description of foods

编码	食物类别和名称	食物描述	样品处理	数据来源	采样日期	采样地点	产地
核果类							
06-2-115	蜜桃		去皮、去核，数斤混合打匀			送检	河北
06-2-116	桃（糖水罐头）	主要原料：桃、水、白砂糖等。佳康牌	数罐混合打匀		2001.11	送检	河北
06-2-207	布朗	见附图	去皮、去核，数斤混合打匀		2002.9	北京市崇文门菜市场	
06-2-208	西梅		去皮、去核，数斤混合打匀		2002.9	北京市家乐福超市	
06-2-312	冬枣	见附图	去核，数斤混合打匀		2002.9	北京市家乐福超市	山东
06-2-313	小枣（干）		去核，数斤混合打匀		2003.7	北京市崇文门菜市场	河北
浆果类							
06-3-911	红提子葡萄	红色。见附图	去皮、去籽，数斤混合打匀		2002.9	北京市家乐福超市	山东
06-3-912	无花果（干）			TW-FCT			台湾
柑橘类							
06-4-303	葡萄柚（台湾）[西柚]	见附图	去皮、去籽	TW-FCT			台湾
06-4-304	葡萄柚（以色列）[西柚]		去皮、去籽，数斤混合打匀		2002.9	北京市家乐福超市	以色列
热带、亚热带水果							
06-5-021	桂圆（干）	干制桂圆，带壳	去皮、去核，数斤加水浸湿混合打匀		2001.8	送检	广东
06-5-022	红毛丹	见附图	去皮、去核，数斤混合打匀		2002.9	北京市崇文门菜市场	
06-5-023	火龙果[仙蜜果、红龙果]	见附图	去皮，十余个混合打匀		2002.9	北京市崇文门菜市场	
06-5-024	荔枝（干）	干制荔枝，带壳	去皮、去核，加水浸湿混合打匀		2002.3	送检	福建
06-5-025	榴莲	见附图	去壳，数份数斤混合打匀		2002.9	北京市家乐福超市	泰国
06-5-026	芒果（大头）			YN-FCT			云南
06-5-027	木瓜[番木瓜]	见附图		YN-FCT			云南
06-5-028	酸木瓜			YN-FCT			云南

食物描述 Description of foods

编码	食物类别和名称	食物描述	样品处理	数据来源	采样日期	采样地点	产地
06-5-029	蒲桃 [香果、水石榴]		去皮、去核，数斤混合打匀			送检	贵州
06-5-030	山竹	见附图	去壳、去核，数份数斤混合打匀		2002.9	北京市家乐福超市	
06-5-031	香蕉 (红皮，海南)	见附图	去皮，数斤混合打匀		2002.9	北京市家乐福超市	海南
06-5-032	香蕉 (红皮，泰国)	见附图	去皮，数斤混合打匀		2002.9	北京市家乐福超市	泰国
瓜果类							
06-6-206	小西瓜 [地雷瓜]	见附图	去皮、去籽，数个等量混合打匀		2002.9	北京市家乐福超市	
	坚果、种子类						
树坚果							
07-1-026	山核桃 (熟)	带壳，加盐。商品名：椒盐山核桃。勤俭牌	去壳，数包混合磨碎		2001.6	送检	浙江
07-1-027	栗子 (北京密云) [板栗]	带壳，生	去壳，数斤混合打碎			送检	北京
07-1-028	栗子 (河南) [板栗]	带壳，生	去壳，数斤混合打碎			送检	河南
07-1-029	栗子 (山东) [板栗]	带壳，生	去壳，数斤混合打碎			送检	山东
07-1-030	栗子 (河北迁西) [板栗]	带壳，生	去壳，数斤混合打碎			送检	河北迁西
07-1-031	栗子 (河北邢台) [板栗]	带壳，生	去壳，数斤混合打碎			送检	河北邢台
07-1-032	栗子仁 (熟)	商品名：甘栗仁	数包混合磨碎		2001.8	送检	河北
07-1-033	松子 (熟)	带壳，加盐。商品名：巴西松子	去壳，数包混合磨碎		2001.9	送检	广东
07-1-034	杏仁 (熟，带壳)	加盐。商品名：开口杏仁	去壳，数包混合磨碎		2001.8	送检	广东
07-1-035	杏仁 (熟，去壳)	加盐。商品名：大杏仁。枫叶牧场牌	数包混合磨碎		2001.7	送检	广东
07-1-036	腰果 (熟)	加盐	数包混合磨碎		2001.7	送检	
07-1-037	榛子 (熟)	带壳。商品名：美国榛子。枫叶牌	去壳，数包混合磨碎		2001.7	送检	广东
07-1-038	榛子仁 (熟)	加盐。商品名：五香榛子仁	数包混合磨碎		2001.9	送检	广东
07-1-039	开心果 (熟)	带壳，加盐。正林牌	去壳，数包混合磨碎		2001.6	送检	甘肃
07-1-040	香榧 (熟)	带壳，加盐。幸良贡宝牌	去壳，数包混合磨碎		2001.11	送检	浙江

食物描述 Description of foods

编码	食物类别和名称	食物描述	样品处理	数据来源	采样日期	采样地点	产地
种子							
07-2-020	花生(烤,勤俭牌)	带壳,加盐。商品名：美味花生	去壳,数包混合磨碎		2001.6	送检	四川
07-2-021	花生(烤,密日兴牌)	带壳,加盐	去壳,数包混合磨碎			送检	北京
07-2-022	花生仁(油炸)	加盐	数包混合磨碎			送检	北京
07-2-023	葵花子(奶油香瓜子)	主要原料：葵花子、盐等。加盐。正林牌	去壳,数包混合磨碎		2001.6	送检	甘肃
07-2-024	葵花子(熟)	主要原料：葵花子、盐等。加盐。商品名：美国葵花子。正林牌	去壳,数包混合磨碎		2001.6	送检	甘肃
07-2-025	南瓜子(熟)[白瓜子]	主要原料：南瓜子、盐等。加盐。正林牌	去壳,数包混合磨碎		2001.6	送检	甘肃
07-2-026	西瓜子(熟)[黑瓜子]	主要原料：黑瓜子、盐、酱油等。加盐。正林牌	去壳,数包混合磨碎		2001.6	送检	甘肃
	畜肉类及制品						
猪							
08-1-121	猪肉(前臀尖,杜长大猪)	生,肥瘦肉,去皮	数份等量混合打匀		2002.4	北京市大红门食品公司	河北
08-1-122	猪肉(前臀尖,良杂猪)	生,肥瘦肉,去皮	数份等量混合打匀		2002.4	北京市大红门食品公司	河北
08-1-123	猪肉(后臀尖,杜长大猪)	生,肥瘦肉,去皮	数份等量混合打匀		2002.4	北京市大红门食品公司	河北
08-1-124	猪肉(后臀尖,良杂猪)	生,肥瘦肉,去皮	数份等量混合打匀		2002.4	北京市大红门食品公司	河北
08-1-125	猪肉(硬肋,杜长大猪)	生,肥瘦肉,去皮	数份等量混合打匀		2002.4	北京市大红门食品公司	河北
08-1-126	猪肉(硬肋,良杂猪)	生,肥瘦肉,去皮	数份等量混合打匀		2002.4	北京市大红门食品公司	河北
08-1-127	猪肉(通脊,杜长大猪)	生,瘦	数份等量混合打匀		2002.4	北京市大红门食品公司	河北
08-1-128	猪肉(通脊,良杂猪)	生,瘦	数份等量混合打匀		2002.4	北京市大红门食品公司	河北
08-1-129	猪肉(里脊)	生,瘦	数份等量混合打匀		2002.4	北京市大红门食品公司	河北
08-1-130	猪皮	生	数份等量混合打匀		2002.4	北京市大红门食品公司	河北
08-1-131	猪小排(杜长大猪)	生,瘦,带骨	去骨,数份等量混合打匀		2002.4	北京市大红门食品公司	河北
08-1-132	猪小排(良杂猪)	生,瘦,带骨	去骨,数份等量混合打匀		2002.4	北京市大红门食品公司	河北
08-1-213	猪肚	生	数份等量混合打匀		2002.4	北京市大红门食品公司	河北

食物描述 Description of foods

编码	食物类别和名称	食物描述	样品处理	数据来源	采样日期	采样地点	产地
08-1-214	猪肝	生	数份等量混合打匀		2002.4	北京市大红门食品公司	河北
08-1-215	猪舌 [口条]	生	数份等量混合打匀		2002.4	北京市大红门食品公司	河北
08-1-216	猪肾 [猪腰子]	生	数份等量混合打匀		2002.4	北京市大红门食品公司	河北
08-1-318	火腿心全精肉	生, 腌制。雪舫蒋牌	数包等量混合打匀		2001.11	送检	浙江
08-1-319	火腿心肉	生, 带皮带骨, 腌制。商品名：火腿心。金云牌	去皮、去骨, 数包等量混合打匀		2001.8	送检	浙江
08-1-320	腊肉	主要原料：猪肉、白砂糖、精盐等。生, 腌制	数袋等量混合均匀打碎		2002.3	送检	广东
08-1-321	叉烧肉	主要原料：猪腿肉、糖、盐等。熟。商品名：太湖叉烧肉。三梅牌	数袋等量混合均匀打碎		2001.11	送检	江苏
08-1-322	酱排骨	主要原料：猪胸肉、肋排、盐、糖等。熟。商品名：无锡酱排骨。三梅牌	去骨, 数袋等量混合均匀打碎		2001.11	送检	江苏
08-1-323	香糟块肉	主要原料：猪五花肉、盐、糖等。熟。三梅牌	数袋等量混合均匀打碎		2001.11	送检	江苏
08-1-324	熏烤小里脊	主要原料：里脊肉、精盐、白糖等。熟。双汇牌	数袋等量混合均匀打碎		2001.5	送检	河南
08-1-325	猪肉脯	主要原料：猪后腿肉、白砂糖、精盐等。熟。伊香牌	数袋混合均匀、加水打碎		2001.8	送检	江苏
08-1-326	肉酥	主要原料：猪肉、白砂糖、组织蛋白粉、食盐等。熟。佳家福牌	数袋混合均匀磨碎		2001.11	送检	天津
08-1-327	猪肉松	主要原料：猪肉、白砂糖、食盐等。熟。采枫牌	数袋混合均匀磨碎		2001.8	送检	广东
08-1-328	扒猪脸	熟, 肥瘦肉, 带皮	数斤混合打匀			送检	北京
08-1-329	酱肘子	熟, 瘦, 无骨。天福号牌	数斤混合打匀			送检	北京
08-1-423	脆皮肠	主要原料：牛肉、肥膘、分离蛋白、食盐、白糖等。熟。双汇牌	数包混合打匀		2001.5	送检	河南
08-1-424	热狗肠	主要原料：猪瘦肉、肥膘、分离蛋白、淀粉、食盐、白糖等。熟。双汇牌	数根混合打匀		2001.5	送检	河南
08-1-425	火腿肠	主要原料：猪瘦肉、肥膘、淀粉、分离蛋白、食盐、白砂糖等。熟。双汇牌	数包混合打匀		2001.8	送检	河南

食物描述 Description of foods

编码	食物类别和名称	食物描述	样品处理	数据来源	采样日期	采样地点	产地
08-1-426	火腿	主要原料：猪肉、食盐等。熟。梅林牌	数罐混合打匀		2001.11	送检	上海
08-1-427	火腿 (云南)	熟，罐装。商品名：宣威火腿		YN-FCT			云南
08-1-428	三明治火腿	熟。双汇牌	数罐混合打匀		2001.5	送检	河南
08-1-429	午餐肉	主要原料：猪肉、食盐、淀粉等。熟。梅林牌	数罐混合均匀打碎		2001.11	送检	上海
牛							
08-2-111	牛肉 (背部肉)[上脑]	生，肥瘦肉	数份等量混合打匀		2002.6	北京市劲松大厂牛羊肉门市部	河北
08-2-112	牛肉 (里脊肉)[牛柳]	生，瘦	数份等量混合打匀		2002.6	北京市劲松大厂牛羊肉门市部	河北
08-2-113	牛肉 (臀部肉)[紫盖、白板]	生，瘦	数份等量混合打匀		2002.6	北京市劲松大厂牛羊肉门市部	河北
08-2-114	牛肉 (肩部肉)[肩肉]	生，肥瘦肉	数份等量混合打匀		2002.6	北京市劲松大厂牛羊肉门市部	河北
08-2-115	牛肉 (胸部肉)[牛胸]	生，肥瘦肉	数份等量混合打匀		2002.6	北京市劲松大厂牛羊肉门市部	河北
08-2-116	牛肉 (腹部肉)[牛腩]	生，肥瘦肉	数份等量混合打匀		2002.6	北京市劲松大厂牛羊肉门市部	河北
08-2-117	牛肉 (膝圆肉)[和尚头]	生，瘦	数份等量混合打匀		2002.6	北京市劲松大厂牛羊肉门市部	河北
08-2-118	牛肉 (股内肉) [针扒、米龙、黄瓜条]	生，瘦	数份等量混合打匀		2002.6	北京市劲松大厂牛羊肉门市部	河北
08-2-119	牛肉 (小腿肉) [牛展、牛腱子]	生，瘦	数份等量混合打匀		2002.6	北京市劲松大厂牛羊肉门市部	河北
08-2-210	牛百叶 (黑)	生	数份等量混合打匀		2002.6	北京市劲松大厂牛羊肉门市部	河北
08-2-307	牛肉 (酱，五香)	主要原料：牛肉、姜粉等。熟。正阳门牌	数袋混合均匀磨碎		2001.11	送检	北京
08-2-308	牛肉 (清香)	主要原料：牛肉、混合粉等。熟。正阳门牌	数袋混合均匀磨碎		2001.11	送检	北京
08-2-309	牛腱子 (香叶)	主要原料：牛腱子、精盐、味精等。熟。正阳门牌	数袋混合均匀磨碎		2001.11	送检	北京
08-2-310	牛肉干 (长富牌)	主要原料：黄牛肉、精盐、砂糖、植物油等。熟。长富牌	加水浸软、数袋混合打匀		2001.6	送检	重庆
08-2-311	牛肉干 (沙爹牌)	熟		YN-FCT			云南

食物描述 Description of foods

编码	食物类别和名称	食物描述	样品处理	数据来源	采样日期	采样地点	产地
羊							
08-3-113	羊肉(上脑)	生,肥瘦肉	数份等量混合打匀		2002.9	北京市劲松大厂牛羊肉门市部	
08-3-114	羊肉(腰窝)	生,肥瘦肉	数份等量混合打匀		2002.9	北京市劲松大厂牛羊肉门市部	
08-3-115	羊肉(前腿)	生,瘦	数份等量混合打匀		2002.9	北京市劲松大厂牛羊肉门市部	
08-3-116	羊肉(后腿)	生,瘦	数份等量混合打匀		2002.9	北京市劲松大厂牛羊肉门市部	
08-3-117	羊肉片	生	数袋混合均匀打碎			送检	
08-3-309	烧羊肉(五香)	主要原料：羊肉、花生油、食盐等。熟。正阳门牌	数袋混合均匀打碎		2001.11	送检	北京
08-3-310	羊肉串(生)	主要原料：羊后腿肉、白糖、精盐等。生。宝羊牌	数袋混合均匀打碎		2001.11	送检	青海
驴							
08-4-304	驴肉(五香)	主要原料：驴肉、精盐、白糖、味精等。熟。宴友思牌	数袋混合均匀打碎		2001.8	送检	陕西
其它							
08-9-006	鹿肉(梅花鹿)	生,冷冻	数袋混合均匀打碎		2001.11	送检	吉林
	禽肉类及制品						
鸡							
09-1-112	鸡胸脯肉	生,冷冻,无皮无骨	数袋等量混合均匀打碎		2002.7	北京市宣武区永安路菜市场	
09-1-113	鸡腿	生,冷冻	去皮、去骨,数斤混合打匀		2002.7	北京市宣武区永安路菜市场	
09-1-114	鸡翅	生,冷冻	去骨,数斤混合打匀		2002.7	北京市宣武区永安路菜市场	
09-1-115	鸡块(带浆粉)	主要原料：鸡肉、水解蛋白、浆粉等。生,冷冻。商品名：原味鸡块	数袋等量混合均匀打碎		2001.11	送检	河北
09-1-116	野山鸡	生,冷冻	去皮、去骨,数只等量混合打匀		2001.11	送检	河北
09-1-308	扒鸡(五香脱骨)	主要原料：鸡、蜂蜜、植物油、食盐、酱油等。熟。万事吉牌	去骨,数袋等量混合打匀		2001.11	送检	山东

编码	食物类别和名称	食物描述	样品处理	数据来源	采样日期	采样地点	产地
09-1-309	烤鸡	主要原料：鸡、食盐、陈年老汤等。熟。老唐牌	去骨，数袋等量混合打匀		2001.11	送检	北京
09-1-310	童子鸡(熟)	主要原料：一年内小鸡、啤酒、精盐、味精等。熟。商品名：啤酒童子鸡。清远楼牌	去骨，数袋等量混合打匀		2001.11	送检	河北
鸭							
09-2-214	鸭豉片	主要原料：鸭肉、白砂糖、食盐、曲酒等。生	数包混合打匀		2002.3	送检	广东
09-2-307	烤鸭(老唐牌)	主要原料：鸭、食盐、香油等。熟	去骨，胸脯肉皮肉混合打匀		2001.11	送检	北京
09-2-308	烤鸭(全聚德牌)	熟	去骨，胸脯肉皮肉混合打匀			送检	北京
鹅							
09-3-302	腊鹅	生，腌制。商品名：百禽腊鹅。百丈泉牌	去骨，胸脯肉皮肉混合打匀		2002.3	送检	江西
火鸡							
09-4-301	火鸡腿	熟，无皮	去骨，数个混合打匀		2002.9	北京市家乐福超市	
其它							
09-9-003	乳鸽	主要原料：乳鸽、陈年老汤汁等。生，冷冻。基立牌	去骨，数只混合打匀		2001.11	送检	河北
09-9-004	乳鸽(红烧)	主要原料：乳鸽、食盐、酱油等。熟。中鸽牌	去骨，数只混合打匀		2001.11	送检	河南
	乳类及制品						
液态乳							
10-1-105	牛乳(光明牌)	利乐包装，超高温灭菌。商品名：100%纯牛奶	数包混合均匀		2001.4	送检	上海
10-1-106	牛乳(乐百氏牌)	塑料瓶装，超高温灭菌。商品名：纯牛奶(100%)	数瓶混合均匀		2001.4	送检	广东
10-1-107	牛乳(帕玛拉特牌)	利乐包装，超高温灭菌。商品名：纯牛奶(100%)	数包混合均匀		2001.4	送检	天津
10-1-108	牛乳(三元牌)	利乐包装，超高温灭菌。商品名：纯牛奶	数包混合均匀		2001.4	送检	北京

食物描述 Description of foods

编码	食物类别和名称	食物描述	样品处理	数据来源	采样日期	采样地点	产地
10-1-109	牛乳 (完达山牌)	利乐包装,超高温灭菌。商品名：100%纯牛奶	数盒混合均匀		2001.4	送检	黑龙江
10-1-110	牛乳 (龙丹牌)	利乐包装,超高温灭菌。商品名：纯鲜牛奶(100%)	数包混合均匀		2001.4	送检	黑龙江
10-1-111	牛乳 (蒙牛牌)	利乐包装,超高温灭菌。商品名：纯鲜牛奶	数包混合均匀		2001.4	送检	内蒙古
10-1-112	牛乳 (新南洋牌)	利乐包装,超高温灭菌。商品名：纯鲜牛奶	数包混合均匀		2001.4	送检	北京
10-1-113	牛乳 (帕玛拉特)	利乐包装,超高温灭菌。商品名：保鲜牛奶	数包混合均匀		2001.4	送检	天津
10-1-114	牛乳 (伊利牌)	利乐包装,超高温灭菌。商品名：保鲜纯牛奶	数包混合均匀		2001.6	送检	内蒙古
10-1-115	牛乳 (部分脱脂,帕玛拉特)	利乐包装,超高温灭菌	数盒混合均匀		2001.4	送检	天津
10-1-116	牛乳 (脱脂,帕玛拉特)	利乐包装,超高温灭菌	数盒混合均匀		2001.4	送检	天津
10-1-117	牛乳 (强化锌、钙,帕玛拉特)	主要原料:鲜牛奶、乳酸锌、乳酸亚铁等。利乐包装,超高温灭菌。商品名:保鲜牛奶(加锌、钙)	数盒混合均匀		2001.4	送检	天津
10-1-118	牛奶 (草莓味,卡夫牌)	主要原料：鲜牛奶、水、全脂奶粉、白砂糖等。利乐包装,超高温灭菌	数盒混合均匀		2001.4	送检	北京
10-1-119	牛奶 (巧克力味,卡夫牌)	主要原料：鲜牛奶、水、全脂奶粉、白砂糖等。利乐包装,超高温灭菌	数盒混合均匀		2001.4	送检	北京
10-1-120	牛奶 (巧克力味,三元牌)	主要原料：鲜牛奶、白砂糖等。利乐包装,超高温灭菌	数盒混合均匀		2001.4	送检	北京
10-1-121	学生奶	主要原料：鲜牛奶、水、白砂糖等。商品名：中国学生奶	数瓶混合均匀		2001.6	送检	黑龙江

奶粉

编码	食物类别和名称	食物描述	样品处理	数据来源	采样日期	采样地点	产地
10-2-105	全脂奶粉 (雀巢)	主要原料：鲜牛奶、白砂糖、大豆磷脂、维生素A、维生素D_3等		FNL	2003		
10-2-106	全脂奶粉 (三鹿牌)	主要原料：鲜牛奶等	数袋等量混合均匀		2001.4	送检	河北
10-2-107	全脂奶粉 (伊利牌)	主要原料：牛奶、复合维生素等。无蔗糖	数袋等量混合均匀		2001.5	送检	内蒙古
10-2-108	全脂甜奶粉 (三鹿牌)	主要原料：鲜牛奶、蔗糖等。商品名：全脂加糖奶粉	数袋等量混合均匀		2001.4	送检	河北

编码	食物类别和名称	食物描述	样品处理	数据来源	采样日期	采样地点	产地
10-2-109	全脂甜奶粉（伊利牌）	主要原料：牛奶、白砂糖、复合维生素等。速溶	数袋等量混合均匀		2001.5	送检	内蒙古
10-2-110	低脂奶粉（高钙高铁，雀巢）	主要原料：脱脂奶、乳脂、乳酸钙和碳酸钙、焦磷酸铁、大豆磷脂、维生素C、E、A、D_3等。商品名：雀巢高钙高铁奶粉（低脂）		FNL	2003		
10-2-111	低脂奶粉（高钙高铁，伊利牌）	主要原料：鲜牛奶、脱脂奶粉、钙、铁、维生素C、A、D_3等。商品名：伊利高钙高铁低脂奶粉	数袋等量混合均匀		2001.5	送检	内蒙古
10-2-112	高钙高铁奶粉（可淇牌）	主要原料：鲜牛奶、脱盐乳清粉、脱脂奶粉、矿物质、维生素等		FNL	2003		广东
10-2-113	儿童奶粉（安儿健 A+，美赞臣）	主要原料：全脂奶粉、玉米糖浆固体、脱脂奶粉、蔗糖、乳糖、矿物质、维生素等。商品名：安儿健 A+ 儿童成长奶粉。适于3～6岁儿童		FNL	2003		
10-2-114	儿童奶粉（适体健，美赞臣）	主要原料：脱脂奶粉、全脂奶粉、玉米糖浆固体、蔗糖、植脂末、矿物质、维生素等。商品名：适体健儿童营养奶粉。适于3岁以上儿童		FNL	2003		广东
10-2-115	儿童奶粉（惠氏）	主要原料：脱脂牛奶、麦芽糖糊精、白砂糖、植物油、浓缩乳清蛋白、矿物质、维生素等。商品名：惠氏S-26金装学儿乐奶粉。适于3～7岁儿童		FNL	2003		上海
10-2-116	儿童奶粉（可淇牌）	主要原料：鲜牛奶、脱脂乳清粉、脱脂奶粉、维生素和矿物质等。商品名：可淇成长奶粉。适于3岁以上儿童		FNL	2003		广东
10-2-117	儿童奶粉（三鹿牌）	主要原料：鲜牛奶、脱盐乳清粉、多种维生素和矿物质等。商品名：三鹿助长奶粉。适于儿童、青少年		FNL	2003		河北
10-2-118	儿童奶粉（完达山牌）	主要原料：鲜牛奶、脱脂奶粉、脱脂乳清粉、维生素和矿物质等。商品名：完达山3段配方奶粉。适于3～6岁儿童		FNL	2003		黑龙江
10-2-119	孕妇乳母奶粉（惠氏）	主要原料：脱脂牛奶、麦芽糖糊精、浓缩乳清蛋白、白砂糖、植物油、维生素和矿物质等。商品名：爱儿乐妈妈		FNL	2003		上海
10-2-120	孕妇乳母奶粉（美赞臣）	主要原料：脱脂奶粉、玉米糖浆固体、全脂奶粉、矿物质、维生素、DHA等。商品名：安婴妈妈孕妇及授乳妇女营养奶粉		FNL	2003		

食物描述 Description of foods

编码	食物类别和名称	食物描述	样品处理	数据来源	采样日期	采样地点	产地
10-2-121	中老年奶粉 (可淇牌)	主要原料：鲜牛奶、脱脂奶粉、脱盐乳清粉、麦芽糊精、矿物质、维生素等		FNL	2003		广东
10-2-122	中老年奶粉 (雀巢)	主要原料：脱脂奶、低芥酸籽油、乳脂、玉料油、碳酸钙、大豆卵磷脂、维生素E、A、D_3等		FNL	2003		
10-2-123	中老年奶粉 (三鹿牌)	主要原料：鲜牛奶、脱脂奶粉、多种维生素和矿物质等		FNL	2003		河北
10-2-124	中老年奶粉 (森永牌)	主要原料：脱脂牛乳 (或脂脂乳粉)、精炼玉米油、大豆磷脂、多种维生素、硫酸亚铁、硫酸锌等		FNL	2003		黑龙江
酸奶							
10-3-007	酸奶 (调味)	主要原料：鲜牛奶、白砂糖、乳清蛋白、维生素A、D等。商品名：酸奶小超人。光明牌	黄桃、草莓、菠萝、原味多种口味数盒等量混匀		2001.8	送检	上海
10-3-008	酸奶 (果粒)	主要原料：鲜牛奶、乳粉、水果等。商品名：果粒酸奶。光明牌	黄桃、草莓两种口味数盒等量混匀		2001.8	送检	上海
奶酪							
10-4-012	奶酪 (光明牌)	主要原料：奶酪、牛奶、食盐等	数袋等量混合打匀		2001.8	送检	上海
10-4-013	奶酪 (骑士牌)		数袋等量混合打匀			送检	内蒙古
10-4-014	低脂奶酪	主要原料：奶酪、牛奶、食盐等。光明牌	数袋等量混合打匀		2001.8	送检	上海
10-4-015	硬质干酪			UK-FCT			
奶油							
10-5-008	奶油	主要原料：乳脂肪等。光明牌	数盒混合打匀		2001.8	送检	上海
其它							
10-9-004	全脂甜炼乳 (雀巢)	主要原料：牛奶、白砂糖等。商品名：鹰唛炼乳	数罐等量混合均匀		2001.11	送检	山东
10-9-005	全脂甜炼乳 (燕山牌)	主要原料：牛奶、白砂糖等	数瓶等量混合均匀		2001.11	送检	北京
10-9-006	脱脂甜炼乳			Korea-FCT			

编码	食物类别和名称	食物描述	样品处理	数据来源	采样日期	采样地点	产地
	蛋类及制品						
鸡蛋							
11-1-109	鸡蛋(红皮)	生	去壳，十余个混合打匀		2002.7	北京市宣武区永安路菜市场	
11-1-110	藏鸡蛋	生	去壳，十余个混合打匀			送检	西藏
11-1-111	乌鸡蛋(绿皮)	生。帅尔牌	去壳，十余个混合打匀		2001.4	送检	黑龙江
11-1-204	鸡蛋(煮)			Korea-FCT			
11-1-205	毛蛋	生	去壳，十余个混合打匀			送检	山东
11-1-206	荷包蛋(油煎)			Korea-FCT			
11-1-207	荷包蛋(煮)			Korea-FCT			
鸭蛋							
11-2-104	海鸭蛋	生。海湾牌	去壳，十余个混合打匀		2001.11	送检	广西
11-2-203	咸鸭蛋(煮)	三湖牌	去壳，十余个混合打匀		2001.6	送检	江苏
鹅蛋							
11-3-104	鹅蛋(煮)			Korea-FCT			
	鱼虾蟹贝类						
鱼							
12-1-131	草鱼 [白鲩、草包鱼]	鲜	鲜活鱼去鳞、鳍、头、刺和内脏，数条鱼肉打匀		2002.7	北京市宣武区永安路菜市场	天津
12-1-132	鲢鱼 [白鲢、胖子、连子鱼]	鲜	鲜活鱼去鳞、鳍、头、刺和内脏，数条鱼肉打匀		2002.7	北京市宣武区永安路菜市场	天津
12-1-133	鲫鱼 [喜头鱼、海附鱼]	鲜	鲜活鱼去鳞、鳍、头、刺和内脏，数条鱼肉打匀		2002.7	北京市宣武区永安路菜市场	天津
12-1-241	带鱼(切段)	生，冷冻	去刺，数斤鱼段混合打匀		2001.11	送检	浙江

食物描述 Description of foods

编码	食物类别和名称	食物描述	样品处理	数据来源	采样日期	采样地点	产地
12-1-242	黄鱼(小黄花鱼)	生,冷冻	去鳞、头、刺和内脏,数斤混合打匀		2001.11	送检	浙江
12-1-243	金鲳鱼	生,冷冻	鱼化冻后去鳞、鳍、头、刺和内脏,数条鱼肉打匀		2003.10	送检	浙江
12-1-244	鲭鱼	生,含鱼皮,去鳞、骨和内脏		TW-FCT			台湾
12-1-245	双髻鲨	生,含鱼皮,去鳞、骨和内脏		TW-FCT			台湾
12-1-303	金鲨鱼翅(干)		数盒混均磨碎		2002.3	送检	广东
12-1-304	鱼排	主要原料:白身鱼、面包粉、食盐等。生,冷冻	数份数袋混均磨碎		2001.11	送检	
12-1-305	鱼丸	主要原料:鱼肉、淀粉、食盐等。生,冷冻	数份数袋混均磨碎		2001.11	送检	
12-1-306	鱼子酱	主要原料:海鲭鱼子、番茄酱、植物油、碘盐等。姑香牌	数瓶混合打匀		2002.3	送检	山东
12-1-401	草鱼(熏)	主要原料:草鱼、植物油、食盐、味精、黄酒等。熟,袋装。商品名:太湖熏鱼。三梅牌	数袋混合打匀		2001.11	送检	江苏
12-1-402	丁香鱼(香辣味)	主要原料:丁香鱼、植物油、糖、食盐等。熟,罐装。喜客来牌	数罐混合打匀		2001.11	送检	福建
12-1-403	凤尾鱼(熟)	主要原料:凤尾鱼、植物油、食盐、糖等。熟,罐装。甘竹牌	数罐混合打匀		2001.11	送检	广东
12-1-404	箭鱼(炸)	主要原料:箭鱼、植物油、白砂糖、食盐等。熟,罐装。珍味源牌	数罐混合打匀		2001.11	送检	广东
12-1-405	金枪鱼(盐水浸)			UK-FCT			
12-1-406	金枪鱼(油浸)			UK-FCT			
12-1-407	鲮鱼(豆豉,熟)	主要原料:鲮鱼、植物油、豆豉、食盐、糖等。熟,罐装。商品名:豆豉鲮鱼。甘竹牌	数罐混合打匀		2001.11	送检	广东
12-1-408	鳗鱼(红烧)	主要原料:海鳗、植物油、白砂糖、食盐等。熟,罐装。鹰金钱牌	数罐混合打匀		2001.11	送检	广东
12-1-409	鲭鱼(烤,150℃,10分)	熟,不含鱼骨和内脏		TW-FCT			台湾
12-1-410	鲭鱼(烤,150℃,20分)	熟,不含鱼骨和内脏		TW-FCT			台湾
12-1-411	鲭鱼(烤,150℃,30分)	熟,不含鱼骨和内脏		TW-FCT			台湾

食物描述 Description of foods

编码	食物类别和名称	食物描述	样品处理	数据来源	采样日期	采样地点	产地
12-1-412	鲭鱼 (烤, 180℃, 10分)	熟, 不含鱼骨和内脏		TW-FCT			台湾
12-1-413	鲭鱼 (烤, 210℃, 10分)	熟, 不含鱼骨和内脏		TW-FCT			台湾
12-1-414	鲭鱼 (炸)	熟, 不含鱼骨和内脏, 在180℃沙拉油中炸3分钟		TW-FCT			台湾
12-1-415	鲭鱼 (蒸)	熟, 不含鱼骨和内脏, 以100℃蒸10分钟		TW-FCT			台湾
12-1-416	鲭鱼 (煮)	熟, 不含鱼骨和内脏, 以100℃煮10分钟		TW-FCT			台湾
12-1-417	沙丁鱼 (茄汁, 熟)	主要原料：沙丁鱼、水、植物油、番茄酱、食盐等。熟, 罐装。商品名：茄汁沙丁鱼。红塔牌	数罐混合打匀		2001.11	送检	辽宁
12-1-418	沙丁鱼 (盐水浸)			UK-FCT			
12-1-419	沙丁鱼 (油浸)			UK-FCT			
12-1-420	午餐鱼 (香辣味)	主要原料：蓝圆鲹、色拉油、糖、食盐等。熟, 罐装。喜客来牌	数罐混合打匀		2001.11	送检	福建
12-1-421	鳕鱼 (烤)	鱼片加上黄油后烤制		UK-FCT			
12-1-422	鳕鱼 (炸)	裹面包屑冷冻, 混合油煎炸		UK-FCT			
虾							
12-2-203	虾酱	主要原料：海虾酱、植物蛋白、植物油、食糖、食盐等。姑香牌	数瓶混合打匀		2002.3	送检	山东
12-2-204	虾仁 (红)	冷冻。宏基牌	数包混合打匀		2001.11	送检	浙江
12-2-301	虾仁肉丸	主要原料：猪肉、虾仁等。熟		TW-FCT			台湾
蟹							
12-3-006	海蟹 (小)	冷冻, 无背盖	去硬壳, 数包混合打匀		2001.11	送检	浙江
12-3-301	蟹足棒	主要原料：鱼糜、淀粉、蟹棒、食盐、糖等。生, 冷冻	数份数袋混合打匀		2001.11	送检	浙江
贝							
12-4-117	海蚌 [西施舌]			FJ-FCT			福建

食物描述 Description of foods

编码	食物类别和名称	食物描述	样品处理	数据来源	采样日期	采样地点	产地
12-4-601	文蛤丸	主要原料：文蛤肉、虱目鱼肉等		TW-FCT			台湾
其它							
12-9-014	甲鱼蛋					送检	北京
12-9-301	墨鱼圈	主要原料：墨鱼肉等。生，冷冻	数包混合打匀		2001.11	送检	浙江
12-9-302	墨鱼丸	主要原料：鱼肉、墨鱼肉、淀粉等。生，冷冻	数份数包混合打匀		2001.11	送检	
	婴幼儿食品						
婴幼儿配方粉							
13-1-101	婴儿配方奶粉（爱儿乐，惠氏）	主要原料：脱脂牛奶、脱盐乳清蛋白、植物油、乳糖、矿物质、维生素等。商品名：S-26爱儿乐。适于0~6个月婴儿		FNL	2003		新加坡
13-1-102	婴儿配方奶粉（爱儿乐，惠氏，金装）	主要原料：脱脂牛奶、乳糖、植物油、以α乳清蛋白为主的乳清蛋白、植物油、矿物质、维生素等。商品名：S-26金装爱儿乐。适于0~6个月婴儿		FNL	2003		新加坡
13-1-103	婴儿配方奶粉（爱力大1，美赞臣）	主要原料：玉米糖浆固体、全脂奶粉、精炼植物油、乳糖、脱脂奶粉、浓缩乳清蛋白、矿物质、维生素等。商品名：爱力大1初生婴儿配方奶粉。适于0~12个月婴儿		FNL	2003		
13-1-104	婴儿配方奶粉（安婴儿，美赞臣）	主要原料：乳糖、精炼植物油、脱脂奶粉、浓缩乳清蛋白、大豆卵磷脂、矿物质、维生素等。适于0~12个月婴儿		FNL	2003		
13-1-105	婴儿配方奶粉（安婴儿A+，美赞臣）	主要原料：乳糖、精炼植物油、浓缩乳清蛋白、脱脂奶粉、大豆卵磷脂、矿物质、维生素等。适于0~12个月婴儿		FNL	2003		
13-1-106	婴儿配方奶粉（安婴乐，美赞臣）	主要原料：玉米糖浆固体、牛奶蛋白、精炼植物油、大豆卵磷脂、矿物质、维生素、牛磺酸等。不含乳糖和蔗糖。适于0~12个月乳糖不耐受婴幼儿		FNL	2003		
13-1-107	婴儿配方奶粉（吉利蜜1，森永牌）	主要原料：牛奶、脱盐乳清粉、精炼植物油、大豆磷脂、奶油、多种维生素等。适于0~6个月婴儿		FNL	2003		黑龙江
13-1-108	婴儿配方奶粉（可淇牌）	主要原料：鲜牛奶、脱盐乳清粉、乳糖、植物油、低聚糖、维生素、矿物质等。适于0~6个月婴儿		FNL	2003		广东

编码	食物类别和名称	食物描述	样品处理	数据来源	采样日期	采样地点	产地
13-1-109	婴儿配方奶粉 (力多精1，雀巢)	主要原料：脱脂奶、麦芽糖糊精、乳糖、脱盐乳清蛋白、植物油、矿物质、多种维生素等。强化铁。商品名：力多精1初生婴儿配方奶粉(含铁质)。适于0~6个月婴儿		FNL	2003		黑龙江
13-1-110	婴儿配方奶粉 (美素力1)	主要原料：脱脂奶、脱矿物乳清、植物油、乳糖、低聚乳糖、麦芽糖糊精、多种矿物质和维生素等。金装。适于0~6个月婴儿		FNL	2003		
13-1-111	婴儿配方奶粉 (美素力H)	主要原料：脱脂奶、脱矿物乳清、植物油、蔗糖、麦芽糖糊精、低聚果糖、矿物质、维生素等。全能装。适于0~6个月婴儿		FNL	2003		
13-1-112	婴儿配方奶粉 (美素力，袋装)	主要原料：脱矿物质乳清粉、植物油、乳糖、脱脂奶固体、葡萄糖糖浆、矿物质和维生素等。适于0~6个月婴儿		FNL	2003		
13-1-113	婴儿配方奶粉 (圣元牌)	主要原料：鲜牛奶、脱盐乳清粉、乳脂、精炼植物油、乳糖、低聚果糖、维生素、矿物质等。商品名：圣元优聪配方1段初生婴儿奶粉。适于0~6个月婴儿		FNL	2003		山东
13-1-114	婴儿配方奶粉 (完达山牌)	主要原料：鲜牛奶、乳清粉、多种维生素和微量元素等。商品名：完达山1段配方奶粉。适于0~6个月婴儿		FNL	2003		黑龙江
13-1-115	婴儿奶粉 (高钙，圣元牌)	主要原料：鲜牛奶、脱盐乳清粉、乳糖、精炼植物油、乳钙、多种矿物质和维生素等。强化钙。商品名：圣元优强婴儿补钙奶粉。适于0~6个月婴儿		FNL	2003		山东
13-1-116	婴儿配方豆粉 (爱儿素，惠氏)	主要原料：玉米糖浆、植物油、分离大豆蛋白、白砂糖、矿物质、维生素等。商品名：S-26爱儿素Nursoy。适用于对乳糖不耐受、腹泻恢复期、对牛奶蛋白过敏的婴儿		FNL	2003		爱尔兰
13-1-201	较大婴儿配方奶粉 (爱力大2，美赞臣)	主要原料：全脂奶粉、玉米糖浆固体、脱脂奶粉、蔗糖、乳糖、精炼植物油、矿物质、维生素等。适于6~12个月婴儿		FNL	2003		
13-1-202	较大婴儿配方奶粉 (安婴宝，美赞臣)	主要原料：玉米糖浆固体、全脂奶粉、脱脂奶粉、精炼植物油、乳糖、大豆卵磷脂、矿物质、维生素等。适于6~12个月婴儿		FNL	2003		
13-1-203	较大婴儿配方奶粉 (安婴宝A+，美赞臣)	主要原料：玉米糖浆固体、全脂奶粉、脱脂奶粉、精炼植物油、乳糖、大豆卵磷脂、矿物质、维生素等。适于6~12个月婴儿		FNL	2003		

食物描述 Description of foods

编码	食物类别和名称	食物描述	样品处理	数据来源	采样日期	采样地点	产地
13-1-204	较大婴儿配方奶粉 (健儿乐，惠氏)	主要原料：脱脂牛奶、乳糖、植物油、脱盐乳清粉、白砂糖、矿物质、维生素等。商品名：S-26健儿乐。适于6～12个月婴儿		FNL	2003		新加坡
13-1-205	较大婴儿配方奶粉 (健儿乐，惠氏，金装)	主要原料：脱脂牛奶、乳糖、植物油、脱盐乳清粉、白砂糖、多种矿物质和维生素等。商品名：S-26金装健儿乐。适于6～12个月婴儿		FNL	2003		新加坡
13-1-206	较大婴儿配方奶粉 (可淇牌)	主要原料：鲜牛奶、脱盐乳清粉、乳清蛋白粉、葡萄糖、植物油、矿物质、维生素等。适于6～12个月婴儿		FNL	2003		广东
13-1-207	较大婴儿配方奶粉 (美素乐2)	主要原料：脱脂奶、脱矿物乳清、植物油、乳糖、低聚果糖、麦芽糖糊精、矿物质和维生素等。金装。商品名：美素乐较大婴儿及幼儿配方奶粉2段。适于6～12个月婴儿		FNL	2003		
13-1-208	较大婴儿配方奶粉 (美素乐，全能装)	主要原料：脱脂奶、脱矿物乳清、植物油、乳糖、低聚果糖、麦芽糖糊精、矿物质和维生素等。适于6～12个月婴儿		FNL	2003		
13-1-209	较大婴儿配方奶粉 (美素乐，袋装)	主要原料：脱矿物质乳清粉、脱脂乳固体、植物油、蔗糖、葡萄糖浆固体、矿物质、维生素等。适于6～12个月婴儿		FNL	2003		
13-1-210	较大婴幼儿配方奶粉 (吉利蜜2，森永牌)	主要原料：牛奶、脱脂奶粉、脱盐乳清粉、奶油、精炼植物油、碳酸钙、多种维生素等。适于6个月～3岁婴幼儿		FNL	2003		黑龙江
13-1-211	较大婴幼儿配方奶粉 (力多精2，雀巢)	主要原料：脱脂奶、乳脂、麦芽糖糊精、维生素和矿物质等。商品名：力多精2较大婴儿及幼童奶粉。适于6个月以上婴幼儿		FNL	2003		黑龙江
13-1-212	较大婴儿配方奶粉 (圣元牌)	主要原料：鲜牛奶、脱盐乳清粉、乳脂、精炼植物油、乳糖、低聚果糖、维生素、矿物质等。商品名：圣元优聪配方2段较大婴儿奶粉。适于6～12个月婴儿		FNL	2003		山东
13-1-213	较大婴幼儿奶粉 (高钙，圣元牌)	主要原料：鲜牛奶、脱盐乳清粉、乳糖、精炼植物油、乳钙、多种维生素和矿物质等。强化钙。商品名：圣元优强幼儿补钙奶粉。适于6个月～3岁婴幼儿		FNL	2003		山东
13-1-214	较大婴幼儿配方奶粉 (完达山牌)	主要原料：鲜牛奶、脱脂奶粉、多种维生素和微量元素等。商品名：完达山2段配方奶粉。适于6个月～3岁婴幼儿		FNL	2003		黑龙江

编码	食物类别和名称	食物描述	样品处理	数据来源	采样日期	采样地点	产地
13-1-301	幼儿奶粉 (爱力大3, 美赞臣)	主要原料：脱脂奶粉、全脂奶粉、玉米糖浆固体、蔗糖、精炼植物油、乳糖、矿物质、维生素等。商品名：爱力大3成长配方奶粉。适于1～3岁幼儿		FNL	2003		
13-1-302	幼儿奶粉 (安儿宝, 美赞臣)	主要原料：脱脂奶粉、全脂奶粉、玉米糖浆固体、蔗糖、精炼植物油、乳糖、矿物质、维生素等。高蛋白。商品名：安儿宝高蛋白成长奶粉。适于1～3岁幼儿		FNL	2003		
13-1-303	幼儿奶粉 (安儿宝A+, 美赞臣)	主要原料：脱脂奶粉、全脂奶粉、玉米糖浆固体、蔗糖、精炼植物油、乳糖、矿物质、维生素等。高蛋白。商品名：安儿宝A+高蛋白成长奶粉。适于1～3岁幼儿		FNL	2003		
13-1-304	幼儿奶粉 (惠氏)	主要原料：脱脂牛奶、麦芽糖糊精、植物油、浓缩乳清蛋白、白砂糖、矿物质、维生素等。商品名：S-26幼儿乐。适于1～3岁幼儿		FNL	2003		新加坡
13-1-305	幼儿奶粉 (惠氏, 金装)	主要原料：脱脂牛奶、麦芽糖糊精、植物油、浓缩乳清蛋白、白砂糖、矿物质、维生素等。商品名：S-26金装幼儿乐。适于1～3岁幼儿		FNL	2003		新加坡
13-1-306	幼儿奶粉 (可淇牌)	主要原料：鲜牛奶、脱盐乳清粉、植物油、维生素、矿物质等。商品名：可淇幼儿配方奶粉。适于1～3岁婴幼儿		FNL	2003		广东
13-1-307	幼儿奶粉 (美素高)	主要原料：脱脂奶、脱矿物乳清、植物油、蔗糖、麦芽糖糊清、低聚果糖、维生素和矿物质等。商品名：美素高成长配方奶粉3段。适于1～3岁幼儿		FNL	2003		
13-1-308	幼儿奶粉 (美素高, 全能装)	主要原料：脱脂奶、脱矿物乳清、植物油、蔗糖、麦芽糖糊精、低聚果糖、矿物质、维生素等。全能装。商品名：美素高成长配方奶粉(香草味)。适于1～3岁幼儿		FNL	2003		
13-1-309	幼儿奶粉 (美素高, 袋装)	主要原料：脱脂奶固体、脱矿物质乳清粉、植物油、蔗糖、麦芽糖糊精、多种矿物质、维生素等。袋装。商品名：美素高成长配方奶粉(香草味)。适于1～3岁幼儿		FNL	2003		
13-1-310	幼儿奶粉 (雀巢)	主要原料：脱脂奶、白砂糖、乳脂、蜂蜜、玉米油、大豆卵磷脂、多种维生素、矿物质等。商品名：雀巢成长奶粉		FNL	2003		黑龙江
13-1-311	幼儿奶粉 (雀巢金牌)	主要原料：脱脂奶、玉米糖浆、植物油脂、白砂糖、乳脂、蜂蜜、多种维生素、矿物质等。商品名：雀巢金牌成长奶粉		FNL	2003		黑龙江

食物描述 Description of foods

编码	食物类别和名称	食物描述	样品处理	数据来源	采样日期	采样地点	产地
13-1-312	幼儿奶粉 (森永牌)	主要原料：牛奶、脱脂奶粉、脱盐乳清粉、白砂糖、精炼植物油、碳酸钙、大豆磷脂、多种维生素等。商品名：森永吉利蜜3成长奶粉。适于1岁以上幼儿		FNL	2003		黑龙江
13-1-313	幼儿奶粉 (圣元牌)	主要原料：鲜牛奶、脱盐乳清粉、乳脂、精炼植物油、乳糖、低聚果糖、维生素、矿物质等。商品名：圣元优聪3段幼儿成长奶粉。适于1~3岁幼儿		FNL	2003		山东
婴幼儿断乳期辅助食品							
13-2-001	胡萝卜苹果泥 (亨氏)	主要原料：苹果、胡萝卜、橙汁、维生素C等	数瓶混合打匀		2001.8	送检	山东
13-2-002	鸡肝蔬菜泥 (亨氏)	主要原料：土豆、鸡肝、胡萝卜、青刀豆、奶酪等	数瓶混合打匀		2001.8	送检	山东
13-2-003	香甜胡萝卜泥 (亨氏)	主要原料：胡萝卜等	数瓶混合打匀		2001.8	送检	山东
婴幼儿补充食品							
13-3-009	米粉 (雀巢)	主要原料：大米粉、白砂糖、番茄酱、矿物质和维生素等。适于6个月以上婴幼儿		FNL	2003		
13-3-010	米粉 (高蛋白, 雀巢)	主要原料：脱脂奶、大米粉、白砂糖、乳脂、玉米油、矿物质和维生素等。适于6个月以上婴幼儿		FNL	2003		黑龙江
13-3-011	米粉 (高蛋白, 亨氏)	主要原料：大米、脱脂豆粉、大豆分离蛋白、脱脂奶粉、维生素等。强化维生素A、D和钙, 袋装	数袋等量混合均匀		2001.7	送检	广东
13-3-012	米粉 (苹果, 雀巢)	主要原料：大米粉、白砂糖、苹果泥、磷脂、多种维生素和矿物质等。适于6个月以上婴幼儿		FNL	2003		黑龙江
13-3-013	米粉 (蔬菜, 亨氏)	主要原料：大米、白砂糖、全脂奶粉、大豆分离蛋白胡萝卜、菠菜、番茄、多种维生素和矿物质等。适于6~24个月婴幼儿		FNL	2003		广东
13-3-014	米粉 (蔬菜, 雀巢)	主要原料：大米粉、白砂糖、番茄酱、菠菜、磷脂、多种维生素和矿物质等。适于7个月以上婴幼儿		FNL	2003		黑龙江
13-3-015	米粉 (胡萝卜, 亨氏)	主要原料：大米、白砂糖、胡萝卜、多种维生素和矿物质等。适于4~24个月婴幼儿		FNL	2003		广东
13-3-016	米粉 (胡萝卜, 雀巢)	主要原料：大米粉、白砂糖、胡萝卜泥、磷脂、多种维生素和矿物质等。适于6个月以上婴幼儿		FNL	2003		黑龙江

编码	食物类别和名称	食物描述	样品处理	数据来源	采样日期	采样地点	产地
13-3-017	米粉 (番茄, 亨氏)	主要原料：大米、白砂糖、脱脂奶粉、全脂奶粉、番茄、DHA、多种维生素和矿物质等。含DHA。适于4～24个月婴幼儿		FNL	2003		广东
13-3-018	米粉 (猪肝蔬菜, 亨氏)	主要原料：大米、白砂糖、全脂奶粉、大豆分离蛋白、猪肝、胡萝卜、豌豆、番茄、多种维生素和矿物质等。适于6～24个月婴幼儿		FNL	2003		广东
13-3-019	米粉 (鱼肉蔬菜, 亨氏)	主要原料：大米、白砂糖、鳕鱼、全脂奶粉、大豆分离蛋白、胡萝卜、菠菜、番茄、多种维生素和矿物质等。适于8～24个月婴幼儿		FNL	2003		广东
13-3-020	麦粉 (蜂蜜, 雀巢)	主要原料：小麦面粉、白砂糖、蜂蜜、磷脂、多种维生素和矿物质等。适于6个月以上婴幼儿		FNL	2003		黑龙江
	小吃、甜饼						
小吃							
14-1-038	春卷 (素馅)	主要原料：富强粉、植物油、卷心菜、蘑菇、胡萝卜、青豆角、豆腐干等。生、冷冻	数盒混合打匀		2001.11	送检	天津
14-1-039	黑芝麻汤圆	主要原料：糯米粉、芝麻、植物油、芝麻粉、芝麻酱、花生仁等。生、冷冻	数份数盒等量混合打匀		2001.11	送检	
14-1-040	醪糟	主要原料：水、糯米、白砂糖、曲药等。东汉牌	数瓶混合打匀		2001.9	送检	四川
14-1-041	煎饼	主要原料：玉米、小麦、小米、大豆等。商品名：老区煎饼。嘉会牌	数袋混合打匀		2001.11	送检	山东
14-1-042	过桥米线			YN-FCT			云南
蛋糕、甜点							
14-2-108	蛋糕 (巧克力)			Korea-FCT			
14-2-109	蛋糕 (水果)			Korea-FCT			
14-2-209	月饼 (蛋黄)	主要原料：小麦面粉、植物油、蛋黄、莲蓉等	十余个混合磨碎		2001.8	送检	广东
14-2-210	月饼 (豆沙)	主要原料：小麦面粉、植物油、赤豆等	十余个混合磨碎		2001.8	送检	广东
14-2-211	月饼 (桂花板栗)	主要原料：小麦面粉、植物油、桂花、板栗等	十余个混合磨碎		2001.8	送检	广东

食物描述 Description of foods

编码	食物类别和名称	食物描述	样品处理	数据来源	采样日期	采样地点	产地
14-2-212	月饼 (奶油莲蓉)			ShH-FCT			上海
14-2-332	沙琪玛蛋酥	主要原料：小麦面粉、鸡蛋、棕榈油、白砂糖、麦芽糖、葡萄干等。台尚牌	数包混合均匀磨碎		2001.8	送检	上海
14-2-333	香橙水果馅饼	主要原料：面粉、多种水果馅等	数袋混合打匀			送检	
	速食食品						
	快餐食品						
15-1-001	鸡柳汉堡 (肯德基)		数份等量混合打匀			送检	北京
15-1-002	香芋甜心 (肯德基)	主要原料：芋头等	数份等量混合打匀		2003.8	送检	北京
15-1-003	鸡肉汉堡 (肯德基)	主要原料：鸡肉、玉米、胡萝卜、青豆、生菜等	数份等量混合打匀		2003.8	送检	北京
15-1-004	鸡肉卷 (肯德基)	主要原料：鸡腿肉、黄瓜条、大葱、面饼、面酱等	数份等量混合打匀		2003.8	送检	北京
15-1-005	上校鸡块 (肯德基)		数份等量混合打匀			送检	北京
15-1-006	辣鸡翅 (肯德基)		去骨、数份等量混合打匀			送检	北京
15-1-007	新奥尔良鸡翅 (肯德基)		去骨、数份等量混合打匀		2003.8	送检	北京
15-1-008	劲爆鸡米花 (肯德基)	主要原料：鸡腿肉丁等	数份等量混合打匀		2003.8	送检	北京
15-1-009	甜玉米籽粒 (肯德基)		数份等量混合打匀			送检	北京
15-1-010	薯条 (肯德基)		数份等量混合打匀			送检	北京
15-1-011	比萨饼 (夹奶酪)			USA-FCT			
15-1-012	比萨饼 (夹奶酪、肉和蔬菜)			USA-FCI			
15-1-013	三明治 (夹火腿、干酪)			Korea-FCT			
15-1-014	三明治 (夹鸡蛋、干酪)			Korea-FCT			
15-1-015	三明治 (夹鸡肉片，无调料酱)			USA-FCI			
15-1-016	三明治 (夹烤牛肉片)			USA-FCT			
15-1-017	三明治 (夹鱼肉片)			Korea-FCT			
15-1-018	干酪汉堡包 (夹熏肉，加调料酱)			USA-FCT			

编码	食物类别和名称	食物描述	样品处理	数据来源	采样日期	采样地点	产地
15-1-019	干酪汉堡包(普通型,夹单层肉饼,无调料酱)			USA-FCT			
15-1-020	干酪汉堡包(普通型,夹奶酪、单层肉饼,加调料酱)			USA-FCT			
15-1-021	干酪汉堡包(普通型,夹奶酪、单层肉饼,加调料酱和蔬菜)			USA-FCT			
15-1-022	干酪汉堡包(普通型,夹奶酪、双层肉饼、双层面包,加调料酱和蔬菜)			USA-FCT			
15-1-023	汉堡包(普通型,夹肉饼,加调料酱和蔬菜)			USA-FCT			
15-1-024	热狗(原味)			USA-FCT			
方便食品							
15-2-105	早餐奶	主要原料:牛奶、麦片、鸡蛋等。三元牌	数盒混合均匀		2001.4	送检	北京
15-2-106	八宝粥(康师傅牌)	主要原料:水、糯米、薏仁、麦仁、赤豆、花豆、花生、桂圆、蒟蒻、银耳、白砂糖等。商品名:实粒派桂圆八宝粥	数罐混合打匀		2001.4	送检	天津
15-2-107	八宝粥(亲亲牌)	主要原料:水、糯米、薏仁、麦仁、赤豆、绿豆、花豆、花生仁、桂圆、砂糖等	数罐混合打匀		2001.4	送检	江苏
15-2-108	八宝粥(同茂牌)	主要原料:水、糯米、麦仁、赤豆、绿豆、花豆、花生仁、桂圆、白砂糖、燕窝香料等。商品名:燕窝八宝粥	数罐混合打匀		2001.4	送检	福建
15-2-109	八宝粥(娃哈哈牌)	主要原料:纯净水、糯米、米仁、赤豆、红芸豆、花生仁、莲子、桂圆、银耳、白砂糖等。商品名:桂圆莲子营养八宝粥	数罐混合打匀		2001.4	送检	浙江
15-2-110	八宝粥(无糖,娃哈哈牌)	主要原料:纯净水、糯米、米仁、赤豆、红芸豆、花生仁、魔芋、莲子、银耳、木糖醇等。商品名:无糖营养八宝粥	数罐混合打匀		2001.4	送检	浙江
15-2-111	八宝粥(椰树牌)	主要原料:矿泉水、薏米、糯米、赤豆、绿豆、花生、莲子、桂圆、红枣、白砂糖等。商品名:天然八宝粥	数罐混合打匀		2001.10	送检	海南
15-2-112	黑芝麻糊粉	主要原料:大米、黑米、黑芝麻、花生仁、核桃仁等	数袋等量混合均匀		2001.7	送检	江苏
15-2-113	麦片	主要原料:麦、米、麦芽精、玉米等。超级牌	数袋等量混合均匀磨碎		2001.10	送检	江苏
15-2-114	麦片(原味香奶)	主要原料:麦片、奶粉等	数袋混合均匀磨碎		2001.7	送检	江苏

食物描述 Description of foods

编码	食物类别和名称	食物描述	样品处理	数据来源	采样日期	采样地点	产地
15-2-115	燕麦片	主要原料：天然燕麦等。免煮。寿牌	数袋混合均匀磨碎		2001.11	送检	内蒙古
15-2-116	燕麦片(果仁,甜)	主要原料：燕麦片、糖、奶粉、核桃仁、葡萄干等。约克牌	数袋混合均匀磨碎		2001.11	送检	内蒙古
15-2-117	苦荞麦片(无糖)		数盒等量混合均匀磨碎			送检	贵州
15-2-118	玉米片			USA-FCT			
15-2-119	玉米片(低钠)			USA-FCT			
15-2-202	鸡汁味干脆面(面饼＋调味料)	主要原料：面饼:小麦面粉、植物油、食盐等；调味包:食盐、味精、鸡肉精粉等。康师傅牌	相同个数的面饼与调味包混合磨碎		2001.5	送检	天津
15-2-203	海鲜味方便面(面饼＋调味料＋油料)	主要原料：面饼:小麦面粉、植物油、食盐等；调味包:食盐、味精、海鲜粉等;油包:棕榈油等。商品名:劲拉面海'鲜珍锅煮面。康师傅牌	将面饼和调味包、油料包分别测定,测定结果按样品重量比折算		2001.5	送检	天津
15-2-204	海鲜味方便面(面饼＋调味料)	主要原料：面饼:小麦面粉、植物油、食盐等；调味包:食盐、味精、海鲜粉等。康师傅牌	相同个数的面饼与调味包混合磨碎		2001.5	送检	天津
15-2-205	油料(海鲜味方便面)	主要原料：棕榈油等。康师傅牌	数个油包混合打匀		2001.5	送检	天津
15-2-206	红烧牛肉方便面(面饼＋调味料+蔬菜+肉酱)	主要原料：面饼:小麦面粉、植物油、食盐、鸡蛋等；肉酱包:棕榈油、牛肉等;调味包:食盐、味精等;脱水蔬菜。商品名:珍品红烧牛肉面。康师傅牌	将面饼和调味包和蔬菜包、肉酱包分别测定,测定结果按样品重量比折算		2001.5	送检	天津
15-2-207	红烧牛肉方便面(面饼+调味料+蔬菜)	主要原料：面饼:小麦面粉、植物油、食盐、鸡蛋等；调味包:食盐、味精等;脱水蔬菜。康师傅牌	相同个数的面饼、调味包、蔬菜包混合磨碎		2001.5	送检	天津
15-2-208	肉酱(红烧牛肉方便面)	主要原料：棕榈油、牛肉等。康师傅牌	数个肉酱包混合打匀		2001.5	送检	天津
15-2-209	鳕鱼方便面(面饼+调味料+珍料+调味油+蔬菜)	主要原料:面饼:小麦面粉、植物油、食盐等;调味包:食盐、味精、海鲜粉等;珍料包:精选鱼肉、精制油、食盐等;调味油包:棕榈油等;脱水蔬菜。商品名:料珍多极品鳕鱼面。康师傅牌	将面饼和调味包和蔬菜包、珍料包和调味油包分别测定,测定结果按样品重量比折算		2001.5	送检	天津
15-2-210	鳕鱼方便面(面饼+调味料+蔬菜)	主要原料：面饼:小麦面粉、植物油、食盐等；调味包:食盐、味精、海鲜粉等;脱水蔬菜。康师傅牌	相同个数的面饼、调味包和蔬菜包混合磨碎		2001.5	送检	天津
15-2-211	油酱料(珍料+调味油,鳕鱼方便面)	主要原料：珍料包:精选鱼肉、精制油、食盐等；调味油包:棕榈油等。康师傅牌	相同个数的珍料包和调味油包混合打匀		2001.5	送检	天津
15-2-212	铁板牛肉炒面(面饼+汤料+蔬菜+调味酱)	主要原料:面饼:小麦面粉、植物油、食盐、鸡蛋等;汤包:脱水鸡蛋、水蔬脱菜、食盐、味精;蔬菜包:脱水牛肉丝、脱水蔬菜;调味酱包:棕榈油、酱油、牛肉抽取物等。商品名:新面族炒面套餐-铁板牛肉配翡翠芙蓉汤。康师傅牌	将面饼和汤包和蔬菜包、调味酱包分别测定,测定结果按样品重量比折算		2001.5	送检	天津

编码	食物类别和名称	食物描述	样品处理	数据来源	采样日期	采样地点	产地
15-2-213	铁板牛肉炒面 (面饼+汤料+蔬菜)	主要原料：面饼：小麦面粉、植物油、食盐、鸡蛋等；汤包：脱水鸡蛋、脱水蔬菜、食盐、味精；蔬菜包：脱水牛肉丝、脱水蔬菜。康师傅牌	相同个数的面饼、汤包和蔬菜包混合磨碎		2001.5	送检	天津
15-2-214	调味酱(铁板牛肉炒面)	主要原料：棕榈油、酱油、牛肉抽取物等。康师傅牌	数个调味酱包混合打匀		2001.5	送检	天津
15-2-215	玉米红烧牛肉味方便面 (面饼+调味料+蔬菜+肉酱)	主要原料：面饼：玉米粉、大豆粉、鸡蛋；肉酱包：食用油脂、牛肉；调味包：食盐、牛肉粉；脱水蔬菜。商品名：玉米红烧牛肉面。敖东牌	将面饼和调味包和蔬菜包、肉酱包分别测定，测定结果按样品重量比折算		2001.6	送检	吉林
15-2-216	玉米红烧牛肉味方便面 (面饼+调味料+蔬菜)	主要原料：面饼：玉米粉、大豆粉、鸡蛋；调味包：食盐、牛肉粉；脱水蔬菜。敖东牌	相同个数的面饼、调味包、蔬菜包混合磨碎		2001.6	送检	吉林
15-2-217	肉酱 (玉米红烧牛肉味方便面)	主要原料：食用油脂、牛肉等。敖东牌	数个肉酱包混合打匀		2001.6	送检	吉林
15-2-218	海鲜鸡汁味米线 (米线+调味料+蔬菜+肉酱)	主要原料：面饼：大米粉、食盐；肉酱包：鸡肉、虾肉、棕榈油等；调味包：食盐、味精等；脱水蔬菜。商品名：快餐米线230 (海鲜鸡汁)。沙博士牌	将面饼和调味包和蔬菜包、肉酱包分别测定，测定结果按样品重量比折算		2001.6	送检	江苏
15-2-219	海鲜鸡汁味米线 (米线 + 调味料 + 蔬菜)	主要原料：面饼：大米粉、食盐；调味包：食盐、味精等；脱水蔬菜。沙博士牌	相同个数的面饼、调味包、蔬菜包混合磨碎		2001.6	送检	江苏
15-2-220	肉酱(海鲜鸡汁味米线)	主要原料：鸡肉、虾肉、棕榈油等。沙博士牌	数个肉酱包混合打匀		2001.6	送检	江苏
15-2-221	冬菜虾仁馄饨	主要原料：虾仁、鱼肉、蔬菜、面粉等。熟，冷冻包装		TW-FCT			台湾
15-2-222	韭菜合子	熟		TW-FCT			台湾
15-2-223	糯米饭团	主要原料：油条、肉松、菜脯、糯米饭等。熟		TW-FCT			台湾
15-2-224	什锦炒饭	主要原料：米饭、火腿、蔬菜等。熟，冷冻包装		TW-FCT			台湾
15-2-225	虾仁炒饭	主要原料：米饭、虾仁、蔬菜等。熟，冷冻包装		TW-FCT			台湾
15-2-314	面包条(白)			Korea-FCT			
15-2-315	面包屑			Korea-FCT			
15-2-316	葡萄干面包			Korea-FCT			
15-2-415	饼干(三明治)	主要原料：小麦面粉、植物油、乳清粉、奶粉等。乐之牌	数包混合均匀磨碎		2001.10	送检	江苏
15-2-416	饼干(夹心)	主要原料：小麦面粉、植物油、乳清粉、全脂奶粉等。达能牌	牛奶、草莓、巧克力三种口味等量混合均匀磨碎		2001.9	送检	上海
15-2-417	饼干(甜酥夹心)	主要原料：小麦面粉、植物油、全脂奶粉、玉米淀粉等。商品名：甜酥夹心莱姆柠檬饼干。康师傅牌	数包混合均匀磨碎		2001.5	送检	天津

食物描述 Description of foods

编码	食物类别和名称	食物描述	样品处理	数据来源	采样日期	采样地点	产地
15-2-418	饼干(苏打夹心)	主要原料：小麦面粉、植物油、全脂乳粉、脱脂乳粉、玉米淀粉等	香草巧克力、奶油、柠檬三种口味等量混合均匀磨碎		2001.7	送检	天津
15-2-419	饼干(咸)	主要原料：小麦面粉、植物油等。商品名：达能闲趣。达能牌	数包混合均匀磨碎		2001.9	送检	上海
15-2-420	曲奇饼(加奶油)		数包混合均匀磨碎			送检	
15-2-421	早茶饼	主要原料：小麦面粉、白砂糖、植物油、可可粉、全脂奶粉、食盐等。嘉顿牌	数包混合均匀磨碎		2001.7	送检	广东
15-2-501	饺子(素馅)	主要原料：小麦面粉、时令蔬菜、鸡蛋、虾皮、木耳、植物油、食盐等。生、冷冻	数份数袋混合打匀		2001.11	送检	
15-2-502	饺子(三鲜馅)	主要原料：小麦面粉、虾仁、木耳、鸡蛋、植物油、猪肉、韭菜等。生、冷冻	数份数袋混合打匀		2001.11	送检	
15-2-503	饺子(猪肉白菜馅)	主要原料：小麦面粉、猪肉、白菜、植物油、食盐等。生、冷冻	数份数袋混合打匀		2001.11	送检	天津
15-2-504	饺子(猪肉韭菜馅)	主要原料：小麦面粉、猪肉、韭菜、植物油、食盐等。生、冷冻	数份数袋混合打匀		2001.11	送检	
15-2-505	饺子(猪肉芹菜馅)	主要原料：小麦面粉、猪肉、芹菜、植物油、食盐等。生、冷冻	数份数袋混合打匀		2001.11	送检	天津
15-2-506	饺子(猪肉茴香馅)	主要原料：小麦面粉、猪肉、茴香、植物油、食盐等。生、冷冻	数份数袋混合打匀		2001.11	送检	
15-2-507	饺子(猪肉香菇馅)	主要原料：面粉、猪肉、香菇、鳕鱼等		TW-FCT			台湾
15-2-508	饺子(猪肉虾仁馅)	主要原料：面粉、猪肉、虾仁、香菇等。生、冷冻		TW-FCT			台湾
15-2-509	饺子(鸡肉蘑菇馅)	主要原料：面粉、鸡肉、砂糖、猪肉、菇类、调味料等。生、冷冻		TW-FCT			台湾
15-2-510	饺子(海鳗猪肉馅)	主要原料：面粉、海鳗、猪肉等。生、冷冻		TW-FCT			台湾
15-2-511	饺子(海鳗虾仁馅)	主要原料：面粉、海鳗、虾仁、猪肉等。生、冷冻		TW-FCT			台湾
15-2-512	包子(三鲜馅)	主要原料：小麦面粉、虾仁、木耳、鸡蛋、植物油、猪肉等。生、冷冻。狗不理牌	数包混合打匀		2001.11	送检	天津

编码	食物类别和名称	食物描述	样品处理	数据来源	采样日期	采样地点	产地
15-2-513	包子(猪肉馅)	主要原料：小麦面粉、猪肉、植物油、酱油、食盐等。生、冷冻	数包混合打匀		2001.11	送检	
休闲食品							
15-3-101	米饼(鸡蛋牛奶味)	主要原料：大米粉、植物油、白砂糖、葡萄糖、麦芽糊精、食盐等。奇多牌	数包混合均匀磨碎		2001.6	送检	上海
15-3-102	雪米饼	主要原料：稻米、白砂糖、植物油、食盐、味精等。康师傅牌	数份数包混合均匀磨碎		2001.8	送检	浙江
15-3-103	蛋酥卷	主要原料：鸡蛋、小麦面粉、白砂糖、植物油、食盐、β-胡萝卜素等。康师傅牌	数包混合均匀磨碎		2001.7	送检	天津
15-3-104	巧克力派	主要原料：小麦面粉、白砂糖、鸡蛋、全脂乳粉等	数包混合均匀磨碎		2001.7	送检	
15-3-105	法式卷饼	主要原料：小麦面粉、全脂奶粉、鸡蛋、蛋黄粉、植物油等	数包混合均匀磨碎		2001.9	送检	天津
15-3-106	立体脆	主要原料：玉米粉、植物油、白砂糖、食盐等	数包混合均匀磨碎		2001.7	送检	上海
15-3-107	粟米脆	主要原料：玉米粉、植物油、食盐等。百事牌	数包混合均匀磨碎		2001.10	送检	上海
15-3-108	通心脆	主要原料：薯条、马铃薯粉、植物油等。卡迪那牌	数包混合均匀磨碎		2001.8	送检	北京
15-3-109	洋葱圈	主要原料：小麦面粉、玉米淀粉、棕榈油、精熟马铃薯等。衣心牌	数包混合均匀磨碎		2001.5	送检	辽宁
15-3-201	虾片			Korea-FCT			
15-3-202	锅巴(豆香)	主要原料：大米、黄豆、棕榈油、淀粉、食盐、牛肉粉等。太阳牌	数份混合均匀磨碎		2001.9	送检	陕西
15-3-203	锅巴(小米)	主要原料：小米、棕榈油、淀粉、食盐等。太阳牌	数包混合均匀磨碎		2001.9	送检	陕西
15-3-204	海苔	主要原料：海苔、盐、酱油、调味料、海带等。波力牌	数包混合均匀磨碎		2001.5	送检	江苏
15-3-205	香菇片	主要原料：香菇、白砂糖、食盐、味精、酱油、植物油等。波力牌	数包混合后、加水制匀浆		2001.10	送检	江苏

食物描述 Description of foods

编码	食物类别和名称	食物描述	样品处理	数据来源	采样日期	采样地点	产地
15-3-206	薯片(烧烤味)	主要原料：马铃薯、植物油、白砂糖、食盐等。百事牌	数包混合均匀磨碎		2001.7	送检	上海
15-3-207	薯片(香辣味)	主要原料：马铃薯粉、植物油、糖粉、蓝莓粉、碘盐等。卡迪那牌	数包混合均匀磨碎		2001.5	送检	北京
15-3-208	薯圈	主要原料：马铃薯粉、植物油、糖等。肯肯牌	数包混合均匀磨碎		2001.8	送检	天津
15-3-301	怪味胡豆	主要原料：蚕豆、白糖、植物油、食盐等。天吉牌	数包混合均匀磨碎		2001.11	送检	重庆
15-3-302	奶油五香豆	主要原料：蚕豆、食盐等	数包等量混合均匀磨碎		2001.7	送检	上海
15-3-303	夹心米果	主要原料：精制米、植物油、白砂糖、全脂乳粉、乳清粉、蛋黄粉、食盐等	数包混合均匀磨碎		2001.9	送检	天津
15-3-304	乐芙球	主要原料：小麦面粉、全脂乳粉、植物油、鸡蛋、白砂糖等	草莓、牛奶、巧克力三种口味等量混合均匀磨碎		2001.7	送检	天津
15-3-305	玉米花	主要原料：玉米粒、植物油、食盐等。玉米粒经微波炉爆后食用。欧陆派牌	数包混合均匀磨碎		2001.8	送检	广东
15-3-306	果仁脆枣	主要原料：枣、花生仁等	数包混合均匀磨碎			送检	北京
15-3-307	空心脆枣	主要原料：枣等	数包混合均匀磨碎			送检	北京
15-3-308	鱼肉粒	主要原料：三文鱼、小麦面粉、白砂糖、豆粉等。商品名：日式三文鱼肉粒。乐高牌	几种口味等量混合磨碎		2001.8	送检	广东
15-3-401	果冻(草莓水果冻)	主要原料：水、蔗糖、海藻抽取物、低聚果糖等。亲亲牌	数十个混合打匀		2001.5	送检	辽宁
15-3-402	果冻(蒟蒻冻)	主要原料：水、白砂糖、椰果、果汁、蒟蒻粉等。波力牌	数十个混合打匀		2001.8	送检	江苏
15-3-403	果冻(蒟蒻椰果冻)	主要原料：水、白砂糖、椰果、果汁、蒟蒻粉等。柳川牌	数十个混合打匀		2001.8	送检	江苏
15-3-404	果冻(AD钙果冻)	主要原料：水、蔗糖、海藻抽取物、乳酸钙、维生素A、D等。亲亲牌	数十个混合打匀		2001.5	送检	辽宁
	饮料类						
碳酸饮料							
16-1-009	可口可乐			USA-FCT			

编码	食物类别和名称	食物描述	样品处理	数据来源	采样日期	采样地点	产地
果汁及果汁饮料							
16-2-012	菠萝汁饮料(百果洲牌)	主要原料：菠萝汁、维生素C等	数盒等量混合均匀		2001.9	送检	云南
16-2-013	菠萝汁饮料(大湖牌)	主要原料：水、菠萝汁等	数瓶等混合均匀		2001.10	送检	天津
16-2-014	苹果汁饮料(光明牌)	主要原料：水、苹果汁等	数瓶混合均匀		2001.8	送检	上海
16-2-015	苹果汁饮料(亨氏)	主要原料：苹果汁、维生素C等	数盒混合均匀		2001.8	送检	山东
16-2-016	苹果果肉饮料	主要原料：水、苹果浆、糖、维生素C等。茹梦牌	数盒等量混合均匀打碎		2001.7	送检	北京
16-2-017	橙汁饮料(光明牌)	主要原料：水、甜橙汁等	数瓶等量混合均匀		2001.8	送检	上海
16-2-018	橙汁饮料(茹梦牌)	主要原料：水、白砂糖、橙汁、维生素C等	数盒等量混合均匀		2001.7	送检	重庆
16-2-019	橙汁饮料(汇源牌)		数盒混合均匀			送检	上海
16-2-020	橙汁饮料(三得利牌)		数盒混合均匀			送检	上海
16-2-021	芒果汁饮料			TW-FCT			台湾
16-2-022	沙棘果浆	主要原料：野生沙棘果、果糖等	数瓶混合均匀打碎		2002.3	送检	青海
16-2-023	山楂果肉饮料	主要原料：水、山楂果浆、糖、维生素C等。茹梦牌	数听混合均匀打碎		2001.7	送检	北京
16-2-024	酸枣果汁饮料	主要原料：纯净水、野生酸枣、蔗糖等。福运泉牌	数瓶混合均匀打碎		2001.6	送检	天津
16-2-025	西番莲汁饮料	主要原料：西番莲汁、维生素C等。百果洲牌	数盒混合均匀		2001.9	送检	云南
16-2-026	西柚汁饮料	主要原料：水、西柚汁等。大湖牌	数瓶混合均匀		2001.10	送检	天津
16-2-027	椰子汁饮料	主要原料：矿泉水、椰肉汁、白砂糖等。椰树牌	数罐混合均匀		2001.9	送检	海南
16-2-028	杏仁椰汁饮料	椰树牌	数罐混合均匀			送检	海南
蔬菜汁饮料							
16-3-002	胡萝卜汁饮料	主要原料：水、胡萝卜原浆、蔗糖、麦芽低聚糖等。喜奥牌	数瓶混合均匀		2001.10	送检	河北
含乳饮料							
16-4-003	AD钙奶	椰树牌	数瓶混合均匀			送检	海南

食物描述 Description of foods

编码	食物类别和名称	食物描述	样品处理	数据来源	采样日期	采样地点	产地
16-4-004	健康快车奶饮料	主要原料：水、奶粉、白砂糖、乳酸钙、乳酸、维生素A、D等。乐百氏牌	数瓶混合均匀		2001.4	送检	广东
16-4-005	粒粒果奶饮料	主要原料：水、奶粉、白砂糖、乳酸钙、乳酸、蒟蒻粉、维生素A、D等。乐百氏牌	数瓶混合均匀		2001.4	送检	广东
16-4-006	酸乳饮料	主要原料：鲜牛奶、水、白砂糖、乳酸等。商品名：优酸乳。伊利牌	数盒混合均匀		2001.4	送检	内蒙古
16-4-007	酸乳饮料(发酵)	主要原料：水、奶粉、白砂糖、乳酸菌等。喜乐牌	数瓶混合均匀		2001.6	送检	广东
植物蛋白饮料							
16-5-003	核桃乳(儿童型)		数罐混合均匀			送检	贵州
16-5-004	核桃乳(女性型)		数罐混合均匀			送检	贵州
16-5-005	核桃乳(中老年型)		数罐混合均匀			送检	贵州
16-5-006	核桃乳(佐餐调和型)		数罐混合均匀			送检	贵州
16-5-007	杏仁露	主要原料：水、杏仁、白糖等。露露牌	数罐混合均匀		2001.6	送检	河北
茶叶及茶饮料							
16-6-111	大麦茶	绿茶和烤大麦混合		Japan-FCT			
16-6-202	大麦茶水	绿茶和烤大麦混合、水泡		Korea-FCT			
固体饮料							
16-7-011	高乐高营养饮品	主要原料：糖、低脂肪可可粉、玉米淀粉、小麦面粉、奶蛋白、多种维生素等	数瓶等量混合均匀磨碎		2001.4	送检	天津
16-7-012	菓珍	主要原料：砂糖、麦芽糊精、维生素C、磷酸钙等	数瓶等量混合均匀磨碎		2001.11	送检	天津
16-7-013	桂花酸梅晶	主要原料：白砂糖、乌梅、山楂、甘草、桂花、维生素C、纤维素胶等。怡泰牌	数袋等量混合均匀磨碎		2001.6	送检	江苏
16-7-014	柠檬茶	主要原料：白砂糖、速溶茶粉、维生素C等。雀巢牌	数瓶等量混合均匀磨碎		2001.11	送检	上海
16-7-015	巧克力麦芽营养饮品	主要原料：白砂糖、麦芽精粉、乳及乳清粉、可可粉、矿物质、维生素等。雀巢牌	数袋混合均匀磨碎		2001.4	送检	上海

食物描述 Description of foods

编码	食物类别和名称	食物描述	样品处理	数据来源	采样日期	采样地点	产地
16-7-016	咖啡豆	元帅牌	数袋混合均匀磨碎		2002.3	送检	上海
16-7-017	咖啡粉	普通速溶型		USA-FCT			
16-7-018	咖啡伴侣	雀巢牌	数袋混合均匀磨碎			送检	
冰激凌、棒冰类							
16-8-009	冰激凌（草莓味）	主要原料：水、白砂糖、奶粉、葡萄糖浆、植物油、乳清粉、淀粉等。雀巢牌	数盒混合均匀磨碎		2002.3	送检	广东
16-8-010	冰激凌（苦咖啡味）	主要原料：牛奶、水、白砂糖、植物油、鸡蛋、咖啡、巧克力等。伊利牌	数盒混合均匀磨碎		2002.3	送检	内蒙古
16-8-011	冰激凌（加奶油）	主要原料：奶油、牛奶、脱脂奶粉、乳清粉、白砂糖、卵磷脂等。八喜牌	数盒混合均匀磨碎		2002.3	送检	北京
16-8-012	冰激凌（草莓圣代）	主要原料：冰淇淋、草莓酱等。肯德基牌	数盒混合均匀磨碎		2003.8	送检	北京
16-8-013	冰激凌（巧克力圣代）	主要原料：冰淇淋、巧克力汁等。肯德基牌	数个混合均匀磨碎		2003.8	送检	北京
16-8-014	冰激凌（脆皮甜筒）	肯德基牌	数盒混合均匀磨碎		2003.8	送检	北京
16-8-015	冰激凌（花心筒）	主要原料：水、白砂糖、奶粉、植物油、小麦面粉、花生、玉米糖浆、淀粉等。雀巢牌	数个混合均匀磨碎		2002.3	送检	
16-8-016	冰激凌（金百合）	和路雪牌	数盒混合均匀磨碎		2002.3	送检	北京
16-8-017	雪糕（百乐宝）	主要原料：水、白砂糖、全脂奶粉、植物油、葡萄糖浆、脱脂奶粉等。商品名：百乐宝小牛奶。百乐宝牌	数个混合均匀磨碎		2002.3	送检	北京
16-8-018	雪糕（红豆缘）	主要原料：水、牛奶、白砂糖、植物油、赤豆等。蒙牛牌	数个混合均匀磨碎		2002.3	送检	内蒙古
16-8-019	棒冰（可乐冰）	雀巢牌	数个混合均匀磨碎		2002.3	送检	
16-8-020	棒冰（奇彩旋）	和路雪牌	数个混合均匀磨碎		2002.3	送检	北京
其它							
16-9-002	纯净水（康师傅牌）		数瓶等量混合均匀		2003.7	北京市崇文门菜市场	天津
16-9-003	纯净水（乐百氏牌）		数瓶等量混合均匀		2003.7	北京市崇文门菜市场	广东
16-9-004	纯净水（娃哈哈牌）		数瓶等量混合均匀		2003.7	北京市崇文门菜市场	浙江

食物描述 Description of foods

编码	食物类别和名称	食物描述	样品处理	数据来源	采样日期	采样地点	产地
16-9-005	纯净水 (椰树牌)		数瓶等量混合均匀		2003.7	北京市崇文门菜市场	北京
16-9-006	饮用水 (农夫山泉牌)	商品名：饮用天然水	数瓶等量混合均匀		2003.7	北京市崇文门菜市场	浙江
16-9-007	饮用水 (雀巢)	商品名：优质饮用水	数瓶等量混合均匀		2003.7	北京市崇文门菜市场	上海
16-9-008	矿泉水 (获特满牌)	商品名：矿物质饮品	数瓶等量混合均匀		2003.7	北京市崇文门菜市场	上海
16-9-009	矿泉水 (康师傅牌)	商品名：矿物质水	数瓶等量混合均匀		2003.7	北京市崇文门菜市场	天津
16-9-010	矿泉水 (蓝涧牌)		数瓶等量混合均匀		2003.7	北京市崇文门菜市场	北京
16-9-011	矿泉水 (乐百氏牌)		数瓶等量混合均匀		2003.7	北京市崇文门菜市场	广东
16-9-012	矿泉水 (雀巢)		数瓶等量混合均匀		2003.7	北京市崇文门菜市场	天津
16-9-013	矿泉水 (椰树牌)		数瓶等量混合均匀		2003.7	北京市崇文门菜市场	海南
	含酒精饮料						
发酵酒							
17-1-115	啤酒 (4.3%, 青岛牌)		数罐混合均匀		2001.6	送检	山东
17-1-116	啤酒 (4%, 燕京牌)	主要原料：天然矿泉水、大麦、麦芽等	数罐混合均匀		2003.7		北京
17-1-117	啤酒 (5.1%, 生力牌)		数罐混合均匀		2001.6	送检	河北
17-1-205	葡萄酒 (干白, 11%, 长城牌)		数瓶等量混合均匀		2001.7	送检	河北
17-1-206	葡萄酒 (干白, 12%, 张裕牌)		数瓶等量混合均匀		2003.7		山东
17-1-207	葡萄酒 (半干白, 11.5%, 王朝牌)		数瓶等量混合均匀		2003.7		天津
17-1-208	葡萄酒 (干红, 11.5%, 长城牌)		数瓶等量混合均匀		2001.7	送检	河北
17-1-209	葡萄酒 (干红, 11.5%, 王朝牌)		数瓶等量混合均匀		2003.7		天津
17-1-210	葡萄酒 (干红, 12%, 张裕牌)		数瓶等量混合均匀		2003.7		山东
17-1-211	黑加仑酒 (8%)	奥维牌	数瓶混合均匀		2002.3	送检	安徽
17-1-212	雪利酒	普通型		UK-FCT			
17-1-309	花雕酒 (16.5%)	主要原料：水、糯米、小麦等。鹅池牌	数瓶等量混合均匀		2001.9	送检	浙江

食物描述 Description of foods

编码	食物类别和名称	食物描述	样品处理	数据来源	采样日期	采样地点	产地
蒸馏酒							
17-2-127	董酒 (浓香型, 46%)	主要原料：高粱、山泉水等	数瓶等量混合均匀		2001.9	送检	贵州
17-2-128	二锅头 (56%)	红星牌	数瓶等量混合均匀		2003.7		北京
17-2-129	汾酒 (清香型, 53%)		数瓶等量混合均匀		2001.9	送检	山西
17-2-130	古井贡酒 (浓香型, 38%)	主要原料：高粱、小麦、大麦、豌豆等	数瓶等量混合均匀		2001.11	送检	安徽
17-2-131	剑南春 (52%)	主要原料：高粱、大米、糯米、玉米、小麦等	数瓶等量混合均匀		2001.10	送检	四川
17-2-132	剑南春 (浓香型, 38%)	主要原料：高粱、大米、糯米、玉米、小麦等	数瓶等量混合均匀		2001.10	送检	四川
17-2-133	京酒 (浓香型, 38%)	主要原料：高粱、大米、糯米、玉米、小麦等	数瓶等量混合均匀		2003.7		宜宾
17-2-134	茅台酒 (53%)	主要原料：高粱、小麦等	数瓶等量混合均匀		2003.7		贵州
17-2-135	五粮液 (52%)	主要原料：高粱、大米、糯米、玉米、小麦等	数瓶等量混合均匀		2003.7		宜宾
17-2-136	竹叶青酒 (45%)		数瓶等量混合均匀		2001.9	送检	山西
17-2-137	金奖白兰地 (38%)	张裕牌	数瓶等量混合均匀		2001.8	送检	山东
17-2-138	伏特加			USA-FCT			
17-2-139	威士忌			USA-FCT			
露酒							
17-3-105	苹果酒 (干型)			UK-FCT			
17-3-106	苹果酒 (甜)			UK-FCT			
17-3-107	果汁朗姆酒 (9.9%)			Korea-FCT			
17-3-108	鸡尾酒	波旁酒和苏打水混合		Korea-FCT			
17-3-109	马提尼酒 (32%)			USA-FCT			
17-3-110	曼哈顿酒 (30.6%)			Korea-FCT			
17-3-111	酸味威士忌 (16.8%)			USA-FCT			

食物描述 Description of foods

编码	食物类别和名称	食物描述	样品处理	数据来源	采样日期	采样地点	产地
	糖、果脯和蜜饯、蜂蜜						
糖果							
18-2-101	夹心糖	雅客牌	数包混合磨碎		2001.7	送检	福建
18-2-102	水果味软糖	主要原料：白砂糖、麦芽糖饴、果胶、动物胶等。芭比牌	数包混合磨碎		2001.9	送检	天津
18-2-201	牛奶糖	主要原料：白砂糖、麦芽糖、奶油、氢化油、炼乳、奶粉、盐、碳酸氢钠等。喔喔牌	数包混合磨碎		2002.3	送检	上海
18-2-202	酸奶软糖	主要原料：白砂糖、葡萄糖浆、氢化植物油、乳酸、果汁等	数包混合磨碎		2001.8	送检	广东
18-2-203	太妃糖	主要原料：白糖、炼乳、奶油、葡萄糖浆、植物油等。金帝牌	数包混合磨碎		2002.6	送检	广东
18-2-301	花生牛轧糖	主要原料：白砂糖、麦芽糖浆、花生、奶油、植物油、食盐等。圆缘牌	数包混合磨碎		2001.10	送检	江苏
18-2-302	花生芝麻糖	主要原料：花生、芝麻、白砂糖、麦芽糖浆、植物油等。圆缘牌	数包混合磨碎		2001.10	送检	江苏
18-2-303	四味粽子糖	主要原料：白砂糖、淀粉糖浆、松仁、玫泥等	数包混合磨碎		2001.8	送检	江苏
18-2-401	巧克力(充气)	主要原料：白砂糖、全脂奶粉、可可脂等。可可脂含量28%。金帝牌	数包混合磨碎		2002.4	送检	广东
18-2-402	巧克力(果仁)	主要原料：白砂糖、全脂奶粉、脱脂奶粉、榛子仁、杏仁、可可脂等。可可脂含量27%。金帝牌	数包混合磨碎		2002.6	送检	广东
18-2-403	巧克力(黑)			USA-FCT			
18-2-404	巧克力(牛奶)	主要原料：白砂糖、全脂奶粉、脱脂奶粉、可可脂等。可可脂含量38%。金帝牌	数包混合磨碎		2002.4	送检	广东
果脯和蜜饯							
18-3-012	冰糖酸角	主要原料：酸角、冰糖、白砂糖等	去核、数包混合打匀		2001.9	送检	广东
18-3-013	甘草杏	主要原料：杏、白砂糖、食盐、甘草等。亨兴牌	去核、数包混合打匀		2001.10	送检	广东
18-3-014	清凉杏肉		数包混合打匀			送检	北京

食物描述 Description of foods

编码	食物类别和名称	食物描述	样品处理	数据来源	采样日期	采样地点	产地
18-3-015	雪梅	主要原料：黄杏胚、食盐、甘草等。汾煌牌	去核、数包混合打匀		2001.8	送检	广东
18-3-016	九制梅肉	主要原料：鲜果胚、糖、食盐等。无核	数包混合打匀		2001.9	送检	广东
18-3-017	九制西梅	主要原料：西梅、白砂糖、食盐、甘草等。展翠牌	去核、数包混合打匀		2001.10	送检	广东
18-3-018	九制应子	主要原料：李干、白砂糖、食盐、甘草等。展翠牌	去核、数包混合打匀		2001.10	送检	广东
18-3-019	梅脯	主要原料：梅、蔗糖、柿霜等。无核。洱宝牌	数包混合打匀		2001.11	送检	云南
18-3-020	阿胶枣		数包混合打匀			送检	北京
18-3-021	黑贡枣	主要原料：油枣、白砂糖、枣花蜜等。无核。德泰牌	数包混合打匀		2001.8	送检	山西
18-3-022	野酸枣		数包混合打匀			送检	北京
18-3-023	多味山楂		数包混合均匀磨碎			送检	北京
18-3-024	山楂脯		数包混合打匀			送检	北京
18-3-025	地瓜干	主要原料：甘薯、白砂糖等。商品名：小地瓜	数包混合均匀磨碎			送检	北京
蜂蜜							
18-4-001	蜂蜜						
18-4-002	蜂蜜（槐花）	源牌	数袋混合打匀		2002.3	送检	辽宁
18-4-003	蜂蜜（天麻）			YN-FCT			云南
18-4-004	蜂蜜（硬蜜）			YN-FCT			云南
18-4-005	蜂蜜（油菜花）			YN-FCT			云南

油脂类

编码	食物类别和名称	食物描述	样品处理	数据来源	采样日期	采样地点	产地
植物油							
19-2-020	核桃油	邦太牌	数桶等量混合均匀		2001.7	送检	云南
19-2-021	花生油	鲁花牌	数桶等量混合均匀		2001.10	送检	山东
19-2-022	葵花子油	绿洲果实牌	数桶等量混合均匀		2001.11	送检	北京
19-2-023	粟米油［玉米胚芽油］	金龙鱼牌	数桶等量混合均匀		2001.8	送检	广东
19-2-024	米糠油	豫达牌	数桶等量混合均匀		2001.11	送检	河南

食物描述 Description of foods

编码	食物类别和名称	食物描述	样品处理	数据来源	采样日期	采样地点	产地
19-2-025	油茶籽油	百味美牌	数桶等量混合均匀		2001.8	送检	湖南
19-2-026	芝麻油 [香油]	古币牌	数瓶等量混合均匀		2001.11	送检	北京
19-2-027	大豆色拉油	福临门牌	数桶等量混合均匀		2001.11	送检	天津
19-2-028	色拉油	绿宝牌	数桶等量混合均匀		2001.11	送检	北京
	调味品类						
酱油							
20-1-011	黄豆酱油	主要原料：水、脱脂大豆、小麦面粉、麸皮、食盐、味精等。淘大牌	数瓶等量混合均匀		2001.11	送检	上海
20-1-012	老抽	主要原料：水、脱脂大豆、小麦面粉、麸皮、食盐、白砂糖等。商品名：金标老抽。淘大牌	数瓶等量混合均匀		2001.11	送检	上海
20-1-013	生抽	主要原料：水、脱脂大豆、小麦面粉、麸皮、食盐、味精等。商品名：上等生抽。淘大牌	数瓶等量混合均匀		2001.11	送检	上海
酱							
20-3-116	海鲜酱 (阿香婆)	主要原料：辣椒、鲜虾、花生、芝麻、核桃、糖、味精等	数瓶混合打匀		2001.9	送检	陕西
20-3-117	牛肉酱 (阿香婆)	主要原料：番茄、辣椒、牛肉、花生、芝麻、核桃、糊精、味精等	数瓶混合打匀		2001.9	送检	陕西
20-3-118	花生酱	主要原料：花生、糖、食盐、氢化植物油等。四季宝牌	数瓶混合打匀		2001.11	送检	山东
20-3-119	花生酱 (加巧克力)	主要原料：花生、麦芽糖、白砂糖、植物油、可可粉、脱脂奶粉、食盐等。四季宝牌	数瓶混合打匀		2001.11	送检	山东
20-3-120	芝麻酱	火鸟牌	数瓶混合打匀		2001.11	送检	北京
20-3-121	千岛沙拉酱	主要原料：色拉油、糖、鸡蛋、番茄酱、水、醋、食盐、味精等。好乐门牌	数瓶混合打匀		2001.11	送检	北京
20-3-122	沙拉酱	主要原料：色拉油、蛋黄、食醋、食盐、白砂糖、味精等。丘比牌	数瓶混合打匀		2001.11	送检	北京
20-3-123	奶油攀司	主要原料：全脂奶粉、白砂糖、植物油脂、磷脂等。大昌牌	数管混合打匀		2001.11	送检	上海

食物描述 Description of foods

编码	食物类别和名称	食物描述	样品处理	数据来源	采样日期	采样地点	产地
20-3-207	草莓酱	主要原料：草莓、砂糖、果胶等。丘比牌	数瓶混合打匀		2001.11	送检	北京
20-3-208	番茄沙司	主要原料：水、番茄酱、白砂糖、醋、食盐、淀粉等。味好美牌	数瓶混合打匀		2001.11	送检	上海
腐乳							
20-4-006	腐乳(香辣味)		数瓶等量混合打匀			送检	北京
20-4-007	腐乳(白.石宝寨牌)[酱豆腐]	主要原料：大豆、白酒、食盐等	数盒等量混合打匀		2002.3	送检	重庆
20-4-008	腐乳(白.王致和牌)[酱豆腐]		数瓶等量混合打匀			送检	北京
咸菜类							
20-5-036	剁辣椒	主要原料：鲜红辣椒、精盐等。Y.G 牌	数瓶等量混合均匀磨碎		2002.3	送检	湖南
20-5-037	酱八宝菜		数包混合均匀磨碎			送检	北京
20-5-038	酱甘露		数包混合均匀磨碎			送检	北京
20-5-039	酱花生米		数包混合均匀磨碎			送检	北京
20-5-040	酱籽萝		数包混合均匀磨碎			送检	北京
20-5-041	麻仁金丝	主要原料：苤蓝、甜面酱、麻仁、姜丝、糖、水等。袋装。六必居牌	数袋混合均匀磨碎			送检	北京
20-5-042	雪菜	主要原料：雪菜、植物油、碘盐、辣椒等。粘香牌	数包混合打匀		2002.3	送检	山东
20-5-043	腌大头菜	散装。六必居牌	数份等量混合打匀		2002.7	北京市崇文门菜市场	北京
20-5-044	腌芥菜头	散装。六必居牌	数份等量混合打匀		2002.7	北京市崇文门菜市场	北京
20-5-045	腌韭菜花		数包混合均匀磨碎			送检	北京
20-5-046	腌萝卜条	散装。六必居牌	数份等量混合打匀		2002.7	北京市崇文门菜市场	北京
20-5-047	榨菜(鱼泉牌)	主要原料：榨菜、植物油等	数包混合打匀		2001.6	送检	重庆
20-5-048	榨菜(正林牌)	主要原料：青菜头、芝麻油、盐、味精等	数包混合打匀		2001.7	送检	四川
香辛料							
20-6-011	咖喱粉	罐装		Japan-FCT			

食物描述 Description of foods

编码	食物类别和名称	食物描述	样品处理	数据来源	采样日期	采样地点	产地
盐、味精及其它							
20-7-202	鸡粉	主要原料：食盐、鸡肉粉、麦芽糊精、水解蛋白、淀粉、白砂糖、味精、鸡油等。罐装。家乐牌	数罐等量混匀磨碎		2001.11	送检	广东
20-7-203	鸡精	主要原料：食盐、鸡肉粉、水解蛋白、麦芽糊精、淀粉、白砂糖等。罐装。美极牌	数罐等量混匀磨碎		2001.11	送检	广东
20-7-401	料酒	商品名：料酒王	数瓶等量混合均匀磨碎			送检	北京
	其它						
21-9-014	蜂蛹[蜂胚、蜂仔]			YN-FCT			云南
21-9-015	蜂蛹 (油蜂)			YN-FCT			云南
21-9-016	蜂蛹 (大黄蜂)			YN-FCT			云南
21-9-017	葛根	见附图		YN-FCT			云南
21-9-018	花椒叶 (干)	花椒树的嫩叶, 晒干		YN-FCT			云南
21-9-019	花粉 (油菜)			YN-FCT			云南
21-9-020	花粉 (油松)[松花粉]			YN-FCT			云南
21-9-021	花粉 (荞麦)			YN-FCT			云南
21-9-022	牛蛙	人工养殖		YN-FCT			云南
21-9-023	仙人掌 (食用)		十数片各取 1/4, 去皮, 混合打匀		2003.9	送检	海南
21-9-024	仙人掌果 [仙桃]		数十个去皮, 打碎, 去籽		2003.9	送检	海南
21-9-025	仙人掌籽		数十个仙人掌果去皮, 打碎, 去果肉		2003.9	送检	海南

表一 食物一般营养成分

Table 1 Nutrient Content of Foods

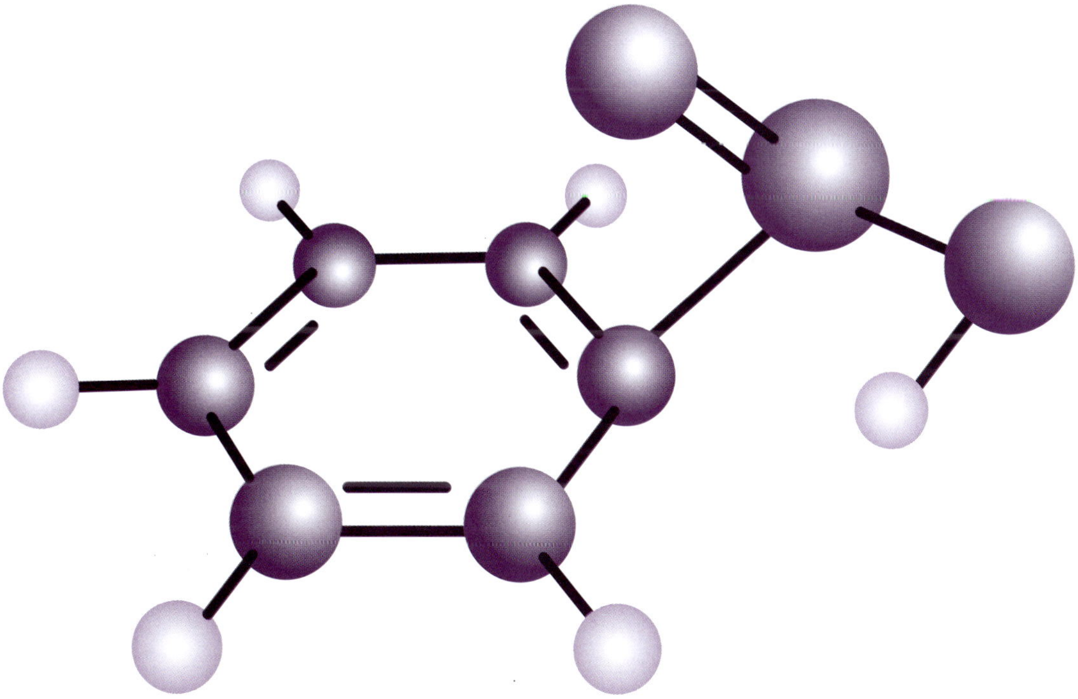

Notes

谷类及制品

Cereals and Cereal Products

谷类是我国的主要粮食作物，品种繁多，据统计多达4万种以上。广义上的谷类应包括：稻米、小麦、玉米、小米、大麦、青稞、高粱、薏米、燕麦、荞麦、莜麦、糜子等。本节包括了以上谷类及以此为原料的家庭主食食品。按照谷类作物品种的不同，分为小麦、稻米、玉米、大麦、小米和黄米、其它等几个亚类。

按常规，小麦面粉的质量标准分为4个等级：特制一等粉、特制二等粉、标准粉和普通面粉。用于制作面条和面包的一般为前三种。面粉的质量取决于小麦的品种和制作方法，质量等级的判断主要根据面粉的灰分、粗细度、面筋质含量等来判定（灰分：特一粉≤0.7%，标准粉≤1.10%；面筋质：特一粉≥26.0%，标准粉≥24.0%）。

稻米按照粒形、粒质分为籼米、粳米和糯米三类。籼型非糯性稻米谷粒呈长椭圆形或细长形，出米率低，米饭膨胀性大，但粘性较小。粳型非糯性稻米谷粒呈卵圆形或椭圆形，出米率高，米饭膨胀性小，但粘性大。以上两种稻谷根据收获季节又分为早稻和晚稻。糯稻谷又分籼型和粳型糯米，其特点是粘性大。稻谷的分类等级标准主要根据出糙率、水分含量、黄粒限度等指标来判断。

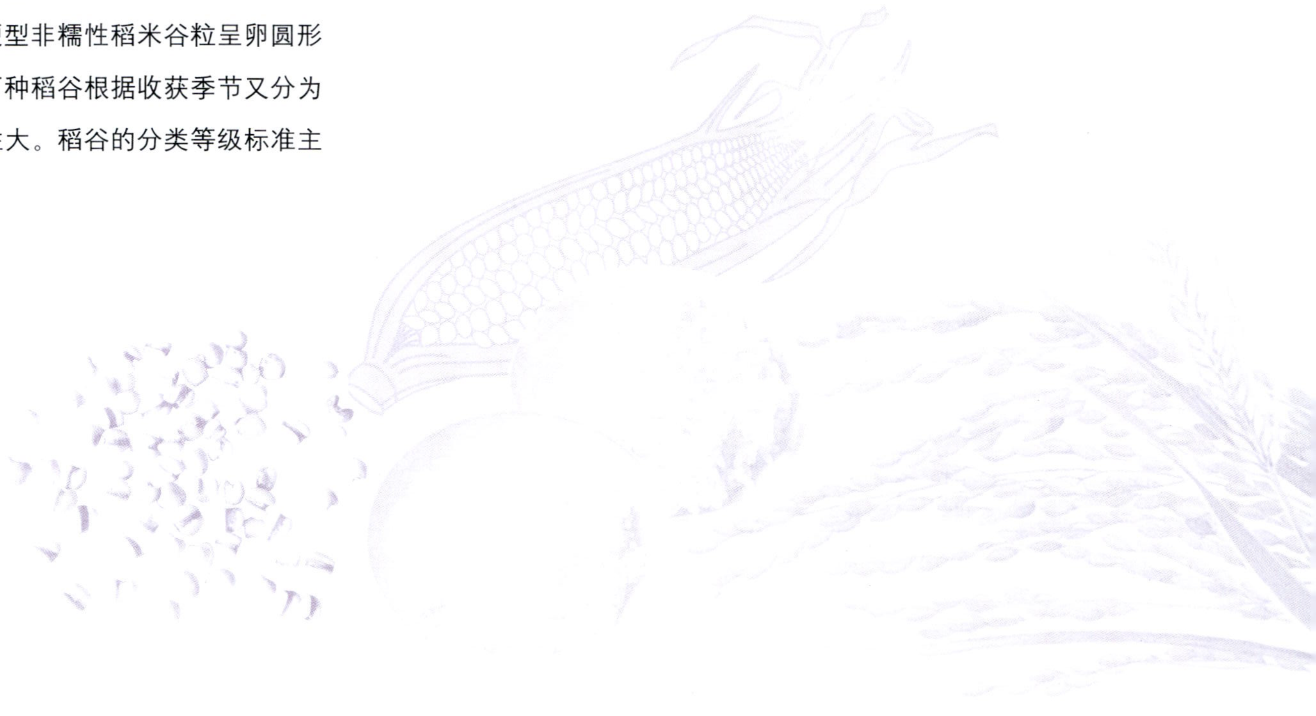

谷类及制品 Cereals and cereal products

（以每100g可食部计）

编码 Code	食物名称 Food name	食部 Edible	水分 Water	能量 Energy		蛋白质 Protein	脂肪 Fat	碳水化合物 CHO	膳食纤维 (Dietary fiber)			胆固醇 Cholesterol	灰分 Ash	维生素A		硫胺素 Thiamin	核黄素 Riboflavin	维生素B_6 Vit B_6
									总 Total	可溶性 Soluble	不溶性 Insoluble			Vit A	胡萝卜素 Carotene			
		%	g	kcal	kJ	g	g	g	g	g	g	mg	g	μgRE	μg	mg	mg	mg
小麦																		
01-1-206	小麦面粉（标准粉）	100	9.9	354	1482	15.7	2.5	70.9	3.7	—	—	—	1.0	(0)	(0)	0.46	0.05	0.07
01-1-207	小麦面粉（富强粉、特一粉）	100	10.8	361	1509	12.3	1.5	74.9	0.4	—	—	—	0.5	(0)	(0)	0.11	0.03	0.06
01-1-208	小麦面粉（特制）	100	10.4	366	1531	13.3	2.2	73.5	—	—	0.3	—	0.6	(0)	(0)	0.09	0.04	0.07
01-1-313	挂面（富强粉）	100	10.2	361	1511	13.0	1.5	74.7	0.8	—	—	—	0.6	(0)	(0)	0.13	0.04	0.80
01-1-314	龙须面（素）	100	10.4	356	1490	10.8	1.8	75.7	1.5	—	—	—	1.3	(0)	(0)	0.07	0.03	—
01-1-315	龙须面（鸡蛋）	100	10.2	345	1445	14.0	1.8	71.5	3.2	—	—	—	2.5	42	(0)	0.17	0.05	—
01-1-316	面条（富强粉，切面）	100	29.0	272	1140	8.9	0.4	60.7	2.4	—	—	—	1.0	(0)	(0)	0.07	0.02	0.09
01-1-317	面条（富强粉，煮）	100	72.7	104	433	3.9	0.4	22.8	1.7	—	—	—	0.2	(0)	(0)	0.02	0.01	0.05
01-1-410	花卷（加牛奶）	100	30.8	274	1145	6.5	3.2	58.9	4.2	—	—	—	0.6	—	(0)	0.03	0.03	0.03
01-1-411	馒头（富强粉）	100	40.3	226	946	7.1	1.3	50.9	4.4	—	—	—	0.4	(0)	(0)	0.12	0.02	0.06
01-1-503	面筋（肉馅）	100	49.2	364	1522	16.2	33.2	0.1	—	—	—	23	1.4	67	—	0.06	0.10	—
稻米																		
01-2-106	粳米（极品精米）	100	13.9	337	1412	6.4	1.2	78.1	2.8	—	—	—	0.4	(0)	(0)	0.06	0.02	—
01-2-107	粳米（西域王米）	100	13.3	352	1472	7.5	1.8	77.0	—	—	0.6	—	0.4	(0)	(0)	0.07	0.04	—
01-2-108	粳米（小站稻米）	100	12.9	342	1429	6.9	0.7	79.2	2.3	—	—	—	0.3	(0)	(0)	0.04	0.02	—
01-2-214	籼米	100	13.1	328	1374	7.5	1.1	78.0	5.9	—	—	—	0.3	(0)	(0)	0.07	0.02	0.07
01-2-215	香米	100	13.5	335	1400	8.4	0.7	77.2	3.5	—	—	—	0.2	(0)	(0)	0.03	0.02	—
01-2-408	籼米饭（蒸）	100	70.1	113	474	3.0	0.4	26.4	2.0	—	—	—	0.1	(0)	(0)	0.01	0.01	—
01-2-409	籼米粥	100	85.0	58	242	1.3	0.2	13.4	0.7	—	—	—	0.1	(0)	(0)	Tr	Tr	—
01-2-410	米粉	100	12.7	346	1446	0.4	0.8	85.8	1.6	—	—	—	0.3	Tr	—	0.01	0.01	Tr
01-2-411	河粉	100	11.2	356	1491	7.7	1.5	79.2	1.2	—	—	—	0.4	Tr	—	0.02	0.02	0.04

谷类及制品 Cereals and cereal products

（以每100g可食部计）

编码 Code	食物名称 Food name	维生素B₁₂ Vit B_{12} μg	叶酸 Folate μg	烟酸 Niacin mg	维生素C Vit C mg	维生素E (Vit E) Total mg	维生素E (Vit E) α-TE mg	钙 Ca mg	磷 P mg	钾 K mg	钠 Na mg	镁 Mg mg	铁 Fe mg	锌 Zn mg	硒 Se μg	铜 Cu mg	锰 Mn mg	碘 I μg
小麦																		
01-1-206	小麦面粉（标准粉）	(0)	23.3	1.91	(0)	0.32	Tr	31	167	190	3.1	50	0.6	0.20	7.42	0.06	0.10	Tr
01-1-207	小麦面粉（富强粉、特一粉）	(0)	10.3	0.94	(0)	0.32	Tr	27	114	128	2.7	32	0.7	0.39	6.79	0.03	0.04	2.9
01-1-208	小麦面粉（特制）	(0)	4.6	1.01	(0)	Tr	Tr	23	167	356	60.3	105	0	0.94	8.41	Tr	0.02	3.4
01-1-313	挂面（富强粉）	(0)	8.1	1.26	(0)	Tr	Tr	21	112	122	110.6	48	1.0	0.08	3.46	0.04	0.05	1.8
01-1-314	龙须面（素）	(0)	8.9	—	(0)	—	—	15	86	77	249.8	19	2.2	1.19	2.51	0.14	0.49	Tr
01-1-315	龙须面（鸡蛋）	Tr	12.9	0.90	(0)	0.21	0.03	12	140	529	711.2	25	1.5	0.83	3.34	0.17	0.47	—
01-1-316	面条（富强粉，切面）	(0)	23.3	1.10	(0)	Tr	Tr	24	92	102	11.5	29	0.4	0.12	2.34	0.02	0.04	Tr
01-1-317	面条（富强粉，煮）	(0)	2.1	0.56	(0)	Tr	Tr	4	24	15	26.9	10	0.2	0.10	1.16	0.01	0.01	Tr
01-1-410	花卷（加牛奶）	—	19.1	0.61	(0)	0.85	0.36	9	71	211	97.0	14	0.7	0.36	1.94	0.04	0.19	Tr
01-1-411	馒头（富强粉）	(0)	8.7	0.79	(0)	Tr	Tr	58	43	146	165.0	20	0.4	0.21	2.66	0.02	0.03	Tr
01-1-503	面筋（肉馅）	—	19.1	2.70	—	0.92	un	113	224	167	663.8	18	4.9	1.42	6.18	0.08	0.07	16.4
稻米																		
01-2-106	粳米（极品精米）	(0)	11.5	0.67	(0)	Tr	Tr	3	69	86	2.7	25	0.2	1.76	4.17	0.23	1.14	—
01-2-107	粳米（西域王米）	(0)	14.9	1.00	(0)	Tr	Tr	5	66	119	2.0	17	0.8	1.02	2.92	0.24	0.43	2.8
01-2-108	粳米（小站稻米）	(0)	8.7	0.82	(0)	Tr	Tr	3	82	111	2.2	16	0.3	1.94	10.10	0.35	0.44	—
01-2-214	籼米	(0)	19.7	0.94	(0)	Tr	Tr	12	112	109	1.7	28	0.1	0.15	2.76	0.01	0.02	Tr
01-2-215	香米	(0)	22.3	0.42	(0)	Tr	Tr	3	58	112	1.8	7	0.2	1.85	4.09	0.13	0.80	—
01-2-408	籼米饭（蒸）	(0)	6.9	1.70	(0)	Tr	Tr	6	15	21	1.7	10	0.1	0.14	1.13	0.01	0.02	Tr
01-2-409	籼米粥	(0)	1.6	—	(0)	Tr	Tr	7	20	13	2.8	7	0.1	0.12	0.74	0.01	0.01	Tr
01-2-410	米粉	(0)	Tr	—	(0)	Tr	Tr	11	45	19	52.2	6	2.4	0.36	0.45	0	0.08	Tr
01-2-411	河粉	(0)	8.4	—	(0)	0.23	0.07	51	105	83	8.2	23	1.0	1.57	4.19	0.24	0.71	Tr

谷类及制品 Cereals and cereal products

(以每 100g 可食部计)

编码 Code	食物名称 Food name	食部 Edible %	水分 Water g	能量 Energy kcal	能量 Energy kJ	蛋白质 Protein g	脂肪 Fat g	碳水化合物 CHO g	膳食纤维 (Dietary fiber) 总 Total g	可溶性 Soluble g	不溶性 Insoluble g	胆固醇 Cholesterol mg	灰分 Ash g	维生素 A Vit A μgRE	胡萝卜素 Carotene μg	硫胺素 Thiamin mg	核黄素 Riboflavin mg	维生素 B_6 Vit B_6 mg
玉米																		
01-3-108	玉米粒(黄，干)	100	11.8	298	1248	8.0	0.8	79.2	14.4	—	—	—	0.2	17	100	0.03	0.02	—
01-3-109	玉米面(黄)	100	11.2	339	1419	8.5	1.5	78.4	5.5	—	—	—	0.4	7	40	0.07	0.04	0.08
01-3-110	玉米糁(黄)	100	12.5	297	1243	7.4	1.2	78.7	14.5	—	—	—	0.2	—	—	0.03	0.03	0.05
01-3-202	玉米面面条	100	12.3	348	1456	6.6	0.3	80.5	—	—	0.6[a]	—	0.4	—	—	—	—	—
大麦																		
01-4-102	黑大麦	100	10.9	297	1243	10.2	2.2	74.3	—	—	15.2[a]	—	2.4	—	—	0.54	0.14	—
小米																		
01-5-104	小米(黄)	100	9.7	355	1485	8.9	3.0	77.7	4.6	—	—	—	0.7	—	—	0.32	0.06	—
其它																		
01-9-010	荞麦面	100	14.2	329	1377	11.3	2.8	70.2	5.5	—	—	—	1.5	3	20	0.26	0.10	—
01-9-011	莜麦面	100	8.8	380	1589	13.7	8.6	67.7	5.8	—	—	—	1.2	—	—	0.20	0.09	—
01-9-201	高粱面面条	100	23.4	304	1271	7.0	0.2	68.7	—	—	0.3[a]	—	0.7	—	—	—	—	—

谷类及制品 Cereals and cereal products

(以每100g可食部计)

编码 Code	食物名称 Food name	维生素B_{12} Vit B_{12} μg	叶酸 Folate μg	烟酸 Niacin mg	维生素C Vit C mg	维生素E (Vit E) Total mg	维生素E (Vit E) α-TE mg	钙 Ca mg	磷 P mg	钾 K mg	钠 Na mg	镁 Mg mg	铁 Fe mg	锌 Zn mg	硒 Se μg	铜 Cu mg	锰 Mn mg	碘 I μg
玉米																		
01-3-108	玉米粒(黄，干)	(0)	10.4	0.56	(0)	0.38	Tr	—	—	—	—	—	—	—	1.24	—	—	—
01-3-109	玉米面(黄)	(0)	—	0.80	(0)	0.98	0.05	22	196	249	2.3	84	0.4	0.08	2.68	0.01	0.02	Tr
01-3-110	玉米糁(黄)	(0)	8.9	0.76	(0)	0.96	0.04	49	143	177	1.7	151	0.2	0.05	1.09	0.01	0.01	Tr
01-3-202	玉米面面条	(0)	—	—	(0)	—	—	—	—	—	—	—	—	—	—	—	—	—
大麦																		
01-4-102	黑大麦	(0)	—	5.40	(0)	—	—	20	390	241	17.0	69	6.5	2.33	3.99	1.09	1.17	—
小米																		
01-5-104	小米(黄)	(0)	22.4	1.04	(0)	1.62	0.39	8	158	335	0.6	50	1.6	2.81	2.72	0.41	0.38	Tr
其它																		
01-9-010	荞麦面	(0)	29.1	3.47	(0)	5.31	0.70	71	243	304	0.9	151	7.0	1.94	2.16	0.39	0.59	—
01-9-011	莜麦面	(0)	22.4	0.29	(0)	0.39	0.29	40	259	255	1.8	62	3.8	2.18	2.90	0.41	1.71	—
01-9-201	高粱面面条	(0)	—	—	(0)	—	—	—	—	—	—	—	—	—	—	—	—	—

Notes

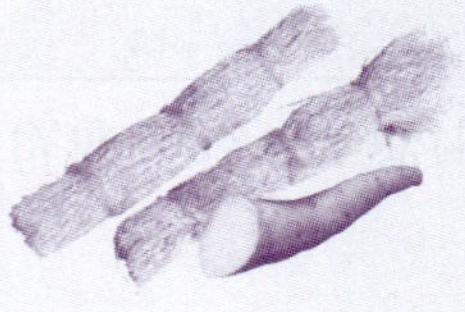

薯类、淀粉及制品

Tubers, Starches and Products

本类食物以提供碳水化合物为主，分为以下两个亚类。

1.薯类：如马铃薯、甘薯、木薯等。

2.淀粉类：如各种淀粉、粉丝、粉条、藕粉等。

马铃薯、甘薯、木薯被称为世界三大薯类。马铃薯俗称土豆、洋芋、洋山芋，属茄科一年生块茎类植物。世界上79%的国家种植马铃薯，仅次于小麦、水稻和玉米。甘薯又名山芋、红芋、红薯、白薯等。木薯别称树薯、木番薯等，原产地为非洲南部，为热带和亚热带多年生植物，在温带为一年生灌木。薯类是为居民提供淀粉的主要食物之一。

薯类、淀粉及制品 Tubers, starches and products

(以每100g可食部计)

编码 Code	食物名称 Food name	食部 Edible	水分 Water	能量 Energy		蛋白质 Protein	脂肪 Fat	碳水化合物 CHO	膳食纤维 (Dietary fiber)			胆固醇 Cholesterol	灰分 Ash	维生素A		硫胺素 Thiamin	核黄素 Riboflavin	维生素B_6 Vit B_6
									总 Total	可溶性 Soluble	不溶性 Insoluble			Vit A	胡萝卜素 Carotene			
		%	g	kcal	kJ	g	g	g	g	g	g	mg	g	μgRE	μg	mg	mg	mg
薯类																		
02-1-104	马铃薯[土豆、洋芋]	94	78.6	79	329	2.6	0.2	17.8	1.2	0.1	1.1	—	0.8	1	6	0.10	0.02	0.27
02-1-105	马铃薯(烤)	100	80.8	70	293[c]	1.8	0.1	16.4	—	—	0.4[b]	—	0.9	0	0	0.08	0.01	—
02-1-106	马铃薯(蒸)	100	80.6	69	289[c]	3.0	Tr	15.3	—	—	0.2[b]	—	1.1	0	0	0.11	0.04	—
02-1-107	马铃薯(煮)	100	81.5	65	272[c]	3.2	Tr	14.2	—	—	0.2[b]	—	1.1	0	0	0.09	0.04	—
02-1-108	马铃薯全粉	100	5.6	355	1486	8.4	0.5	82.7	—	—	3.5[a]	—	2.8	Tr	Tr	0.11	0.25	0.42
02-1-205	甘薯(红心)[山芋、红薯]	90	83.4	57	238	0.7	0.2	15.3	2.2	—	—	—	0.4	(125)	(750)	0.05	0.01	0.15
淀粉类																		
02-2-108	淀粉(小麦)	100	13.1	351	1469	0.2	0.5	86.0	(0)	(0)	(0)	—	0.2	0	0	0	0	(0)
02-2-109	淀粉(大米)	100	9.7	366	1531	0.2	0.7	89.3	(0)	(0)	(0)	—	0.1	0	0	0	0	(0)
02-2-110	淀粉(马铃薯)	100	17.4	332	1389[c]	0.1	0.1	82.0	—	—	0[b]	—	0.4	0	0	0	0	—
02-2-111	淀粉(甘薯)	100	15.1	342	1431[c]	0.1	0.2	84.4	—	—	0[b]	—	0.2	0	0	0	0	—
02-2-112	煎炸粉	100	11.9	331	1385[c]	12.1	1.4	73.6	—	—	0.7[b]	—	1.0	0	0	0.23	0.07	—

薯类、淀粉及制品 Tubers, starches and products

(以每 100g 可食部计)

编码 Code	食物名称 Food name	维生素 B_{12} Vit B_{12} μg	叶酸 Folate μg	烟酸 Niacin mg	维生素 C Vit C mg	维生素 E (Vit E) Total mg	α-TE mg	钙 Ca mg	磷 P mg	钾 K mg	钠 Na mg	镁 Mg mg	铁 Fe mg	锌 Zn mg	硒 Se μg	铜 Cu mg	锰 Mn mg	碘 I μg
薯类																		
02-1-104	马铃薯 [土豆、洋芋]	(0)	12.4	—	14.0	Tr	Tr	7	46	347	5.9	24	0.4	0.30	0.47	0.09	0.10	1.2
02-1-105	马铃薯 (烤)	—	—	0.80	15.0	—	—	2	60	357	6.0	—	0.7	—	—	—	—	—
02-1-106	马铃薯 (蒸)	—	—	0.90	30.0	—	—	4	67	484	3.0	—	0.7	—	—	—	—	—
02-1-107	马铃薯 (煮)	—	—	0.80	26.0	—	—	4	64	480	2.0	—	0.6	—	—	—	—	—
02-1-108	马铃薯全粉	(0)	—	—	25.9	Tr	Tr	35	170	980	71.0	100	0.8	12.50	1.40	0.35	0.33	25.0
02-1-205	甘薯 (红心) [山芋、红薯]	(0)	19.6	0.20	4.0	Tr	Tr	18	26	88	70.9	17	0.2	0.16	0.22	0.05	0.08	0.4
淀粉类																		
02-2-108	淀粉 (小麦)	(0)	(0)	0	0	(0)	(0)	14	33	8	3.0	5	0.6	0.10	—	0.02	—	—
02-2-109	淀粉 (大米)	(0)	(0)	0	0	(0)	(0)	29	20	2	11.0	8	1.5	0.10	—	0.06	—	—
02-2-110	淀粉 (马铃薯)	—	—	0	0	—	—	22	40	32	5.0	—	1.8	—	—	—	—	—
02-2-111	淀粉 (甘薯)	—	—	0.10	0	—	—	62	14	7	3.0	—	2.6	—	—	—	—	—
02-2-112	煎炸粉	—	—	3.20	0	—	—	11	102	299	18.0	—	2.0	—	—	—	—	—

Notes

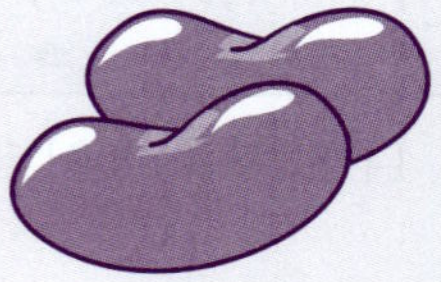

干豆类及制品

Dried Legumes and Legume Products

豆类作物主要有大豆、绿豆、赤豆、芸豆、蚕豆、豌豆等。按照营养成分含量的多少可将豆类分为两大类：一类是大豆，含有较高的蛋白质（35%～40%）和脂肪（15%～20%），而碳水化合物相对较少（20%～30%）；另一类是除大豆外的其它豆类，含有较高的碳水化合物（55%～65%），中等的蛋白质（20%～30%）和少量的脂肪（低于5%）。本节按照其品种的不同分为大豆、绿豆、赤豆、芸豆、蚕豆、其它等几个亚类。

豆类制品主要指大豆制品，即以大豆为原料经过制作或精炼提取的产品。大豆制品的品种众多，按照生产工艺可分为两类：一类是发酵豆制品，包括腐乳、臭豆腐、豆瓣酱、酱油等；另一类是非发酵豆制品，包括水豆腐、干豆腐（百页）、卤制、油炸、熏干制品、冷冻豆制品等。列在本节的大豆制品主要指非发酵豆制品，有关发酵豆制品的食物成分在“调味品类”介绍。

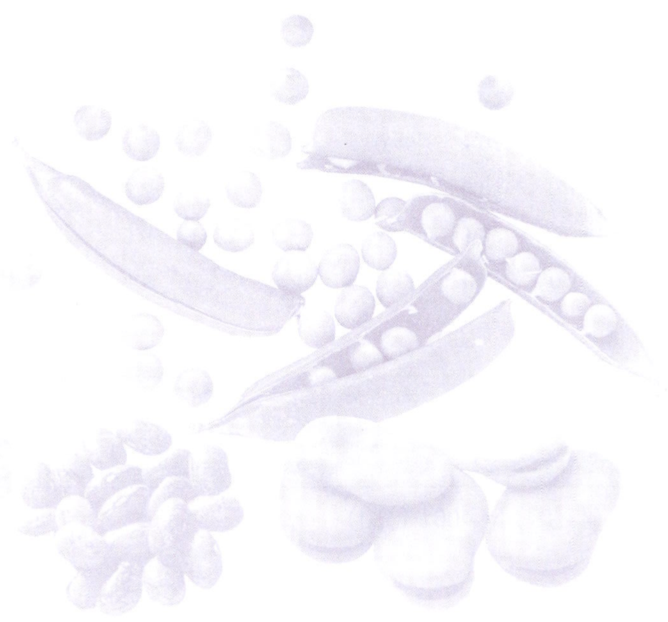

干豆类及制品 Dried legumes and legume products

(以每100g可食部计)

编码 Code	食物名称 Food name	食部 Edible %	水分 Water g	能量 Energy kcal	能量 Energy kJ	蛋白质 Protein g	脂肪 Fat g	碳水化合物 CHO g	膳食纤维 (Dietary fiber) 总 Total g	可溶性 Soluble g	不溶性 Insoluble g	胆固醇 Cholesterol mg	灰分 Ash g	维生素A Vit A μgRE	胡萝卜素 Carotene μg	硫胺素 Thiamin mg	核黄素 Riboflavin mg	维生素B_6 Vit B_6 mg
大豆																		
03-1-104	黄豆	100	9.2	389	1626	33.1	15.9	37.3	—	—	9.0[a]	—	4.5	7	40	0.11	0.22	0.46
03-1-206	豆奶粉 (维维牌)	100	2.4	419	1753	19.4	9.4	65.2	—	—	1.0[a]	—	3.6	1525	—	1.01	1.32	—
03-1-207	豆奶粉 (多力牌)	100	2.6	398	1663	12.3	6.5	76.4	4.0	—	—	—	2.2	—	—	0.10	0.08	0.10
03-1-208	豆奶粉 (大磨牌)	100	4.3	432	1807	27.4	13.0	51.6	—	—	0.3	—	3.7	—	—	0.46	1.01	—
03-1-306	豆腐 (北豆腐)	100	78.6	111	462	9.2	8.1	3.0	2.8	—	—	—	1.1	—	—	0.05	0.02	0.03
03-1-307	豆腐 (南豆腐)	100	83.6	84	352	5.7	5.8	3.9	1.6	—	—	—	1.0	—	—	0.06	0.02	0.05
03-1-405	豆浆	100	93.8	30	126	3.0	1.6	1.2	0.3	—	—	—	0.4	—	—	0.02	0.02	—
03-1-406	豆浆 (甜)	100	91.8	33	139	2.4	0.5	4.9	—	—	0.1	—	0.4	—	—	0.04	0.02	—
03-1-527	豆腐皮	100	9.4	431	1803	51.6	23.0	12.5	(8.1)	—	—	—	3.5	47	280	0.22	0.12	—
03-1-528	腐竹	100	7.1	476	1990	54.2	27.2	8.1	4.6	—	—	—	3.4	—	—	0.02	0.17	—
03-1-529	豆腐干	100	30.1	414	1731	19.6	35.2	11.4	6.8	—	—	—	3.7	—	—	0.02	0.08	—
赤豆																		
03-3-204	红豆沙	100	37.9	240	1005	4.5	0.1	57.1	—	—	1.8[a]	—	0.4	—	—	0.02	0.02	0.01
03-3-205	红豆馅	100	33.0	255	1069	4.5	0.2	61.7	—	—	2.8[a]	—	0.6	—	—	0.02	0.04	0.02
蚕豆																		
03-5-203	蚕豆 (煮)	100	83.7	62	259[c]	4.8	0.5	10.1	3.6	—	—	0	0.9	14	—	0.13	0.09	0.03
其它																		
03-9-204	豇豆 (煮)	100	64.8	133	556[c]	9.5	0.6	24.0	—	—	1.8[b]	—	1.1	2	9	0.26	0.28	—
03-9-303	豌豆 (煮)	100	70.5	107	448[c]	8.9	0.3	19.2	—	—	2.4[b]	—	1.1	6	33	0.22	0.09	—
03-9-401	鹰嘴豆 [桃豆]	100	11.3	316	1323	21.2	4.2	60.1	—	—	11.6[a]	—	3.3	14	86	0.41	0.25	—

干豆类及制品 Dried legumes and legume products

(以每100g可食部计)

编码 Code	食物名称 Food name	维生素B_{12} Vit B_{12} μg	叶酸 Folate μg	烟酸 Niacin mg	维生素C Vit C mg	维生素E (Vit E) Total mg	维生素E (Vit E) α-TE mg	钙 Ca mg	磷 P mg	钾 K mg	钠 Na mg	镁 Mg mg	铁 Fe mg	锌 Zn mg	硒 Se μg	铜 Cu mg	锰 Mn mg	碘 I μg
大豆																		
03-1-104	黄豆	(0)	181.1	1.53	—	—	—	123	418	1276	13.8	211	35.8	4.61	2.03	1.17	2.03	—
03-1-206	豆奶粉(维维牌)	—	—	3.59	32.0	30.10	un	635	393	571	221.3	47	8.3	6.25	—	—	—	—
03-1-207	豆奶粉(多力牌)	—	86.5	0.49	—	6.68	0.95	268	241	540	151.4	60	1.7	0.95	1.10	0.29	0.46	—
03-1-208	豆奶粉(大磨牌)	—	92.2	—	16.0	22.18	8.19	281	486	720	99.2	152	4.5	7.14	3.96	1.12	1.31	14.3
03-1-306	豆腐(北豆腐)	—	39.8	0.11	(Tr)	8.40	1.00	105	112	106	7.3	63	1.5	0.74	2.46	0.06	0.07	—
03-1-307	豆腐(南豆腐)	—	25.8	Tr	(Tr)	5.72	0.71	113	76	154	3.1	36	1.2	0.43	1.23	0.04	0.03	—
03-1-405	豆浆	—	5.0	0.14	(Tr)	1.06	0.17	5	42	117	3.7	15	0.4	0.28	Tr	0.16	0.16	Tr
03-1-406	豆浆(甜)	—	—	0.15	(Tr)	1.27	un	27	21	54	—	15	0.5	0.27	0.10	0.08	—	—
03-1-527	豆腐皮	Tr	Tr	0.91	(Tr)	46.55	5.67	239	494	877	7.4	179	11.7	4.08	2.26	1.17	2.71	5.0
03-1-528	腐竹	—	48.4	0.80	(Tr)	28.43	3.19	50	655	670	27.1	140	3.8	4.71	1.51	0.86	2.38	—
03-1-529	豆腐干	—	9.1	0.47	(Tr)	29.63	5.89	352	408	153	690.2	109	4.8	1.77	3.20	0.11	0.92	—
赤豆																		
03-3-204	红豆沙	—	—	—	(Tr)	2.69	un	19	65	21	26.3	7	1.1	0.60	0.41	0.06	0.22	—
03-3-205	红豆馅	Tr	—	—	0	3.66	un	16	90	59	28.6	10	1.3	0.64	0.39	0.12	0.27	—
蚕豆																		
03-5-203	蚕豆(煮)	0	58.0	1.20	19.8	—	—	18	73	193	41.0	31	1.5	0.47	1.00	0.06	0.26	—
其它																		
03-9-204	豇豆(煮)	—	—	0.80	1.0	—	—	29	87	(400)	Tr	—	3.4	—	—	—	—	—
03-9-303	豌豆(煮)	—	—	1.90	14.0	—	—	29	129	230	1.0	—	2.3	—	—	—	—	—
03-9-401	鹰嘴豆[桃豆]	(0)	—	—	3.5	11.61	un	150	450	830	6.0	210	3.4	1.50	—	0.44	2.20	—

Notes

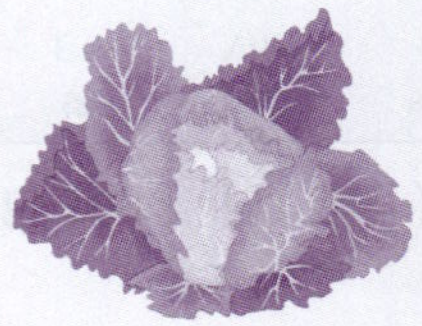

蔬菜类及制品

Vegetables and Vegetable Products

关于蔬菜的定义和分类，科学界与消费者的认识常常有所不同。结合农学院蔬菜学上的分类和膳食营养调查的实际应用，本节把蔬菜分为8个亚类，其中包括了相应的脱水蔬菜和罐头制品等。

1.根菜类：包括萝卜、胡萝卜等。

2.鲜豆类：包括菜豆、蚕豆、豌豆、绿豆芽、黄豆芽等。

3.茄果、瓜菜类：包括茄子、番茄、甜椒、黄瓜、南瓜等。

4.葱蒜类：包括大蒜、大葱、洋葱、韭菜等。

5.嫩茎、叶、花菜类：包括大白菜、油菜、菜花、竹笋等。

6.水生蔬菜类：包括慈菇、菱角、藕、茭白等。

7.薯芋类：包括豆薯、山药、芋头、姜等。

8.野生蔬菜类：包括地肤、香椿、苜蓿、蕨菜等。

本节收录了许多新品种蔬菜。

蔬菜类及制品 Vegetables and vegetable products

（以每100g可食部计）

编码 Code	食物名称 Food name	食部 Edible	水分 Water	能量 Energy		蛋白质 Protein	脂肪 Fat	碳水化合物 CHO	膳食纤维 (Dietary fiber) 总 Total	可溶性 Soluble	不溶性 Insoluble	胆固醇 Cholesterol	灰分 Ash	维生素A Vit A	胡萝卜素 Carotene	硫胺素 Thiamin	核黄素 Riboflavin	维生素B_6 Vit B_6
		%	g	kcal	kJ	g	g	g	g	g	g	mg	g	μgRE	μg	mg	mg	mg
根菜类																		
04-1-111	白萝卜 [莱菔]	95	94.6	13	52	0.7	0.1	4.0	1.8	—	—	—	0.6	Tr	Tr	0.02	0.01	0.06
04-1-112	白萝卜 (圆)	94	94.8	13	53	0.7	0.2	3.6	1.6	0.4	1.0	—	0.7	Tr	Tr	0.02	0.01	0.07
04-1-113	青萝卜	95	91.0	23	98	1.2	0.2	6.9	2.7	—	—	—	0.7	15	88	0.01	0.02	0.08
04-1-114	变萝卜 [红皮萝卜]	96	94.2	15	61	0.8	0.1	4.2	1.6	0.5	1.1	—	0.7	Tr	Tr	0.01	0.02	0.04
04-1-115	樱桃萝卜	46	95.4	9	36	0.9	0.1	3.0	2.0	—	—	—	0.6	3	18	0.01	0.03	0.05
04-1-204	胡萝卜	97	90.0	25	106	1.0	0.2	8.1	3.2	—	—	—	0.7	685	4107	—	0.02	0.16
04-1-402	根芹 [根洋芹、球根塘蒿]	67	86.2	27	113	2.2	0.1	10.0	5.7	1.1	4.6	—	1.5	3	19	0.04	0.07	0.32
04-1-403	紫菜头	89	86.4	33	140	1.8	0.2	10.6	4.5	0.2	4.2	—	1.0	Tr	Tr	0.02	0.03	0.04
鲜豆菜和豆苗类																		
04-2-118	扁豆	96	89.5	23	96	2.3	0.2	7.4	4.4	(0.5)	(3.9)	—	0.6	11	65	0.05	0.06	0.10
04-2-119	豇豆	97	90.1	18	76	2.2	(0.3)	7.3	4.3	—	—	—	0.7	88	526	0.06	0.05	0.06
04-2-120	四季豆 [菜豆、芸豆]	96	91.2	15	63	2.0	0.2	6.0	4.7	—	—	—	0.6	16	96	0.02	0.05	0.05
04-2-121	四棱豆 [杨桃豆、翅豆]	96	93.0	11	48	2.0	0.2	4.2	3.8	—	—	—	0.6	68	407	0.05	0.04	—
04-2-122	甜脆荷兰豆 [甜豆]	100	88.0	17	70	3.0	0.3	8.1	7.6	0.8	6.8	—	0.6	42	253	0.08	0.06	0.08
04-2-205	黄豆芽	100	89.8	32	134	4.4	1.6	3.6	3.6	—	—	—	0.6	2	9	0.05	0.07	0.06
04-2-206	绿豆芽	100	95.3	13	54	1.7	0.1	2.6	1.3	(0.1)	(1.2)	—	0.3	2	11	0.02	0.02	0.03
04-2-207	黑豆苗	100	91.7	25	104	4.4	0.8	2.6	2.6	1.0	1.6	—	0.5	20	122	0.05	0.07	0.13
04-2-208	豌豆苗	100	91.2	26	110	4.8	0.8	2.6	2.6	—	—	—	0.6	56	333	0.11	0.16	0.05
茄果、瓜菜类																		
04-3-115	茄子 (白皮，长)	97	92.5	14	59	1.3	0.1	5.5	3.5	—	—	—	0.6	3	15	0.05	0.03	0.05
04-3-116	茄子 (紫皮，长)	95	93.4	13	52	1.1	0.1	4.8	3.0	—	—	—	0.6	—	—	0.03	0.03	0.05

蔬菜类及制品 Vegetables and vegetable products

（以每 100g 可食部计）

编码 Code	食物名称 Food name	维生素 B_{12} Vit B_{12} μg	叶酸 Folate μg	烟酸 Niacin mg	维生素C Vit C mg	维生素E (Vit E) Total mg	维生素E (Vit E) α-TE mg	钙 Ca mg	磷 P mg	钾 K mg	钠 Na mg	镁 Mg mg	铁 Fe mg	锌 Zn mg	硒 Se μg	铜 Cu mg	锰 Mn mg	碘 I μg
根菜类																		
04-1-111	白萝卜 [莱菔]	(0)	6.8	0.14	19.0	Tr	Tr	47	16	167	54.3	12	0.2	0.14	0.12	0.01	0.05	Tr
04-1-112	白萝卜 (圆)	(0)	21.6	0.31	16.0	Tr	Tr	25	31	14	117.5	9	0.3	0.12	0.22	0.01	0.04	—
04-1-113	青萝卜	(0)	26.3	0.62	7.0	Tr	Tr	47	31	248	56.0	15	0.3	0.16	0.10	0.02	0.06	—
04-1-114	变萝卜 [红皮萝卜]	(0)	25.8	0.22	5.6	Tr	Tr	39	27	16	111.2	24	0.3	0.23	0.27	0.02	0.04	1.0
04-1-115	樱桃萝卜	(0)	79.5	0.22	14.0	Tr	Tr	18	23	202	82.6	15	0.4	0.18	0.28	0.01	0.06	—
04-1-204	胡萝卜	(0)	4.8	—	9.0	0.31	0.31	27	38	119	120.7	18	0.3	0.22	0.60	0.07	0.08	Tr
04-1-402	根芹 [根洋芹、球根塘蒿]	(0)	53.9	1.26	1.0	Tr	Tr	79	166	441	75.9	33	0.5	0.58	1.03	0.23	0.33	—
04-1-403	紫菜头	(0)	43.3	0.24	1.0	Tr	Tr	16	32	26	306.0	27	0.5	0.31	0.06	0.08	0.31	Tr
鲜豆菜和豆苗类																		
04-2-118	扁豆	(0)	15.6	0.24	2.0	Tr	Tr	57	49	163	3.9	31	0.5	0.26	Tr	0.05	0.13	2.2
04-2-119	豇豆	(0)	75.4	—	13.0	0.39	un	62	55	171	9.5	55	0.8	0.38	0.66	0.12	0.27	Tr
04-2-120	匹季豆 [菜豆、芸豆]	(0)	27.7	0.26	Tr	Tr	Tr	43	47	196	4.4	27	0.6	0.33	0.04	0.05	0.26	Tr
04-2-121	四棱豆 [杨桃豆、翅豆]	(0)	5.3	0.68	3.0	0.39	un	61	29	160	5.7	25	0.5	0.31	0.29	0.08	0.51	0.7
04-2-122	甜脆荷兰豆 [甜豆]	(0)	58.4	0.58	24.0	0.22	un	65	59	18	4.4	25	0.7	0.39	0.16	0.07	0.62	5.7
04-2-205	黄豆芽	(0)	30.1	0.32	4.0	0.64	un	30	60	175	28.3	36	0.6	0.37	0.34	0.09	0.22	0.4
04-2-206	绿豆芽	(0)	6.1	0.35	4.0	Tr	Tr	14	19	32	25.8	18	0.3	0.20	0.27	0.05	0.05	0.2
04-2-207	黑豆苗	(0)	140.7	0.41	9.0	0.77	un	58	55	119	14.9	23	1.0	0.36	0.71	0.12	0.22	0.6
04-2-208	豌豆苗	(0)	99.5	0.49	8.0	0.10	0.10	15	60	145	20.9	14	0.5	0.42	0.56	0.07	0.08	0.1
茄果、瓜菜类																		
04-3-115	茄子 (白皮，长)	(0)	20.4	0.44	—	Tr	Tr	10	30	238	1.9	16	0.5	0.20	0.16	0.05	0.12	1.0
04-3-116	茄子 (紫皮，长)	(0)	6.3	—	—	Tr	Tr	50	21	147	5.0	11	0.5	0.20	0.09	0.04	0.09	Tr

蔬菜类及制品 Vegetables and vegetable products

(以每100g可食部计)

编码 Code	食物名称 Food name	食部 Edible	水分 Water	能量 Energy		蛋白质 Protein	脂肪 Fat	碳水化合物 CHO	膳食纤维 (Dietary fiber) 总 Total	可溶性 Soluble	不溶性 Insoluble	胆固醇 Cholesterol	灰分 Ash	维生素A Vit A	胡萝卜素 Carotene	硫胺素 Thiamin	核黄素 Riboflavin	维生素B_6 Vit B_6
		%	g	kcal	kJ	g	g	g	g	g	g	mg	g	μgRE	μg	mg	mg	mg
04-3-117	茄子 (紫皮，圆)	98	93.3	19	79	0.8	0.2	5.3	1.8	—	—	—	0.4	4	23	0.03	0.02	0.04
04-3-118	香瓜茄	96	93.6	17	72	0.6	Tr	5.5	1.8	1.1	0.6	—	0.3	3	19	0.03	0.02	0.04
04-3-119	番茄 [西红柿]	97	95.2	11	46	0.9	0.2	3.3	1.9	—	—	—	0.4	63	375	0.02	0.01	0.06
04-3-120	樱桃番茄 [小西红柿]	98	92.5	22	91	1.0	0.2	5.8	1.8	—	—	—	0.5	55	332	0.03	0.02	—
04-3-121	辣椒 (小红尖辣椒)	89	76.4	32	136	4.1	0.4	17.7	14.6	2.8	11.8	—	1.4	—	—	0.16	0.16	0.83
04-3-122	辣椒 (小红尖辣椒，干)	88	10.2	197	825	15.4	12.0	57.4	50.5	—	—	—	5.0	563	3376	0.48	0.71	—
04-3-123	辣椒 (青，尖)	91	93.4	17	70	0.8	0.3	5.2	2.5	—	—	—	0.3	16	98	0.02	0.02	0.17
04-3-124	甜椒 [灯笼椒、柿子椒]	82	94.6	16	66	1.0	0.2	3.8	1.3	—	—	—	0.4	13	76	0.02	0.02	0.12
04-3-125	彩椒	83	91.5	19	81	1.3	0.2	6.4	3.3	—	—	—	0.6	132	794	0.05	0.05	—
04-3-126	秋葵 [黄秋葵、羊角豆]	98	91.2	16	68	1.8	0.2	6.2	4.4	2.6	1.8	—	0.6	40	238	0.06	0.05	0.06
04-3-221	冬瓜	80	96.9	8	34	0.3	0.2	2.4	1.1	—	—	—	0.2	Tr	Tr	Tr	Tr	0.02
04-3-222	飞碟瓜	91	94.1	13	52	1.0	0.1	4.4	2.5	0.9	1.6	—	0.4	8	47	0.02	0.02	0.05
04-3-223	黄金西葫芦	91	93.7	11	47	1.8	0.1	3.6	2.8	—	—	—	0.8	27	164	0.01	0.03	0.05
04-3-224	黄茎瓜	100	95.4	18	76	1.2	0.9	2.0	—	—	0.7[a]	—	0.5	113	680	0.03	0.02	0.10
04-3-225	迷你黄瓜 [荷兰乳黄瓜]	92	95.8	12	51	1.0	0.2	2.5	0.9	—	—	—	0.5	6	38	0.02	0.02	0.04
04-3-226	秋黄瓜 [旱黄瓜]	92	96.0	12	49	0.9	0.2	2.5	0.9	—	—	—	0.4	7	40	0.02	0.01	0.04
04-3-227	南瓜 (栗面)	74	88.8	31	129	1.4	0.1	8.8	2.7	0.1	2.6	—	0.9	253	1518	0.03	0.04	0.15
04-3-228	丝瓜	83	94.1	16	68	1.3	0.2	4.0	1.7	—	—	—	0.4	26	155	0.02	0.04	0.11
葱蒜类																		
04-4-206	大葱	82	91.8	23	95	1.6	0.3	5.8	2.4	0.2	2.2	—	0.5	11	64	0.06	0.03	0.16
04-4-207	细香葱 [香葱、四季葱]	89	91.1	21	88	1.4	0.3	6.6	3.4	—	—	—	0.6	21	123	0.03	0.05	0.06
04-4-404	韭菜	90	92.0	18	75	2.4	0.4	4.5	3.3	—	—	—	0.7	266	1596	0.04	0.05	0.20

蔬菜类及制品 Vegetables and vegetable products

(以每100g可食部计)

编码 Code	食物名称 Food name	维生素B_{12} Vit B_{12} μg	叶酸 Folate μg	烟酸 Niacin mg	维生素C Vit C mg	维生素E (Vit E) Total mg	α-TE mg	钙 Ca mg	磷 P mg	钾 K mg	钠 Na mg	镁 Mg mg	铁 Fe mg	锌 Zn mg	硒 Se μg	铜 Cu mg	锰 Mn mg	碘 I μg
04-3-117	茄子(紫皮，圆)	(0)	9.3	0.50	—	Tr	Tr	7	15	153	4.6	10	0.3	0.12	0.16	0.04	0.10	1.1
04-3-118	香瓜茄	(0)	6.4	0.28	60.0	Tr	Tr	10	12	17	3.8	9	0.2	0.08	0.10	0.03	0.03	Tr
04-3-119	番茄[西红柿]	(0)	5.5	0.49	14.0	0.42	0.28	4	24	179	9.7	12	0.2	0.12	Tr	0.04	0.06	2.5
04-3-120	樱桃番茄[小西红柿]	(0)	61.8	0.92	33.0	0.98	0.75	6	26	262	10.0	12	0.3	0.20	0.20	0.04	0.06	0.1
04-3-121	辣椒(小红尖辣椒)	(0)	37.5	2.51	86.0	8.11	un	29	115	18	11.5	59	0.6	0.33	0.96	0.20	0.30	2.8
04-3-122	辣椒(小红尖辣椒，干)	(0)	19.4	9.53	—	27.51	un	152	300	991	55.7	170	6.9	1.01	1.70	0.55	1.07	Tr
04-3-123	辣椒(青，尖)	(0)	3.6	0.62	59.0	0.38	0.38	11	20	154	7.0	15	0.3	0.21	0.02	0.05	0.05	0.6
04-3-124	甜椒[灯笼椒、柿子椒]	(0)	3.6	0.39	130.0	0.41	0.41	—	—	—	—	—	—	—	0.38	—	—	—
04-3-125	彩椒	(0)	83.4	1.09	104.0	1.60	un	9	26	278	6.8	18	0.5	0.18	0.12	0.06	0.09	—
04-3-126	秋葵[黄秋葵、羊角豆]	(0)	90.9	0.42	7.2	Tr	Tr	101	41	19	8.7	38	0.2	0.24	0.54	0.03	0.13	Tr
04-3-221	冬瓜	(0)	9.4	0.22	16.0	0.04	0.04	12	11	57	2.8	10	0.1	0.10	0.02	0.01	0.02	Tr
04-3-222	飞碟瓜	(0)	38.4	0.25	3.0	0.12	un	32	29	119	4.3	16	0.4	0.20	0.15	0.04	0.04	0.7
04-3-223	黄金西葫芦	(0)	—	—	13.3	0.13	un	33	47	20	3.0	18	0.4	0.22	0.10	0.04	0.08	0.3
04-3-224	黄茎瓜	(0)	—	—	Tr	0.20	un	—	17	—	—	—	—	0.29	0.20	—	—	—
04-3-225	迷你黄瓜[荷兰乳黄瓜]	(0)	2.1	—	—	Tr	Tr	20	21	173	2.2	12	0.3	0.17	0.92	0.03	0.06	Tr
04-3-226	秋黄瓜[旱黄瓜]	(0)	Tr	—	—	Tr	Tr	9	23	141	2.2	9	0.2	0.17	0.10	0.03	0.07	0.2
04-3-227	南瓜(栗面)	(0)	31.7	0.52	5.0	1.92	1.92	16	56	445	11.0	9	0.4	0.22	0.49	0.04	0.03	—
04-3-228	丝瓜	(0)	22.6	0.32	4.0	0.08	0.08	37	33	121	3.7	19	0.3	0.22	0.20	0.05	0.07	0.4
葱蒜类																		
04-4-206	大葱	(0)	11.5	0.50	3.0	Tr	Tr	63	25	110	8.9	16	0.6	0.29	0.21	0.03	0.34	Tr
04-4-207	细香葱[香葱、四季葱]	(0)	21.5	0.49	9.0	0.18	0.18	72	29	123	13.6	19	1.3	0.22	0.74	0.01	0.11	0.5
04-4-404	韭菜	(0)	61.2	0.86	2.0	0.57	un	44	45	241	5.8	24	0.7	0.25	1.33	0.05	0.21	Tr

蔬菜类及制品 Vegetables and vegetable products

(以每 100g 可食部计)

编码 Code	食物名称 Food name	食部 Edible	水分 Water	能量 Energy		蛋白质 Protein	脂肪 Fat	碳水化合物 CHO	膳食纤维 (Dietary fiber)			胆固醇 Cholesterol	灰分 Ash	维生素 A		硫胺素 Thiamin	核黄素 Riboflavin	维生素B_6 Vit B_6
									总 Total	可溶性 Soluble	不溶性 Insoluble			Vit A	胡萝卜素 Carotene			
		%	g	kcal	kJ	g	g	g	g	g	g	mg	g	μgRE	μg	mg	mg	mg
嫩茎、叶、花菜类																		
04-5-117	大白菜 (白口)	85	95.6	13	52	1.0	0.1	2.9	1.0	—	—	—	0.4	2	10	0.02	0.01	—
04-5-118	大白菜 (青口)	83	95.6	9	36	1.1	0.1	2.6	1.8	—	—	—	0.6	5	31	0.02	0.02	0.08
04-5-119	酸白菜 [酸菜]	100	94.9	5	20	0.7	0.2	2.6	2.6	—	—	—	1.6	—	—	0.01	0.01	—
04-5-120	小白菜 [青菜]	94	94.8	10	43	1.4	0.3	2.4	1.9	—	—	—	1.1	309	1853	0.01	0.05	0.07
04-5-121	奶白菜	100	92.6	17	69	2.7	0.2	3.3	2.3	0.8	1.5	—	1.2	190	1141	0.02	0.10	0.05
04-5-122	鸡毛菜	100	93.5	15	61	2.7	0.2	2.6	2.1	—	—	—	1.0	138	826	0.04	0.09	0.09
04-5-123	娃娃菜	97	95.0	8	33	1.9	—	2.4	2.3	—	—	—	0.7	8	48	0.04	0.03	—
04-5-124	乌塌菜 [塌菜、塌棵菜]	96	94.5	8	34	1.8	0.1	2.6	2.6	0.8	1.8	—	1.0	261	1568	0.01	0.08	0.09
04-5-125	油菜	96	95.6	10	41	1.3	0.5	2.0	2.0	—	—	—	0.9	181	1083	0.02	0.05	0.08
04-5-126	油菜心	100	95.1	11	45	1.3	0.4	2.7	2.2	—	—	—	0.5	—	—	0.02	0.06	0.11
04-5-210	结球甘蓝 (绿) [圆白菜]	86	94.5	12	51	0.9	0.2	4.0	2.3	—	—	—	0.4	2	12	0.02	0.02	0.06
04-5-211	结球甘蓝 (紫)	86	91.8	19	81	1.2	0.2	6.2	3.0	—	—	—	0.6	—	—	0.04	0.03	0.07
04-5-212	抱子甘蓝	87	86.7	23	95	3.5	—	8.8	6.6	—	—	—	1.0	5	31	0.06	0.05	0.17
04-5-213	羽衣甘蓝	100	87.2	32	132	5.0	0.4	5.7	(3.7)	(0.5)	(3.2)	—	1.7	728	4368	0.07	0.18	0.26
04-5-214	盖菜	94	94.8	9	38	1.5	—	2.8	2.0	—	—	—	0.9	81	487	0.02	0.07	0.12
04-5-215	芥蓝 [甘蓝菜、盖蓝菜]	98	91.0	16	67	3.1	0.3	4.1	3.9	—	—	—	1.5	—	—	0.03	0.12	0.06
04-5-216	菜花 [花椰菜]	82	93.2	15	61	1.7	0.2	4.2	2.7	0.6	2.1	—	0.7	2	11	0.04	0.04	0.11
04-5-217	西兰花 [绿菜花]	83	91.6	19	81	3.5	0.6	3.7	3.7	—	—	—	0.6	25	151	0.06	0.08	0.17
04-5-327	番杏 [新西兰菠菜、夏菠菜]	100	94.0	10	42	1.8	(0.1)	3.1	2.6	—	—	—	1.2	105	628	0.03	0.09	0.16
04-5-328	樱桃萝卜缨	100	94.0	9	37	2.0	0.1	2.7	2.7	0.4	2.3	—	1.2	240	1440	0.04	0.09	0.11
04-5-329	白凤菜	100	93.4	10	40	1.6	—	4.0	3.2	—	—	—	1.0	178	1066	0.03	0.06	0.07

蔬菜类及制品 Vegetables and vegetable products

(以每100g可食部计)

编码 Code	食物名称 Food name	维生素 B_{12} Vit B_{12} μg	叶酸 Folate μg	烟酸 Niacin mg	维生素C Vit C mg	维生素E (Vit E) Total mg	维生素E (Vit E) α-TE mg	钙 Ca mg	磷 P mg	钾 K mg	钠 Na mg	镁 Mg mg	铁 Fe mg	锌 Zn mg	硒 Se μg	铜 Cu mg	锰 Mn mg	碘 I μg
嫩茎、叶、花菜类																		
04-5-117	大白菜(白口)	(0)	14.8	0.32	8.0	0.06	0.06	29	21	109	39.9	12	0.3	0.15	0.04	0.01	0.08	0.6
04-5-118	大白菜(青口)	(0)	5.3	—	11.0	Tr	Tr	66	12	156	38.2	14	0.2	0.23	0.29	0.01	0.07	0.4
04-5-119	酸白菜[酸菜]	(0)	3.9	Tr	—	—	—	48	38	104	43.1	21	0.3	0.03	0.16	Tr	0.01	Tr
04-5-120	小白菜[青菜]	(0)	57.2	—	64.0	0.40	0.40	117	26	116	132.2	30	1.3	0.23	0.39	0.02	0.15	—
04-5-121	奶白菜	(0)	116.8	0.59	37.4	0.16	0.16	66	55	126	170.2	41	1.0	0.28	0.43	0.05	0.24	0.5
04-5-122	鸡毛菜	(0)	165.8	0.61	24.0	0.30	0.30	78	25	230	62.7	35	2.1	0.31	0.24	0.03	0.26	1.4
04-5-123	娃娃菜	(0)	86.4	0.61	12.0	Tr	Tr	78	58	278	19.3	17	0.4	0.35	0.16	0.03	0.13	—
04-5-124	乌塌菜[塌菜、塌棵菜]	(0)	96.8	0.21	33.9	0.28	0.28	43	35	213	59.5	29	1.6	0.25	0.77	0.02	0.15	0.4
04-5-125	油菜	(0)	103.9	0.55	—	Tr	Tr	148	23	175	73.7	25	0.9	0.31	0.73	0.03	0.23	Tr
04-5-126	油菜心	(0)	66.6	0.41	Tr	0.16	0.16	74	26	166	33.4	25	0.6	0.19	0.26	0.04	0.07	Tr
04-5-210	结球甘蓝(绿)[圆白菜]	(0)	—	0.24	16.0	Tr	Tr	28	18	46	42.1	14	0.2	0.12	0.27	0.01	0.09	Tr
04-5-211	结球甘蓝(紫)	(0)	41.9	0.15	26.0	Tr	Tr	65	22	177	27.0	15	0.4	0.16	0.24	0.02	0.15	0.2
04-5-212	抱子甘蓝	(0)	44.4	0.54	38.0	Tr	Tr	59	60	350	35.5	24	0.6	0.35	0.65	0.05	0.19	—
04-5-213	羽衣甘蓝	(0)	113.4	1.09	63.0	1.12	0.86	66	82	395	66.8	53	1.6	0.56	—	0.06	0.40	—
04-5-214	盖菜	(0)	101.0	0.21	14.0	0.75	un	76	33	150	73.5	28	0.5	0.47	0.56	0.04	0.15	0.7
04-5-215	芥蓝[甘蓝菜、盖蓝菜]	(0)	98.7	0.68	37.0	Tr	Tr	121	52	345	40.2	40	1.0	0.40	0.39	0.03	0.31	0.6
04-5-216	菜花[花椰菜]	(0)	13.5	0.32	32.0	Tr	Tr	31	32	206	39.2	18	0.4	0.17	2.86	0.02	0.09	Tr
04-5-217	西兰花[绿菜花]	(0)	29.8	0.73	56.0	0.76	0.61	50	61	179	46.7	22	0.9	0.46	0.43	0.03	0.16	Tr
04-5-327	番杏[新西兰菠菜、夏菠菜]	(0)	116.7	0.23	Tr	0.23	0.23	136	25	107	445.2	38	0.8	0.36	0.32	0.04	0.76	0.9
04-5-328	樱桃萝卜缨	(0)	122.2	0.26	14.0	1.40	1.40	56	50	126	111.3	45	3.9	0.40	0.58	0.03	0.51	—
04-5-329	白凤菜	(0)	37.2	0.77	6.0	0.12	0.12	41	29	192	152.0	63	1.8	0.23	0.77	0.09	0.70	—

蔬菜类及制品 Vegetables and vegetable products

(以每100g可食部计)

编码 Code	食物名称 Food name	食部 Edible %	水分 Water g	能量 Energy kcal	能量 Energy kJ	蛋白质 Protein g	脂肪 Fat g	碳水化合物 CHO g	膳食纤维 (Dietary fiber) 总 Total g	可溶性 Soluble g	不溶性 Insoluble g	胆固醇 Cholesterol mg	灰分 Ash g	维生素A Vit A μgRE	胡萝卜素 Carotene μg	硫胺素 Thiamin mg	核黄素 Riboflavin mg	维生素B_6 Vit B_6 mg
04-5-330	紫背天葵 [红风菜、血皮菜]	100	93.1	12	52	1.9	—	3.8	2.6	—	—	—	1.2	308	1847	0.05	0.08	0.08
04-5-331	芹菜 (茎)	100	95.4	11	44	0.4	0.2	3.1	1.3	0.3	1.0	—	0.9	3	18	0.01	0.02	0.06
04-5-332	西芹 [西洋芹菜、美芹]	85	93.6	12	51	0.6	0.1	4.8	2.6	0.4	2.2	—	0.9	5	29	0.01	0.03	0.05
04-5-333	生菜	94	96.7	10	42	1.6	0.4	1.1	1.1	—	—	—	0.2	4	26	0.02	0.01	0.05
04-5-334	油麦菜	81	95.9	8	33	1.1	0.4	2.1	2.1	—	—	—	0.5	125	751	0.03	0.07	—
04-5-335	叶甜菜 (白梗)	100	94.2	7	31	1.6	0.1	2.8	2.8	0.6	2.2	—	1.3	—	—	0.01	0.08	0.04
04-5-336	莴笋叶 [莴苣菜]	100	95.0	12	51	1.0	0.2	2.9	1.3	—	—	—	0.9	4	24	0.03	Tr	0.07
04-5-337	蕹菜 [空心菜、藤藤菜]	100	92.3	11	44	2.2	0.2	4.0	4.0	—	—	—	1.3	286	1714	0.03	0.05	0.08
04-5-338	观达菜 [根达菜、牛皮菜]	100	91.8	18	74	1.9	0.3	4.5	—	—	2.8[a]	—	1.5	78	470	0.01	0.24	—
04-5-339	球茎茴香 [甜茴香、意大利茴香]	70	93.2	10	44	1.2	Tr	4.7	3.3	0.9	2.2	—	0.9	1	6	0.03	0.06	Tr
04-5-415	芦笋 (绿) [石刁柏、龙须菜]	90	93.3	13	56	2.6	0.1	3.3	2.8	—	—	—	0.7	3	20	0.07	0.08	0.11
04-5-416	芦笋 (紫)	93	93.1	18	74	2.7	0.2	3.4	2.1	0.7	1.3	—	0.6	46	273	0.10	0.13	0.02
04-5-417	结球菊苣	89	93.8	12	49	1.8	0.2	3.4	2.7	—	—	—	0.8	17	104	0.04	0.04	0.05
04-5-418	软化白菊苣	97	94.7	13	56	1.5	0.2	3.1	1.7	—	—	—	0.5	2	14	0.04	0.02	0.05
水生蔬菜类																		
04-6-010	藕 [莲藕]	88	86.4	42	177	1.2	0.2	11.5	2.6	0.3	2.2	—	0.7	Tr	Tr	0.04	0.01	0.05
薯芋类																		
04-7-203	芋头 [芋艿、毛芋]	88	85.0	54	225	1.3	0.2	12.7	—	—	(1.0)	—	0.8	2	14	0.05	0.02	0.10
04-7-204	芋头 (煮)	100	83.0	60	251[c]	2.9	0.1	13.0	—	—	0.3[b]	—	1.0	0	0	0.06	0.03	—
野生蔬菜类																		
04-8-081	苦苣菜 [苦菜、天精菜]	100	90.3	29	121	3.1	0.6	4.5	—	—	1.7[a]	—	1.5	9055	54330	0.11	0.16	—

（以每100g可食部计）

编码 Code	食物名称 Food name	维生素 B_{12} Vit B_{12} μg	叶酸 Folate μg	烟酸 Niacin mg	维生素C Vit C mg	维生素E (Vit E) Total mg	α-TE mg	钙 Ca mg	磷 P mg	钾 K mg	钠 Na mg	镁 Mg mg	铁 Fe mg	锌 Zn mg	硒 Se μg	铜 Cu mg	锰 Mn mg	碘 I μg
04-5-330	紫背天葵 [红风菜、血皮菜]	(0)	23.7	0.27	3.0	0.20	un	69	31	367	19.3	72	0.8	0.37	0.92	0.09	0.80	—
04-5-331	芹菜 (茎)	(0)	13.6	0.22	2.0	Tr	Tr	15	13	128	166.4	16	0.2	0.14	0.07	0.03	0.04	0.3
04-5-332	西芹 [西洋芹菜、美芹]	(0)	29.8	0.22	4.0	Tr	Tr	36	35	15	313.3	15	0.2	0.10	0.10	0.02	0.06	Tr
04-5-333	生菜	(0)	31.6	—	Tr	Tr	Tr	14	12	91	16.1	7	0.2	0.12	0.04	0.01	0.06	Tr
04-5-334	油麦菜	(0)	77.9	0.56	2.0	0.45	0.45	60	26	164	32.0	23	0.5	0.24	0.16	0.02	0.06	Tr
04-5-335	叶甜菜 (白梗)	(0)	63.9	0.23	7.4	0.34	0.34	48	26	24	356.5	48	0.6	0.22	0.30	0.06	0.15	0.2
04-5-336	莴笋叶 [莴苣菜]	(0)	22.7	—	Tr	Tr	Tr	9	37	305	35.6	19	0.2	0.19	0.21	0.05	0.03	0.3
04-5-337	蕹菜 [空心菜、藤藤菜]	(0)	78.9	0.22	5.0	0.10	0.10	115	37	304	107.6	46	1.0	0.27	—	0.05	0.52	0.4
04-5-338	观达菜 [根达菜、牛皮菜]	(0)	—	—	6.4	0.50	un	76	17	290	220.0	64	1.3	0.18	1.40	0.02	0.48	—
04-5-339	球茎茴香 [甜茴香、意大利茴香]	(0)	57.6	0.22	3.3	Tr	Tr	76	35	24	90.5	23	0.4	0.18	Tr	0.09	0.12	0.4
04-5-415	芦笋 (绿) [石刁柏、龙须菜]	(0)	145.5	1.12	7.0	0.19	0.11	9	51	304	12.4	18	1.4	0.55	0.62	0.10	0.12	0.1
04-5-416	芦笋 (紫)	(0)	150.9	0.95	8.3	0.54	0.34	13	49	26	9.2	14	0.4	0.42	0.07	0.12	0.12	Tr
04-5-417	结球菊苣	(0)	95.9	0.23	2.0	0.20	0.02	78	53	365	24.9	20	0.8	0.39	0.33	0.10	0.25	—
04-5-418	软化白菊苣	(0)	42.4	0.07	1.0	0.14	0.01	11	53	216	33.6	20	0.2	0.24	0.21	0.06	0.14	Tr
水生蔬菜类																		
04-6-010	藕 [莲藕]	(0)	10.3	0.12	19.0	0.32	0.32	18	45	293	34.3	14	0.3	0.24	0.17	0.09	0.89	2.4
薯芋类																		
04-7-203	芋头 [芋艿、毛芋]	(0)	31.3	0.28	1.5	Tr	Tr	11	50	25	5.5	19	0.3	0.19	0.91	0.06	0.30	—
04-7-204	芋头 (煮)	—	—	0.50	Tr	—	—	16	58	317	1.0	—	0.5	—	—	—	—	—
野生蔬菜类																		
04-8-081	苦苣菜 [苦菜、天精菜]	(0)	67.0	0.70	3.0	2.73	un	230	53	350	17.3	58	6.5	0.61	—	0.09	—	—

蔬菜类及制品 Vegetables and vegetable products

(以每 100g 可食部计)

编码 Code	食物名称 Food name	食部 Edible	水分 Water	能量 Energy		蛋白质 Protein	脂肪 Fat	碳水化合物 CHO	膳食纤维 (Dietary fiber)			胆固醇 Cholesterol	灰分 Ash	维生素 A		硫胺素 Thiamin	核黄素 Riboflavin	维生素 B_6 Vit B_6
									总 Total	可溶性 Soluble	不溶性 Insoluble			Vit A	胡萝卜素 Carotene			
		%	g	kcal	kJ	g	g	g	g	g	g	mg	g	μgRE	μg	mg	mg	mg
04-8-082	苜蓿 [草头、金花菜]	95	90.2	32	134	5.0	0.7	2.9	—	—	1.4[a]	—	1.2	915	5490	0.02	0.17	—
04-8-083	鱼腥草 (叶) [蕺菜、臭菜]	100	84.9	13	54	2.1	—	10.7	9.6	—	—	—	2.3	Tr	Tr	0.03	0.12	0.38
04-8-084	鱼腥草 (根)	86	77.4	39	164	2.1	—	19.5	11.8	—	—	—	1.0	7	41	0.09	0.06	—

蔬菜类及制品 Vegetables and vegetable products

(以每100g可食部计)

编码 Code	食物名称 Food name	维生素B_{12} Vit B_{12} μg	叶酸 Folate μg	烟酸 Niacin mg	维生素C Vit C mg	维生素E (Vit E) Total mg	维生素E (Vit E) α-TE mg	钙 Ca mg	磷 P mg	钾 K mg	钠 Na mg	镁 Mg mg	铁 Fe mg	锌 Zn mg	硒 Se μg	铜 Cu mg	锰 Mn mg	碘 I μg
04-8-082	苜蓿 [草头、金花菜]	(0)	—	1.00	102.0	2.82	un	112	22	32	26.2	11	2.8	0.25	0.11	0.04	0.13	—
04-8-083	鱼腥草 (叶) [蕺菜、臭菜]	(0)	41.6	1.04	16.0	1.28	un	57	31	494	21.6	145	2.3	0.40	1.25	0.09	1.00	—
04-8-084	鱼腥草 (根)	(0)	41.2	0.78	3.0	0.26	0.26	74	55	469	42.4	27	2.3	0.69	0.43	0.11	1.28	—

Notes

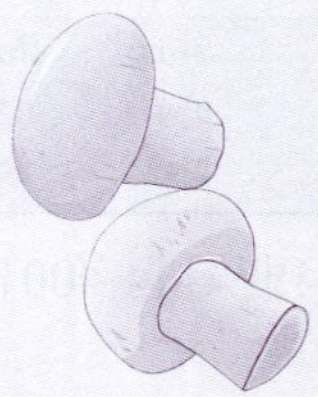

菌藻类

Fungi and Algae

菌类和藻类是两个不同的类别，它们均不同于一般的动植物性食物，由于都含有丰富的蛋白质，习惯上常将其放在一起。

1. 菌类：食用菌又称真菌食物，属真菌类的担子菌纲，包括蘑菇、香菇、平菇、木耳等。它既不同于植物性食物，也不同于动物性食物。食用菌营养丰富，且具有“高蛋白、低脂肪”的特点。新鲜蘑菇含蛋白质较少，干蘑菇则高达40%左右。

2. 藻类：海藻类系海洋生或海边生植物，含有丰富的蛋白质和维生素B类。可用作食品的海洋藻类有100多种。根据海藻的生活习性，把海藻分为浮游藻和底栖藻两大类型。浮游藻由一个细胞组成，所以也称为海洋单细胞藻。这类生物是一群具有叶绿素，能够进行光合作用，并生产有机物的自养型生物。它们是海洋中最重要的初级生产者，又是养殖鱼、虾、贝的饵料。现在，在中国海记录到的浮游藻有1817种。栖息在海底的藻类称为底栖藻。根据海藻的颜色，把它们分为三大类：绿藻类、褐藻类和红藻类。褐藻类已被大量用来制作工业上有广泛用途的褐藻胶。

本节只提供了少量藻类食物的数据。

菌藻类 Fungi and algae

(以每100g可食部计)

编码 Code	食物名称 Food name	食部 Edible %	水分 Water g	能量 Energy kcal	能量 Energy kJ	蛋白质 Protein g	脂肪 Fat g	碳水化合物 CHO g	膳食纤维 (Dietary fiber) 总 Total g	可溶性 Soluble g	不溶性 Insoluble g	胆固醇 Cholesterol mg	灰分 Ash g	维生素A Vit A μgRE	胡萝卜素 Carotene μg	硫胺素 Thiamin mg	核黄素 Riboflavin mg	维生素B6 Vit B_6 mg
菌类																		
05-1-028	白蘑菇 [双孢蘑菇、洋蘑菇]	100	91.4	27	113[c]	3.5	0.4	3.8	1.8	—	—	—	0.9	0	—	0.02	0.30	0.02
05-1-029	北风菌 [荷叶离褶伞、一窝羊]	77	94.6	14	59	1.7	0.1	2.9	—	—	1.2[a]	—	0.7	Tr	Tr	0.05	0.38	—
05-1-030	草菇 [大黑头细花草、稻菇]	100	94.6	14	59	1.1	0.4	3.1	1.4	—	—	—	0.9	—	—	0.02	0.03	—
05-1-031	茶树菇 (干) [柱状田头菇、茶薪菇]	100	12.2	279	1166	23.1	2.6	56.1	15.4	—	—	—	6.0	Tr	Tr	0.32	1.48	—
05-1-032	干巴菌	91	86.5	26	109	3.8	0.4	8.0	—	—	6.3[a]	—	1.3	Tr	Tr	0.06	1.84	—
05-1-033	红奶浆菌 [多汁乳菇、谷熟菌]	94	94.0	13	54	1.5	0.4	3.3	—	—	2.4[a]	—	0.8	Tr	Tr	0.03	0.27	—
05-1-034	黄蘑 (干)	100	11.0	225	940	24.6	6.4	46.9	29.7	—	—	—	11.1	19	114	0.48	1.46	0.16
05-1-035	黄伞菇 (干) [多脂鳞伞、黄丝菌]	100	10.8	237	993	22.8	3.2	57.5	28.1	—	—	—	5.7	Tr	Tr	0.17	1.93	0.12
05-1-036	鸡腿菇 (干) [毛头鬼伞]	100	10.8	257	1075	26.7	2.0	51.8	18.8	—	—	—	8.7	—	—	0.14	1.79	—
05-1-037	鸡油菌 [黄丝菌、杏菌]	92	91.4	21	88	2.0	0.3	5.1	—	—	2.6[a]	—	1.2	249	1490	0.03	0.39	—
05-1-038	鸡枞 [蚁枞、伞把菇、鸡枞菌]	96	94.5	16	68	2.5	0.2	2.5	—	—	1.3[a]	—	0.4	Tr	Tr	0.02	0.25	—
05-1-039	鸡枞 (干)	100	13.6	251	1048	32.8	3.7	44.8	23.3	—	—	—	5.1	12	70	0.26	1.22	0.36
05-1-040	鸡枞 (油炸) [油鸡枞]	100	16.5	635	2657	4.8	66.3	10.2	—	—	5.4[a]	—	2.2	—	Tr	0.03	0.24	—
05-1-041	鸡枞花	86	95.0	16	67	2.3	0.3	1.8	—	—	0.8[a]	—	0.6	Tr	Tr	0.20	0.14	—
05-1-042	白牛肝菌 [美味牛肝菌]	93	90.2	32	134	4.0	0.4	4.5	—	—	1.5[a]	—	0.9	Tr	Tr	0.14	1.11	—
05-1-043	白牛肝菌 (干) [美味牛肝菌]	100	11.6	253	1057	27.8	1.6	53.3	21.5	—	—	—	5.7	18	108	0.32	1.72	0.06
05-1-044	黑牛肝菌 [铜色牛肝菌]	95	90.6	29	121	3.6	0.2	4.8	—	—	1.6[a]	—	0.8	Tr	Tr	0.07	0.31	—

菌藻类 Fungi and algae

(以每 100g 可食部计)

编码 Code	食物名称 Food name	维生素 B_{12} Vit B_{12} μg	叶酸 Folate μg	烟酸 Niacin mg	维生素 C Vit C mg	维生素 E (Vit E) Total mg	维生素 E (Vit E) α-TE mg	钙 Ca mg	磷 P mg	钾 K mg	钠 Na mg	镁 Mg mg	铁 Fe mg	锌 Zn mg	硒 Se μg	铜 Cu mg	锰 Mn mg	碘 I μg
菌类																		
05-1-028	白蘑菇 [双孢蘑菇、洋蘑菇]	—	—	3.50	0.1	—	—	6	93	350	57.0	11	1.0	0.60	—	—	—	—
05-1-029	北风菌 [荷叶离褶伞、一窝羊]	—	—	0.70	—	7.28	7.28	3	36	254	1.4	5	1.5	0.47	0.17	0.26	0.09	—
05-1-030	草菇 [大黑头细花草、稻菇]	Tr	—	1.39	—	0.70	un	5	24	53	332.1	5	1.1	0.33	0.90	0.10	0.09	Tr
05-1-031	茶树菇 (干) [柱状田头菇、茶薪菇]	—	107.8	39.39	—	—	—	4	908	2165	6.0	124	9.3	8.38	7.24	2.76	0.73	17.1
05-1-032	干巴菌	—	—	1.20	—	45.14	un	10	104	328	2.1	11	21.0	0.78	—	0.30	0.67	—
05-1-033	红奶浆菌 [多汁乳菇、谷熟菌]	—	—	1.20	—	—	—	4	27	245	1.2	5	5.9	0.42	0.13	0.26	0.11	—
05-1-034	黄蘑 (干)	—	201.5	12.43	—	4.05	un	33	857	4647	31.9	122	51.3	7.04	6.78	0.47	2.51	—
05-1-035	黄伞菇 (干) [多脂鳞伞、黄丝菌]	—	101.9	41.38	—	—	—	4	566	3128	6.4	96	7.6	5.58	13.56	5.39	0.67	12.6
05-1-036	鸡腿菇 (干) [毛头鬼伞]	—	351.8	24.99	—	5.01	un	9	764	4053	68.2	119	6.5	3.95	15.39	1.40	0.72	—
05-1-037	鸡油菌 [黄丝菌、杏菌]	—	—	1.90	—	4.84	4.76	12	44	339	2.8	10	2.2	0.54	0.32	0.31	0.15	—
05-1-038	鸡枞 [蚁枞、伞把菇、鸡枞菌]	—	—	5.50	—	—	—	4	38	102	3.1	8	1.8	0.46	0.14	0.58	0.12	—
05-1-039	鸡枞 (干)	—	347.3	34.21	—	4.17	un	8	1005	1312	23.9	116	31.8	7.16	33.44	2.39	2.13	—
05-1-040	鸡枞 (油炸) [油鸡枞]	—	—	9.20	—	—	—	28	232	367	1265.7	33	31.1	3.26	2.73	1.28	1.16	—
05-1-041	鸡枞花	—	—	1.60	—	11.46	un	8	73	173	2.7	9	4.7	0.44	0.15	0.36	0.12	—
05-1-042	白牛肝菌 [美味牛肝菌]	—	—	2.10	—	8.93	un	5	68	301	2.1	10	2.1	0.98	0.25	0.32	0.19	—
05-1-043	巨牛肝菌 (干) [美味牛肝菌]	—	124.4	43.08	—	4.42	un	2	528	1571	9.1	47	9.2	5.80	758.80	1.19	3.88	—
05-1-044	黑牛肝菌 [铜色牛肝菌]	—	—	6.60	—	—	—	2	60	291	1.3	8	2.1	1.19	0.34	0.37	0.17	—

菌藻类 Fungi and algae

(以每100g可食部计)

编码 Code	食物名称 Food name	食部 Edible %	水分 Water g	能量 Energy kcal	能量 Energy kJ	蛋白质 Protein g	脂肪 Fat g	碳水化合物 CHO g	膳食纤维 (Dietary fiber) 总 Total g	可溶性 Soluble g	不溶性 Insoluble g	胆固醇 Cholesterol mg	灰分 Ash g	维生素A Vit A μgRE	胡萝卜素 Carotene μg	硫胺素 Thiamin mg	核黄素 Riboflavin mg	维生素B_6 Vit B_6 mg
05-1-045	黄皮牛肝菌 [黄皮疣柄牛肝菌、黄癞头]	97	89.7	24	100	4.3	0.1	5.3	—	—	3.9[a]	—	0.6	Tr	Tr	0.03	0.57	—
05-1-046	乳牛肝菌(干) [粘盖牛肝菌、松树菌]	100	10.5	178	746	15.3	2.8	66.0	43.0	—	—	—	5.4	59	357	0.86	1.72	—
05-1-047	牛眼睛菌 [马勃菌]	93	86.6	32	134	5.1	0.3	6.6	—	—	4.4[a]	—	1.4	Tr	Tr	—	0.25	—
05-1-048	平菇 [糙皮侧耳、青蘑]	100	94.4	14	59	1.7	0.1	3.2	1.6	—	—	—	0.6	2	10	0.03	0.08	0.09
05-1-049	青头菌 [变绿红菇、绿菇]	95	93.3	15	63	2.7	0.1	3.1	—	—	2.2[a]	—	0.8	Tr	Tr	0.01	0.46	—
05-1-050	松蘑(干) [松茸、松口蘑]	100	10.6	202	847	12.5	3.0	66.5	35.1	—	—	—	7.4	16	97	0.08	1.48	0.12
05-1-051	杏鲍菇	100	89.6	31	129	1.3	0.1	8.3	—	—	2.1[a]	—	0.7	Tr	Tr	0.03	0.14	0.03
05-1-052	血红菇(干)	100	7.8	252	1054	22.4	6.7	56.0	30.5	—	—	—	7.1	Tr	Tr	0.13	4.30	0.06
05-1-053	元蘑(干) [亚侧耳、冬蘑、黄蘑]	100	7.8	146	609	12.3	1.5	70.3	49.6	—	—	—	8.1	34	202	0.16	10.75	0.08
05-1-054	竹荪(干) [竹笙、竹参]	100	13.9	155	648	17.8	3.1	60.3	—	—	46.4[a]	—	4.9	Tr	Tr	0.03	1.75	—
05-1-055	榛蘑(干) [小蜜环菌]	100	8.0	271	1135	17.7	10.8	54.6	28.8	—	—	—	8.9	81	483	0.14	0.71	0.09
藻类																		
05-2-009	螺旋藻(干)	100	6.5	356	1487	64.7	3.1	18.2	—	—	1.0[a]	—	7.5	6468	38810	0.28	1.41	—
05-2-010	裙带菜(干) [海芥菜、海木耳]	100	9.2	119	498	25.0	1.7	41.5	40.6	8.3	31.1	—	22.6	372	2230	0.02	0.07	Tr
05-2-011	海带菜	100	68.3	89	373	1.4	7.5	15.3	11.3	—	—	—	7.5	67	402	0.04	0.03	0.07

菌藻类 Fungi and algae

（以每100g可食部计）

编码 Code	食物名称 Food name	维生素B_{12} Vit B_{12} μg	叶酸 Folate μg	烟酸 Niacin mg	维生素C Vit C mg	维生素E (Vit E) Total mg	α-TE mg	钙 Ca mg	磷 P mg	钾 K mg	钠 Na mg	镁 Mg mg	铁 Fe mg	锌 Zn mg	硒 Se μg	铜 Cu mg	锰 Mn mg	碘 I μg
05-1-045	黄皮牛肝菌[黄皮疣柄牛肝菌、黄癞头]	—	—	3.20	—	Tr	Tr	2	49	224	1.6	8	1.4	1.07	0.37	0.35	0.28	—
05-1-046	乳牛肝菌(干)[粘盖牛肝菌、松树菌]	—	144.7	67.66	—	6.85	un	12	391	1481	11.2	55	20.3	5.43	42.45	0.35	1.85	—
05-1-047	牛眼睛菌[马勃菌]	—	—	1.60	—	—	—	8	141	532	1.8	21	4.1	1.81	0.29	0.14	0.32	—
05-1-048	平菇[糙皮侧耳、青蘑]	—	14.7	—	—	0.37	un	4	54	208	13.2	13	0.7	0.57	0.25	0.08	0.05	0.8
05-1-049	青头菌[变绿红菇、绿菇]	—	—	4.00	—	Tr	Tr	4	52	269	1.1	8	1.4	0.67	0.22	0.34	0.10	—
05-1-050	松蘑(干)[松茸、松口蘑]	—	97.1	23.42	—	5.48	un	7	390	2402	31.6	50	156.5	5.49	102.60	1.76	1.13	—
05-1-051	杏鲍菇	—	42.8	3.68	—	0.60	un	13	66	242	3.5	9	0.5	0.39	1.80	0.06	0.04	Tr
05-1-052	血红菇(干)	—	39.5	26.85	—	—	—	9	327	3520	2.9	61	25.2	6.03	11.82	2.84	1.09	9.3
05-1-053	元蘑(干)[亚侧耳、冬蘑、黄蘑]	—	173.6	33.02	—	3.63	un	6	369	3877	13.4	131	7.8	1.89	1.45	0.30	3.39	—
05-1-054	竹荪(干)[竹笙、竹参]	—	—	9.10	—	—	—	18	289	11882	50.0	114	17.8	2.20	4.17	2.51	8.47	—
05-1-055	榛蘑(干)[小蜜环菌]	—	288.2	26.91	—	3.35	un	9	893	4629	18.7	100	22.4	6.00	2.38	1.36	1.55	—
藻类																		
05-2-009	螺旋藻(干)	—	—	10.00	Tr	27.11	Tr	137	1317	1506	1624.0	402	88.0	2.62	5.24	0.54	1.24	—
05-2-010	裙带菜(干)[海芥菜、海木耳]	—	29.6	Tr	—	Tr	Tr	947	305	335	4411.6	1022	16.4	2.62	15.88	0.12	0.95	15878.0
05-2-011	海带菜	—	1.6	Tr	—	2.37	un	201	27	44	2511.7	46	2.3	4.93	0.50	0.07	0.33	923.0

Notes

水果类及制品

Fruit and Fruit Products

我国水果品种繁多。依据果实的形态和生理特征将此类食物分为6个亚类，其罐头、凉果等制品也包括在本节中。

1.仁果类：仁果类水果在植物学上多属于蔷薇科，其食用部分主要是由肉质的花托发育而成，子房形成果芯，果芯内有数个小型种子，如苹果、梨、山楂、海棠果等。

2.核果类：核果类水果在植物学上也属于蔷薇科，此类果实大都由外、中、内果皮构成。外果皮较薄，中果皮肉质为主要食用部分，内果皮木质化，坚硬成核，核中有仁。常见的有桃、杏、梅、李、樱桃、枣等。

3.浆果类：这类果实浆汁多，其种子小而数量多，散布在果肉内，包括葡萄、草莓、猕猴桃、沙棘、醋栗、石榴、无花果、柿子、桑葚等。

4.柑橘类：属于芸香科柑橘类属植物，其果实外果皮为革质，中果皮较疏松，内果皮多形成囊瓣。常见的有橙、柑橘、柚、柠檬等。

5.亚热带和热带水果：包括香蕉、菠萝、芒果、椰子、番石榴、荔枝、枇杷、洋桃等。

6.瓜果类：指西瓜、甜瓜、哈密瓜、黄金瓜等一般作为水果食用的瓜类食物。

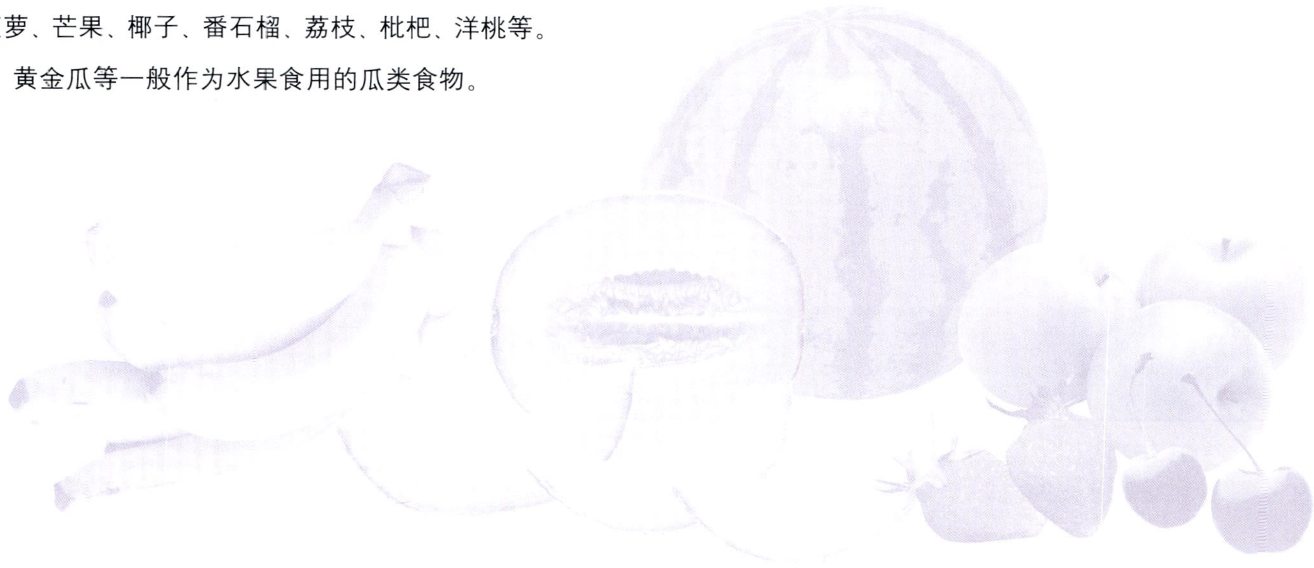

水果类及制品 Fruit and fruit products

(以每100g可食部计)

编码 Code	食物名称 Food name	食部 Edible %	水分 Water g	能量 Energy kcal	能量 Energy kJ	蛋白质 Protein g	脂肪 Fat g	碳水化合物 CHO g	膳食纤维 (Dietary fiber) 总 Total g	可溶性 Soluble g	不溶性 Insoluble g	胆固醇 Cholesterol mg	灰分 Ash g	维生素A Vit A μgRE	胡萝卜素 Carotene μg	硫胺素 Thiamin mg	核黄素 Riboflavin mg	维生素B_6 Vit B_6 mg
仁果类																		
06-1-907	蛇果	84	84.4	55	232	0.1	0.2	14.9	1.6	—	—	—	0.4	3	16	0.01	Tr	0.02
核果类																		
06-2-115	蜜桃	88	87.9	45	188	0.6	0.1	11.0	—	—	0.6[a]	—	0.4	Tr	Tr	0.01	0.02	—
06-2-116	桃 (糖水罐头)	100	84.9	59	249	0.3	0.2	14.5	0.4	—	—	—	0.1	—	—	Tr	0.04	—
06-2-207	布朗	87	88.0	41	173	0.6	0.2	10.7	1.4	—	—	—	0.5	8	46	0.01	0.01	0.03
06-2-208	西梅	76	88.5	39	163	0.7	0.1	10.3	1.5	0.6	0.7	—	0.4	1	8	0.01	0.01	0.05
06-2-312	冬枣	93	69.5	105	439	1.8	0.2	27.8	3.8	1.4	2.2	—	0.7	Tr	Tr	0.08	0.09	—
06-2-313	小枣 (干)	81	28.3	266	1114	2.7	0.7	66.8	4.5	—	—	—	1.5	Tr	Tr	0.17	0.14	—
浆果类																		
06-3-911	红提子葡萄	86	85.6	52	218	0.4	0.2	13.1	0.9	0.9	Tr	—	0.7	2	9	0.02	0.01	0.08
06-3-912	无花果 (干)	100	11.5	361	1510[c]	3.6	4.3	77.8	13.3	—	—	—	2.9	1	—	0.13	0.07	0.94
柑橘类																		
06-4-303	葡萄柚 (台湾) [西柚]	73	90.9	33	138[c]	0.7	0.3	7.8	1.2	—	—	—	0.3	47	—	0.05	0.01	0.01
06-4-304	葡萄柚 (以色列) [西柚]	65	88.8	37	153	0.7	0.1	10.0	1.8	—	—	—	0.4	11	65	0.05	0.02	0.04
热带、亚热带水果																		
06-5-021	桂圆 (干)	34	14.0	309	1292	5.6	0.2	76.2	5.1	—	—	—	4.0	—	—	0.01	0.58	—
06-5-022	红毛丹	79	80.0	79	330	1.0	1.2	17.5	1.5	1.0	0.5	—	0.3	Tr	Tr	0.01	0.04	0.05
06-5-023	火龙果 [仙蜜果、红龙果]	69	84.8	51	215	1.1	0.2	13.3	2.0	0.4	1.6	—	0.6	Tr	Tr	0.03	0.02	0.04
06-5-024	荔枝 (干)	56	15.0	317	1327	4.5	1.2	77.4	5.3	—	—	—	1.9	—	—	0	0.32	—
06-5-025	榴莲	37	64.5	147	613	2.6	3.3	28.3	1.7	Tr	1.7	—	1.3	3	20	0.20	0.13	0.14

水果类及制品 Fruit and fruit products

(以每100g可食部计)

编码 Code	食物名称 Food name	维生素 B_{12} Vit B_{12} μg	叶酸 Folate μg	烟酸 Niacin mg	维生素C Vit C mg	维生素E (Vit E) Total mg	α-TE mg	钙 Ca mg	磷 P mg	钾 K mg	钠 Na mg	镁 Mg mg	铁 Fe mg	锌 Zn mg	硒 Se μg	铜 Cu mg	锰 Mn mg	碘 I μg
仁果类																		
06-1-907	蛇果	(0)	—	0.04	2.0	Tr	Tr	5	21	14	3.1	6	0.1	0.08	Tr	0.02	0.01	Tr
核果类																		
06-2-115	蜜桃	(0)	—	0.50	Tr	—	—	4	8	77	1.7	4	0.2	0.15	Tr	0.06	0.08	—
06-2-116	桃 (糖水罐头)	(0)	—	0.20	Tr	—	—	3	9	63	2.7	5	0.1	0.25	—	0.05	0.03	—
06-2-207	布朗	(0)	—	0.43	2.0	Tr	Tr	5	11	14	2.2	7	0.2	0.10	0.10	0.02	0.03	Tr
06-2-208	西梅	(0)	1.5	0.18	1.4	0.18	0.18	11	16	155	3.2	10	0.1	0.04	0.11	0.02	0.04	Tr
06-2-312	冬枣	(0)	29.9	0.51	243.0	0.19	0.19	16	29	195	33.0	17	0.2	0.19	0.14	0.08	0.13	6.7
06-2-313	小枣 (干)	(0)	—	—	Tr	Tr	Tr	62	61	486	12.2	24	1.2	0.50	0.60	0.48	0.22	2.6
浆果类																		
06-3-911	红提子葡萄	(0)	2.9	0.07	Tr	0.34	0.03	2	20	186	4.4	5	0.2	0.06	0.08	0.04	0.04	2.0
06-3-912	无花果 (干)	—	—	0.79	5.2	un	1.68	363	67	898	10.0	96	4.5	0.80	—	—	—	—
柑橘类																		
06-4-303	葡萄柚 (台湾) [西柚]	—	—	0.20	38.0	—	—	21	17	60	7.0	9	0.1	0.10	—	—	—	—
06-4-304	葡萄柚 (以色列) [西柚]	(0)	16.8	0.18	36.0	0.17	0.17	5	16	180	4.1	10	0.3	0.01	0.03	0.02	0.02	Tr
热带、亚热带水果																		
06-5-021	桂圆 (干)	(0)	12.1	2.67	—	—	—	8	135	891	3.2	39	1.1	0.61	0.19	0.89	0.42	—
06-5-022	红毛丹	(0)	18.8	0.31	35.0	Tr	Tr	11	20	13	2.3	12	0.3	0.24	0.11	0.21	0.35	1.3
06-5-023	火龙果 [仙蜜果、红龙果]	(0)	28.1	0.22	3.0	0.14	0.14	7	35	20	2.7	30	0.3	0.29	0.03	0.04	0.19	0.4
06-5-024	荔枝 (干)	(0)	—	2.25	—	—	—	12	114	—	—	—	—	0.01	—	0.05	0.06	—
06-5-025	榴莲	(0)	116.9	1.19	2.8	2.28	2.28	4	38	261	2.9	27	0.3	0.16	3.26	0.12	0.22	5.6

水果类及制品 Fruit and fruit products

(以每100g可食部计)

编码 Code	食物名称 Food name	食部 Edible	水分 Water	能量 Energy		蛋白质 Protein	脂肪 Fat	碳水化合物 CHO	膳食纤维 (Dietary fiber) 总 Total	可溶性 Soluble	不溶性 Insoluble	胆固醇 Cholesterol	灰分 Ash	维生素A Vit A	胡萝卜素 Carotene	硫胺素 Thiamin	核黄素 Riboflavin	维生素B_6 Vit B_6
		%	g	kcal	kJ	g	g	g	g	g	g	mg	g	μgRE	μg	mg	mg	mg
06-5-026	芒果(大头)	68	86.1	50	209	0.5	0.1	12.9	—	—	1.1[a]	—	0.4	347	2080	0.03	0.01	—
06-5-027	木瓜[番木瓜]	89	91.7	30	126	0.6	Tr	7.2	—	—	0.5[a]	—	0.5	—	—	0.01	0.02	—
06-5-028	酸木瓜	79	87.8	35	146	0.3	0.2	11.1	—	—	3.0[a]	—	0.6	Tr	Tr	0.02	0.01	—
06-5-029	蒲桃[香果、水石榴]	69	88.9	38	160	0.6	Tr	10.1	—	—	1.1	—	0.4	2	10	0.24	0.10	—
06-5-030	山竹	25	81.2	69	290	0.4	0.2	18.0	1.5	0.9	0.4	—	0.2	Tr	Tr	0.08	0.02	0.03
06-5-031	香蕉(红皮,海南)	70	77.1	82	344	1.1	0.2	20.8	1.8	—	—	—	0.8	6	36	0.02	0.02	0.19
6-5-032	香蕉(红皮,泰国)	67	78.1	78	326	1.1	0.2	19.7	1.8	—	—	—	0.9	6	38	0.01	0.02	0.20
瓜果类																		
06-6-206	小西瓜[地雷瓜]	62	92.1	29	123	0.8	0.1	6.7	0.4	—	—	—	0.3	10	58	0.02	0.02	0.05

水果类及制品 Fruit and fruit products

(以每100g可食部计)

编码 Code	食物名称 Food name	维生素 B_{12} Vit B_{12} μg	叶酸 Folate μg	烟酸 Niacin mg	维生素C Vit C mg	维生素E (Vit E) Total mg	α-TE mg	钙 Ca mg	磷 P mg	钾 K mg	钠 Na mg	镁 Mg mg	铁 Fe mg	锌 Zn mg	硒 Se μg	铜 Cu mg	锰 Mn mg	碘 I μg
06-5-026	芒果 (大头)	(0)	—	0.40	14.0	—	—	7	12	153	3.6	10	0.5	0.14	0.25	0.10	0.24	—
06-5-027	木瓜 [番木瓜]	(0)	—	1.30	31.0	Tr	Tr	22	11	182	10.4	17	0.6	0.12	0.37	0.03	0.05	—
06-5-028	酸木瓜	—	—	0.20	106.0	—	—	20	11	260	1.9	11	0.8	0.55	0.20	0.06	0.08	—
06-5-029	蒲桃 [香果、水石榴]	(0)	—	—	3.1	0.19	un	121	111	10	—	24	2.2	1.52	—	0.73	0.07	—
06-5-030	山竹	(0)	7.4	0.30	1.2	0.36	un	11	9	48	3.8	19	0.3	0.06	0.54	0.03	0.10	1.1
06-5-031	香蕉 (红皮, 海南)	(0)	11.2	0.51	4.9	0.20	0.20	9	17	208	3.2	33	0.2	0.04	0.07	0.10	0.07	Tr
6-5-032	香蕉 (红皮, 泰国)	(0)	9.7	C.47	5.7	0.19	0.19	9	15	189	3.1	34	0.2	0.07	0.06	0.09	0.12	0.1
瓜果类																		
06-6-206	小西瓜 [地雷瓜]	(0)	1.7	0.13	2.0	Tr	Tr	6	9	177	4.8	9	0.2	0.08	0.11	0.02	0.02	1.7

Notes

坚果、种子类

Nuts and Seeds

坚果又称壳果，这类食物食用部分多为坚硬果核内的种仁子叶或胚乳，富含淀粉和油脂。植物的干种子在商业上常与坚果放在一起，本节也采用这种方法，并将此类食物分成两个亚类。

1. 树坚果：包括杏仁、腰果、榛子、山核桃、松子、核桃、板栗、白果（银杏）等。

2. 种子：包括花生、葵花子、南瓜子、西瓜子等。

坚果、种子类 Nuts and seeds

(以每100g可食部计)

编码 Code	食物名称 Food name	食部 Edible %	水分 Water g	能量 Energy kcal	能量 Energy kJ	蛋白质 Protein g	脂肪 Fat g	碳水化合物 CHO g	膳食纤维 (Dietary fiber) 总 Total g	可溶性 Soluble g	不溶性 Insoluble g	胆固醇 Cholesterol mg	灰分 Ash g	维生素A Vit A μgRE	胡萝卜素 Carotene μg	硫胺素 Thiamin mg	核黄素 Riboflavin mg	维生素B_6 Vit B_6 mg
树坚果																		
07-1-026	山核桃 (熟)	45	2.8	618	2586	8.3	64.5	21.3	20.2	—	—	—	3.1	23	137	0.11	0.07	0.07
07-1-027	栗子 (北京密云) [板栗]	80	53.3	182	762	4.4	1.6	39.6	—	—	2.0[a]	—	1.1	7	40	—	—	—
07-1-028	栗子 (河南) [板栗]	80	51.2	186	777	4.4	1.4	41.9	—	—	3.1[a]	—	1.1	8	48	—	—	—
07-1-029	栗子 (山东) [板栗]	80	57.3	164	688	4.4	1.0	36.3	—	—	1.9[a]	—	1.0	9	56	—	—	—
07-1-030	栗子 (河北迁西) [板栗]	80	53.6	178	745	3.8	0.9	40.7	—	—	2.1[a]	—	1.0	7	44	—	—	—
07-1-031	栗子 (河北邢台) [板栗]	80	53.6	179	750	4.3	1.1	39.9	—	—	1.8[a]	—	1.1	7	44	—	—	—
07-1-032	栗子仁 (熟)	100	47.3	174	727	4.5	1.5	45.7	10.2	—	—	—	1.0	—	—	0.08	0.12	—
07-1-033	松子 (熟)	69	3.4	530	2218	12.9	40.4	40.3	11.6	—	—	—	3.0	—	—	0.14	0.17	0.21
07-1-034	杏仁 (熟, 带壳)	63	1.7	626	2619	25.1	58.4	11.0	11.0	—	—	—	3.8	—	—	0.06	0.66	—
07-1-035	杏仁 (熟, 去壳)	100	3.1	605	2530	28.0	54.4	11.1	10.3	—	—	0	3.4	—	—	0.09	0.52	0.15
07-1-036	腰果 (熟)	100	2.1	594	2484	24.0	50.9	20.4	10.5	0.1	10.4	0	2.6	—	—	0.24	0.13	0.43
07-1-037	榛子 (熟)	66	2.2	617	2579	12.5	57.3	25.6	12.9	Tr	12.9	—	2.4	—	—	0.17	0.11	0.59
07-1-038	榛子仁 (熟)	100	2.2	610	2552	15.6	52.9	26.7	8.8	—	—	—	2.6	—	—	0.19	0.12	—
07-1-039	开心果 (熟)	82	0.8	614	2570	20.6	53.0	21.9	8.2	Tr	8.2	—	3.7	—	—	0.45	0.10	—
07-1-040	香榧 (熟)	61	1.1	618	2586	12.4	57.0	26.9	13.0	—	—	—	2.6	—	—	0.04	0.10	—
种子																		
07-2-020	花生 (烤, 勤俭牌)	72	2.5	566	2366	26.4	46.3	21.2	—	—	10.4	—	3.6	8	47	0.25	0.08	0.43
07-2-021	花生 (烤, 密日兴牌)	71	3.1	459	1921	16.6	22.3	55.9	—	—	7.9[a]	—	2.1	86	518	0.20	0.08	—
07-2-022	花生仁 (油炸)	100	1.3	549	2296	22.2	47.1	26.2	—	—	17.2[a]	—	3.2	—	—	0.30	0.08	—
07-2-023	葵花子 (奶油香瓜子)	51	1.4	591	2472	22.7	54.1	17.9	—	—	14.6	—	3.9	—	—	0.54	0.12	0.45
07-2-024	葵花子 (熟)	48	2.7	567	2372	28.5	49.0	15.1	12.1	3.9	8.2	—	4.7	9	52	0.94	0.12	0.86
07-2-025	南瓜子 (熟) [白瓜子]	69	3.2	597	2497	26.6	52.8	12.9	—	—	9.1	—	4.5	14	81	0.20	0.10	0.12

坚果、种子类 Nuts and seeds

（以每100g可食部计）

编码 Code	食物名称 Food name	维生素 B_{12} Vit B_{12} μg	叶酸 Folate μg	烟酸 Niacin mg	维生素C Vit C mg	维生素E (Vit E) Total mg	α-TE mg	钙 Ca mg	磷 P mg	钾 K mg	钠 Na mg	镁 Mg mg	铁 Fe mg	锌 Zn mg	硒 Se μg	铜 Cu mg	锰 Mn mg	碘 I μg
树坚果																		
07-1-026	山核桃(熟)	(0)	69.8	0.83	—	14.75	2.14	132	279	4	855.5	130	6.0	7.07	1.15	1.33	11.39	18.8
07-1-027	栗子(北京密云)[板栗]	(0)	—	—	23.2	3.94	un	16	72	—	—	—	0.4	5.60	1.20	—	—	—
07-1-028	栗子(河南)[油栗]	(0)	—	—	24.2	3.06	un	19	95	—	—	—	0.2	8.00	1.40	—	—	—
07-1-029	栗子(山东)[油栗]	(0)	—	—	18.9	3.49	un	19	90	—	—	—	0.4	—	1.80	—	—	—
07-1-030	栗子(河北迁西)[板栗]	(0)	—	—	26.1	4.82	un	17	84	—	—	—	0.6	7.13	—	—	—	—
07-1-031	栗子(河北邢台)[板栗]	(0)	—	—	15.4	3.14	un	19	73	—	—	—	0.6	5.60	0.95	—	—	—
07-1-032	栗子仁(熟)	(0)	19.5	1.14	—	9.28	0.93	9	105	468	8.7	52	1.1	0.76	Tr	0.45	2.01	—
07-1-033	松子(熟)	(0)	—	1.36	—	28.25	16.04	14	453	1007	666.0	272	3.9	4.32	0.59	1.01	1.36	9.7
07-1-034	杏仁(熟,带壳)	(0)	—	2.61	—	35.54	32.91	240	565	668	195.8	218	2.7	2.21	3.33	1.00	1.93	—
07-1-035	杏仁(熟,去壳)	Tr	10.8	2.77	—	27.17	25.23	174	341	693	342.2	277	5.3	3.72	1.72	1.43	2.45	8.4
07-1-036	腰果(熟)	Tr	24.6	1.28	—	6.70	0.62	19	639	680	35.7	595	7.4	5.30	10.93	2.57	1.19	—
07-1-037	榛子(熟)	Tr	20.7	1.02	—	22.81	20.26	95	369	1001	9.4	172	3.8	2.25	2.02	1.13	1.96	6.3
07-1-038	榛子仁(熟)	(0)	56.4	1.16	—	22.18	19.70	86	336	807	153.0	168	4.2	2.22	1.12	1.39	2.90	4.4
07-1-039	开心果(熟)	(0)	34.5	1.05	—	19.36	2.85	108	468	735	756.4	118	4.4	3.11	6.50	0.83	1.69	37.9
07-1-040	香榧(熟)	(0)	36.9	—	—	114.16	un	83	248	664	215.6	291	1.8	1.94	1.50	0.38	0.74	—
种子																		
07-2-020	花生(烤,勤俭牌)	(0)	63.8	12.13	—	13.88	7.78	79	376	541	79.4	200	2.1	3.61	2.19	1.23	1.56	9.4
07-2-021	花生(烤,旺日兴牌)	(0)	—	10.00	—	8.05	un	23	299	344	171.1	51	2.6	2.61	5.44	0.34	—	14.7
07-2-022	花生仁(油炸)	(0)	—	—	—	8.70	un	20	474	551	207.8	84	1.6	3.16	—	0.56	—	—
07-2-023	葵花子(奶油香瓜子)	(0)	238.4	2.46	—	21.79	18.99	77	925	423	604.3	412	6.7	7.62	12.49	2.53	2.57	31.4
07-2-024	葵花子(熟)	(0)	304.5	2.10	—	11.70	9.71	112	1032	399	634.7	509	6.4	7.45	56.68	2.42	3.48	38.5
07-2-025	南瓜子(熟)[白瓜子]	(0)	143.8	2.96	—	31.06	2.64	26	1034	610	145.1	424	9.1	7.77	2.42	1.32	4.38	11.0

坚果、种子类 Nuts and seeds

(以每 100g 可食部计)

编码 Code	食物名称 Food name	食部 Edible	水分 Water	能量 Energy		蛋白质 Protein	脂肪 Fat	碳水化合物 CHO	膳食纤维 (Dietary fiber)			胆固醇 Cholesterol	灰分 Ash	维生素 A		硫胺素 Thiamin	核黄素 Riboflavin	维生素B_6 Vit B_6
									总 Total	可溶性 Soluble	不溶性 Insoluble			Vit A	胡萝卜素 Carotene			
		%	g	kcal	kJ	g	g	g	g	g	g	mg	g	μgRE	μg	mg	mg	mg
07-2-026	西瓜子 (熟) [黑瓜子]	38	10.7	532	2228	29.0	46.0	9.5	—	—	8.9	—	4.8	Tr	Tr	0.06	0.06	0.39

坚果、种子类 Nuts and seeds

(以每100g 可食部计)

编码 Code	食物名称 Food name	维生素 B_{12} Vit B_{12} μg	叶酸 Folate μg	烟酸 Niacin mg	维生素 C Vit C mg	维生素 E (Vit E) Total mg	α-TE mg	钙 Ca mg	磷 P mg	钾 K mg	钠 Na mg	镁 Mg mg	铁 Fe mg	锌 Zn mg	硒 Se μg	铜 Cu mg	锰 Mn mg	碘 I μg
07-2-026	西瓜子 (熟) [黑瓜子]	(0)	223.4	1.12	—	21.10	un	44	1080	880	599.4	437	7.7	5.02	22.64	1.87	2.12	20.7

Notes

畜肉类及制品

Meat and Meat Products

常见的家畜有猪、牛、羊、驴、马等。本节按以上种类分为亚类。

畜体的各部位主要分为头部、躯干和四肢，各部位的命名主要以骨为基础，附录中给出了牛的解剖部位图。肉和肉制品包括动物的骨骼肌，也包括它们的腺体和器官（如舌头、肝、心脏、肾和脑等）。肉脯、火腿肠等肉制品也包括在此节中。

肉的质量分级一般基于三个因素：胴体的成熟度、脂肪花纹度和肌肉坚实度。颜色也是一个参考依据。这些因素导致肉的产量、嫩度、风味、烹调过程中营养素的损失以及总体质量大不相同。

畜肉类及制品 Meat and meat products

(以每100g可食部计)

编码 Code	食物名称 Food name	食部 Edible %	水分 Water g	能量 Energy kcal	能量 Energy kJ	蛋白质 Protein g	脂肪 Fat g	碳水化合物 CHO g	膳食纤维 (Dietary fiber) 总 Total g	可溶性 Soluble g	不溶性 Insoluble g	胆固醇 Cholesterol mg	灰分 Ash g	维生素A Vit A μgRE	胡萝卜素 Carotene μg	硫胺素 Thiamin mg	核黄素 Riboflavin mg	维生素 B_6 Vit B_6 mg
猪																		
08-1-121	猪肉 (前臀尖, 杜长大猪)	100	58.6	289	1209	15.3	25.3	0	—	—	—	80	0.8	8	(0)	0.27	0.12	—
08-1-122	猪肉 (前臀尖, 良杂猪)	100	53.7	334	1397	14.2	30.4	0.9	—	—	—	41	0.8	9	(0)	0.24	0.11	—
08-1-123	猪肉 (后臀尖, 杜长大猪)	100	71.2	165	691	20.8	9.1	0	—	—	—	43	1.1	Tr	(0)	0.31	0.13	0.22
08-1-124	猪肉 (后臀尖, 良杂猪)	100	68.8	175	730	20.0	10.5	0	—	—	—	66	1.1	Tr	(0)	0.45	0.10	0.15
08-1-125	猪肉 (硬肋, 杜长大猪)	100	36.5	557	2331	10.8	57.1	0	—	—	—	61	0.6	12	(0)	0.21	0.08	0.06
08-1-126	猪肉 (硬肋, 良杂猪)	100	38.4	536	2243	11.6	54.4	0	—	—	—	81	0.6	12	(0)	0.15	0.08	0.08
08-1-127	猪肉 (通脊, 杜长大猪)	100	70.7	159	667	22.3	7.8	0	—	—	—	151	1.2	Tr	(0)	0.28	0.10	—
08-1-128	猪肉 (通脊, 良杂猪)	100	73.2	140	587	20.7	6.4	0	—	—	—	64	1.1	Tr	(0)	0.20	0.08	0.24
08-1-129	猪肉 (里脊)	100	74.7	150	626	19.6	7.9	0	—	—	—	—	1.2	Tr	(0)	0.32	0.20	0.20
08-1-130	猪皮	100	46.9	363	1517	27.4	28.1	0	—	—	—	100	0.5	3	(0)	0.03	0.14	—
08-1-131	猪小排 (杜长大猪)	70	60.0	295	1234	16.8	25.3	0	—	—	—	120	0.8	7	(0)	0.31	0.26	0.11
08-1-132	猪小排 (良杂猪)	61	55.4	351	1467	14.1	32.7	0	—	—	—	68	0.8	6	(0)	0.30	0.32	0.08
08-1-213	猪肚	100	79.3	97	405	14.1	3.5	2.2	—	—	—	290	0.9	2	(0)	0.10	0.22	0.05
08-1-214	猪肝	100	72.6	126	528	19.2	4.7	1.8	—	—	—	180	1.7	6502	(0)	0.22	2.02	0.29
08-1-215	猪舌 [口条]	100	70.2	184	770	18.1	12.4	0	—	—	—	230	0.9	Tr	(0)	0.27	0.41	0.14
08-1-216	猪肾 [猪腰子]	100	80.6	82	342	15.8	1.8	0.6	—	—	—	430	1.2	39	(0)	0.19	1.18	—
08-1-318	火腿心全精肉	100	35.2	322	1346	37.0	19.3	0	—	—	—	—	13.5	Tr	—	0.20	0.35	—
08-1-319	火腿心肉	81	25.6	528	2209	22.2	48.8	0	—	—	—	—	8.4	Tr	—	0.18	0.26	—
08-1-320	腊肉	100	8.2	692	2895	18.2	68.0	1.8	—	—	—	—	3.8	Tr	—	0.23	0.16	0.08
08-1-321	叉烧肉	100	60.4	196	819	20.9	9.8	6.0	—	—	—	37	2.9	Tr	—	0.05	0.09	—
08-1-322	酱排骨	80	39.0	366	1529	21.7	26.7	9.6	—	—	—	19	3.0	72	—	0.03	0.12	—
08-1-323	香糟块肉	100	34.8	542	2266	15.5	53.3	0	—	—	—	21	1.4	62	—	0.14	0.08	—

畜肉类及制品 Meat and meat products

(以每100g可食部计)

编码 Code	食物名称 Food name	维生素 B_{12} Vit B_{12} μg	叶酸 Folate μg	烟酸 Niacin mg	维生素C Vit C mg	维生素E (Vit E) Total mg	维生素E (Vit E) α-TE mg	钙 Ca mg	磷 P mg	钾 K mg	钠 Na mg	镁 Mg mg	铁 Fe mg	锌 Zn mg	硒 Se μg	铜 Cu mg	锰 Mn mg	碘 I μg
猪																		
08-1-121	猪肉 (前臀尖, 杜长大猪)	—	Tr	4.20	(Tr)	0.57	0.57	1	69	—	—	—	—	2.45	6.67	Tr	Tr	—
08-1-122	猪肉 (前臀尖, 良杂猪)	—	Tr	3.14	(Tr)	0.69	0.69	1	97	308	53.9	20	1.1	1.91	5.25	Tr	0.02	—
08-1-123	猪肉 (后臀尖, 杜长大猪)	—	Tr	8.02	(Tr)	—	—	2	134	—	—	—	—	2.24	9.92	Tr	Tr	—
08-1-124	猪肉 (后臀尖, 良杂猪)	—	Tr	4.57	(Tr)	0.34	0.34	1	208	334	47.9	21	0.9	2.29	6.36	Tr	0.02	—
08-1-125	猪肉 (硬肋, 杜长大猪)	—	Tr	2.81	(Tr)	—	—	3	84	—	—	—	—	1.23	5.26	Tr	Tr	—
08-1-126	猪肉 (硬肋, 良杂猪)	—	Tr	2.70	(Tr)	1.03	0.78	1	105	—	—	—	—	1.33	5.31	Tr	Tr	—
08-1-127	猪肉 (通脊, 杜长大猪)	—	Tr	9.67	(Tr)	0.22	0.22	2	92	—	—	—	—	1.54	8.13	Tr	Tr	—
08-1-128	猪肉 (通脊, 良杂猪)	—	Tr	6.98	(Tr)	0.15	0.15	2	141	338	46.5	23	0.9	2.20	6.72	Tr	0.02	—
08-1-129	猪肉 (里脊)	—	Tr	6.37	(Tr)	0.33	0.33	6	184	317	43.2	28	1.5	2.01	8.32	0.01	Tr	—
08-1-130	猪皮	4.53	5.4	0.63	(Tr)	Tr	Tr	13	37	62	72.4	56	1.7	0.67	4.68	Tr	Tr	—
08-1-131	猪小排 (杜长大猪)	—	1.0	4.11	(Tr)	0.46	0.46	14	101	—	—	—	—	2.42	8.46	Tr	Tr	—
08-1-132	猪小排 (良杂猪)	—	0.5	3.09	(Tr)	0.72	0.72	36	117	230	62.6	14	1.4	2.20	5.94	Tr	Tr	—
08-1-213	猪肚	—	3.8	2.85	(Tr)	0.28	0.28	11	152	171	75.1	12	2.4	1.93	11.68	0.01	Tr	—
08-1-214	猪肝	—	425.1	10.11	(Tr)	Tr	Tr	6	243	235	68.6	24	23.2	3.68	26.12	0.02	0.01	—
08-1-215	猪舌 [口条]	—	1.7	4.25	(Tr)	Tr	Tr	13	213	216	79.4	14	0.1	2.89	13.94	0.01	Tr	—
08-1-216	猪肾 [猪腰子]	—	9.2	—	(Tr)	Tr	Tr	12	210	217	134.2	22	0.1	3.15	157.24	0.03	0.01	—
08-1-318	火腿心全精肉	4.70	22.9	9.49	(Tr)	0.26	0.03	22	391	836	8612.0	17	5.0	9.48	12.11	0.26	0.13	56.3
08-1-319	火腿心肉	1.26	4.8	5.07	(Tr)	Tr	Tr	15	62	367	2268.2	11	2.1	1.87	14.34	0.06	0.21	—
08-1-320	腊肉	2.25	Tr	—	(Tr)	Tr	Tr	293	137	416	763.9	35	0.1	0.06	13.70	0.01	0.01	12.3
08-1-321	叉烧肉	Tr	Tr	3.83	(0)	0.97	0.54	5	136	100	726.4	12	3.6	8.50	6.65	0.12	0.06	57.4
08-1-322	酱排骨	—	10.1	2.51	(0)	0.62	0.62	10	103	226	825.5	13	2.4	3.43	9.18	0.07	0.03	28.3
08-1-323	香糟块肉	Tr	Tr	Tr	(0)	0.46	0.46	30	122	103	747.8	16	5.4	2.12	8.82	0.23	0.19	12.8

畜肉类及制品 Meat and meat products

（以每100g可食部计）

编码 Code	食物名称 Food name	食部 Edible	水分 Water	能量 Energy		蛋白质 Protein	脂肪 Fat	碳水化合物 CHO	膳食纤维 (Dietary fiber) 总 Total	可溶性 Soluble	不溶性 Insoluble	胆固醇 Cholesterol	灰分 Ash	维生素A Vit A	胡萝卜素 Carotene	硫胺素 Thiamin	核黄素 Riboflavin	维生素B6 Vit B_6
		%	g	kcal	kJ	g	g	g	g	g	g	mg	g	μgRE	μg	mg	mg	mg
08-1-324	熏烤小里脊	100	63.2	153	641	17.7	3.9	11.8	—	—	—	94	3.4	Tr	—	0.34	0.18	0.18
08-1-325	猪肉脯	100	11.2	378	1580	28.0	8.8	46.6	—	—	—	71	5.4	84	—	0.22	0.27	—
08-1-326	肉酥	100	2.4	509	2128	30.7	27.1	35.5	—	—	—	—	4.3	Tr	—	0.09	0.15	—
08-1-327	猪肉松	100	14.0	373	1562	41.8	10.2	28.6	—	—	—	70	5.4	Tr	—	0.09	0.24	—
08-1-328	扒猪脸	100	48.6	347	1453	18.8	29.6	1.4	—	—	—	—	1.6	22	—	0.03	0.13	—
08-1-329	酱肘子	100	58.9	202	846	29.6	8.5	1.8	—	—	—	—	1.2	Tr	—	0.17	0.18	0.13
08-1-423	脆皮肠	100	50.9	302	1262	16.6	24.0	4.8	—	—	—	50	3.7	3	—	0.09	0.08	—
08-1-424	热狗肠	100	51.3	307	1284	13.2	25.2	6.9	—	—	—	47	3.5	Tr	—	0.11	0.09	0.07
08-1-425	火腿肠	100	61.5	215	900	12.1	14.6	8.8	—	—	—	13	3.0	56	—	0.04	0.11	0.01
08-1-426	火腿	100	76.6	99	416	15.5	3.4	1.7	—	—	—	39	2.8	Tr	—	0.08	0.14	0.08
08-1-427	火腿（云南）	100	22.1	565	2365	11.4	56.1	3.7	—	—	0[a]	89	6.7	Tr	—	0.09	0.05	—
08-1-428	三明治火腿	100	73.2	115	481	12.5	4.5	6.1	—	—	—	36	3.7	Tr	—	0.14	0.09	—
08-1-429	午餐肉	100	55.2	320	1339	9.0	30.1	3.3	—	—	—	—	2.4	Tr	—	0.09	0.09	0.06
牛																		
08-2-111	牛肉（背部肉）[上脑]	100	66.4	193	808	17.4	12.4	3.0	—	—	—	56	0.8	Tr	(0)	0.04	0.08	—
08-2-112	牛肉（里脊肉）[牛柳]	100	72.0	134	561	22.3	5.0	0	—	—	—	44	1.1	Tr	(0)	0.04	0.10	0.33
08-2-113	牛肉（臀部肉）[紫盖、白板]	100	72.8	117	491	22.6	2.6	0.9	—	—	—	22	1.1	Tr	(0)	0.05	0.09	0.26
08-2-114	牛肉（肩部肉）[肩肉]	100	53.3	342	1430	14.1	31.7	0	—	—	—	51	0.9	1	(0)	0.02	0.06	—
08-2-115	牛肉（胸部肉）[牛胸]	100	58.8	326	1362	16.6	28.8	0	—	—	—	56	0.8	Tr	(0)	0.02	0.09	—
08-2-116	牛肉（腹部肉）[牛腩]	100	57.6	332	1390	17.1	29.3	0	—	—	—	44	1.0	Tr	(0)	0.02	0.06	0.10
08-2-117	牛肉（膝圆肉）[和尚头]	100	74.6	106	444	22.4	1.8	0.1	—	—	—	43	1.1	Tr	(0)	0.04	0.10	0.24
08-2-118	牛肉（股内肉）[针扒、米龙、黄瓜条]	100	72.5	119	497	22.8	2.9	0.4	—	—	—	—	1.4	Tr	(0)	0.04	0.08	0.30

(以每100g可食部计)

编码 Code	食物名称 Food name	维生素 B_{12} Vit B_{12} μg	叶酸 Folate μg	烟酸 Niacin mg	维生素C Vit C mg	维生素E (Vit E) Total mg	α-TE mg	钙 Ca mg	磷 P mg	钾 K mg	钠 Na mg	镁 Mg mg	铁 Fe mg	锌 Zn mg	硒 Se μg	铜 Cu mg	锰 Mn mg	碘 I μg
08-1-324	熏烤小里脊	Tr	0.5	5.39	(0)	0.45	0.45	6	263	718	814.2	16	6.7	4.10	12.50	0.28	0.31	28.1
08-1-325	猪肉脯	—	5.7	18.48	(0)	1.10	0.49	17	233	381	1638.2	47	3.9	3.08	6.86	0.20	0.43	—
08-1-326	肉酥	—	—	3.93	(0)	4.47	0.74	11	256	278	1540.7	25	3.7	4.38	19.88	0.05	0.26	35.4
08-1-327	猪肉松	—	5.3	4.70	(0)	2.00	1.34	3	255	460	1929.2	24	3.3	4.43	9.16	0.19	0.19	—
08-1-328	扒猪脸	—	—	1.20	(0)	—	—	15	81	75	392.7	8	1.4	1.45	13.96	0.12	0.04	—
08-1-329	酱肘子	—	—	—	(0)	0.74	un	15	140	57	197.0	11	1.9	4.07	—	0.12	0.04	—
08-1-423	脆皮肠	—	6.6	3.82	(0)	0.54	0.54	13	287	542	992.7	19	3.9	2.24	6.51	0.17	0.13	49.6
08-1-424	热狗肠	Tr	12.5	2.36	(0)	0.74	0.39	10	211	613	861.9	12	3.2	1.36	7.06	0.11	0.10	38.8
08-1-425	火腿肠	—	—	1.78	(0)	0.65	0.36	19	157	130	1119.5	6	1.8	0.70	4.84	0.13	0.18	—
08-1-426	火腿	Tr	27.2	5.53	(0)	0.48	0.34	6	301	174	1471.3	11	1.0	2.09	7.96	0.07	0.03	3.6
08-1-427	火腿 (云南)	—	—	2.30	(0)	—	—	171	141	330	5557.5	194	41.2	4.43	4.31	1.57	0.74	—
08-1-428	三明治火腿	—	5.7	3.72	(0)	0.36	0.14	11	238	532	898.6	16	3.0	1.48	7.35	0.15	—	32.2
08-1-429	午餐肉	Tr	—	3.54	(0)	0.75	0.35	6	84	131	528.7	8	0.6	1.38	7.80	0.06	0.07	5.4
牛																		
08-2-111	牛肉 (背部肉) [上脑]	—	3.8	2.28	(Tr)	0.17	0.17	—	—	—	—	—	0.7	4.65	1.84	0.01	Tr	—
08-2-112	牛肉 (里脊肉) [牛柳]	—	4.9	6.24	(Tr)	Tr	Tr	3	241	140	75.1	29	0.4	4.73	3.57	0.01	Tr	0.5
08-2-113	牛肉 (臀部肉) [紫盖、白板]	—	4.4	4.86	(Tr)	Tr	Tr	2	159	325	40.2	22	1.4	5.48	3.63	0.01	0.02	—
08-2-114	牛肉 (肩部肉) [肩肉]	—	3.6	1.66	(Tr)	0.19	0.19	—	—	—	—	—	0.5	2.59	2.32	0.01	Tr	—
08-2-115	牛肉 (胸部肉) [牛胸]	—	4.0	1.90	(Tr)	0.23	0.23	—	—	—	—	—	0.7	4.55	1.75	0.01	Tr	—
08-2-116	牛肉 (腹部肉) [牛腩]	—	4.4	2.20	(Tr)	Tr	Tr	—	—	—	—	—	0.6	2.69	3.20	0.01	Tr	—
08-2-117	牛肉 (膝圆肉) [和尚头]	—	6.2	3.44	(Tr)	Tr	Tr	1	154	316	43.5	21	1.2	4.82	3.06	0.01	0.02	—
08-2-118	牛肉 (股内肉) [针扒、米龙、黄瓜条]	—	0.9	4.82	(Tr)	Tr	Tr	2	141	275	37.8	20	1.0	4.81	2.98	0.01	0.02	—

畜肉类及制品 Meat and meat products

(以每100g可食部计)

编码 Code	食物名称 Food name	食部 Edible %	水分 Water g	能量 Energy kcal	能量 Energy kJ	蛋白质 Protein g	脂肪 Fat g	碳水化合物 CHO g	膳食纤维 (Dietary fiber) 总 Total g	可溶性 Soluble g	不溶性 Insoluble g	胆固醇 Cholesterol mg	灰分 Ash g	维生素A Vit A μgRE	胡萝卜素 Carotene μg	硫胺素 Thiamin mg	核黄素 Riboflavin mg	维生素B_6 Vit B_6 mg
08-2-119	牛肉(小腿肉) [牛展、牛腱子]	100	73.4	122	509	23.0	3.3	0	—	—	—	61	1.0	Tr	(0)	0.03	0.13	—
08-2-210	牛百叶(黑)	100	85.6	70	292	13.2	1.9	0	—	—	—	71	0.4	Tr	(0)	0.02	0.15	—
08-2-307	牛肉(酱,五香)	100	55.5	229	959	33.2	10.7	0	—	—	—	41	2.1	Tr	—	0.02	0.12	—
08-2-308	牛肉(清香)	100	63.6	200	835	25.8	10.7	0	—	—	—	39	3.7	Tr	—	0.02	0.09	0.08
08-2-309	牛腱子(香叶)	100	53.9	205	856	35.6	5.5	3.2	—	—	—	47	1.8	Tr	—	0.03	0.14	0.07
08-2-310	牛肉干(长富牌)	100	14.6	342	1431	41.8	5.1	32.2	—	—	—	—	6.3	Tr	—	0.29	0.14	0.11
08-2-311	牛肉干(沙爹牌)	100	16.8	327	1368	40.1	3.6	33.6	—	—	0[a]	—	5.9	—	—	0.07	0.13	—
羊																		
08-3-113	羊肉(上脑)	100	78.0	94	393	19.0	2.0	0	—	—	—	—	1.0	3	(0)	0.06	0.14	0.10
08-3-114	羊肉(腰窝)	100	73.5	135	565	18.9	6.6	0	—	—	—	—	1.0	6	(0)	0.02	0.14	0.08
08-3-115	羊肉(前腿)	100	77.1	97	407	19.8	2.0	0	—	—	—	—	1.1	3	(0)	0.12	0.15	0.12
08-3-116	羊肉(后腿)	100	75.1	111	465	20.6	3.2	0	—	—	—	—	1.1	5	(0)	0.06	0.14	0.09
08-3-117	羊肉片	100	74.9	118	492	18.0	4.0	2.4	—	—	—	—	0.7	16	(0)	—	—	—
08-3-309	烧羊肉(五香)	100	59.4	183	766	33.6	5.4	0	—	—	—	43	2.2	Tr	—	0.03	0.16	0.08
08-3-310	羊肉串(生)	100	74.5	118	492	13.0	4.8	5.6	—	—	—	24	2.1	146	(0)	0.07	0.17	0.15
驴																		
08-4-304	驴肉(五香)	100	64.9	167	698	28.2	6.0	0	—	—	—	49	3.0	79	(0)	0.01	0.16	—
其它																		
08-9-006	鹿肉(梅花鹿)	100	78.0	92	384	19.7	1.3	0.3	—	—	—	5	0.7	Tr	(0)	0.05	0.24	0.10

(以每100g可食部计)

编码 Code	食物名称 Food name	维生素 B_{12} Vit B_{12} μg	叶酸 Folate μg	烟酸 Niacin mg	维生素C Vit C mg	维生素E (Vit E) Total mg	维生素E (Vit E) α-TE mg	钙 Ca mg	磷 P mg	钾 K mg	钠 Na mg	镁 Mg mg	铁 Fe mg	锌 Zn mg	硒 Se μg	铜 Cu mg	锰 Mn mg	碘 I μg
08-2-119	牛肉(小腿肉) [牛展、牛腱子]	—	2.8	3.69	(Tr)	Tr	Tr	5	181	182	83.1	22	0.3	5.07	2.54	0.01	Tr	—
08-2-210	牛百叶(黑)	—	15.7	—	(Tr)	Tr	Tr	40	104	162	60.6	17	2.1	7.03	3.80	0.01	0.04	—
08-2-307	牛肉(酱,五香)	Tr	5.6	5.33	(0)	1.41	1.20	11	163	327	926.0	18	3.1	13.60	9.96	0.15	0.21	24.5
08-2-308	牛肉(清香)	Tr	8.7	7.22	(0)	0.32	0.32	5	227	217	935.0	6	2.6	8.08	15.36	0.08	0.02	49.7
08-2-309	牛腱子(香叶)	Tr	22.9	—	(0)	0.37	0.37	9	160	229	880.4	18	6.0	8.82	2.97	0.12	0.11	24.5
08-2-310	牛肉干(长富牌)	Tr	12.3	4.81	(0)	Tr	Tr	34	183	112	1529.0	31	10.0	5.51	25.64	0.16	0.20	48.4
08-2-311	牛肉干(沙爹牌)	—	—	6.40	9.0	—	—	29	188	265	1402.5	43	7.3	5.81	3.92	1.44	1.34	—
羊																		
08-3-113	羊肉(上脑)	—	1.7	3.30	(Tr)	0.44	0.44	3	164	359	106.6	20	2.4	2.68	6.79	0.07	0.02	5.2
08-3-114	羊肉(腰窝)	—	Tr	2.17	(Tr)	0.46	0.46	3	158	372	109.2	26	1.8	2.88	6.25	0.08	0.01	6.6
08-3-115	羊肉(前腿)	—	Tr	3.13	(Tr)	0.63	0.63	3	170	338	92.8	29	3.0	2.22	5.78	0.09	0.01	7.7
08-3-116	羊肉(后腿)	—	Tr	3.68	(Tr)	0.58	0.58	3	169	352	93.8	19	4.0	3.07	9.06	0.10	0.02	4.1
08-3-117	羊肉片	—	—	—	(Tr)	0.53	un	12	145	108	92.0	9	2.3	2.14	6.18	0.12	0.08	—
08-3-309	烧羊肉(五香)	Tr	5.0	5.63	(0)	1.62	0.85	11	167	213	759.1	18	3.0	8.26	15.22	0.11	0.13	37.8
08-3-310	羊肉串(生)	2.29	7.0	3.32	(Tr)	0.61	0.33	17	222	278	616.2	17	2.5	2.26	2.08	0.10	0.41	22.7
驴																		
08-4-304	驴肉(五香)	—	5.7	2.93	(0)	0.83	0.64	5	317	201	877.2	18	5.8	7.80	3.80	0.20	0.13	77.9
其它																		
08-9-006	鹿肉(梅花鹿)	—	18.8	—	(Tr)	Tr	Tr	4	177	196	32.7	12	2.3	2.23	4.65	0.01	—	1.5

Notes

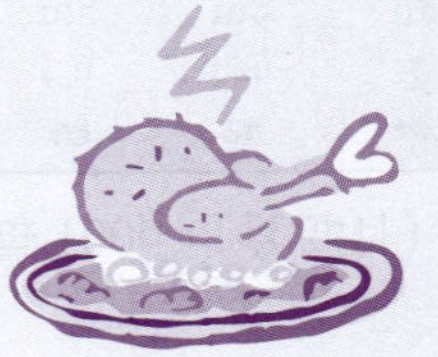

禽肉类及制品

Poultry and Poultry Products

常见的家禽有鸡、鸭、鹅、火鸡等。按此常规将家禽及其制品分成相应的亚类。

家禽的分割与家畜类大致相同，主要分为头部、躯干、翅膀和内脏等。

市场上对家禽的等级一般基于生长年限和体重，主要考虑的是烹调加工方面的鲜嫩度。

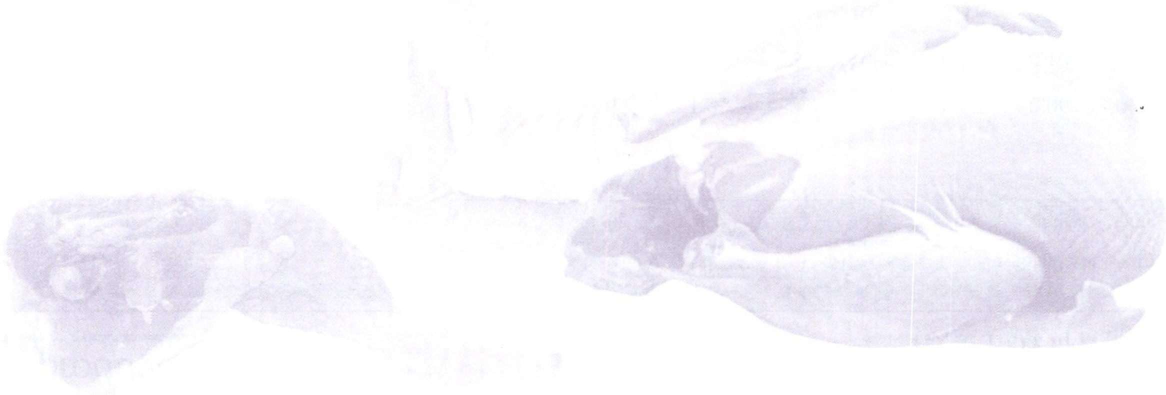

禽肉类及制品 Poultry and poultry products

(以每100g可食部计)

编码 Code	食物名称 Food name	食部 Edible %	水分 Water g	能量 Energy kcal	能量 Energy kJ	蛋白质 Protein g	脂肪 Fat g	碳水化合物 CHO g	膳食纤维 (Dietary fiber) 总 Total g	可溶性 Soluble g	不溶性 Insoluble g	胆固醇 Cholesterol mg	灰分 Ash g	维生素A Vit A μgRE	胡萝卜素 Carotene μg	硫胺素 Thiamin mg	核黄素 Riboflavin mg	维生素B_6 Vit B_6 mg
鸡																		
09-1-112	鸡胸脯肉	100	71.7	118	493	24.6	1.9	0.6	—	—	—	65	1.2	3	(0)	0.07	0.06	0.50
09-1-113	鸡腿	74	71.7	146	609	20.2	7.2	0	—	—	—	99	0.9	22	(0)	0.06	0.10	0.14
09-1-114	鸡翅	69	63.3	202	843	19.0	11.5	5.5	—	—	—	81	0.7	28	(0)	Tr	0.05	0.26
09-1-115	鸡块 (带浆粉)	100	58.2	206	861	12.2	9.1	18.8	—	—	—	22	1.7	Tr	(0)	0.05	0.05	0.15
09-1-116	野山鸡	63	70.3	126	527	20.4	2.0	6.6	—	—	—	—	0.7	75	(0)	0.03	0.14	0.35
09-1-308	扒鸡 (五香脱骨)	77	59.7	206	862	23.4	10.8	3.8	—	—	—	36	2.3	138	—	0.03	0.11	—
09-1-309	烤鸡	72	55.4	265	1107	28.1	16.9	0	—	—	—	26	4.6	165	—	0.03	0.16	—
09-1-310	童子鸡 (熟)	57	66.8	226	946	15.8	18.1	0	—	—	—	22	1.7	21	—	0.04	0.10	0.19
鸭																		
09-2-214	鸭豉片	100	11.3	603	2521	18.3	56.1	6.1	—	—	—	—	8.2	Tr	(0)	0.26	0.11	0.09
09-2-307	烤鸭 (老唐牌)	60	57.0	309	1292	20.3	25.3	0	—	—	—	78	2.4	170	—	0.06	0.19	—
09-2-308	烤鸭 (全聚德牌)	65	33.4	530	2216	18.1	50.8	0	—	—	—	—	0.7	107	—	0.13	0.25	—
鹅																		
09-3-302	腊鹅	54	15.8	410	1717	24.6	21.5	29.6	—	—	—	—	8.5	Tr	(0)	0.13	0.54	—
火鸡																		
09-4-301	火鸡腿	85	72.5	100	416	16.7	0.7	6.6	—	—	—	—	3.5	Tr	(0)	0.02	0.14	0.08
其它																		
09-9-003	乳鸽	56	57.5	352	1473	11.3	34.1	0	—	—	—	—	1.5	46	(0)	0.08	0.36	0.11
09-9-004	乳鸽 (红烧)	82	59.0	255	1066	16.9	20.8	0	—	—	—	—	4.0	—	—	0.04	0.36	—

禽肉类及制品 Poultry and poultry products

(以每100g可食部计)

编码 Code	食物名称 Food name	维生素 B_{12} Vit B_{12} μg	叶酸 Folate μg	烟酸 Niacin mg	维生素C Vit C mg	维生素E (Vit E) Total mg	维生素E (Vit E) α-TE mg	钙 Ca mg	磷 P mg	钾 K mg	钠 Na mg	镁 Mg mg	铁 Fe mg	锌 Zn mg	硒 Se μg	铜 Cu mg	锰 Mn mg	碘 I μg
鸡																		
09-1-112	鸡胸脯肉	—	0.7	11.96	(Tr)	0.41	0.41	1	170	333	44.8	28	1.0	0.26	11.75	0.01	0.01	6.8
09-1-113	鸡腿	—	15.9	3.25	(Tr)	Tr	Tr	3	271	221	73.6	21	1.8	1.11	9.70	0.01	0.01	—
09-1-114	鸡翅	—	Tr	4.36	(Tr)	0.44	0.29	8	94	205	50.8	17	0.9	0.42	8.72	Tr	0.01	—
09-1-115	鸡块(带浆粉)	Tr	10.3	4.69	(Tr)	0.40	0.21	6	202	230	329.8	13	0.5	0.54	6.38	0.05	0.03	4.5
09-1-116	野山鸡	4.41	18.5	7.54	(Tr)	0.27	0.27	92	173	155	37.8	8	0.9	1.19	11.09	0.07	0.03	3.5
09-1-308	扒鸡(五香脱骨)	—	7.0	4.70	(0)	0.84	0.53	222	307	131	633.2	13	1.7	1.43	10.90	0.05	0.09	37.0
09-1-309	烤鸡	—	8.0	—	(0)	0.35	0.24	36	135	207	560.0	11	2	1.58	19.28	0.05	0.11	89.7
09-1-310	童子鸡(熟)	Tr	8.4	5.55	(0)	0.32	0.18	111	221	145	910.1	7	0.5	1.21	8.27	0.03	0.36	25.1
鸭																		
09-2-214	鸭豉片	2.62	—	3.27	(Tr)	Tr	Tr	—	—	—	—	—	0.1	0.38	15.41	0.01	0.01	—
09-2-307	烤鸭(老唐牌)	—	—	3.00	(0)	1.06	0.60	7	102	187	776.4	6	1.3	2.76	16.30	0.20	0.10	—
09-2-308	烤鸭(全聚德牌)	—	—	2.70	(0)	—	—	11	147	103	29.9	8	1.6	1.69	24.83	—	—	—
鹅																		
09-3-302	腊鹅	6.07	24.1	5.63	(0)	Tr	Tr	36	317	388	2880.0	27	7.8	3.25	14.32	1.02	0.16	12.3
火鸡																		
09-4-301	火鸡腿	—	8.7	1.29	(0)	Tr	Tr	17	161	253	1071.0	16	1.2	2.50	13.12	0.08	0.04	33.6
其它																		
09-9-003	乳鸽	7.87	1.2	2.48	(0)	0.84	0.52	866	573	163	653.8	21	2.0	2.40	11.97	0.09	0.04	16.3
09-9-004	乳鸽(红烧)	8.25	—	3.27	(0)	—	—	1614	1050	385	1809.8	61	8.8	6.33	24.44	0.42	0.29	61.1

Notes

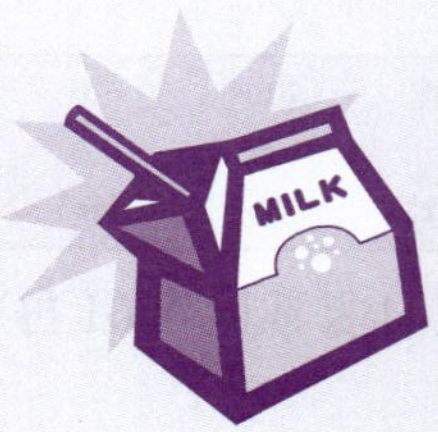

乳类及制品

Milk and Milk Products

乳类食品按来源，主要分为牛乳、羊乳、马乳和人乳。市场产品以牛乳为主。参考国家有关标准，本节将乳类食品分为6个亚类。

1. 液态乳：分为巴氏杀菌乳和灭菌乳。前者消毒温度在100℃以下，只能短期存放；后者经超高温瞬时灭菌（135℃以上），可以室温较长时间保存。两种纯牛奶的质量标准都要求蛋白质含量不低于2.9%。灭菌调味乳的蛋白质不低于2.3%，脂肪含量一般比纯牛乳低0.2%～0.5%左右。

2. 奶粉：是指将原料乳灭菌、浓缩，然后经喷雾、干燥制成的粉状产品。通常分为四种：全脂奶粉、脱脂乳粉、全脂加糖乳粉、调味乳粉。一般来讲，全脂奶粉蛋白质等成分是液体乳浓缩的7～8倍，调味奶粉是5倍左右。目前强化乳粉较多，均包括在此类。

3. 酸奶：根据口味常分为三种：纯酸牛奶，是以牛乳或乳粉为原料，脱脂或不脱脂，经发酵制成的产品，乳酸菌含量一般在10^7以上；调味酸奶 指添加了糖或调味剂等辅料的酸奶；果味酸奶指添加了天然果料等辅料的酸奶。

4. 奶酪：也称干酪，指原料乳经消毒后，再用乳酸菌发酵的产品。产品富含蛋白质和脂肪。

5. 奶油：又称黄油，是指将消毒乳离心分离为稀奶油和脱脂乳，然后以发酵或不发酵的稀奶油为原料制成的固态产品。另外还有含水量较少的产品称为无水奶油。

6. 其它：包括炼乳、奶片、奶皮等。

乳类及制品 Milk and milk products

(以每100g可食部计)

编码 Code	食物名称 Food name	食部 Edible %	水分 Water g	能量 Energy kcal	能量 Energy kJ	蛋白质 Protein g	脂肪 Fat g	碳水化合物 CHO g	膳食纤维 (Dietary fiber) 总 Total g	可溶性 Soluble g	不溶性 Insoluble g	胆固醇 Cholesterol mg	灰分 Ash g	维生素A Vit A μgRE	胡萝卜素 Carotene μg	硫胺素 Thiamin mg	核黄素 Riboflavin mg	维生素B_6 Vit B_6 mg
液态乳																		
10-1-105	牛乳(光明牌)	100	88.0	61	256	3.1	3.2	5.0	(0)	(0)	(0)	3	0.7	28	—	0.02	0.10	0.03
10-1-106	牛乳(乐百氏牌)	100	87.4	67	279	3.3	3.8	4.8	(0)	(0)	(0)	4	0.7	11	—	0.02	0.09	0.03
10-1-107	牛乳(帕玛拉特牌)	100	87.9	61	256	3.0	3.1	5.3	(0)	(0)	(0)	6	0.7	14	—	0.02	0.08	0.03
10-1-108	牛乳(三元牌)	100	86.9	69	289	3.4	3.9	5.1	(0)	(0)	(0)	1	0.7	30	—	0.02	0.10	0.02
10-1-109	牛乳(完达山牌)	100	88.3	60	251	2.9	3.2	4.9	(0)	(0)	(0)	7	0.7	17	—	0.03	0.09	—
10-1-110	牛乳(龙丹牌)	100	87.5	66	277	2.9	3.8	5.1	(0)	(0)	(0)	6	0.7	11	—	0.02	0.10	0.03
10-1-111	牛乳(蒙牛牌)	100	87.2	67	280	3.1	3.7	5.3	(0)	(0)	(0)	1	0.7	14	—	0.02	0.11	0.03
10-1-112	牛乳(新南洋牌)	100	87.4	67	279	3.1	3.8	5.1	(0)	(0)	(0)	5	0.7	17	—	0.02	0.11	0.02
10-1-113	牛乳(帕玛拉特)	100	88.1	61	254	2.9	3.2	5.1	(0)	(0)	(0)	5	0.7	15	—	0.02	0.13	0.02
10-1-114	牛乳(伊利牌)	100	86.9	68	283	3.2	3.7	5.4	(0)	(0)	(0)	—	0.8	16	—	0.02	0.13	—
10-1-115	牛乳(部分脱脂，帕玛拉特)	100	90.1	43	181	2.9	1.3	5.0	(0)	(0)	(0)	5	0.7	6	—	0.03	0.09	—
10-1-116	牛乳(脱脂，帕玛拉特)	100	91.4	33	136	2.9	0.2	4.8	(0)	(0)	(0)	2	0.7	Tr	—	0.03	0.08	—
10-1-117	牛乳(强化锌、钙，帕玛拉特)	100	88.2	60	251	3.0	3.1	5.0	(0)	(0)	(0)	2	0.7	15	—	0.02	0.11	—
10-1-118	牛奶(草莓味，卡夫牌)	100	83.4	79	331	2.7	3.0	10.3	(0)	(0)	(0)	4	0.6	18	—	0.02	0.11	—
10-1-119	牛奶(巧克力味，卡夫牌)	100	83.3	80	335	2.8	3.2	10.0	(0)	(0)	(0)	5	0.7	17	—	0.02	0.11	0.02
10-1-120	牛奶(巧克力味，三元牌)	100	84.4	74	310	2.3	2.8	9.9	(0)	(0)	(0)	1	0.6	18	—	0.02	0.08	—
10-1-121	学生奶	100	86.1	66	277	2.6	2.6	8.1	(0)	(0)	(0)	—	0.6	30	—	0.02	0.14	—
奶粉																		
10-2-105	全脂奶粉(雀巢)	100	—	504	2109	24.0	28.0	39.0	—	—	—	—	5.8	630	—	—	1.10	—
10-2-106	全脂奶粉(三鹿牌)	100	2.2	516	2158	25.4	29.6	37.1	—	—	—	58	5.8	8	3	0.23	1.20	0.12

乳类及制品 Milk and milk products

(以每100g可食部计)

编码 Code	食物名称 Food name	维生素 B_{12} Vit B_{12} μg	叶酸 Folate μg	烟酸 Niacin mg	维生素C Vit C mg	维生素E (Vit E) Total mg	α-TE mg	钙 Ca mg	磷 P mg	钾 K mg	钠 Na mg	镁 Mg mg	铁 Fe mg	锌 Zn mg	硒 Se μg	铜 Cu mg	锰 Mn mg	碘 I μg
液态乳																		
10-1-105	牛乳 (光明牌)	—	11.0	0.13	(Tr)	0.07	0.07	85	87	132	24.8	8	0.1	0.25	1.70	0.01	—	3.5
10-1-106	牛乳 (乐百氏牌)	—	Tr	0.13	(Tr)	0.09	0.09	104	100	142	38.4	12	0.6	0.85	1.08	0.01	0.01	Tr
10-1-107	牛乳 (帕玛拉特牌)	—	Tr	0.10	(Tr)	0.05	0.05	113	99	166	68.2	11	0.4	0.67	0.22	0.01	0.01	0.6
10-1-108	牛乳 (三元牌)	—	1.7	0.13	(Tr)	0.18	0.13	88	88	177	35.1	10	0.3	0.42	1.70	0.01	0.01	2.3
10-1-109	牛乳 (完达山牌)	—	2.9	0.08	(Tr)	0.10	0.06	91	87	161	292.1	9	0.1	0.28	0.60	0.01	—	1.2
10-1-110	牛乳 (龙丹牌)	—	4.3	0.11	(Tr)	0.15	0.08	82	83	145	41.5	9	0.1	0.46	0.80	Tr	0.01	1.2
10-1-111	牛乳 (蒙牛牌)	—	10.7	0.11	(Tr)	0.10	0.10	98	94	159	48.9	11	0.2	0.51	1.10	Tr	Tr	1.4
10-1-112	牛乳 (新南洋牌)	—	5.8	0.11	(Tr)	0.08	0.08	92	59	163	46.1	11	0.3	0.45	1.20	Tr	0.02	1.5
10-1-113	牛乳 (帕玛拉特)	—	2.0	0.08	(Tr)	0.07	0.07	93	99	181	62.1	11	0.4	0.58	1.25	0.01	0.01	0.9
10-1-114	牛乳 (伊利牌)	—	4.7	0.08	(Tr)	Tr	Tr	110	103	348	49.5	12	0.1	0.45	1.51	0.02	—	—
10-1-115	牛乳 (部分脱脂, 帕玛拉特)	—	0.4	0.07	(Tr)	Tr	Tr	66	91	185	279.5	8	0.2	0.30	1.49	0.02	Tr	3.6
10-1-116	牛乳 (脱脂, 帕玛拉特)	—	0.6	0.07	(Tr)	Tr	Tr	75	96	204	117.2	9	0.3	0.54	1.05	0.01	—	4.6
10-1-117	牛乳 (强化锌、钙, 帕玛拉特)	—	Tr	0.08	(Tr)	0.06	0.06	93	103	171	62.1	11	1.0	1.10	1.38	Tr	0.01	Tr
10-1-118	牛奶 (草莓味, 卡夫牌)	—	1.2	0.09	(Tr)	0.14	0.10	78	83	157	28.3	9	0.3	0.37	1.30	0	0.01	Tr
10-1-119	牛奶 (巧克力味, 卡夫牌)	—	6.2	0.12	(Tr)	0.07	0.07	81	92	154	31.4	13	0.5	0.31	1.63	0.02	0.02	Tr
10-1-120	牛奶 (巧克力味, 三元牌)	—	7.8	0.09	(Tr)	0.25	0.20	101.2	75	165	36.3	12	0.5	0.37	1.07	0.03	0.03	0.9
10-1-121	学生奶	—	0.3	0.06	(Tr)	Tr	Tr	87	78	140	47.3	8	0.1	1.53	0.85	Tr	Tr	—
奶粉																		
10-2-105	全脂奶粉 (雀巢)	—	—	—	—	—	—	930	720	—	—	—	—	—	—	—	—	—
10-2-106	全脂奶粉 (三鹿牌)	5.91	—	0.60	—	0.01	un	667	796	1500	491.2	92	4.9	5.74	1.38	0.10	0.09	30.2

乳类及制品 Milk and milk products

(以每100g可食部计)

编码 Code	食物名称 Food name	食部 Edible %	水分 Water g	能量 Energy kcal	能量 Energy kJ	蛋白质 Protein g	脂肪 Fat g	碳水化合物 CHO g	膳食纤维 (Dietary fiber) 总 Total g	可溶性 Soluble g	不溶性 Insoluble g	胆固醇 Cholesterol mg	灰分 Ash g	维生素A Vit A μgRE	胡萝卜素 Carotene μg	硫胺素 Thiamin mg	核黄素 Riboflavin mg	维生素B_6 Vit B_6 mg
10-2-107	全脂奶粉 (伊利牌)	100	3.0	504	2109	22.0	26.0	45.5	—	—	—	65	3.5	525	—	0.04	0.17	—
10-2-108	全脂甜奶粉 (三鹿牌)	100	2.5	477	1995	21.2	21.1	50.5	—	—	—	32	4.7	141	—	0.11	0.73	—
10-2-109	全脂甜奶粉 (伊利牌)	100	3.2	476	1992	19.0	21.0	52.8	—	—	—	28	4.0	579	—	0.70	—	—
10-2-110	低脂奶粉 (高钙高铁, 雀巢)	100	—	413	1729	27.0	11.7	50.0	—	—	—	—	—	570	—	—	1.40	—
10-2-111	低脂奶粉 (高钙高铁, 伊利牌)	100	3.1	423	1768	27.0	11.0	53.9	—	—	—	49	5.0	675	—	0.30	1.60	—
10-2-112	高钙高铁奶粉 (可淇牌)	100	4.0	437	1828	17.0	13.0	63.0	—	—	—	—	—	630	—	0.80	1.00	—
10-2-113	儿童奶粉 (安儿健A+, 美赞臣)	100	—	427	1785	17.9	11.1	64.0	—	—	—	—	—	594	—	0.40	0.98	0.36
10-2-114	儿童奶粉 (适体健, 美赞臣)	100	—	407	1703	16.0	9.0	68.0	2.5	—	—	—	—	375	170	0.50	0.50	0.50
10-2-115	儿童奶粉 (惠氏)	100	—	451	1876	17.0	15.0	62.0	—	—	—	—	—	487	95	0.41	0.72	0.45
10-2-116	儿童奶粉 (可淇牌)	100	4.0	457	1912	17.0	17.0	59.0	—	—	—	—	—	420	100	0.60	0.60	0.35
10-2-117	儿童奶粉 (三鹿牌)	100	2.9	462	1933	18.3	17.5	57.8	—	—	—	37	3.5	362	—	1.33	1.71	—
10-2-118	儿童奶粉 (完达山牌)	100	—	458	1916	17.0	18.0	57.0	—	—	—	—	—	540	—	0.40	0.80	0.80
10-2-119	孕妇乳母奶粉 (惠氏)	100	—	405	1723	16.0	6.8	70.0	—	—	—	—	—	610	85	0.65	0.81	0.98
10-2-120	孕妇乳母奶粉 (美赞臣)	100	—	380	1588	23.3	3.9	62.4	—	—	—	—	—	960	—	0.67	0.80	1.00
10-2-121	中老年奶粉 (可淇牌)	100	4.0	432	1807	18.0	12.0	63.0	—	—	—	—	—	540	—	0.55	1.00	—
10-2-122	中老年奶粉 (雀巢)	100	—	429	1790	30.0	14.4	44.8	—	—	—	—	7.3	390	—	0.23	1.40	—
10-2-123	中老年奶粉 (三鹿牌)	100	2.9	403	1688	25.2	5.8	62.6	—	—	—	41	3.5	574	—	1.33	1.71	—
10-2-124	中老年奶粉 (森永牌)	100	3.0	418	1750	22.0	10.0	60.0	—	—	—	—	5.0	600	100	1.00	1.00	1.00
酸奶																		
10-3-007	酸奶 (调味)	100	81.2	88	370	3.0	3.2	11.9	—	—	—	—	0.7	—	—	0.03	0.14	0.02
10-3-008	酸奶 (果粒)	100	78.5	97	407	3.3	2.9	14.6	0.1	—	—	—	0.7	—	—	0.03	0.18	0.02

（以每100g可食部计）

编码 Code	食物名称 Food name	维生素 B_{12} Vit B_{12} μg	叶酸 Folate μg	烟酸 Niacin mg	维生素C Vit C mg	维生素E (Vit E) Total mg	α-TE mg	钙 Ca mg	磷 P mg	钾 K mg	钠 Na mg	镁 Mg mg	铁 Fe mg	锌 Zn mg	硒 Se μg	铜 Cu mg	锰 Mn mg	碘 I μg
10-2-107	全脂奶粉 (伊利牌)	—	5.9	0.09	—	—	—	750	550	209	220.6	91	3.9	3.97	11.78	0.20	0.01	—
10-2-108	全脂甜奶粉 (三鹿牌)	—	—	0.90	—	0.48	un	589	668	1589	282.8	67	3.7	5.13	1.25	0.05	0.09	—
10-2-109	全脂甜奶粉 (伊利牌)	—	—	—	—	—	—	620	460	1795	184.1	76	4.3	2.63	6.19	0.19	0.05	—
10-2-110	低脂奶粉 (高钙高铁, 雀巢)	—	—	—	60.0	—	—	1745	1325	1325	—	100	10.0	7.00	—	—	—	—
10-2-111	低脂奶粉 (高钙高铁, 伊利牌)	1.50	—	—	65.0	—	—	1350	950	1338	406.9	35	12.0	5.00	8.36	0.20	0.13	—
10-2-112	高钙高铁奶粉 (可淇牌)	—	—	—	40.0	10.00	un	1000	480	800	350.0	50	9.0	6.00	—	—	—	—
10-2-113	儿童奶粉 (安儿健 A+, 美赞臣)	2.20	57.0	5.20	51.0	un	5.23	730	450	730	210.0	55	8.1	4.40	—	0.35	0.04	28.0
10-2-114	儿童奶粉 (适体健, 美赞臣)	1.00	165.0	6.60	38.0	un	4.23	500	500	1150	250.0	60	6.3	4.40	10.00	0.36	1.25	90.0
10-2-115	儿童奶粉 (惠氏)	2.00	90.0	4.10	45.0	un	3.77	495	450	721	248.0	59	5.6	5.40	—	0.20	—	45.0
10-2-116	儿童奶粉 (可淇牌)	2.00	50.0	3.50	40.0	10.00	un	850	425	—	—	40	9.0	6.00	—	—	—	—
10-2-117	儿童奶粉 (三鹿牌)	—	—	7.80	65.0	un	4.50	756	469	1261	115.7	47	10.2	12.20	5.10	0.05	0.12	—
10-2-118	儿童奶粉 (完达山牌)	1.00	50.0	3.60	40.0	un	8.05	800	550	800	300.0	78	8.0	6.00	—	0.34	0.03	—
10-2-119	孕妇乳母奶粉 (惠氏)	2.40	339.0	7.70	102.0	un	6.71	407	386	772	346.0	130	8.1	5.30	—	0.49	0.81	53.0
10-2-120	孕妇乳母奶粉 (美赞臣)	3.20	530.0	8.00	24.0	un	8.05	1700	650	1000	360.0	75	7.1	15.00	—	—	—	60.0
10-2-121	中老年奶粉 (可淇牌)	—	—	—	40.0	12.00	un	1000	500	—	—	—	9.0	6.00	21.00	—	—	—
10-2-122	中老年奶粉 (雀巢)	1.80	—	—	—	10.50	un	1740	890	1390	410.0	100	—	—	—	—	—	—
10-2-123	中老年奶粉 (三鹿牌)	—	—	5.90	45.8	un	8.52	1148	774	2526	175.4	78	9.2	9.30	21.50	0.13	0.02	54.2
10-2-124	中老年奶粉 (森永牌)	3.00	—	16.60	60.0	un	13.42	800	630	—	—	75	7.0	4.00	—	—	—	60.0
酸奶																		
10-3-007	酸奶 (调味)	—	11.3	0.06	(Tr)	—	—	160	168	272	69.6	12	1.6	0.63	1.42	0.01	0.03	—
10-3-008	酸奶 (果粒)	0.10	15.6	0.08	1.0	—	—	61	103	241	53.8	8	0.1	0.39	1.19	0.01	0.02	—

乳类及制品 Milk and milk products

(以每100g可食部计)

编码 Code	食物名称 Food name	食部 Edible	水分 Water	能量 Energy		蛋白质 Protein	脂肪 Fat	碳水化合物 CHO	膳食纤维 (Dietary fiber)			胆固醇 Cholesterol	灰分 Ash	维生素A		硫胺素 Thiamin	核黄素 Riboflavin	维生素B_6 Vit B_6
									总 Total	可溶性 Soluble	不溶性 Insoluble			Vit A	胡萝卜素 Carotene			
		%	g	kcal	kJ	g	g	g	g	g	g	mg	g	μgRE	μg	mg	mg	mg
奶酪																		
10-4-012	奶酪 (光明牌)	100	43.0	348	1454	16.5	28.4	6.5	(0)	(0)	(0)	—	5.6	—	—	0.07	0.45	0.03
10-4-013	奶酪 (骑士牌)	100	31.7	386	1614	23.0	25.4	16.3	(0)	(0)	(0)	—	3.6	—	—	0.19	0.30	—
10-4-014	低脂奶酪	100	48.0	241	1009	21.6	11.6	12.6	(0)	(0)	(0)	37	6.2	—	—	0.06	0.49	0.03
10-4-015	硬质干酪	100	37.3	411	1702	24.9	34.5	0.1	0	—	—	100	—	330	215	0.03	0.41	0.15
奶油																		
10-5-008	奶油	100	11.0	785	3285	1.1	86.0	1.7	(0)	(0)	(0)	155	0.2	840	—	0.02	0.02	Tr
其它																		
10-9-004	全脂甜炼乳 (雀巢)	100	15.9	380	1588	7.5	10.0	64.9	(0)	(0)	(0)	7	1.7	—	—	0.07	0.41	—
10-9-005	全脂甜炼乳 (燕山牌)	100	17.1	374	1565	8.2	10.0	62.8	(0)	(0)	(0)	3	1.9	—	—	0.08	0.32	—
10-9-006	脱脂甜炼乳	100	29.0	270	1130[c]	10.3	0.2	58.0	0	—	—	—	2.5	0	0	0.10	0.50	—

乳类及制品 Milk and milk products

(以每100g可食部计)

编码 Code	食物名称 Food name	维生素 B_{12} Vit B_{12} μg	叶酸 Folate μg	烟酸 Niacin mg	维生素C Vit C mg	维生素E (Vit E) Total mg	维生素E (Vit E) α-TE mg	钙 Ca mg	磷 P mg	钾 K mg	钠 Na mg	镁 Mg mg	铁 Fe mg	锌 Zn mg	硒 Se μg	铜 Cu mg	锰 Mn mg	碘 I μg
奶酪																		
10-4-012	奶酪 (光明牌)	0.90	2.8	Tr	(Tr)	Tr	Tr	445	389	315	1598.0	20	0.2	2.35	5.08	0.02	0.01	—
10-4-013	奶酪 (骑士牌)	—	—	0.05	(Tr)	—	—	796	307	42	531.8	35	2.2	5.03	—	0.06	0.10	11.0
10-4-014	低脂奶酪	0.23	11.5	Tr	(Tr)	Tr	Tr	522	606	368	1684.8	29	0.2	3.41	6.82	0.03	0.02	—
10-4-015	硬质干酪	2.40	31.0	0.10	Tr	un	0.52	731	500	76	687.0	29	0.3	4.10	6.00	0.05	Tr	30.0
奶油																		
10-5-008	奶油	Tr	3.0	Tr	(Tr)	2.23	2.23	2	—	31	1.7	0	0.1	—	1.00	Tr	0.01	—
其它																		
10-9-004	全脂甜炼乳 (雀巢)	—	7.8	0.21	(Tr)	0.30	0.30	334	243	308	88.6	21	0.2	1.04	18.74	0.12	0.06	13.7
10-9-005	全脂甜炼乳 (燕山牌)	—	13.1	0.22	(Tr)	Tr	Tr	317	246	428	103.9	23	0.2	1.15	7.89	0.03	0.05	8.9
10-9-006	脱脂甜炼乳	—	—	0.20	2.0	—	—	330	300	520	180.0	—	0.3	—	—	—	—	—

Notes

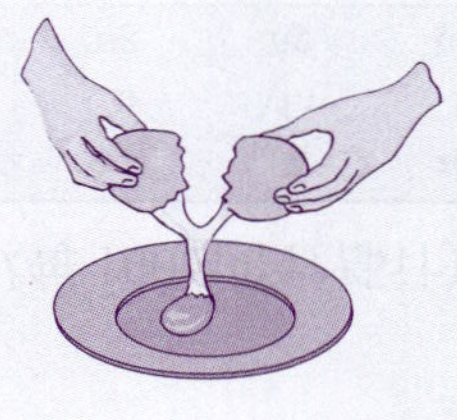

蛋类及制品

Eggs and Egg Products

市场上常见的禽蛋类包括鸡蛋、鸭蛋、鹅蛋、鹌鹑蛋等。本节依此分成相应的亚类。

居民最常消费的是鸡蛋。鸡蛋分级用对光检查法，主要是检查其新鲜程度。鸡蛋壳的颜色取决于鸡的品种，而鸡蛋黄的颜色取决于饲料，如果饲料中类胡萝卜素和维生素A含量高，则蛋黄颜色深。

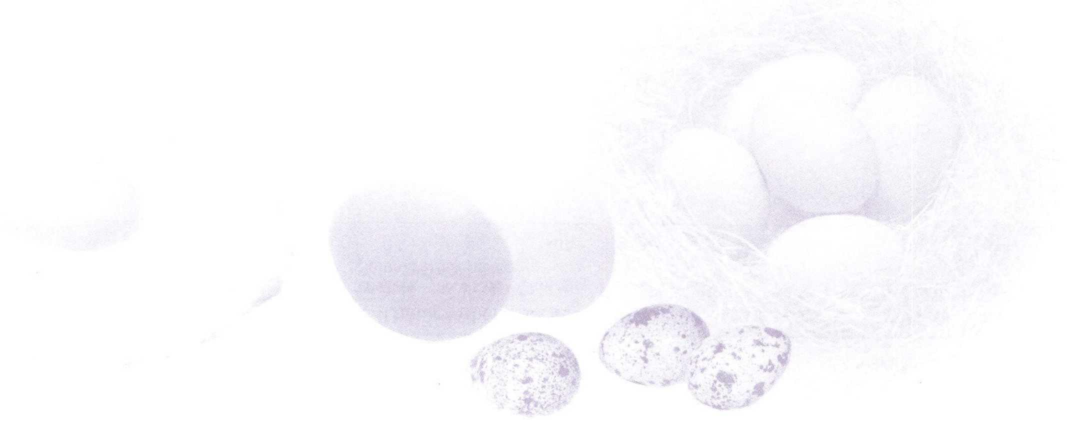

蛋类及制品 Eggs and egg products

(以每100g可食部计)

编码 Code	食物名称 Food name	食部 Edible %	水分 Water g	能量 Energy kcal	能量 Energy kJ	蛋白质 Protein g	脂肪 Fat g	碳水化合物 CHO g	膳食纤维 (Dietary fiber) 总 Total g	可溶性 Soluble g	不溶性 Insoluble g	胆固醇 Cholesterol mg	灰分 Ash g	维生素A Vit A μgRE	胡萝卜素 Carotene μg	硫胺素 Thiamin mg	核黄素 Riboflavin mg	维生素B_6 Vit B_6 mg
鸡蛋																		
11-1-109	鸡蛋(红皮)	87	77.1	143	600	12.2	10.5	0	(0)	(0)	(0)	—	0.8	—	—	0.05	0.11	0.03
11-1-110	藏鸡蛋	86	72.7	162	677	12.6	11.3	2.4	(0)	(0)	(0)	—	1.0	—	—	0.07	0.44	—
11-1-111	乌鸡蛋(绿皮)	88	69.7	170	712	12.6	10.6	6.1	(0)	(0)	(0)	—	1.0	—	—	0.09	0.43	0.03
11-1-204	鸡蛋(煮)	86	76.3	151	632[c]	12.1	10.5	0.1	0	—	—	—	1.0	(147)	(18)	0.04	0.39	—
11-1-205	毛蛋	87	72.3	176	735	14.2	13.2	0	—	—	—	—	1.2	161	—	0.04	0.65	—
11-1-206	荷包蛋(油煎)	100	68.6	199	833[c]	13.5	15.0	1.4	0	—	—	—	1.6	248	—	0.06	0.52	—
11-1-207	荷包蛋(煮)	100	74.9	164	686[c]	12.3	11.7	0.2	(0)	—	—	—	0.9	160	21	0.06	0.40	—
鸭蛋																		
11-2-104	海鸭蛋	87	55.6	243	1015	12.7	13.8	16.9	(0)	(0)	(0)	—	1.0	—	—	0.13	0.40	0.02
11-2-203	咸鸭蛋(煮)	84	70.0	177	739	13.8	13.5	0	(0)	(0)	(0)	—	4.2	—	—	0.15	0.28	0.03
鹅蛋																		
11-3-104	鹅蛋(煮)	85	71.9	182	761[c]	12.7	13.6	1.0	0	—	—	—	0.8	174	18	0.06	0.32	—

蛋类及制品 Eggs and egg products

(以每100g可食部计)

编码 Code	食物名称 Food name	维生素B_{12} Vit B_{12} μg	叶酸 Folate μg	烟酸 Niacin mg	维生素C Vit C mg	维生素E (Vit E) Total mg	α-TE mg	钙 Ca mg	磷 P mg	钾 K mg	钠 Na mg	镁 Mg mg	铁 Fe mg	锌 Zn mg	硒 Se μg	铜 Cu mg	锰 Mn mg	碘 I μg
鸡蛋																		
11-1-109	鸡蛋(红皮)	—	70.7	—	(0)	0.84	0.61	44	182	121	125.7	11	1.0	0.38	13.83	Tr	0.01	—
11-1-110	藏鸡蛋	—	—	—	—	1.54	un	57	177	73	119.2	13	2.8	1.52	5.70	0.08	0.03	—
11-1-111	乌鸡蛋(绿皮)	—	118.9	0.05	(0)	3.73	2.67	42	273	514	106.7	11	3.8	2.05	28.31	0.05	Tr	20.0
11-1-204	鸡蛋(煮)	—	—	0.10	0	—	—	35	206	130	130.0	—	1.7	—	—	—	—	—
11-1-205	毛蛋	—	—	0.87	—	1.49	un	204	155	66	75.8	—	1.8	1.64	29.00	—	—	—
11-1-206	荷包蛋(油煎)	—	—	0.10	0	—	—	55	194	132	353.0	—	1.6	—	—	—	—	—
11-1-207	荷包蛋(煮)	—	—	0.10	0	—	—	55	200	100	110.0	—	2.2	—	—	—	—	—
鸭蛋																		
11-2-104	海鸭蛋	—	89.7	Tr	(0)	1.66	0.92	118	6	119	105.1	1	3.1	0.25	41.51	0.02	0.06	45.7
11-2-203	咸鸭蛋(煮)	—	88.2	0.04	(0)	2.85	2.22	52	212	226	1131.0	22	2.1	1.50	32.76	0.20	0.07	30.0
鹅蛋																		
11-3-104	鹅蛋(煮)	—	—	0.10	0	—	—	41	70	76	45.0	—	2.5	—	—	—	—	—

Notes

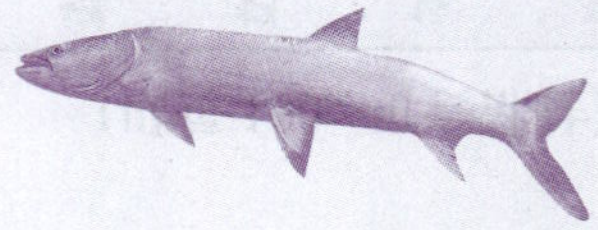

鱼虾蟹贝类

Fish, Shellfish and Mollusc

从水中获得的食品习惯上被称为水产品。此处包括的主要是一些水产动物性食物，按其品种分成以下几个亚类。

1.鱼：包括草鱼、鲤鱼、鳟鱼等各种鱼和鱼罐头、鱼片干等加工制品。

2.虾：包括白米虾、对虾、基围虾等各种虾和虾仁、虾脑酱等加工制品。

3.蟹：包括海蟹、河蟹等各种蟹。

4.贝：包括鲍鱼、蛏、扇贝、牡蛎及各种蛤蜊、蚶、螺等。

5.其它：包括海参、海蜇、鱿鱼等软体动物。

上述水产食物的营养成分受季节、成熟度以及饲料等因素的影响很大。

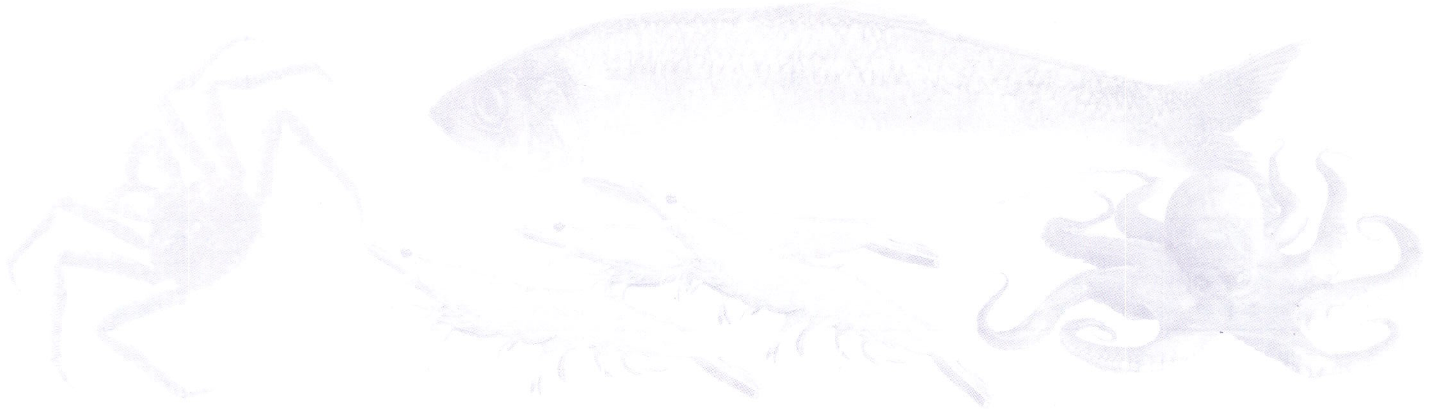

鱼虾蟹贝类 Fish, shellfish and mollusc

(以每100g可食部计)

编码 Code	食物名称 Food name	食部 Edible	水分 Water	能量 Energy		蛋白质 Protein	脂肪 Fat	碳水化合物 CHO	膳食纤维 (Dietary fiber) 总 Total	可溶性 Soluble	不溶性 Insoluble	胆固醇 Cholesterol	灰分 Ash	维生素A Vit A	胡萝卜素 Carotene	硫胺素 Thiamin	核黄素 Riboflavin	维生素B_6 Vit B_6
		%	g	kcal	kJ	g	g	g	g	g	g	mg	g	μgRE	μg	mg	mg	mg
鱼																		
12-1-131	草鱼 [白鲩、草包鱼]	58	78.2	96	403	17.7	2.6	0.5	—	—	—	47	1.0	Tr	(0)	Tr	0.04	0.10
12-1-132	鲢鱼 [白鲢、胖子、连子鱼]	61	82.8	84	352	16.3	2.1	0	—	—	—	38	1.1	Tr	(0)	0.01	0.05	0.10
12-1-133	鲫鱼 [喜头鱼、海附鱼]	54	78.6	89	373	18.0	1.6	0.7	—	—	—	21	1.1	Tr	(0)	0.08	0.06	0.10
12-1-241	带鱼 (切段)	70	78.8	108	453	17.6	4.2	0	—	—	—	52	1.1	19	(0)	0.02	0.08	0.02
12-1-242	黄鱼 (小黄花鱼)	62	79.4	114	477	17.0	5.1	0	—	—	—	76	1.6	94	(0)	0.03	0.08	0.04
12-1-243	金鲳鱼	66	77.4	99	415	18.7	2.7	0	—	—	—	—	1.2	Tr	(0)	0.01	0.09	0.05
12-1-244	鲭鱼	49	45.2	417	1745	14.4	39.4	0.2	—	—	—	60	0.8	183	—	0.03	0.47	0.32
12-1-245	双髻鲨	38	73.6	117	490[c]	27.4	0.1	(0)	—	—	—	58	1.4	82	—	0.02	0.07	0.52
12-1-303	金鲨鱼翅 (干)	100	12.0	350	1463	84.1	0.5	2.3	—	—	—	—	1.1	Tr	(0)	0.01	0.02	—
12-1-304	鱼排	100	61.2	160	669	10.1	2.4	24.5	—	—	—	24	1.8	Tr	—	0.04	0.05	0.03
12-1-305	鱼丸	100	72.5	107	447	11.1	1.3	12.7	—	—	—	77	2.4	5	—	0.02	0.04	0.02
12-1-306	鱼子酱	100	55.9	201	841	9.6	7.1	24.7	—	—	—	—	2.7	Tr	—	0.07	0.04	0.11
12-1-401	草鱼 (熏)	100	45.6	283	1184	24.0	16.5	9.6	—	—	—	9	4.3	127	—	0.03	0.04	—
12-1-402	丁香鱼 (香辣味)	100	30.3	403	1686	19.0	28.2	18.3	—	—	—	—	4.2	Tr	—	0.04	0.05	—
12-1-403	凤尾鱼 (熟)	100	19.5	520	2175	23.5	43.0	9.7	—	—	—	57	4.3	8	48	0.02	0.07	0.02
12-1-404	箭鱼 (炸)	100	47.8	271	1133	20.8	16.1	10.7	—	—	—	60	4.6	21	124	0.02	0.05	0.03
12-1-405	金枪鱼 (盐水浸)	81	74.6	99	422	23.5	0.6	0	0	—	—	51	—	—	Tr	0.02	0.11	0.47
12-1-406	金枪鱼 (油浸)	79	63.3	189	794	27.1	9.0	0	0	—	—	50	—	—	Tr	0.02	0.12	0.51
12-1-407	鲮鱼 (豆豉, 熟)	100	18.8	472	1973	25.5	33.1	17.9	—	—	—	25	4.7	13	75	0.02	0.08	0.06
12-1-408	鳗鱼 (红烧)	100	55.4	211	884	21.3	9.8	9.5	—	—	—	50	4.0	Tr	Tr	0.03	0.09	—
12-1-409	鲭鱼 (烤, 150℃, 10分)	100	45.8	412	1724[c]	16.5	37.8	(0)	—	—	—	77	1.3	164	—	0.18	0.28	0.28
12-1-410	鲭鱼 (烤, 150℃, 20分)	100	45.7	396	1657[c]	19.1	34.8	(0)	—	—	—	72	1.2	132	—	0.25	0.47	0.30

(以每 100g 可食部计)

编码 Code	食物名称 Food name	维生素 B_{12} Vit B_{12} μg	叶酸 Folate μg	烟酸 Niacin mg	维生素 C Vit C mg	维生素 E (Vit E) Total mg	维生素 E (Vit E) α-TE mg	钙 Ca mg	磷 P mg	钾 K mg	钠 Na mg	镁 Mg mg	铁 Fe mg	锌 Zn mg	硒 Se μg	铜 Cu mg	锰 Mn mg	碘 I μg
鱼																		
12-1-131	草鱼 [白鲩、草包鱼]	—	15.5	2.48	(Tr)	Tr	Tr	17	152	325	36.0	26	1.3	0.38	11.67	0.01	0.01	—
12-1-132	鲢鱼 [白鲢、胖子、连子鱼]	—	27.4	3.08	(Tr)	0.30	0.30	53	184	277	57.5	23	1.5	0.67	14.43	0.04	0.01	—
12-1-133	鲫鱼 [喜头鱼、海附鱼]	—	Tr	2.38	(Tr)	0.34	0.34	79	157	290	41.2	41	1.3	0.53	22.96	0.01	Tr	—
12-1-241	带鱼 (切段)	2.02	—	1.45	(Tr)	0.42	0.42	431	282	361	246.4	30	1.1	2.23	26.63	0.07	0.09	—
12-1-242	黄鱼 (小黄花鱼)	—	—	0.72	(Tr)	0.82	0.82	191	217	198	194.3	23	0.7	0.88	26.71	0.04	0.06	—
12-1-243	金鳇鱼	2.60	—	0.93	(Tr)	0.10	0.10	20	170	319	104.1	26	0.5	0.36	32.80	0.04	0.03	8.1
12-1-244	鲭鱼	3.77	—	6.05	0	un	0.74	7	160	308	56.0	24	1.4	1.00	—	—	—	—
12-1-245	双髻鲨	1.79	—	6.90	1.7	un	0	4	259	492	83.0	32	0.8	0.60	—	—	—	—
12-1-303	金鲨鱼翅 (干)	Tr	—	Tr	(Tr)	Tr	Tr	252	115	226	79.6	17	5.1	2.25	72.46	0.04	0.09	10.9
12-1-304	鱼排	—	—	0.47	—	Tr	Tr	13	92	136	383.3	4	1.0	0.62	9.33	0.06	0.09	16.3
12-1-305	鱼丸	Tr	—	Tr	—	0.14	0.14	97	272	360	854.2	11	1.2	1.59	14.02	0.11	0.08	—
12-1-306	鱼子酱	2.68	5.7	0.41	—	3.89	un	23	88	271	394.6	4	2.7	1.35	18.98	0.08	0.27	7.4
12-1-401	草鱼 (熏)	—	4.4	3.29	(0)	6.46	un	448	285	315	1291.8	36	25.7	1.39	8.78	0.07	0.41	55.8
12-1-402	丁香鱼 (香辣味)	—	5.7	2.05	(0)	23.25	un	542	616	363	1417.2	94	4.2	2.57	18.57	0.25	0.37	56.7
12-1-403	凤尾鱼 (熟)	Tr	4.5	1.45	(0)	15.65	5.85	665	643	161	525.4	42	1.3	1.78	39.60	0.12	0.20	17.0
12-1-404	箭鱼 (炸)	Tr	4.9	1.20	(0)	8.70	un	211	167	60	403.6	24	0.7	0.72	23.29	0.02	0.09	15.6
12-1-405	金枪鱼 (盐水浸)	4.00	4.0	14.40	Tr	un	0.55	8	170	230	320.0	27	1.0	0.70	78.00	0.05	Tr	13.0
12-1-406	金枪鱼 (油浸)	5.00	5.0	16.10	Tr	un	1.94	12	200	260	290.0	33	1.6	1.10	90.00	0.20	0.05	14.0
12-1-407	鲮鱼 (豆豉, 熟)	3.88	5.6	1.63	(0)	31.32	un	179	262	399	1291.7	47	9.2	2.18	24.82	0.16	0.23	18.4
12-1-408	鳗鱼 (红烧)	—	0.5	1.47	(0)	5.91	un	37	120	174	1252.0	16	2.2	2.46	24.45	0.04	0.05	56.8
12-1-409	鲭鱼 (烤, 150℃, 10 分)	12.33	—	6.98	0	un	0.51	5	219	333	58.0	27	1.7	1.10	—	—	—	—
12-1-410	鲭鱼 (烤, 150℃, 20 分)	14.65	—	6.95	0	un	0.48	5	246	370	82.0	31	2.0	1.30	—	—	—	—

鱼虾蟹贝类 Fish, shellfish and mollusc

(以每 100g 可食部计)

编码 Code	食物名称 Food name	食部 Edible %	水分 Water g	能量 Energy kcal	能量 Energy kJ	蛋白质 Protein g	脂肪 Fat g	碳水化合物 CHO g	膳食纤维 (Dietary fiber) 总 Total g	膳食纤维 可溶性 Soluble g	膳食纤维 不溶性 Insoluble g	胆固醇 Cholesterol mg	灰分 Ash g	维生素 A Vit A μgRE	维生素 A 胡萝卜素 Carotene μg	硫胺素 Thiamin mg	核黄素 Riboflavin mg	维生素 B_6 Vit B_6 mg
12-1-411	鲭鱼 (烤, 150℃, 30 分)	100	32.0	536	2243[c]	19.9	50.0	(0)	—	—	—	77	1.4	163	—	0.22	0.44	0.33
12-1-412	鲭鱼 (烤, 180℃, 10 分)	100	47.3	373	1561[c]	20.2	31.8	(0)	—	—	—	80	1.3	114	—	0.30	0.45	0.32
12-1-413	鲭鱼 (烤, 210℃, 10 分)	100	39.0	472	1975[c]	19.0	43.4	(0)	—	—	—	64	1.3	170	—	0.22	0.36	0.38
12-1-414	鲭鱼 (炸)	100	28.3	555	2322[c]	17.2	53.4	0.1	—	—	—	51	1.0	103	—	0.14	0.31	0.23
12-1-415	鲭鱼 (蒸)	100	47.0	392	1639[c]	14.6	36.5	0.7	—	—	—	76	1.0	142	—	0.20	0.34	0.24
12-1-416	鲭鱼 (煮)	100	49.3	375	1569[c]	14.9	34.5	0.4	—	—	—	72	0.8	125	—	0.18	0.32	0.31
12-1-417	沙丁鱼 (茄汁, 熟)	100	70.4	155	650	13.8	9.8	3.0	—	—	—	39	3.0	208	1248	0.04	0.12	0.09
12-1-418	沙丁鱼 (盐水浸)	79	66.2	172	721	21.5	9.6	0	0	—	—	60	—	6	Tr	0.01	0.26	0.16
12-1-419	沙丁鱼 (油浸)	82	58.6	220	918	23.3	14.1	0	0	—	—	65	—	7	Tr	0.01	0.29	0.18
12-1-420	午餐鱼 (香辣味)	100	37.5	383	1601	24.4	30.2	3.3	—	—	—	—	4.6	Tr	—	0.04	0.09	—
12-1-421	鳕鱼 (烤)	85	76.6	96	408	21.4	1.2	Tr	0	—	—	(56)	—	2	Tr	0.03	0.05	0.19
12-1-422	鳕鱼 (炸)	98	55.9	235	983	12.4	14.3	15.6	(0.4)	—	—	—	—	Tr	—	0.07	0.06	0.09
虾																		
12-2-203	虾酱	100	72.3	112	467	10.8	7.6	0	—	—	—	—	14.3	65	—	0.05	0.14	0.05
12-2-204	虾仁 (红)	100	87.8	48	202	10.4	0.7	0	—	—	—	—	1.1	Tr	—	0.01	0.02	0.01
12-2-301	虾仁肉丸	100	70.0	151	632[c]	4.6	7.4	16.7	1.3	—	—	17	1.3	4	—	0.08	0.04	0.06
蟹																		
12-3-006	海蟹 (小)	42	79.2	81	339	14.2	1.1	3.6	—	—	—	40	1.9	Tr	(0)	0.03	0.10	0.04
12-3-301	蟹足棒	100	67.4	123	514	9.0	0.6	20.5	—	—	—	17	2.6	5	—	Tr	0.04	—
贝																		
12-4-117	海蚌 [西施舌]	47	87.7	42	174	9.5	0.3	0.2	0	0	0	101	2.3	10	(0)	0	0.03	—
12-4-601	文蛤丸	100	56.6	209	874[c]	16.2	9.2	15.8	—	—	—	65	2.3	2	—	0.01	0.05	0.23

(以每100g可食部计)

编码 Code	食物名称 Food name	维生素B12 Vit B_{12} μg	叶酸 Folate μg	烟酸 Niacin mg	维生素C Vit C mg	维生素E (Vit E) Total mg	维生素E (Vit E) α-TE mg	钙 Ca mg	磷 P mg	钾 K mg	钠 Na mg	镁 Mg mg	铁 Fe mg	锌 Zn mg	硒 Se μg	铜 Cu mg	锰 Mn mg	碘 I μg
12-1-411	鲭鱼(烤, 150℃, 30分)	10.95	—	7.85	0	un	0.90	15	266	359	78.7	30	2.0	1.40	—	—	—	—
12-1-412	鲭鱼(烤, 180℃, 10分)	10.92	—	7.93	0	un	0.30	8	279	395	82.0	32	2.6	1.10	—	—	—	—
12-1-413	鲭鱼(烤, 210℃, 10分)	13.88	—	8.24	0	un	0.84	7	256	358	74.0	31	1.7	0.80	—	—	—	—
12-1-414	鲭鱼(炸)	3.91	—	6.30	0	un	2.27	8	262	301	75.0	27	1.7	1.10	—	—	—	—
12-1-415	鲭鱼(蒸)	6.86	—	5.70	0	un	0.50	5	211	235	52.4	22	2.0	0.90	—	—	—	—
12-1-416	鲭鱼(煮)	4.27	—	4.98	0	un	0.73	6	175	211	51.0	20	1.8	1.00	—	—	—	—
12-1-417	沙丁鱼(茄汁, 熟)	12.00	35.4	5.18	—	5.16	2.06	17	137	268	820.2	20	0.6	0.32	34.64	0.08	—	29.2
12-1-418	沙丁鱼(盐水浸)	13.00	8.0	6.10	Tr	—	—	540	510	320	530.0	45	2.3	2.30	41.00	0.16	0.20	23.0
12-1-419	沙丁鱼(油浸)	15.00	8.0	6.90	Tr	un	0.31	500	520	410	450.0	46	2.3	2.20	49.00	0.11	0.19	23.0
12-1-420	午餐鱼(香辣味)	—	Tr	4.78	(0)	17.35	un	725	801	576	1321.2	63	1.6	2.03	38.10	0.13	0.24	29.5
12-1-421	鳕鱼(烤)	2.00	12.0	2.30	Tr	un	0.59	11	190	350	340.0	26	0.1	0.50	34.00	0.02	0.01	(130.0)
12-1-422	鳕鱼(炸)	—	6.0	1.20	Tr	un	(3.45)	43	190	230	480.0	19	0.4	0.40	17.00	0.08	0.12	—
虾																		
12-2-203	虾酱	10.38	11.0	0.76	—	3.96	un	308	177	196	4584.6	25	11.6	1.52	31.94	0.35	0.57	166.6
12-2-204	虾仁(红)	—	—	Tr	(Tr)	0.70	0.70	23	157	98	272.1	9	0.6	0.62	10.86	0.07	0.05	—
12-2-301	虾仁肉丸	0.53	—	2.40	0	un	0.14	7	31	58	429.0	10	0.7	0.50	—	—	—	—
蟹																		
12-3-006	海蟹(小)	—	15.6	1.46	(Tr)	0.58	0.58	—	293	370	321.5	238	1.1	3.15	25.60	0.40	0.69	—
12-3-301	蟹足棒	Tr	—	Tr	—	0.63	0.28	144	117	164	1242.0	10	0.6	0.72	7.56	0.08	0.27	—
贝																		
12-4-117	海蚌[西施舌]	—	—	Tr	(Tr)	1.51	1.51	63	100	159	793.0	46	3.0	2.34	46.24	0.13	0.10	—
12-4-601	文蛤丸	4.62	—	3.79	0	un	0.38	21	165	226	565.0	23	8.4	1.00	—	—	—	—

(以每100g可食部计)

编码 Code	食物名称 Food name	食部 Edible	水分 Water	能量 Energy		蛋白质 Protein	脂肪 Fat	碳水化合物 CHO	膳食纤维 (Dietary fiber)			胆固醇 Cholesterol	灰分 Ash	维生素A		硫胺素 Thiamin	核黄素 Riboflavin	维生素B_6 Vit B_6
									总 Total	可溶性 Soluble	不溶性 Insoluble			Vit A	胡萝卜素 Carotene			
		%	g	kcal	kJ	g	g	g	g	g	g	mg	g	μgRE	μg	mg	mg	mg
其它																		
12-9-014	甲鱼蛋	100	75.2	128	534	12.5	7.3	3.0	(0)	(0)	(0)	—	2.0	73	—	1.05	1.58	—
12-9-301	墨鱼圈	100	84.8	72	300	13.0	2.2	0	—	—	—	157	0.9	8	—	0.05	0.05	0.03
12-9-302	墨鱼丸	100	71.0	128	535	13.4	4.7	8.0	—	—	—	32	2.9	4	—	0.01	0.03	0.02

(以每100g可食部计)

编码 Code	食物名称 Food name	维生素B12 Vit B_{12} μg	叶酸 Folate μg	烟酸 Niacin mg	维生素C Vit C mg	维生素E (Vit E) Total mg	α-TE mg	钙 Ca mg	磷 P mg	钾 K mg	钠 Na mg	镁 Mg mg	铁 Fe mg	锌 Zn mg	硒 Se μg	铜 Cu mg	锰 Mn mg	碘 I μg
其它																		
12-9-014	甲鱼蛋	—	—	0.03	(Tr)	3.60	un	103	268	156	103.9	11	1.3	0.97	35.23	0.05	0.02	18.5
12-9-301	墨鱼圈	—	—	—	—	1.27	un	9	163	159	93.7	20	0.6	2.56	24.30	0.54	0.04	—
12-9-302	墨鱼丸	—	—	0.86	—	0.50	0.50	24	120	275	825.2	6	0.9	0.98	13.39	0.14	0.09	—

Notes

婴幼儿食品

Infant Foods

参照有关标准，将婴幼儿食品分为以下几个亚类。

1．婴幼儿配方粉：指适用于0～12个月龄的婴幼儿食用的粉状食品，其营养成分能满足0～6个月龄正常婴幼儿的营养需要。另外，也有较大婴儿的配方粉，适于6～36个月龄婴幼儿食用。

2．婴幼儿断奶期辅助食品：指当母乳或婴儿配方食品不能满足婴儿营养需要时为婴幼儿断奶时期生产的配方食品。适于4个月龄以上的婴幼儿食用，包括即食类和非即食类。

3．婴幼儿补充食品：指为补充婴幼儿在断奶期某些营养素不足而生产的食品，包括以谷物为主料，以蔬菜、水果、蛋类或肉类为配料，强化或未强化营养素的产品。

本节所登载的食物成分数据源自实测值和标签摘录，仅作为相关营养调查和研究项目的参考数据。如另有它用，以厂家当年的新产品为准。

婴幼儿食品 Infant foods

(以每 100g 可食部计)

编码 Code	食物名称 Food name	食部 Edible %	水分 Water g	能量 Energy kcal	能量 Energy kJ	蛋白质 Protein g	脂肪 Fat g	碳水化合物 CHO g	膳食纤维 (Dietary fiber) 总 Total g	可溶性 Soluble g	不溶性 Insoluble g	胆固醇 Cholesterol mg	灰分 Ash g	维生素 A Vit A μgRE	胡萝卜素 Carotene μg	硫胺素 Thiamin mg	核黄素 Riboflavin mg	维生素 B_6 Vit B_6 mg
婴幼儿配方粉																		
13-1-101	婴儿配方奶粉 (爱儿乐, 惠氏)	100	—	524	2220	12.0	28.0	56.0	—	—	—	—	—	591	165	0.79	1.18	0.47
13-1-102	婴儿配方奶粉 (爱儿乐, 惠氏, 金装)	100	—	520	2203	11.0	28.0	56.0	—	—	—	—	—	591	165	0.79	1.18	0.47
13-1-103	婴儿配方奶粉 (爱力大 1, 美赞臣)	100	—	488[c]	2043	12.5	22.0	59.0	—	—	—	—	—	561	—	0.38	0.69	0.31
13-1-104	婴儿配方奶粉 (安婴儿, 美赞臣)	100	—	528[c]	2210	11.0	29.0	56.0	—	—	—	—	—	480	—	0.39	0.94	0.35
13-1-105	婴儿配方奶粉 (安婴儿 A+, 美赞臣)	100	—	528[c]	2210	11.0	29.0	56.0	—	—	—	—	—	480	—	0.39	0.94	0.35
13-1-106	婴儿配方奶粉 (安婴乐, 美赞臣)	100	—	520[c]	2176	11.0	28.0	55.6	—	—	—	—	—	480	—	0.42	0.47	0.31
13-1-107	婴儿配方奶粉 (吉利蜜 1, 森永牌)	100	2.7	515	2156	12.6	27.0	55.5	—	—	—	—	2.2	480	45	0.40	0.80	0.30
13-1-108	婴儿配方奶粉 (可淇牌)	100	4.0	497	2079	12.0	25.0	56.0	—	—	—	—	—	450	100	0.40	0.50	0.19
13-1-109	婴儿配方奶粉 (力多精 1, 雀巢)	100	3.0	507	2121	12.5	25.8	56.2	—	—	—	—	2.5	540	—	0.46	0.76	0.38
13-1-110	婴儿配方奶粉 (美素力 1)	100	(3.0)[1]	510	2130	11.1	27.0	55.0	1.9	—	—	—	—	495	310	0.34	0.70	0.30
13-1-111	婴儿配方奶粉 (美素力 H)	100	(2.8)[2]	515	2150	10.8	27.0	57.0	—	—	—	—	—	495	310	0.34	0.70	0.30
13-1-112	婴儿配方奶粉 (美素力, 袋装)	100	(2.8)[2]	515	2150	10.8	27.0	57.0	—	—	—	—	—	495	310	0.34	0.70	0.30
13-1-113	婴儿配方奶粉 (圣元牌)	100	—	522	2184	12.5	28.0	55.0	—	—	—	—	—	475	—	0.40	0.80	0.30
13-1-114	婴儿配方奶粉 (完达山牌)	100	4.5	508	2123	13.3	27.5	51.7	—	—	—	—	3.0	600	—	0.50	0.80	0.28
13-1-115	婴儿奶粉 (高钙, 圣元牌)	100	—	513	2145	12.8	27.0	54.6	—	—	—	—	—	475	—	0.40	0.50	0.30

1. 水分含量范围: ≤ 3.0g/100g　　2. 水分含量范围: ≤ 2.8g/100g

(以每100g可食部计)

编码 Code	食物名称 Food name	维生素 B_{12} Vit B_{12} μg	叶酸 Folate μg	烟酸 Niacin mg	维生素C Vit C mg	维生素E (Vit E) Total mg	维生素E (Vit E) α-TE mg	钙 Ca mg	磷 P mg	钾 K mg	钠 Na mg	镁 Mg mg	铁 Fe mg	锌 Zn mg	硒 Se μg	铜 Cu mg	锰 Mn mg	碘 I μg
婴幼儿配方粉																		
13-1-101	婴儿配方奶粉 (爱儿乐, 惠氏)	1.60	63.0	(4.00)[1]	71.0	un	5.85	362	262	551	126.0	50	6.3	4.70	—	(0.49)[4]	(0.07)[6]	(90.0)[8]
13-1-102	婴儿配方奶粉 (爱儿乐, 惠氏, 金装)	1.60	63.0	3.94	71.0	un	5.85	386	220	512	126.0	35	6.3	4.70	(9.50)[3]	(0.49)[4]	(0.07)[6]	(90.0)[8]
13-1-103	婴儿配方奶粉 (爱力大1, 美赞臣)	2.40	44.0	4.80	57.0	un	5.17	400	290	690	197.0	51	8.8	5.00	8.00	0.29	0.08	62.0
13-1-104	婴儿配方奶粉 (安婴儿, 美赞臣)	2.00	39.0	6.30	59.0	un	6.31	350	230	590	140.0	42	9.4	3.00	—	0.33	0.06	79.0
13-1-105	婴儿配方奶粉 (安婴儿A+, 美赞臣)	2.00	84.0	6.30	106.0	un	6.31	350	230	590	140.0	42	9.4	5.30	14.80	0.33	0.06	79.0
13-1-106	婴儿配方奶粉 (安婴乐, 美赞臣)	1.60	83.0	5.20	62.0	un	6.71	430	290	570	250.0	42	9.4	5.20	—	0.39	0.14	130.0
13-1-107	婴儿配方奶粉 (吉利蜜1, 森永牌)	2.00	100.0	5.00	50.0	un	3.36	360	210	540	160.0	45	7.0	(4.80)[2]	—	(0.31)[5]	(0.02)[7]	(90.0)[8]
13-1-108	婴儿配方奶粉 (可淇牌)	1.00	22.0	4.00	40.0	2.60	un	350	230	680	280.0	30	8.0	4.00	—	0.40	—	80.0
13-1-109	婴儿配方奶粉 (力多精1, 雀巢)	1.50	46.0	0.38	51.0	4.10	un	430	310	500	170.0	45	7.6	4.10	4.40	0.35	0.05	(90.0)[8]
13-1-110	婴儿配方奶粉 (美素力1)	1.20	80.0	5.90	70.0	10.00	un	385	230	500	155.0	46	6.0	4.60	13.00	0.38	0.26	57.0
13-1-111	婴儿配方奶粉 (美素力H)	0.80	80.0	5.90	65.0	un	6.71	385	230	500	155.0	46	6.0	4.60	—	0.39	0.05	54.0
13-1-112	婴儿配方奶粉 (美素力, 袋装)	0.80	80.0	5.90	65.0	un	6.71	385	230	500	155.0	46	6.0	4.60	—	0.39	0.05	54.0
13-1-113	婴儿配方奶粉 (圣元牌)	2.00	50.0	4.00	70.0	un	4.70	400	330	610	220.0	48	7.6	3.50	15.00	0.33	0.10	40.0
13-1-114	婴儿配方奶粉 (完达山牌)	1.25	30.0	4.00	40.0	un	4.19	420	330	680	220.0	50	8.5	5.00	6.00	0.40	0.08	80.0
13-1-115	婴儿奶粉 (高钙, 圣元牌)	1.00	50.0	4.00	70.0	un	4.70	400	330	—	—	58	7.6	3.50	10.00	0.33	0.05	40.0

1. 烟酸含量范围: ≥ 4.00mg/100g
2. 锌含量范围: 2.60～7.00mg/100g
3. 硒含量范围: 6.00～13.00μg/100g
4. 铜含量范围: 0.32～0.65mg/100g
5. 铜含量范围: 0.21～0.41mg/100g
6. 锰含量范围: 0.02～0.12mg/100g
7. 锰含量范围: ≥ 0.02mg/100g
8. 碘含量范围: 30.0～150.0μg/100g

婴幼儿食品 Infant foods

（以每 100g 可食部计）

编码 Code	食物名称 Food name	食部 Edible	水分 Water	能量 Energy		蛋白质 Protein	脂肪 Fat	碳水化合物 CHO	膳食纤维 (Dietary fiber) 总 Total	可溶性 Soluble	不溶性 Insoluble	胆固醇 Cholesterol	灰分 Ash	维生素 A Vit A	胡萝卜素 Carotene	硫胺素 Thiamin	核黄素 Riboflavin	维生素 B_6 Vit B_6
		%	g	kcal	kJ	g	g	g	g	g	g	mg	g	μgRE	μg	mg	mg	mg
13-1-116	婴儿配方豆粉 (爱儿素, 惠氏)	100	—	513	2174	14.0	27.0	53.5	—	—	—	—	—	577	162	0.77	1.15	0.46
13-1-201	较大婴儿配方奶粉 (爱力大 2, 美赞臣)	100	—	458[c]	1917	16.1	16.8	60.0	—	—	—	—	—	588	—	0.43	0.93	0.37
13-1-202	较大婴儿配方奶粉 (安婴宝, 美赞臣)	100	—	447[c]	1869	15.2	16.2	60.0	—	—	—	—	—	582	—	0.40	0.95	0.36
13-1-203	较大婴儿配方奶粉 (安婴宝 A+, 美赞臣)	100	—	453[c]	1894	15.9	16.3	61.0	—	—	—	—	—	408	—	0.36	1.04	0.33
13-1-204	较大婴儿配方奶粉 (健儿乐, 惠氏)	100	—	476	2018	18.0	20.0	56.0	—	—	—	—	—	528	148	0.70	1.06	0.42
13-1-205	较大婴儿配方奶粉 (健儿乐, 惠氏, 金装)	100	—	476	2018	18.0	20.0	56.0	—	—	—	—	—	528	148	0.70	1.06	0.42
13-1-206	较大婴儿配方奶粉 (可淇牌)	100	4.0	449	1879	15.0	21.0	50.0	—	—	—	—	—	765	100	0.31	0.31	0.30
13-1-207	较大婴儿配方奶粉 (美素乐 2)	100	(3.0)[1]	475	1990	15.0	21.0	56.0	2.6	—	—	—	—	420	350	0.47	0.90	0.29
13-1-208	较大婴儿配方奶粉 (美素乐, 全能装)	100	3.0	480	2020	15.0	21.5	57.3	—	—	—	—	3.2	369	350	0.47	0.73	0.29
13-1-209	较大婴儿配方奶粉 (美素乐, 袋装)	100	3.0	480	2008	15.0	21.5	57.3	—	—	—	—	3.2	369	350	0.47	0.73	0.29
13-1-210	较大婴幼儿配方奶粉 (吉利蜜 2, 森永牌)	100	3.0	472	1975	18.0	20.0	55.0	—	—	—	—	4.0	450	45	0.50	0.80	0.30
13-1-211	较大婴幼儿配方奶粉 (力多精 2, 雀巢)	100	3.0	464	1941	20.4	19.0	52.8	—	—	—	—	4.8	570	—	0.70	1.10	0.93
13-1-212	较大婴儿配方奶粉 (圣元牌)	100	—	483	2021	15.0	23.0	54.0	—	—	—	—	—	475	—	0.40	0.90	0.40

1. 水分含量范围: ≤ 3.0g/100g

(以每100g可食部计)

编码 Code	食物名称 Food name	维生素B_{12} Vit B_{12} μg	叶酸 Folate μg	烟酸 Niacin mg	维生素C Vit C mg	维生素E (Vit E) Total mg	α-TE mg	钙 Ca mg	磷 P mg	钾 K mg	钠 Na mg	镁 Mg mg	铁 Fe mg	锌 Zn mg	硒 Se μg	铜 Cu mg	锰 Mn mg	碘 I μg
13-1-116	婴儿配方豆粉 (爱儿素, 惠氏)	2.30	62.0	4.62	69.0	un	5.71	515	385	554	146.0	52	9.2	4.60	(9.45)[2]	(0.46)[4]	(0.21)[7]	(90.5)[9]
13-1-201	较大婴儿配方奶粉 (爱力大2, 美赞臣)	2.00	52.0	5.00	61.0	un	5.03	770	460	870	240.0	64	8.2	3.80	6.90	0.29	0.06	37.0
13-1-202	较大婴儿配方奶粉 (安婴宝, 美赞臣)	2.10	52.0	4.90	60.0	un	5.03	790	620	880	250.0	63	8.3	5.00	—	0.27	0.07	46.0
13-1-203	较大婴儿配方奶粉 (安婴宝A+, 美赞臣)	2.70	75.0	5.40	91.0	un	5.17	530	410	720	186.0	51	8.0	5.00	—	0.38	0.10	104.0
13-1-204	较大婴儿配方奶粉 (健儿乐, 惠氏)	1.90	56.0	2.47	63.0	un	5.17	810	493	880	264.0	62	7.0	4.20	—	(0.30)[5]	(0.08)[8]	(90.0)[10]
13-1-205	较大婴儿配方奶粉 (健儿乐, 惠氏, 金装)	1.90	56.0	2.47	63.0	un	5.17	810	493	880	264.0	62	7.0	4.20	(9.50)[3]	(0.30)[5]	(0.08)[8]	(90.0)[10]
13-1-206	较大婴儿配方奶粉 (可淇牌)	1.04	26.0	3.12	52.0	3.12	un	360	180	950	450.0	30	8.5	5.00	—	0.46	—	90.0
13-1-207	较大婴儿配方奶粉 (美素乐2)	1.50	73.0	5.70	88.0	8.70	un	480	355	635	185.0	55	7.3	4.70	12.00	0.47	0.48	53.0
13-1-208	较大婴儿配方奶粉 (美素乐, 全能装)	1.00	73.0	5.70	88.0	un	5.84	555	410	635	230.0	55	7.3	4.70	—	0.47	0.06	53.0
13-1-209	较大婴儿配方奶粉 (美素乐, 袋装)	1.00	73.0	5.70	88.0	un	5.84	555	410	635	230.0	55	7.3	4.70	—	0.47	0.06	53.0
13-1-210	较大婴幼儿配方奶粉 (吉利蜜2, 森永牌)	2.00	100.0	6.00	50.0	un	3.36	600	350	820	250.0	45	7.0	(5.00)[1]	—	(0.46)[6]	—	(90.0)[10]
13-1-211	较大婴幼儿配方奶粉 (力多精2, 雀巢)	0.93	140.0	0.93	—	3.70	un	770	590	1130	330.0	84	7.9	5.60	6.30	0.56	0.06	(90.0)[10]
13-1-212	较大婴儿配方奶粉 (圣元牌)	2.00	50.0	4.00	70.0	un	2.68	600	427	790	290.0	58	6.7	5.00	15.50	0.33	0.15	50.0

1. 锌含量范围: 3.00～7.00mg/100g
2. 硒含量范围: 6.20～12.70μg/100g
3. 硒含量范围: 6.00～13.00μg/100g
4. 铜含量范围: 0.31～0.61mg/100g
5. 铜含量范围: 0.18～0.42mg/100g
6. 铜含量范围: 0.16～0.75mg/100g
7. 锰含量范围: 0.11～0.31mg/100g
8. 锰含量范围: 0.04～0.13mg/100g
9. 碘含量范围: 31.0～150.0μg/100g
10. 碘含量范围: 30.0～150.0μg/100g

婴幼儿食品 Infant foods

(以每 100g 可食部计)

编码 Code	食物名称 Food name	食部 Edible	水分 Water	能量 Energy		蛋白质 Protein	脂肪 Fat	碳水化合物 CHO	膳食纤维 (Dietary fiber)			胆固醇 Cholesterol	灰分 Ash	维生素 A		硫胺素 Thiamin	核黄素 Riboflavin	维生素 B_6 Vit B_6
									总 Total	可溶性 Soluble	不溶性 Insoluble			Vit A	胡萝卜素 Carotene			
		%	g	kcal	kJ	g	g	g	g	g	g	mg	g	μgRE	μg	mg	mg	mg
13-1-213	较大婴幼儿奶粉 (高钙, 圣元牌)	100	—	483	2019	15.0	22.5	55.0	—	—	—	—	—	475	—	0.40	0.60	0.40
13-1-214	较大婴幼儿配方奶粉 (完达山牌)	100	—	454	1899	18.0	18.0	55.0	—	—	—	—	4.5	540	—	0.50	0.80	0.30
13-1-301	幼儿奶粉 (爱力大 3, 美赞臣)	100	—	454[c]	1900	16.6	16.3	60.0	—	—	—	—	—	600	—	0.45	0.95	0.38
13-1-302	幼儿奶粉 (安儿宝, 美赞臣)	100	—	447[c]	1870	17.8	15.0	61.0	—	—	—	—	—	501	—	0.40	0.65	0.34
13-1-303	幼儿奶粉 (安儿宝 A+, 美赞臣)	100	—	450[c]	1881	17.8	15.0	61.0	—	—	—	—	—	501	—	0.40	0.65	0.34
13-1-304	幼儿奶粉 (惠氏)	100	—	454	1925	15.8	15.8	62.1	—	—	—	—	—	378	95	0.41	0.72	0.45
13-1-305	幼儿奶粉 (惠氏, 金装)	100	—	456	1925	15.8	16.0	62.1	—	—	—	—	—	511	95	0.41	0.72	0.45
13-1-306	幼儿奶粉 (可淇牌)	100	4.0	462	1933	16.5	18.0	58.5	—	—	—	—	—	540	100	0.40	0.40	0.30
13-1-307	幼儿奶粉 (美素高)	100	2.8	440	1900	22.1	18.4	49.1	2.7	—	—	—	4.7	450	300	0.73	0.96	1.05
13-1-308	幼儿奶粉 (美素高, 全能装)	100	(3.0)[1]	448	1900	22.1	18.4	48.6	—	—	—	—	—	450	500	0.73	0.96	1.05
13-1-309	幼儿奶粉 (美素高, 袋装)	100	(3.0)[1]	450	1900	22.1	18.4	48.6	—	—	—	—	—	450	500	0.73	0.96	1.05
13-1-310	幼儿奶粉 (雀巢)	100	3.0	464	1941	21.6	19.0	51.6	—	—	—	—	4.8	557	—	0.97	1.10	—
13-1-311	幼儿奶粉 (雀巢金牌)	100	3.0	463	1940	18.5	18.0	56.8	—	—	—	—	4.2	560	—	0.97	1.10	—
13-1-312	幼儿奶粉 (森永牌)	100	3.0	458	1914	20.0	17.5	55.0	—	—	—	—	4.5	480	45	0.80	0.80	1.00
13-1-313	幼儿奶粉 (圣元牌)	100	—	453	1893	17.5	18.5	54.0	—	—	—	—	—	426	—	0.40	0.80	0.40
婴幼儿断乳期辅助食品																		
13-2-001	胡萝卜苹果泥 (亨氏)	100	89.0	39	162	0.5	0.1	10.1	1.1	—	—	—	0.3	301	1807	0.01	0.02	—
13-2-002	鸡肝蔬菜泥 (亨氏)	100	82.5	76	319	4.0	2.2	10.7	0.6	—	—	—	0.6	1192	—	0.04	0.21	—
13-2-003	香甜胡萝卜泥 (亨氏)	100	90.7	27	114	1.0	0.2	7.6	2.2	—	—	—	0.5	1014	6085	0.02	0.03	—

1. 水分含量范围: ≤ 3.0g/100g

婴幼儿食品 Infant foods

(以每100g可食部计)

编码 Code	食物名称 Food name	维生素 B_{12} Vit B_{12} μg	叶酸 Folate μg	烟酸 Niacin mg	维生素C Vit C mg	维生素E (Vit E) Total mg	α-TE mg	钙 Ca mg	磷 P mg	钾 K mg	钠 Na mg	镁 Mg mg	铁 Fe mg	锌 Zn mg	硒 Se μg	铜 Cu mg	锰 Mn mg	碘 I μg
13-1-213	较大婴幼儿奶粉 (高钙, 圣元牌)	1.00	50.0	4.00	—	un	2.68	700	400	721	246.0	41	6.7	5.00	—	0.33	0.05	50.0
13-1-214	较大婴幼儿配方奶粉 (完达山牌)	1.50	38.0	4.00	40.0	un	3.36	600	520	800	300.0	65	8.5	5.00	—	0.42	0.04	80.0
13-1-301	幼儿奶粉 (爱力大3, 美赞臣)	2.50	57.0	5.20	63.0	un	5.30	830	430	870	230.0	63	7.5	4.60	9.20	0.39	0.07	44.0
13-1-302	幼儿奶粉 (安儿宝, 美赞臣)	2.70	54.0	5.40	45.0	un	5.10	750	470	900	250.0	67	8.0	4.50	—	0.40	0.05	31.0
13-1-303	幼儿奶粉 (安儿宝A+, 美赞臣)	2.70	54.0	5.40	45.0	un	5.10	750	480	900	250.0	67	8.1	4.50	—	0.40	0.05	31.0
13-1-304	幼儿奶粉 (惠氏)	1.80	(37.0)[1]	5.20	54.0	un	3.77	450	360	811	212.0	50	6.8	4.50	—	(0.48)[3]	(0.50)[5]	(90.0)[6]
13-1-305	幼儿奶粉 (惠氏, 金装)	1.80	28.0	5.20	54.0	un	3.77	450	360	811	212.0	50	6.8	4.50	—	(0.48)[3]	(0.50)[5]	(84.5)[7]
13-1-306	幼儿奶粉 (可淇牌)	2.00	40.0	3.00	50.0	5.00	un	750	417	700	320.0	45	9.0	5.00	—	0.45	—	100.0
13-1-307	幼儿奶粉 (美素高)	2.40	50.0	9.25	115.0	un	6.17	890	740	930	270.0	90	10.0	6.00	10.00	0.28	1.00	80.0
13-1-308	幼儿奶粉 (美素高, 全能装)	2.40	50.0	9.30	115.0	9.20	un	890	740	930	270.0	90	10.0	6.00	10.00	0.28	1.00	80.0
13-1-309	幼儿奶粉 (美素高, 袋装)	2.40	50.0	9.30	115.0	9.20	un	890	740	930	270.0	90	8.0	6.00	10.00	0.28	1.00	80.0
13-1-310	幼儿奶粉 (雀巢)	0.90	140.0	1.40	71.0	5.60	un	780	640	1010	305.0	70	8.3	14.00	—	0.19	0.03	(90.0)[6]
13-1-311	幼儿奶粉 (雀巢金牌)	0.93	140.0	1.40	71.0	5.60	un	720	552	865	275.0	60	8.3	14.00	—	0.19	0.03	(90.0)[6]
13-1-312	幼儿奶粉 (森永牌)	2.00	100.0	10.00	45.0	un	6.04	700	410	960	290.0	70	8.0	(5.00)[2]	—	(0.46)[4]	—	(90.0)[6]
13-1-313	幼儿奶粉 (圣元牌)	2.00	50.0	4.00	70.0	un	2.68	600	517	859	300.0	61	6.7	5.00	15.50	0.33	0.15	50.0
	婴幼儿断乳期辅助食品																	
13-2-001	胡萝卜苹果泥 (亨氏)	—	4.9	0.28	94.0	—	—	6	13	92	42.7	6	0.2	0.17	Tr	0.14	0.23	—
13-2-002	鸡肝蔬菜泥 (亨氏)	—	71.9	1.09	—	Tr	Tr	22	118	119	51.4	9	1.2	0.71	6.12	0.04	0.40	—
13-2-003	香甜胡萝卜泥 (亨氏)	—	23.2	0.66	64.0	—	—	10	23	132	110.2	4	0.3	0.18	Tr	0.03	0.19	—

1. 叶酸含量范围: 21.0～52.0μg/100g
2. 锌含量范围: 3.00～7.00mg/100g
3. 铜含量范围: 0.32～0.63mg/100g
4. 铜含量范围: 0.16～0.75mg/100g
5. 锰含量范围: 0.41～0.59mg/100g
6. 碘含量范围: 30.0～150.0μg/100g
7. 碘含量范围: 34.0～135.0μg/100g

婴幼儿食品 Infant foods

(以每100g可食部计)

编码 Code	食物名称 Food name	食部 Edible	水分 Water	能量 Energy		蛋白质 Protein	脂肪 Fat	碳水化合物 CHO	膳食纤维 (Dietary fiber) 总 Total	膳食纤维 (Dietary fiber) 可溶性 Soluble	膳食纤维 (Dietary fiber) 不溶性 Insoluble	胆固醇 Cholesterol	灰分 Ash	维生素A Vit A	维生素A 胡萝卜素 Carotene	硫胺素 Thiamin	核黄素 Riboflavin	维生素B_6 Vit B_6
		%	g	kcal	kJ	g	g	g	g	g	g	mg	g	μgRE	μg	mg	mg	mg
婴幼儿补充食品																		
13-3-009	米粉 (雀巢)	100	—	376	1574	6.1	2.5	83.9	—	—	1.6	—	3.1	300	—	0.70	0.40	—
13-3-010	米粉 (高蛋白, 雀巢)	100	2.5	409	1711	15.0	9.0	67.0	—	—	—	—	3.9	300	—	0.65	0.60	—
13-3-011	米粉 (高蛋白, 亨氏)	100	3.1	375	1570	15.7	2.0	75.9	2.3	—	—	—	3.3	1131	—	0.52	0.70	—
13-3-012	米粉 (苹果, 雀巢)	100	2.5	374	1566	5.4	2.8	81.9	—	—	—	—	3.5	300	—	0.70	0.40	—
13-3-013	米粉 (蔬菜, 亨氏)	100	3.0	394	1649	10.0	3.0	81.8	—	—	—	—	2.2	379	—	0.50	0.50	0.40
13-3-014	米粉 (蔬菜, 雀巢)	100	2.5	373	1561	6.7	3.2	79.4	—	—	—	—	3.3	300	—	0.70	0.40	—
13-3-015	米粉 (胡萝卜, 亨氏)	100	3.5	386	1616	5.0	1.5	88.2	—	—	—	—	1.8	379	—	0.50	0.50	0.30
13-3-016	米粉 (胡萝卜, 雀巢)	100	2.5	374	1564	6.4	4.1	77.8	—	—	—	—	3.5	300	—	0.70	0.40	—
13-3-017	米粉 (番茄, 亨氏)	100	3.0	391	1635	6.2	2.0	87.0	—	—	—	—	1.8	379	—	0.50	0.50	0.30
13-3-018	米粉 (猪肝蔬菜, 亨氏)	100	3.5	391	1636	10.0	3.0	81.0	—	—	—	—	2.5	379	—	0.50	0.50	0.40
13-3-019	米粉 (鱼肉蔬菜, 亨氏)	100	3.5	383	1603	14.5	1.5	77.9	—	—	—	—	2.6	379	—	0.50	0.50	0.50
13-3-020	麦粉 (蜂蜜, 雀巢)	100	3.0	376	1574	8.4	3.4	80.2	—	—	2.2	—	3.1	300	—	0.70	0.40	—

婴幼儿食品 Infant foods

(以每100g可食部计)

编码 Code	食物名称 Food name	维生素 B_{12} Vit B_{12} μg	叶酸 Folate μg	烟酸 Niacin mg	维生素C Vit C mg	维生素E (Vit E) Total mg	α-TE mg	钙 Ca mg	磷 P mg	钾 K mg	钠 Na mg	镁 Mg mg	铁 Fe mg	锌 Zn mg	硒 Se μg	铜 Cu mg	锰 Mn mg	碘 I μg
婴幼儿补充食品																		
13-3-009	米粉 (雀巢)	0.80	22.0	0.30	35.0	3.70	un	600	470	1000	10.0	—	8.0	5.50	—	—	—	20.0
13-3-010	米粉 (高蛋白, 雀巢)	1.15	35.0	0.40	30.0	3.30	un	600	500	835	164.0	—	8.0	5.50	—	—	—	50.0
13-3-011	米粉 (高蛋白, 亨氏)	—	42.8	4.50	—	4.00	un	669	687	581	30.2	64	9.0	4.75	4.08	0.37	0.36	—
13-3-012	米粉 (苹果, 雀巢)	0.75	22.0	0.30	35.0	3.70	un	585	460	1130	15.0	—	8.0	5.50	—	—	—	20.0
13-3-013	米粉 (蔬菜, 亨氏)	1.20	—	4.00	—	5.00	un	550	380	—	—	—	10.0	4.00	—	—	—	—
13-3-014	米粉 (蔬菜, 雀巢)	0.75	22.0	0.30	35.0	3.70	un	585	430	1100	20.0	—	8.0	5.50	—	—	—	20.0
13-3-015	米粉 (胡萝卜, 亨氏)	1.00	—	4.00	—	5.00	un	400	280	—	—	—	10.0	4.00	—	—	—	—
13-3-016	米粉 (胡萝卜, 雀巢)	0.75	22.0	0.30	35.0	3.70	un	585	460	1100	40.0	—	8.0	5.50	—	—	—	20.0
13-3-017	米粉 (番茄, 亨氏)	1.00	—	4.00	—	5.00	un	400	280	—	—	—	10.0	4.00	—	—	—	—
13-3-018	米粉 (猪肝蔬菜, 亨氏)	1.20	—	4.00	—	5.00	un	600	420	—	—	—	15.0	5.60	—	—	—	—
13-3-019	米粉 (鱼肉蔬菜, 亨氏)	1.20	—	4.50	—	5.00	un	680	480	—	—	—	10.0	4.00	—	—	—	—
13-3-020	麦粉 (蜂蜜, 雀巢)	0.75	22.0	0.30	35.0	3.70	un	610	455	1000	2.0	—	8.0	5.50	—	—	—	20.0

Notes

小吃、甜饼

Ethnic Foods and Cakes

本类食物是指各种传统的特色或风味小吃和甜点。小吃包括京八件、炒肝、凉皮等；甜点包括月饼、蛋糕及各种酥饼等。

这些食物由于受地域、民族和市场因素的影响，在配方和成分上存在很大的不固定性。

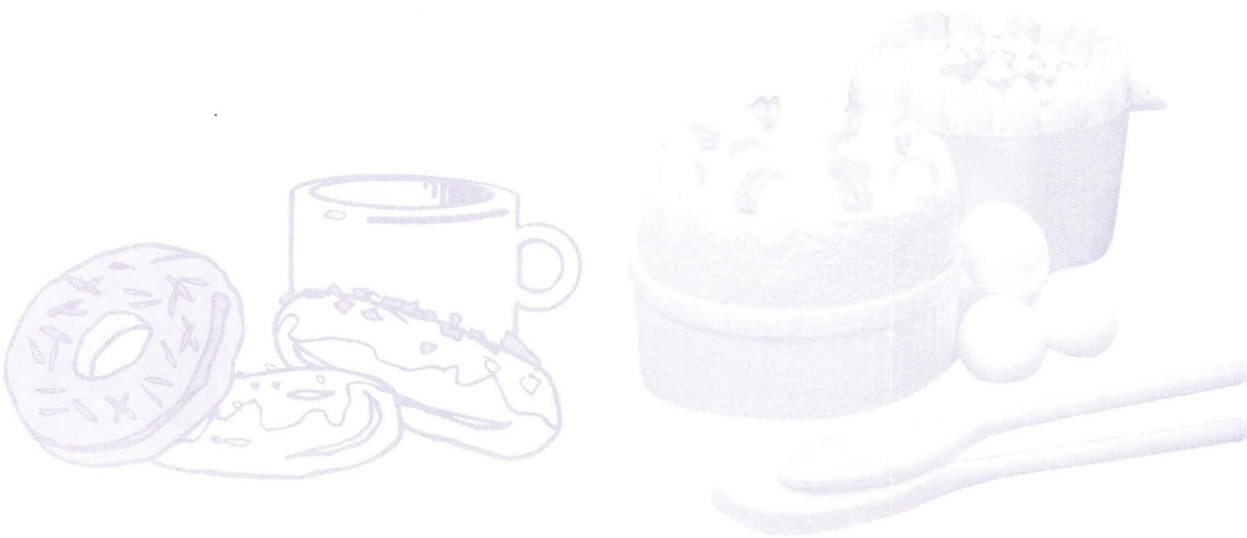

小吃、甜饼 Ethnic foods and cakes

(以每100g可食部计)

编码 Code	食物名称 Food name	食部 Edible %	水分 Water g	能量 Energy kcal	能量 Energy kJ	蛋白质 Protein g	脂肪 Fat g	碳水化合物 CHO g	膳食纤维 (Dietary fiber) 总 Total g	可溶性 Soluble g	不溶性 Insoluble g	胆固醇 Cholesterol mg	灰分 Ash g	维生素 A Vit A μgRE	胡萝卜素 Carotene μg	硫胺素 Thiamin mg	核黄素 Riboflavin mg	维生素B_6 Vit B_6 mg
小吃																		
14-1-038	春卷 (素馅)	100	55.2	182	762	4.9	4.6	33.8	3.5	—	—	—	1.5	—	—	0.04	0.03	0.05
14-1-039	黑芝麻汤圆	100	37.2	311	1300	4.4	13.8	44.2	2.0	—	—	4	0.4	—	—	0.04	0.03	0.06
14-1-040	醪糟	100	74.7	100	418	2.6	0.2	22.4	0.5	—	—	—	0.1	(0)	(0)	0.02	0.02	—
14-1-041	煎饼	100	16.0	317	1327	9.5	3.5	70.0	8.1	—	—	—	1.0	—	—	0.26	0.06	—
14-1-042	过桥米线	100	79.4	92	385	4.0	3.8	11.8	—	—	1.4	6	1.0	12	73	0.12	Tr	—
蛋糕、甜点																		
14-2-108	蛋糕 (巧克力)	100	24.1	437	1828[c]	4.7	30.4	40.2	—	—	0.2[b]	—	0.6	78	51	0.03	0.10	—
14-2-109	蛋糕 (水果)	100	25.3	347	1452[c]	2.9	9.1	61.6	—	—	—	—	1.0	4	—	0.05	0.10	—
14-2-209	月饼 (蛋黄)	100	23.0	399	1669	6.0	20.0	50.2	1.5	—	—	—	0.8	45	—	0.05	0.13	0.11
14-2-210	月饼 (豆沙)	100	22.3	325	1362	5.4	6.9	64.8	4.4	—	—	—	0.6	Tr	Tr	0.02	0.03	—
14-2-211	月饼 (桂花板栗)	100	20.8	331	1386	5.7	6.6	66.3	4.0	—	—	—	0.6	43	Tr	0.02	0.05	—
14-2-212	月饼 (奶油莲芸)	100	20.5	361	1510	5.5	13.0	60.4	—	—	4.9[a]	—	0.6	12	Tr	0.03	0.03	—
14-2-332	沙琪玛蛋酥	100	8.0	506	2116	5.9	30.4	55.1	3.0	—	—	—	0.6	Tr	—	0.03	0.05	—
14-2-333	香橙水果馅饼	100	10.7	445	1864	4.8	19.0	64.2	—	—	0.4[a]	—	1.3	18	—	—	—	—

小吃、甜饼 Ethnic foods and cakes

(以每100g可食部计)

编码 Code	食物名称 Food name	维生素B_{12} Vit B_{12} μg	叶酸 Folate μg	烟酸 Niacin mg	维生素C Vit C mg	维生素E (Vit E) Total mg	α-TE mg	钙 Ca mg	磷 P mg	钾 K mg	钠 Na mg	镁 Mg mg	铁 Fe mg	锌 Zn mg	硒 Se μg	铜 Cu mg	锰 Mn mg	碘 I μg
小吃																		
14-1-038	春卷(素馅)	Tr	7.2	0.33	—	3.59	un	31	54	171	535.8	7	0.7	0.46	3.84	0.05	0.12	—
14-1-039	黑芝麻汤圆	Tr	8.2	1.23	—	2.09	un	69	71	102	23.2	19	1.6	1.31	2.34	0.20	0.28	3.5
14-1-040	醪糟	—	11.3	Tr	—	—	—	1	10	12	19.0	3	0.1	0.39	0.57	0.02	0.11	—
14-1-041	煎饼	Tr	22.6	1.42	—	1.69	un	46	221	240	18.1	62	3.6	1.43	6.02	0.11	0.27	7.9
14-1-042	过桥米线	—	—	0.60	3.0	—	—	13	35	38	310.4	8	0.2	0.31	0.23	0.04	0.06	—
蛋糕、甜点																		
14-2-108	蛋糕(巧克力)	—	—	0.20	0	un	1.01	41	87	66	129.0	—	0.7	—	—	—	—	—
14-2-109	蛋糕(水果)	—	—	0.80	Tr	un	1.06	33	52	153	270.0	—	2.1	—	—	—	—	—
14-2-209	月饼(蛋黄)	—	46.1	Tr	—	6.36	un	35	170	223	108.8	19	2.0	0.97	10.80	0.17	0.23	—
14-2-210	月饼(豆沙)	—	16.4	Tr	—	7.02	un	16	108	262	79.4	28	1.6	0.71	2.00	0.14	0.26	—
14-2-211	月饼(桂花板栗)	—	6.4	—	—	3.19	un	46	89	186	104.0	15	1.7	0.76	1.98	0.31	0.21	—
14-2-212	月饼(奶油莲芸)	—	—	0.90	1.0	2.68	un	23	110	153	27.6	21	1.5	0.67	0.40	0.24	1.29	—
14-2-332	沙琪玛蛋酥	—	4.3	0.30	—	3.61	3.02	6	30	155	114.2	5	0.7	0.28	5.05	0.02	0.02	—
14-2-333	香橙水果馅饼	—	—	—	8.1	—	—	53	—	—	300.0	—	1.0	—	—	—	—	—

Notes

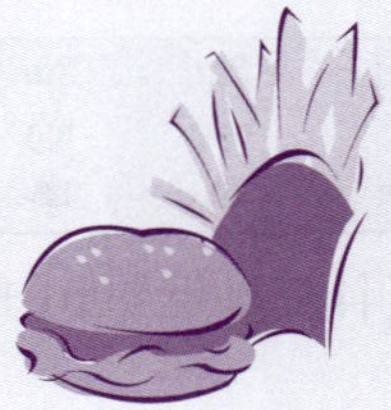

速食食品

Fast Foods

速食食品的定义和范围尚不明确，分类也不统一。本节参考了国内外的定义，分为以下3个亚类。

1. 快餐食品：通常是由几种食物组成的、作为主食的方便食品。如中国特有的快餐和国外的麦当劳、肯德基、比萨饼等。

2. 方便食品：一般是指部分或完全加工成熟食、食用前只需稍微处理或完全不处理即可食用的食品。食品工业中的速食米饭、方便面、方便粥、早餐谷物、冷冻饺子、春卷、饮料、饼干、面包（糕点）、罐头食品等均属于此类食品。

3. 休闲食品：常指传统意义上的零食类速食食品。没有统一分类，按其原料可分为谷物膨化类、果仁类、瓜子类炒货、糖制品、果蔬类、鱼肉类等。

为避免交叉，一些食物如饮料、各种罐头、蛋糕、瓜子、糖制品、鱼肉干等已归到其它相关联的类别中，这里不在重复。

速食食品 Fast foods

(以每100g可食部计)

编码 Code	食物名称 Food name	食部 Edible %	水分 Water g	能量 Energy kcal	能量 Energy kJ	蛋白质 Protein g	脂肪 Fat g	碳水化合物 CHO g	膳食纤维 (Dietary fiber) 总 Total g	可溶性 Soluble g	不溶性 Insoluble g	胆固醇 Cholesterol mg	灰分 Ash g	维生素A Vit A μgRE	胡萝卜素 Carotene μg	硫胺素 Thiamin mg	核黄素 Riboflavin mg	维生素B_6 Vit B_6 mg
快餐食品																		
15-1-001	鸡柳汉堡(肯德基)	100	46.5	269	1126	13.9	13.6	23.8	—	—	1.0[a]	—	2.2	—	—	—	—	—
15-1-002	香芋甜心(肯德基)	100	36.7	280	1169	2.8	7.5	51.8	—	—	1.6	31	1.2	Tr	—	0.08	0.02	0.13
15-1-003	鸡肉汉堡(肯德基)	100	43.3	292	1220	7.9	16.3	31.0	—	—	2.7	51	1.5	44	—	0.07	0.05	0.06
15-1-004	鸡肉卷(肯德基)	100	49.2	253	1057	10.1	13.1	25.2	—	—	1.6	49	2.4	64	—	0.15	0.09	0.07
15-1-005	上校鸡块(肯德基)	100	46.5	261	1092	16.9	12.5	21.1	—	—	0.9[a]	—	3.0	10	—	—	—	—
15-1-006	辣鸡翅(肯德基)	67	41.3	337	1411	19.4	23.6	12.8	—	—	1.0[a]	—	2.9	82	—	—	—	—
15-1-007	新奥尔良鸡翅(肯德基)	70	54.1	240	1003	22.1	13.8	6.8	—	—	—	125	3.2	332	—	0.05	0.08	0.16
15-1-008	劲爆鸡米花(肯德基)	100	44.0	302	1262	18.4	18.9	16.2	—	—	1.7	68	2.5	68	—	0.07	0.11	0.09
15-1-009	甜玉米籽粒(肯德基)	100	67.2	119	496	3.2	0.2	28.6	—	—	2.6[a]	—	0.8	—	—	—	—	—
15-1-010	薯条(肯德基)	100	37.7	298	1248	4.3	15.5	40.5	—	—	5.1[a]	—	2.0	—	—	—	—	—
15-1-011	比萨饼(夹奶酪)	100	47.8	225	941	12.2	5.1	32.5	—	—	—	15	2.4	117	—	0.29	0.26	0.07
15-1-012	比萨饼(夹奶酪、肉和蔬菜)	100	47.7	235	982	16.5	6.8	27.0	—	—	—	26	2.1	74	—	0.27	0.22	0.12
15-1-013	三明治(夹火腿、干酪)	100	50.8	244	1021[c]	14.2	10.6	22.9	—	—	0.1[b]	—	1.6	52	—	0.21	0.33	—
15-1-014	三明治(夹鸡蛋、干酪)	100	56.3	234	979[c]	10.7	13.3	17.8	—	—	0.2[b]	—	2.0	124	—	0.18	0.39	—
15-1-015	三明治(夹鸡肉片，无调料酱)	100	47.3	284	1187	13.3	16.2	21.3	—	—	—	33	2.0	17	—	0.18	0.13	0.11
15-1-016	三明治(夹烤牛肉片)	100	48.6	247	1034	15.5	9.9	24.1	—	—	—	37	1.9	8	—	0.27	0.22	0.19
15-1-017	三明治(夹鱼肉片)	100	47.4	276	1155[c]	10.7	14.4	26.0	—	—	0.4[b]	—	1.6	19	—	0.21	0.14	—
15-1-018	干酪汉堡包(夹熏肉，加调料酱)	100	43.6	311	1303	16.4	18.9	19.0	—	—	—	57	2.1	42	—	0.16	0.21	0.16
15-1-019	干酪汉堡包(普通型，夹单层肉饼，无调料酱)	100	37.3	316	1323	14.5	14.9	31.1	—	—	—	49	2.2	45	—	0.39	0.39	0.09

速食食品 Fast foods

(以每100g可食部计)

编码 Code	食物名称 Food name	维生素 B_{12} Vit B_{12} μg	叶酸 Folate μg	烟酸 Niacin mg	维生素C Vit C mg	维生素E (Vit E) Total mg	维生素E (Vit E) α-TE mg	钙 Ca mg	磷 P mg	钾 K mg	钠 Na mg	镁 Mg mg	铁 Fe mg	锌 Zn mg	硒 Se μg	铜 Cu mg	锰 Mn mg	碘 I μg
快餐食品																		
15-1-001	鸡柳汉堡(肯德基)	—	—	—	Tr	—	—	16	—	—	350.2	—	1.3	—	—	—	—	—
15-1-002	香芋甜心(肯德基)	1.90	1.2	0.54	—	0.38	0.38	12	80	229	194.5	14	0.8	0.98	—	0.11	0.61	—
15-1-003	鸡肉汉堡(肯德基)	1.90	4.1	1.58	Tr	14.96	un	22	92	102	489.7	14	0.7	0.52	—	0.06	0.24	—
15-1-004	鸡肉卷(肯德基)	1.60	19.9	2.25	Tr	6.16	un	34	101	131	816.1	14	1.3	0.56	—	0.06	0.24	—
15-1-005	上校鸡块(肯德基)	—	—	—	—	—	—	32	—	—	370.6	—	1.6	—	—	—	—	—
15-1-006	辣鸡翅(肯德基)	—	—	—	—	—	—	16	—	—	499.3	—	1.6	—	—	—	—	—
15-1-007	新奥尔良鸡翅(肯德基)	2.00	—	3.41	—	0.52	0.41	13	189	160	1263.3	12	0.9	1.39	—	0.10	0.05	—
15-1-008	劲爆鸡米花(肯德基)	1.70	2.8	3.96	—	2.62	1.99	6	166	218	895.3	16	0.8	1.38	—	0.08	0.16	—
15-1-009	甜玉米籽粒(肯德基)	—	—	—	2.9	—	—	8	—	—	11.5	—	0.9	—	—	—	—	—
15-1-010	薯条(肯德基)	—	—	—	—	—	—	31	—	—	58.2	—	2.1	—	—	—	—	—
15-1-011	比萨饼(夹奶酪)	0.53	55.0	3.94	2.0	—	—	185	179	174	533.0	25	0.9	1.29	21.40	0.13	0.37	—
15-1-012	比萨饼(夹奶酪、肉和蔬菜)	0.46	41.0	2.48	2.0	—	—	128	166	226	484.0	23	1.9	1.41	13.80	0.15	0.15	—
15-1-013	三明治(夹火腿、干酪)	—	—	1.80	2.0	—	—	89	104	199	528.0	—	2.2	—	—	—	—	—
15-1-014	三明治(夹鸡蛋、干酪)	—	—	1.40	1.0	—	—	154	207	129	551.0	—	2.0	—	—	—	—	—
15-1-015	三明治(夹鸡肉片，无调料酱)	0.21	55.0	3.74	4.9	—	—	33	128	194	526.0	19	2.6	1.03	22.20	0.13	0.26	—
15-1-016	三明治(夹烤牛肉片)	0.88	41.0	4.22	1.5	—	—	39	172	227	570.0	22	3.0	2.44	21.00	0.07	0.09	—
15-1-017	三明治(夹鱼肉片)	—	—	2.20	2.0	—	—	53	134	215	389.0	—	1.7	—	—	—	—	—
15-1-018	干酪汉堡包(夹熏肉，加调料酱)	1.20	44.0	3.40	1.1	—	—	83	205	170	535.0	23	2.4	3.50	16.90	0.08	0.17	—
15-1-019	干酪汉堡包(普通型，夹单层肉饼，无调料酱)	0.95	53.0	3.63	0	—	—	138	192	161	490.0	21	2.4	2.32	22.20	0.09	0.22	—

速食食品 Fast foods

(以每 100g 可食部计)

编码 Code	食物名称 Food name	食部 Edible	水分 Water	能量 Energy		蛋白质 Protein	脂肪 Fat	碳水化合物 CHO	膳食纤维 (Dietary fiber) 总 Total	可溶性 Soluble	不溶性 Insoluble	胆固醇 Cholesterol	灰分 Ash	维生素 A Vit A	胡萝卜素 Carotene	硫胺素 Thiamin	核黄素 Riboflavin	维生素B_6 Vit B_6
		%	g	kcal	kJ	g	g	g	g	g	g	mg	g	μgRE	μg	mg	mg	mg
15-1-020	干酪汉堡包 (普通型,夹奶酪、单层肉饼,加调料酱)	100	47.7	263	1101	14.1	12.5	23.5	—	—	—	33	2.2	76	—	0.22	0.20	0.10
15-1-021	干酪汉堡包 (普通型,夹奶酪、单层肉饼,加调料酱和蔬菜)	100	55.2	235	983	11.6	12.9	18.3	—	—	—	34	2.1	53	—	0.21	0.15	0.10
15-1-022	干酪汉堡包 (普通型,夹奶酪、双层肉饼,双层面包,加调料酱和蔬菜)	100	46.6	285	1191	13.0	15.5	23.3	—	—	—	41	1.6	34	—	0.25	0.19	0.12
15-1-023	汉堡包 (普通型,夹肉饼,加调料酱和蔬菜)	100	49.4	256	1073	11.7	12.3	24.8	—	—	—	24	1.8	4	—	0.21	0.18	0.11
15-1-024	热狗 (原味)	100	54.0	250	1044	10.6	14.8	18.4	—	—	—	45	2.2	0	—	0.24	0.28	0.05
方便食品																		
15-2-105	早餐奶	100	86.3	68	284	2.3	3.1	7.7	Tr	Tr	Tr	5	0.6	43	—	0.02	0.06	0.03
15-2-106	八宝粥 (康师傅牌)	100	84.5	81	340	1.5	4.4	9.4	0.5	—	—	Tr	0.2	—	—	0.01	0.01	—
15-2-107	八宝粥 (亲亲牌)	100	84.9	76	320	2.1	4.0	8.8	0.8	—	—	Tr	0.2	—	—	0.02	0.01	—
15-2-108	八宝粥 (同茂牌)	100	88.2	46	193	1.3	0.2	10.2	0.4	—	—	Tr	0.1	—	—	0.01	0.01	—
15-2-109	八宝粥 (娃哈哈牌)	100	84.3	64	266	1.7	0.9	12.8	0.6	—	—	Tr	0.3	—	—	0.01	0.01	—
15-2-110	八宝粥 (无糖,娃哈哈牌)	100	88.1	45	189	1.6	0.8	9.4	1.4	0.4	1.0	Tr	0.2	—	—	0.01	0.01	—
15-2-111	八宝粥 (椰树牌)	100	81.6	69	290	1.7	1.0	15.5	2.1	—	—	—	0.2	—	—	0.01	0.01	—
15-2-112	黑芝麻糊粉	100	2.3	408	1706	6.9	7.5	82.3	4.2	—	—	—	1.0	—	—	0.09	0.07	3.60
15-2-113	麦片	100	4.0	393	1642	6.5	9.7	76.3	6.5	—	—	—	3.5	—	—	0.18	0.23	0.20
15-2-114	麦片 (原味香奶)	100	1.8	406	1698	4.7	9.0	82.8	6.3	—	—	—	1.7	—	—	0.06	0.06	0.03
15-2-115	燕麦片	100	9.0	353	1478	14.4	9.7	65.3	13.2	—	—	—	1.6	—	—	0.55	0.11	—
15-2-116	燕麦片 (果仁,甜)	100	5.4	402	1682	8.9	11.1	73.5	6.9	—	—	—	1.1	—	—	0.29	0.07	—
15-2-117	苦荞麦片 (无糖)	100	4.3	411	1721	7.2	8.0	77.9	—	—	0.2[a]	—	2.6	—	—	0.30	0.16	—
15-2-118	玉米片	100	3.0	365	1528	7.0	0.8	86.0	3.5	—	—	0	3.2	537	—	1.30	1.53	1.80

速食食品 Fast foods

(以每100g可食部计)

编码 Code	食物名称 Food name	维生素B12 Vit B_{12} μg	叶酸 Folate μg	烟酸 Niacin mg	维生素C Vit C mg	维生素E (Vit E) Total mg	α-TE mg	钙 Ca mg	磷 P mg	钾 K mg	钠 Na mg	镁 Mg mg	铁 Fe mg	锌 Zn mg	硒 Se μg	铜 Cu mg	锰 Mn mg	碘 I μg
15-1-020	干酪汉堡包(普通型,夹奶酪、单层肉饼，加调料酱)	0.83	48.0	3.29	1.7	un	0.47	98	156	197	545.0	18	2.2	1.85	17.50	0.09	0.16	—
15-1-021	干酪汉堡包(普通型,夹奶酪、单层肉饼，加调料酱和蔬菜)	0.80	42.0	4.14	1.5	—	—	118	140	149	634.0	17	1.7	1.70	13.30	0.08	0.19	—
15-1-022	干酪汉堡包(普通型,夹奶酪、双层肉饼、双层面包,加调料酱和蔬菜)	0.91	40.0	3.66	1.2	un	0.87	74	153	171	404.0	16	2.1	1.81	17.30	0.07	0.12	—
15-1-023	汉堡包(普通型, 夹肉饼, 加调料酱和蔬菜)	0.80	47.0	3.35	1.5	—	—	57	113	206	458.0	20	2.4	1.87	18.70	0.09	0.23	—
15-1-024	热狗(原味)	0.52	49.0	3.72	0.1	—	—	24	99	146	684.0	13	2.4	2.02	26.50	0.08	0.09	—
方便食品																		
15-2-105	早餐奶	—	3.8	0.19	—	0.20	un	54	69	132	64.6	7	0.3	0.32	1.30	0.02	0.02	3.5
15-2-106	八宝粥(康师傅牌)	—	4.8	0.27	—	0.54	un	2	18	184	13.9	6	1.4	0.24	0.26	0.06	0.12	Tr
15-2-107	八宝粥(亲亲牌)	—	4.8	0.51	—	0.67	un	3	26	325	9.8	8	2.1	0.56	—	0.12	0.18	0.5
15-2-108	八宝粥(同茂牌)	—	4.6	0.20	—	0.26	un	2	16	173	8.6	3	1.3	0.33	0.14	0.06	0.16	0.7
15-2-109	八宝粥(娃哈哈牌)	—	3.3	0.22	—	0.41	un	4	22	181	12.2	6	0.9	0.27	0.24	0.04	0.09	1.2
15-2-110	八宝粥(无糖，娃哈哈牌)	—	7.8	0.27	—	0.54	un	11	34	195	4.7	9	1.0	0.41	Tr	0.06	0.06	1.1
15-2-111	八宝粥(椰树牌)	—	8.7	—	—	0.64	un	3	21	85	12.0	7	0.3	0.22	0.22	0.06	0.13	4.3
15-2-112	黑芝麻糊粉	—	23.2	0.90	—	5.64	un	104	113	133	38.1	53	2.8	0.71	1.62	0.20	0.25	—
15-2-113	麦片	—	14.0	2.21	—	—	—	756	397	576	318.4	72	3.1	1.94	5.92	0.28	2.38	6.8
15-2-114	麦片(原味香奶)	—	16.0	0.27	—	8.24	un	18	121	365	138.6	16	1.5	0.57	3.42	0.07	1.43	—
15-2-115	燕麦片	—	30.1	1.34	—	0.75	0.57	46	359	356	12.1	91	4.3	1.71	7.26	0.38	2.53	3.9
15-2-116	燕麦片(果仁，甜)	—	28.2	0.81	—	3.02	un	38	172	410	26.5	58	2.6	1.10	3.88	0.40	1.53	2.2
15-2-117	苦荞麦片(无糖)	—	—	—	—	1.50	un	470	450	420	120.0	110	4.1	2.10	—	0.16	—	—
15-2-118	玉米片	5.40	365.0	17.90	22.0	un	0.14	7	50	90	725.0	11	30.0	0.27	8.30	0.07	0.16	—

速食食品 Fast foods

（以每100g可食部计）

编码 Code	食物名称 Food name	食部 Edible %	水分 Water g	能量 Energy kcal	能量 Energy kJ	蛋白质 Protein g	脂肪 Fat g	碳水化合物 CHO g	膳食纤维 (Dietary fiber) 总 Total g	可溶性 Soluble g	不溶性 Insoluble g	胆固醇 Cholesterol mg	灰分 Ash g	维生素A Vit A μgRE	胡萝卜素 Carotene μg	硫胺素 Thiamin mg	核黄素 Riboflavin mg	维生素B_6 Vit B_6 mg
15-2-119	玉米片(低钠)	100	3.0	384	1608	7.7	0.3	88.8	1.1	—	—	0	0.2	10	—	0.01	0.18	0.06
15-2-202	鸡汁味干脆面(面饼+调味料)	100	2.3	505	2115	11.4	27.0	55.2	—	—	1.0	—	4.1	—	—	0.20	0.03	0.12
15-2-203	海鲜味方便面(面饼+调味料+油料)	100	6.2	451	1889	10.4	19.2	60.1	—	—	0.9	—	4.1	13	78	0.08	0.03	0.07
15-2-204	海鲜味方便面(面饼+调味料)	100	6.7	un	un	10.4	—	78.7	—	—	0.9	—	4.2	13	80	0.08	0.03	0.07
15-2-205	油料(海鲜味方便面)	100	0.3	un	un	10.2	—	89.5	(0)	(0)	(0)	—	—	2	11	Tr	Tr	Tr
15-2-206	红烧牛肉方便面(面饼+调味料+蔬菜+肉酱)	100	4.5	447	1869	10.2	17.9	62.6	1.4	—	—	—	4.8	79	475	0.24	0.04	0.08
15-2-207	红烧牛肉方便面(面饼+调味料+蔬菜)	100	3.8	un	un	10.4	—	81.4	—	—	—	—	4.4	79	475	0.25	0.04	0.08
15-2-208	肉酱(红烧牛肉方便面)	100	5.1	un	un	6.8	—	76.0	—	—	—	—	12.1	—	—	0.06	0.06	0.10
15-2-209	鳕鱼方便面(面饼+调味料+珍料+调味油+蔬菜)	100	5.0	470	1968	10.2	24.2	53.7	—	—	0.8	—	6.9	12	70	0.09	0.02	0.05
15-2-210	鳕鱼方便面(面饼+调味料+蔬菜)	100	2.4	un	un	10.2	—	80.5	—	—	1.3	—	6.9	13	80	0.16	0.03	0.08
15-2-211	油酱料(珍料+调味油料，鳕鱼方便面)	100	77.6	un	un	10.2	—	10.4	—	—	—	—	1.8	—	—	Tr	Tr	Tr
15-2-212	铁板牛肉炒面(面饼+汤料+蔬菜+调味酱)	100	6.0	438	1833	11.7	18.8	59.3	3.8	0.6	3.1	—	4.2	63	345	0.13	0.04	0.09
15-2-213	铁板牛肉炒面(面饼+汤料+蔬菜)	100	3.9	un	un	12.0	—	81.3	4.4	0.7	3.6	—	2.8	63	345	0.10	0.03	0.08
15-2-214	调味酱(铁板牛肉炒面)	100	8.0	un	un	10.1	—	68.8	(0)	(0)	(0)	—	13.1	—	—	0.29	0.10	0.13
15-2-215	玉米红烧牛肉味方便面(面饼+调味料+蔬菜+肉酱)	100	18.6	330	1380	5.8	4.1	68.5	—	—	1.1	—	3.0	—	—	0.29	0.04	0.10
15-2-216	玉米红烧牛肉味方便面(面饼+调味料+蔬菜)	100	22.6	un	un	6.0	—	68.3	—	—	—	—	3.1	—	—	0.03	0.04	—
15-2-217	肉酱(玉米红烧牛肉味方便面)	100	16.2	un	un	3.6	—	78.2	—	—	—	—	2.0	—	—	2.83	0.03	—

速食食品 Fast foods

(以每100g可食部计)

编码 Code	食物名称 Food name	维生素 B_{12} Vit B_{12} μg	叶酸 Folate μg	烟酸 Niacin mg	维生素C Vit C mg	维生素E (Vit E) Total mg	α-TE mg	钙 Ca mg	磷 P mg	钾 K mg	钠 Na mg	镁 Mg mg	铁 Fe mg	锌 Zn mg	硒 Se μg	铜 Cu mg	锰 Mn mg	碘 I μg
15-2-119	玉米片 (低钠)	0	33.0	0.42	0	un	0.14	43	49	73	10.0	13	2.2	0.27	5.10	0.09	0.08	—
15-2-202	鸡汁味干脆面 (面饼+调味料)	—	Tr	1.56	—	3.65	un	86	413	123	976.8	36	3.5	1.07	1.67	0.26	1.05	6.3
15-2-203	海鲜味方便面 (面饼+调味料+油料)	—	Tr	0.90	—	1.66	un	10	101	95	382.8	20	3.5	0.51	3.91	0.20	0.35	10.3
15-2-204	海鲜味方便面 (面饼+调味料)	—	Tr	0.89	—	1.17	un	11	104	99	396.7	21	3.6	0.53	4.05	0.21	0.36	10.7
15-2-205	油料 (海鲜味方便面)	—	Tr	—	—	15.63	un	—	—	—	—	—	—	—	—	—	—	—
15-2-206	红烧牛肉方便面 (面饼+调味料+蔬菜+肉酱)	—	11.6	0.94	—	3.12	un	22	124	128	465.5	24	2.6	0.75	6.99	0.23	0.62	25.1
15-2-207	红烧牛肉方便面 (面饼+调味料+蔬菜)	Tr	11.9	0.89	—	2.27	un	23	131	135	491.3	25	2.8	0.79	6.99	0.24	0.65	26.5
15-2-208	肉酱 (红烧牛肉方便面)	—	6.3	1.80	—	10.71	un	—	—	—	—	—	—	—	—	—	—	—
15-2-209	鳕鱼方便面 (面饼+调味料+珍料+调味油+蔬菜)	—	Tr	0.76	—	0.65	un	8	119	139	828.8	25	2.6	0.80	10.90	0.25	0.59	14.2
15-2-210	鳕鱼方便面 (面饼+调味料+蔬菜)	—	Tr	1.28	—	1.08	un	8	119	139	828.8	25	2.6	0.80	10.90	0.25	0.59	14.2
15-2-211	油酱料 (珍料+调味油料，鳕鱼方便面)	—	Tr	Tr	—	Tr	Tr	—	—	—	—	—	—	—	—	—	—	—
15-2-212	铁板牛肉炒面 (面饼+汤料+蔬菜+调味酱)	—	2.4	1.16	Tr	2.76	un	10	113	121	561.8	21	2.3	0.61	7.05	0.18	0.62	15.3
15-2-213	铁板牛肉炒面 (面饼+汤料+蔬菜)	Tr	2.8	1.15	Tr	1.39	un	12	130	139	596.4	24	2.6	0.70	8.14	0.21	0.71	17.6
15-2-214	调味酱 (铁板牛肉炒面)	—	Tr	1.21	Tr	11.70	un	—	—	—	—	—	—	—	—	—	—	—
15-2-215	玉米红烧牛肉味方便面 (面饼+调味料+蔬菜+肉酱)	—	0.2	0.28	—	—	—	57	224	69	673.7	71	8.5	0.86	1.10	0.06	0.89	—
15-2-216	玉米红烧牛肉味方便面 (面饼+调味料+蔬菜)	—	Tr	0.31	—	—	—	—	—	—	—	—	—	—	—	—	—	—
15-2-217	肉酱 (玉米红烧牛肉味方便面)	—	2.7	Tr	—	—	—	—	—	—	—	—	—	—	—	—	—	—

速食食品 Fast foods

(以每100g可食部计)

编码 Code	食物名称 Food name	食部 Edible %	水分 Water g	能量 Energy kcal	能量 Energy kJ	蛋白质 Protein g	脂肪 Fat g	碳水化合物 CHO g	膳食纤维 (Dietary fiber) 总 Total g	可溶性 Soluble g	不溶性 Insoluble g	胆固醇 Cholesterol mg	灰分 Ash g	维生素A Vit A μgRE	胡萝卜素 Carotene μg	硫胺素 Thiamin mg	核黄素 Riboflavin mg	维生素B_6 Vit B_6 mg
15-2-218	海鲜鸡汁味米线 (米线+调味料+蔬菜+肉酱)	100	58.1	167	699	4.5	1.0	35.5	—	—	0.5	—	0.9	—	—	0.01	0.01	Tr
15-2-219	海鲜鸡汁味米线 (米线+调味料+蔬菜)	100	58.8	un	un	3.9	—	37.2	—	—	0.5	—	0.1	—	—	0.01	0.01	—
15-2-220	肉酱 (海鲜鸡汁味米线)	100	7.9	un	un	7.2	—	69.0	—	—	—	—	15.9	—	—	0.01	0.02	—
15-2-221	冬菜虾仁馄饨	100	58.9	180	753[c]	9.1	4.3	26.5	2.3	—	—	44	1.2	1	—	0.08	0.06	0.01
15-2-222	韭菜合子	100	59.7	211	883[c]	7.5	11.3	20.3	1.4	—	—	36	1.2	219	—	0.04	0.04	0.03
15-2-223	糯米饭团	100	37.0	333	1393[c]	5.9	17.6	38.3	1.1	—	—	(0)	1.2	13	—	0.06	0.02	0.06
15-2-224	什锦炒饭	100	58.7	188	787[c]	5.0	5.6	29.7	2.0	—	—	37	1.0	69	—	0.05	0.07	0.01
15-2-225	虾仁炒饭	100	64.8	138	577[c]	4.7	1.7	26.3	2.7	—	—	11	2.5	0	—	0.02	0.02	Tr
15-2-314	面包条 (白)	100	33.8	283	1184[c]	8.3	5.2	51.1	—	—	0.4[b]	—	1.6	2	12	0.13	0.05	—
15-2-315	面包屑	100	8.1	355	1485[c]	14.2	3.7	72.4	—	—	0.2[b]	—	1.6	0	0	0.13	0.03	—
15-2-316	葡萄干面包	100	38.0	260	1088[c]	6.6	3.7	50.1	—	—	0.2[b]	—	1.6	0	0	0.05	0.06	—
15-2-415	饼干 (三明治)	100	2.0	515	2156	7.1	30.4	57.9	4.6	—	—	—	2.6	127	652	0.10	0.17	—
15-2-416	饼干 (夹心)	100	1.4	449	1877	6.2	15.9	75.3	5.1	—	—	0	1.2	—	—	0.03	0.12	0.03
15-2-417	饼干 (甜酥夹心)	100	2.3	557	2329	5.6	35.1	55.6	—	—	1.0	—	1.4	—	—	0.08	0.07	0.04
15-2-418	饼干 (苏打夹心)	100	1.6	463	1936	7.6	19.3	69.8	5.2	—	—	—	1.7	—	—	0.06	0.11	—
15-2-419	饼干 (咸)	100	1.4	496	2075	8.4	25.6	62.7	4.7	—	—	5	1.9	26	—	0.05	0.07	0.03
15-2-420	曲奇饼 (加奶油)	100	1.5	526	2201	6.4	27.2	64.0	—	—	0.1[a]	—	1.0	8	—	—	—	—
15-2-421	早茶饼	100	3.4	440	1840	8.1	14.5	72.2	3.0	—	—	—	1.8	—	—	0.04	0.10	—
15-2-501	饺子 (素馅)	100	53.4	198	827	6.8	5.6	32.7	2.7	—	—	—	1.5	—	—	0.04	0.06	—
15-2-502	饺子 (三鲜馅)	100	50.7	240	1002	8.8	12.3	26.6	3.2	—	—	2	1.6	—	—	0.06	0.07	0.05
15-2-503	饺子 (猪肉白菜馅)	100	54.2	218	914	7.5	10.8	26.0	3.2	—	—	—	1.5	—	—	0.05	0.06	0.08
15-2-504	饺子 (猪肉韭菜馅)	100	51.2	250	1046	7.0	14.4	26.0	2.9	—	—	2	1.4	17	100	0.06	0.06	0.05

速食食品 Fast foods

(以每100g可食部计)

编码 Code	食物名称 Food name	维生素B_{12} Vit B_{12} μg	叶酸 Folate μg	烟酸 Niacin mg	维生素C Vit C mg	维生素E (Vit E) Total mg	维生素E (Vit E) α-TE mg	钙 Ca mg	磷 P mg	钾 K mg	钠 Na mg	镁 Mg mg	铁 Fe mg	锌 Zn mg	硒 Se μg	铜 Cu mg	锰 Mn mg	碘 I μg
15-2-218	海鲜鸡汁味米线 (米线+调味料+蔬菜+肉酱)	—	4.7	Tr	—	2.20	2.20	5	36	3	13.3	9	0.5	0.23	1.13	0.14	0.18	67.0
15-2-219	海鲜鸡汁味米线 (米线+调味料+蔬菜)	—	4.8	Tr	—	Tr	Tr	—	—	—	—	—	—	—	—	—	—	—
15-2-220	肉酱 (海鲜鸡汁味米线)	—	2.7	Tr	—	2.32	2.32	—	—	—	—	—	—	—	—	—	—	—
15-2-221	冬菜虾仁馄饨	0.33	—	1.10	0	un	0.30	33	90	127	316.0	20	1.1	0.60	—	—	—	—
15-2-222	韭菜合子	0.22	—	3.10	0	un	0.72	59	66	180	287.0	20	1.5	0.90	—	—	—	—
15-2-223	糯米饭团	0.44	—	0.80	0	un	0.76	15	78	86	393.0	22	0.6	0.70	—	—	—	—
15-2-224	什锦炒饭	0.06	—	0.60	4.5	un	0.60	23	62	57	220.0	9	0.4	0.50	—	—	—	—
15-2-225	虾仁炒饭	0.18	—	0.50	1.0	un	0.47	24	44	44	222.0	10	0.6	0.40	—	—	—	—
15-2-314	面包条 (白)	—	—	1.90	0	—	—	22	86	165	66.0	—	0.7	—	—	—	—	—
15-2-315	面包屑	—	—	1.30	0	—	—	29	111	107	535.0	—	0.9	—	—	—	—	—
15-2-316	葡萄干面包	—	—	0.60	0	—	—	42	75	190	370.0	—	1.2	—	—	—	—	—
15-2-415	饼干 (三明治)	—	32.6	0.60	—	7.69	3.20	178	180	291	408.3	19	1.7	0.48	2.66	0.13	0.28	8.3
15-2-416	饼干 (夹心)	—	14.8	0.40	—	3.41	un	45	77	242	303.4	18	1.3	0.38	2.37	0.11	0.18	3.4
15-2-417	饼干 (甜酥夹心)	—	4.9	0.73	—	5.29	un	17	84	114	324.0	13	3.0	0.24	4.93	0.18	0.30	7.4
15-2-418	饼干 (苏打夹心)	—	22.6	0.82	—	5.40	un	26	106	195	394.4	18	1.3	0.66	6.10	0.17	0.21	—
15-2-419	饼干 (咸)	—	19.5	0.68	—	3.82	un	16	82	223	697.2	15	2.0	0.64	4.21	0.14	0.39	Tr
15-2-420	曲奇饼 (加奶油)	—	—	—	Tr	—	—	70	—	—	140.0	—	1.0	—	—	—	—	—
15-2-421	早茶饼	—	4.5	0.63	—	—	—	61	77	144	436.0	13	1.3	0.58	2.90	0.10	0.45	—
15-2-501	饺子 (素馅)	—	13.1	0.29	—	1.54	un	74	76	147	449.2	21	0.5	0.42	6.44	0.07	0.10	17.3
15-2-502	饺子 (三鲜馅)	—	10.7	1.68	—	1.12	un	22	58	172	611.6	12	1.3	0.65	4.77	0.05	0.09	10.6
15-2-503	饺子 (猪肉白菜馅)	—	—	0.54	—	0.39	un	21	96	148	383.2	20	0.5	0.60	3.08	0.04	0.13	12.3
15-2-504	饺子 (猪肉韭菜馅)	—	—	0.54	—	0.57	un	26	81	176	397.6	21	1.3	0.59	4.16	0.04	0.21	9.3

速食食品 Fast foods

(以每100g可食部计)

编码 Code	食物名称 Food name	食部 Edible %	水分 Water g	能量 Energy kcal	能量 Energy kJ	蛋白质 Protein g	脂肪 Fat g	碳水化合物 CHO g	膳食纤维 (Dietary fiber) 总 Total g	可溶性 Soluble g	不溶性 Insoluble g	胆固醇 Cholesterol mg	灰分 Ash g	维生素A Vit A μgRE	胡萝卜素 Carotene μg	硫胺素 Thiamin mg	核黄素 Riboflavin mg	维生素B_6 Vit B_6 mg
15-2-505	饺子(猪肉芹菜馅)	100	52.6	253	1059	7.0	16.8	22.1	3.6	—	—	6	1.5	7	42	0.05	0.08	0.05
15-2-506	饺子(猪肉茴香馅)	100	51.1	223	932	7.3	9.1	31.1	3.2	—	—	8	1.4	—	—	0.05	0.08	0.05
15-2-507	饺子(猪肉香菇馅)	100	59.7	231	967[c]	12.3	15.3	11.5	1.1	—	—	39	1.2	14	—	0.29	0.12	0.18
15-2-508	饺子(猪肉虾仁馅)	100	50.4	267	1117[c]	10.0	15.4	22.7	1.1	—	—	31	1.5	77	—	0.23	0.07	0.22
15-2-509	饺子(鸡肉蘑菇馅)	100	61.0	186	778[c]	7.4	7.4	22.8	1.9	—	—	8	1.5	5	—	0.14	0.08	0.14
15-2-510	饺子(海鳗猪肉馅)	100	55.9	249	1042[c]	14.3	17.7	8.5	—	—	—	73	3.6	24	—	0.20	0.12	0.04
15-2-511	饺子(海鳗虾仁馅)	100	54.7	266	1113[c]	12.3	20.0	9.7	—	—	—	103	3.3	15	—	0.15	0.09	0.04
15-2-512	包子(三鲜馅)	100	53.6	223	935	7.4	8.6	29.1	—	—	—	—	1.3	—	—	0.04	0.07	0.05
15-2-513	包子(猪肉馅)	100	52.8	227	949	7.3	10.0	28.6	1.7	—	—	3	1.3	—	—	0.06	0.06	0.04
休闲食品																		
15-3-101	米饼(鸡蛋牛奶味)	100	1.7	536	2244	4.2	29.9	63.2	—	—	0.6	—	1.0	—	—	0.05	0.03	0.07
15-3-102	雪米饼	100	2.5	463	1936	5.5	17.6	73.5	2.9	—	—	—	0.9	—	—	0.02	0.02	—
15-3-103	蛋酥卷	100	2.1	523	2187	8.1	35.3	53.7	10.6	—	—	—	0.8	177	1063	0.02	0.15	—
15-3-104	巧克力派	100	11.1	425	1780	4.3	17.7	65.7	3.5	—	—	—	1.2	Tr	—	0.03	0.07	—
15-3-105	法式卷饼	100	2.0	535	2239	7.6	34.0	54.7	5.0	—	—	—	1.7	135	—	0.04	0.22	—
15-3-106	立体脆	100	2.6	475	1987	6.0	24.7	63.8	6.6	—	—	—	2.9	—	—	0.87	0.07	—
15-3-107	粟米脆	100	1.4	553	2312	5.6	34.7	56.5	2.0	—	—	—	1.8	—	—	0.05	0.04	—
15-3-108	通心脆	100	2.5	500	2092	3.1	29.6	61.6	6.3	—	—	—	3.2	—	—	0.04	0.04	—
15-3-109	洋葱圈	100	3.8	476	1990	4.3	21.3	68.5	1.8	0.2	1.5	—	2.1	Tr	—	0.31	0.04	0.09
15-3-201	虾片	100	2.3	523	2188	5.3	30.9	59.5	—	—	0.2	—	2.0	0	0	0.01	0	—
15-3-202	锅巴(豆香)	100	0.9	528	2210	7.6	30.6	59.2	3.6	—	—	—	1.7	107	—	0.03	0.04	0.05
15-3-203	锅巴(小米)	100	0.9	554	2318	6.0	36.9	54.6	5.1	—	—	—	1.6	114	—	0.11	0.05	—
15-3-204	海苔	100	5.0	177	740	29.4	4.8	50.4	46.4	15.0	31.4	56	10.4	1595	9573	0.24	0.93	—

速食食品 Fast foods

(以每100g可食部计)

编码 Code	食物名称 Food name	维生素B_{12} Vit B_{12} μg	叶酸 Folate μg	烟酸 Niacin mg	维生素C Vit C mg	维生素E (Vit E) Total mg	α-TE mg	钙 Ca mg	磷 P mg	钾 K mg	钠 Na mg	镁 Mg mg	铁 Fe mg	锌 Zn mg	硒 Se μg	铜 Cu mg	锰 Mn mg	碘 I μg
15-2-505	饺子(猪肉芹菜馅)	—	9.7	1.43	—	0.19	un	27	71	205	415.0	16	0.5	0.39	5.32	0.02	0.10	17.8
15-2-506	饺子(猪肉茴香馅)	—	14.7	0.48	—	0.67	un	12	79	163	335.6	11	0.6	0.44	4.12	0.01	0.04	10.9
15-2-507	饺子(猪肉香菇馅)	0.54	—	2.33	0	un	0.02	4	155	194	673.0	19	0.9	1.20	—	—	—	—
15-2-508	饺子(猪肉虾仁馅)	0.28	—	1.66	6.1	un	78.00	7	96	149	415.0	34	1.1	0.90	—	—	—	—
15-2-509	饺子(鸡肉蘑菇馅)	0.29	—	1.59	8.1	un	0.17	9	116	142	286.0	25	0.7	0.70	—	—	—	—
15-2-510	饺子(海鳗猪肉馅)	0.79	—	3.10	—	un	0.46	11	127	183	678.0	16	0.4	0.80	—	—	—	—
15-2-511	饺子(海鳗虾仁馅)	0.80	—	4.80	—	un	1.12	13	103	155	644.0	15	0.4	0.60	—	—	—	—
15-2-512	包子(三鲜馅)	—	11.3	1.55	—	1.79	un	—	—	—	—	—	—	—	—	—	—	—
15-2-513	包子(猪肉馅)	—	6.8	2.05	—	1.03	un	13	70	283	405.8	7	1.1	0.70	4.90	0.04	0.16	3.2
休闲食品																		
15-3-101	米饼(鸡蛋牛奶味)	—	5.1	0.44	—	3.91	3.35	6	65	34	191.6	7	1.4	0.40	2.86	0.14	0.56	Tr
15-3-102	雪米饼	0.10	3.5	0.44	—	—	—	6	26	29	241.3	2	0.3	0.49	0.89	0.11	3.04	—
15-3-103	蛋酥卷	—	10.4	0.45	—	—	—	18	106	150	144.9	8	2.0	0.84	10.36	0.12	0.83	—
15-3-104	巧克力派	—	Tr	0.25	—	5.24	2.05	48	121	144	273.8	23	19.0	0.52	4.12	0.16	0.56	—
15-3-105	法式卷饼	—	17.7	0.28	—	5.54	un	103	151	324	309.8	17	1.4	0.83	5.55	0.15	0.14	17.7
15-3-106	立体脆	—	25.5	1.45	—	—	—	56	191	268	596.7	72	2.5	1.32	2.80	0.15	0.75	—
15-3-107	粟米脆	—	8.0	—	—	—	—	168	46	53	465.2	9	0.9	0.10	1.13	0.10	0.23	—
15-3-108	通心脆	—	22.1	2.12	—	—	—	10	168	364	96.7	21	0.8	0.41	0.91	0.08	0.08	—
15-3-109	洋葱圈	—	15.6	0.64	—	1.50	un	131	70	125	519.0	18	2.4	0.42	2.32	0.22	0.42	2.5
15-3-201	虾片	—	—	0.40	0	—	—	47	60	96	407.0	—	0.5	—	—	—	—	—
15-3-202	锅巴(豆香)	—	25.0	—	—	9.11	5.28	13	84	264	239.3	22	2.7	0.97	1.55	0.20	0.42	14.8
15-3-203	锅巴(小米)	—	11.2	0.81	—	7.36	5.03	14	127	211	486.6	47	4.5	1.37	0.46	0.26	0.47	16.2
15-3-204	海苔	—	—	5.98	186.0	1.26	1.26	336	520	1774	1599.1	265	14.3	4.11	30.48	1.01	2.39	289.6

速食食品 Fast foods

(以每100g可食部计)

编码 Code	食物名称 Food name	食部 Edible	水分 Water	能量 Energy		蛋白质 Protein	脂肪 Fat	碳水化合物 CHO	膳食纤维 (Dietary fiber)			胆固醇 Cholesterol	灰分 Ash	维生素A		硫胺素 Thiamin	核黄素 Riboflavin	维生素B_6 Vit B_6
									总 Total	可溶性 Soluble	不溶性 Insoluble			Vit A	胡萝卜素 Carotene			
		%	g	kcal	kJ	g	g	g	g	g	g	mg	g	μgRE	μg	mg	mg	mg
15-3-205	香菇片	100	9.5	316	1320	9.9	12.4	61.9	20.8	—	—	—	6.3	—	—	0.54	0.24	—
15-3-206	薯片(烧烤味)	100	1.9	548	2295	7.5	37.6	49.2	4.2	2.7	1.5	—	3.8	—	—	0.17	0.06	—
15-3-207	薯片(香辣味)	100	2.1	555	2322	7.4	40.0	46.6	5.3	0.4	4.9	—	3.9	—	—	0.31	0.05	0.44
15-3-208	薯圈	100	2.2	576	2408	1.3	42.6	51.7	5.0	—	—	—	2.2	—	—	—	0.02	—
15-3-301	怪味胡豆	100	2.5	403	1686	12.6	12.1	69.6	8.7	—	—	—	3.2	—	—	0.08	0.19	—
15-3-302	奶油五香豆	100	11.1	220	919	26.2	2.0	54.0	29.8	6.2	23.6	—	6.7	—	—	0.44	0.20	—
15-3-303	夹心米果	100	1.8	593	2482	5.0	41.9	50.4	1.4	—	—	2	0.9	46	—	0.03	0.16	—
15-3-304	乐芙球	100	2.0	573	2398	7.6	45.0	43.9	9.5	—	—	—	1.5	—	—	0.04	0.31	—
15-3-305	玉米花	100	3.6	406	1698	10.8	13.4	70.4	9.9	—	—	—	1.8	Tr	—	0.10	0.11	—
15-3-306	果仁脆枣	100	4.3	484	2025	13.0	25.6	55.1	—	—	4.7	—	2.0	—	—	—	—	—
15-3-307	空心脆枣	100	1.9	376	1573	6.5	1.2	88.6	—	—	3.8	—	1.8	—	—	—	—	—
15-3-308	鱼肉粒	100	6.3	376	1574	27.1	3.3	59.5	—	—	—	35	3.8	Tr	—	0.06	0.21	0.02
15-3-401	果冻(草莓水果冻)	100	82.1	71	296	0.1	0.2	17.2	Tr	Tr	Tr	—	0.4	—	—	—	Tr	—
15-3-402	果冻(蒟蒻冻)	100	74.2	100	419	0	Tr	25.6	0.5	—	—	—	0.2	—	—	Tr	Tr	—
15-3-403	果冻(蒟蒻椰果冻)	100	72.0	109	457	0	Tr	27.8	0.5	—	—	—	0.2	—	—	Tr	Tr	—
15-3-404	果冻(AD钙果冻)	100	82.6	70	292	0.1	0.4	16.6	—	—	—	—	0.4	—	—	Tr	Tr	—

速食食品 Fast foods

(以每100g可食部计)

编码 Code	食物名称 Food name	维生素 B_{12} Vit B_{12} μg	叶酸 Folate μg	烟酸 Niacin mg	维生素C Vit C mg	维生素E (Vit E) Total mg	维生素E (Vit E) α-TE mg	钙 Ca mg	磷 P mg	钾 K mg	钠 Na mg	镁 Mg mg	铁 Fe mg	锌 Zn mg	硒 Se μg	铜 Cu mg	锰 Mn mg	碘 I μg
15-3-205	香菇片	—	53.3	—	2.0	—	—	12	98	304	2349.8	21	12.5	1.97	6.79	0.20	0.34	39.0
15-3-206	薯片 (烧烤味)	—	32.6	2.76	—	—	—	22	107	1082	508.6	55	1.8	0.93	2.72	0.15	0.11	—
15-3-207	薯片 (香辣味)	—	26.3	2.71	—	5.35	4.93	11	129	1464	366.4	68	3.0	1.74	0.82	0.55	0.41	9.3
15-3-208	薯圈	—	11.3	0.88	—	—	—	6	23	178	701.6	7	2.2	0.17	2.99	0.07	0.62	—
15-3-301	怪味胡豆	—	81.9	1.73	—	4.53	un	61	197	524	1102.1	35	6.7	1.01	14.76	0.48	0.83	25.3
15-3-302	奶油五香豆	—	141.0	1.02	—	—	—	74	563	1054	1577.0	139	4.2	1.77	1.31	1.21	0.35	—
15-3-303	夹心米果	—	14.3	0.64	—	9.91	8.73	100	151	217	79.0	26	0.6	0.82	2.84	0.15	0.29	12.9
15-3-304	乐芙球	—	3.8	Tr	—	—	—	52	108	188	276.3	12	2.1	0.86	6.76	0.12	0.23	—
15-3-305	玉米花	—	15.7	1.19	—	4.50	0.95	2	208	496	1.3	93	2.0	2.61	3.70	0.16	0.46	—
15-3-306	果仁脆枣	—	—	—	Tr	—	—	17	—	—	299.7	—	1.3	—	—	—	—	—
15-3-307	空心脆枣	—	—	—	Tr	—	—	25	—	—	816.6	—	1.8	—	—	—	—	—
15-3-308	鱼肉粒	—	4.5	3.14	—	1.04	un	9	266	470	1211.5	25	2.3	0.95	26.67	0.11	0.45	—
15-3-401	果冻 (草莓水果冻)	—	Tr	Tr	—	—	—	35	1	42	38.0	3	0.9	Tr	0.15	0.08	Tr	Tr
15-3-402	果冻 (蒟蒻冻)	—	0.1	Tr	—	—	—	1	22	35	32.5	1	0.2	—	0.12	0.01	0.02	—
15-3-403	果冻 (蒟蒻椰果冻)	—	0.2	Tr	—	—	—	1	23	54	37.2	1	0.2	—	0.12	Tr	0.02	—
15-3-404	果冻 (AD钙果冻)	—	Tr	Tr	—	—	—	6	1	72	49.6	2	0.9	0.01	0.23	0.04	0.09	Tr

Notes

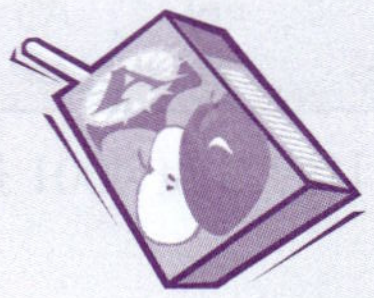

饮料类

Beverages

本类食物包括了软饮料、茶叶、冷饮食品等。软饮料又称非酒精饮料，系指经包装的乙醇含量小于0.5%(m/V)的饮料制品。参考相关的行业标准，将本类食物分成以下几个亚类。

1.碳酸饮料：又称汽水，系指在一定条件下充入二氧化碳气的制品。成品中的二氧化碳气的含量（20℃时体积倍数）不低于2.0倍。碳酸饮料包括果汁型、果味型、可乐型、低热量型、其它型等。

2.果汁（浆）及果汁饮料：指以新鲜或冷藏水果为原料，经加工制成的制品，包括果汁、果浆、浓缩果汁、浓缩果浆、果肉饮料、果汁饮料、果粒果汁饮料、水果饮料浓浆、水果饮料。

3.蔬菜汁及蔬菜汁饮料：用新鲜或冷藏蔬菜（包括可食的根、茎、叶、花、果实、食用菌、食用藻类及蕨类）为原料，经加工制成的制品。包括蔬菜汁、蔬菜汁饮料、复合果蔬汁、发酵蔬菜汁饮料、食用菌饮料、藻类饮料等。

4.含乳饮料：系指以鲜乳或乳制品为原料，经加工制成的制品，包括配制型含乳饮料、发酵型含乳饮料。

5.植物蛋白饮料：指用蛋白质含量较高的植物果实、种子或核果类、坚果类的果仁等为原料，经加工制成的制品，包括豆乳类饮料、椰子乳饮料、杏仁乳类饮料、其它植物蛋白饮料。成品中蛋白质含量不低于0.5%(m/V)。

6.茶及茶饮料：茶饮料是指用水浸泡茶叶，经扣提、过滤、澄清等工艺制成的茶汤或在茶汤中加入水、糖液、酸味剂、食用香精、果汁或植（谷）物抽提液等调制加工而成的制品。包括茶、果汁茶、果味茶及其它茶饮料。茶叶至今无统一的分类，通用的是根据采制工艺和茶叶品质等特点分为绿茶、红茶、乌龙茶、白茶、花茶和紧压茶等6类。

7.固体饮料：以糖、食品添加剂、果汁或植物抽提物等为原料，加工制成的粉末状、颗粒状或块状的制品。成品水分不高于5%(m/m)。

8.冰棒、冰激凌类：主要指冰棍、冰激凌、冰糕、雪糕、布丁冰激凌、奶昔、冰激凌蛋卷、杏仁奶冻、果汁冰等。此类食品，由于制造方法和添加料不同，成分变化较大。其主要原料是稀奶油、脱脂乳、白糖和食用明胶等。本节中这类食物较少。

9.其它：指上述各类不能包括的其它饮料类食品，如矿泉水、纯净水等。

饮料类 Beverages

(以每100g可食部计)

编码 Code	食物名称 Food name	食部 Edible %	水分 Water g	能量 Energy kcal	能量 Energy kJ	蛋白质 Protein g	脂肪 Fat g	碳水化合物 CHO g	膳食纤维 (Dietary fiber) 总 Total g	膳食纤维 可溶性 Soluble g	膳食纤维 不溶性 Insoluble g	胆固醇 Cholesterol mg	灰分 Ash g	维生素A Vit A μgRE	维生素A 胡萝卜素 Carotene μg	硫胺素 Thiamin mg	核黄素 Riboflavin mg	维生素B_6 Vit B_6 mg
碳酸饮料																		
16-1-009	可口可乐	100	89.1	43	181	0.1	0	10.8	0	—	—	0	0.1	0	—	0	0	0
果汁及果汁饮料																		
16-2-012	菠萝汁饮料(百果洲牌)	100	88.1	47	196	0.2	(0.1)	11.4	0.1	—	—	—	0.2	—	—	0.03	0.01	—
16-2-013	菠萝汁饮料(大湖牌)	100	90.9	36	149	0.3	0.2	8.3	0.1	—	—	—	0.3	Tr	Tr	0.05	0.01	—
16-2-014	苹果汁饮料(光明牌)	100	86.7	54	225	0.1	(0.3)	12.8	0.1	—	—	—	0.1	—	—	Tr	Tr	0.02
16-2-015	苹果汁饮料(亨氏)	100	87.9	50	209	0.1	(0.3)	11.7	Tr	Tr	Tr	—	Tr	—	—	Tr	Tr	—
16-2-016	苹果果肉饮料	100	87.3	44	184	0.1	(0.4)	12.1	0.3	—	—	—	0.1	—	—	Tr	Tr	—
16-2-017	橙汁饮料(光明牌)	100	88.6	44	183	0.7	(0.1)	10.2	0.2	—	—	—	0.4	—	—	0.06	0.02	0.07
16-2-018	橙汁饮料(茹梦牌)	100	88.5	47	196	0.3	(0.2)	11.2	0.2	0.2	Tr	—	0.2	—	—	0.02	0.01	—
16-2-019	橙汁饮料(汇源牌)	100	88.2	46	191	0.5	(0)	11.0	—	—	0.1[a]	—	0.3	50	297	0.03	—	0.03
16-2-020	橙汁饮料(三得利牌)	100	88.2	47	197	Tr	(0)	11.8	—	—	0.1[a]	—	Tr	181	1088	Tr	—	0
16-2-021	芒果汁饮料	100	87.9	44	184[c]	0.1	0	12.0	0.2	—	—	—	0.1	14	—	0	0.01	0.01
16-2-022	沙棘果浆	100	18.6	325	1358	0.3	(0.5)	80.2	0.5	—	—	—	0.4	—	—	Tr	0.02	0.01
16-2-023	山楂果肉饮料	100	86.1	55	231	0.1	(0.2)	13.9	0.7	—	—	—	0.1	—	—	Tr	0.01	—
16-2-024	酸枣果汁饮料	100	93.0	27	115	0.1	0	6.7	Tr	Tr	Tr	—	0.2	—	—	Tr	0.01	—
16-2-025	西番莲汁饮料	100	87.6	50	208	0.2	(0.1)	12.0	Tr	Tr	Tr	—	0.1	—	—	Tr	0.01	—
16-2-026	西柚汁饮料	100	91.4	34	142	0.6	0.4	7.3	0.3	—	—	—	0.3	Tr	Tr	0.04	0.01	—
16-2-027	椰子汁饮料	100	90.2	51	213	0.7	2.4	6.6	—	—	—	—	0.1	Tr	Tr	Tr	Tr	—
16-2-028	杏仁椰汁饮料	100	90.2	39	164	0.6	0.1	9.0	—	—	Tr[a]	—	0.1	0	3	0.01	0.01	—
蔬菜汁饮料																		
16-3-002	胡萝卜汁饮料	100	93.4	24	101	0.1	0	6.3	0.4	—	—	—	0.2	7	39	Tr	Tr	—

饮料类 Beverages

(以每100g可食部计)

编码 Code	食物名称 Food name	维生素B_{12} Vit B_{12} μg	叶酸 Folate μg	烟酸 Niacin mg	维生素C Vit C mg	维生素E (Vit E) Total mg	维生素E (Vit E) α-TE mg	钙 Ca mg	磷 P mg	钾 K mg	钠 Na mg	镁 Mg mg	铁 Fe mg	锌 Zn mg	硒 Se μg	铜 Cu mg	锰 Mn mg	碘 I μg
碳酸饮料																		
16-1-009	可口可乐	0	0	0	0	0	0	3	13	1	4.0	1	0	0.01	0.10	0.01	0.02	—
果汁及果汁饮料																		
16-2-012	菠萝汁饮料(百果洲牌)	—	2.3	0.09	22.0	—	—	2	3	59	10.0	3	0.1	0.06	Tr	0.01	0.03	—
16-2-013	菠萝汁饮料(大湖牌)	—	1.7	Tr	Tr	—	—	20	6	196	8.3	19	0.1	0.09	0.28	0.03	2.14	4.7
16-2-014	苹果汁饮料(光明牌)	—	4.0	0.03	Tr	—	—	2	2	93	4.2	4	0	0.03	Tr	0	0.02	—
16-2-015	苹果汁饮料(亨氏)	—	0.1	—	89.0	—	—	3	0	1	8.3	0	0.1	0.03	0.05	0	0.03	—
16-2-016	苹果果肉饮料	—	0.1	—	22.0	—	—	4	2	38	2.2	3	0.1	0.03	Tr	0.04	0.02	Tr
16-2-017	橙汁饮料(光明牌)	—	24.1	0.21	32.0	—	—	3	20	175	1.6	10	0.1	0.03	0.12	0.03	0	0.1
16-2-018	橙汁饮料(茹梦牌)	—	—	—	44.0	—	—	13	7	84	14.9	6	0.3	0.04	Tr	0.01	0.27	Tr
16-2-019	橙汁饮料(汇源牌)	—	11.2	—	35.0	0.24	un	11	13	150	3.0	11	0.1	0.07	0.08	0.02	0.01	0.9
16-2-020	橙汁饮料(三得利牌)	—	5.1	—	59.0	0.39	un	2	0	4	0.8	1	0.1	0.05	Tr	0	0	Tr
16-2-021	芒果汁饮料	—	—	0.28	14.5	—	—	2	2	3	21.0	2	0.2	0	—	—	—	—
16-2-022	沙棘果浆	—	—	0.05	180.0	Tr	Tr	—	—	—	—	—	0.1	0	Tr	—	0.01	2.5
16-2-023	山楂果肉饮料	—	1.2	—	33.0	—	—	11	3	31	2.7	4	0.1	0.03	Tr	0.03	0.02	—
16-2-024	酸枣果汁饮料	—	0.6	—	Tr	Tr	Tr	5	3	43	1.3	3	0.3	Tr	0.04	0.01	0.03	Tr
16-2-025	西番莲汁饮料	—	0.4	0.17	12.0	—	—	2	3	65	9.7	3	0.1	0.06	Tr	0.01	0.03	—
16-2-026	西柚汁饮料	—	2.0	—	37.0	—	—	11	19	190	8.5	9	0.1	0.07	0.18	0.03	0.02	1.5
16-2-027	椰子汁饮料	—	1.8	—	—	Tr	Tr	3	11	53	13.7	4	0.1	0.05	0.38	0.03	0.03	3.6
16-2-028	杏仁椰汁饮料	—	—	0.05	—	—	—	3	10	—	—	3	0.1	0.07	—	0.03	0.03	—
蔬菜汁饮料																		
16-3-002	胡萝卜汁饮料	—	0.9	—	1.0	—	—	5	3	28	47.0	1	0.1	0.02	0.06	0.04	0.02	0.7

饮料类 Beverages

(以每100g可食部计)

编码 Code	食物名称 Food name	食部 Edible %	水分 Water g	能量 Energy kcal	能量 Energy kJ	蛋白质 Protein g	脂肪 Fat g	碳水化合物 CHO g	膳食纤维 (Dietary fiber) 总 Total g	可溶性 Soluble g	不溶性 Insoluble g	胆固醇 Cholesterol mg	灰分 Ash g	维生素A Vit A μgRE	胡萝卜素 Carotene μg	硫胺素 Thiamin mg	核黄素 Riboflavin mg	维生素B_6 Vit B_6 mg
含乳饮料																		
16-4-003	AD钙奶	100	86.0	55	228	1.1	0.1	12.3	—	—	—	—	0.5	144	28	0.03	0.09	—
16-4-004	健康快车奶饮料	100	90.9	38	157	1.1	0.6	6.9	—	—	—	2	0.5	128	—	0.01	0.01	—
16-4-005	粒粒果奶饮料	100	92.8	30	126	1.1	0.6	5.1	—	—	—	1	0.4	90	Tr	0.01	0.01	0.01
16-4-006	酸乳饮料	100	87.8	54	225	1.1	1.3	9.4	—	—	—	2	0.4	4	—	0.02	0.05	0.01
16-4-007	酸乳饮料(发酵)	100	86.6	54	226	0.7	0.3	12.1	—	—	—	—	0.3	Tr	—	0.01	0.01	Tr
植物蛋白饮料																		
16-5-003	核桃乳(儿童型)	100	91.6	44	183	0.8	2.1	5.5	—	—	Tr[a]	—	0.1	—	—	0.02	0.02	—
16-5-004	核桃乳(女性型)	100	90.0	53	222	0.9	2.7	6.2	—	—	Tr[a]	—	0.1	—	—	0.01	0.02	—
16-5-005	核桃乳(中老年型)	100	90.6	52	216	0.9	2.9	5.5	—	—	Tr[a]	—	0.1	—	—	0.02	0.01	—
16-5-006	核桃乳(佐餐调和型)	100	90.8	51	214	0.8	2.9	5.4	—	—	Tr[a]	—	0.1	—	—	0.01	0.01	—
16-5-007	杏仁露	100	90.3	49	205	0.7	2.1	6.8	—	—	—	—	0.1	—	—	0	—	Tr
茶叶及茶饮料																		
16-6-111	大麦茶	—	2.9	305	1276[c]	13.0	3.4	77.6	—	—	7.9[b]	—	3.1	1167	7000	0.16	0.71	—
16-6-202	大麦茶水	100	99.7	1	4	Tr	(0)	0.3	—	—	—	—	Tr	(0)	(0)	0	0	0
固体饮料																		
16-7-011	高乐高营养饮品	100	1.2	394	1650	5.8	2.4	88.4	—	—	1.0	1	2.2	1146	—	1.12	1.28	1.65
16-7-012	菓珍	100	0.2	407	1704	0.1	2.2	96.8	—	—	—	—	0.8	—	—	0.03	0.01	—
16-7-013	桂花酸梅晶	100	2.2	397	1662	0.4	1.6	95.4	0.1	—	—	—	0.4	6	36	0.02	0.05	—
16-7-014	柠檬茶	100	0.2	406	1700	0.2	1.7	97.6	Tr	Tr	Tr	—	0.4	Tr	Tr	0.04	0.03	—
16-7-015	巧克力麦芽营养饮品	100	3.0	390	1631	8.0	4.0	80.6	—	—	0.1	14	4.5	914	—	0.82	1.16	1.39
16-7-016	咖啡豆	100	0.7	203	849	17.1	8.8	68.9	55.1	—	—	—	4.5	17	99	0.08	0.11	—

饮料类 Beverages

（以每100g可食部计）

编码 Code	食物名称 Food name	维生素 B_{12} Vit B_{12} μg	叶酸 Folate μg	烟酸 Niacin mg	维生素C Vit C mg	维生素E (Vit E) Total mg	维生素E (Vit E) α-TE mg	钙 Ca mg	磷 P mg	钾 K mg	钠 Na mg	镁 Mg mg	铁 Fe mg	锌 Zn mg	硒 Se μg	铜 Cu mg	锰 Mn mg	碘 I μg
含乳饮料																		
16-4-003	AD钙奶	—	—	0.05	Tr	0.19	un	121	36	—	—	3	0.3	0.16	—	0.01	0.02	—
16-4-004	健康快车奶饮料	—	Tr	Tr	—	Tr	Tr	68	82	129	207.0	2	0.2	0.13	0.18	0.01	0.01	0.4
16-4-005	粒粒果奶饮料	—	Tr	0.03	—	Tr	Tr	46	95	126	195.8	3	0.2	0.14	2.85	0.01	0.02	Tr
16-4-006	酸乳饮料	—	Tr	Tr	—	Tr	Tr	35	34	106	50.5	4	0.3	0.18	0.20	0.01	0.01	2.9
16-4-007	酸乳饮料（发酵）	—	0.9	0.02	—	Tr	Tr	24	28	33	49.1	2	0.1	0.04	0.15	Tr	Tr	2.4
植物蛋白饮料																		
16-5-003	核桃乳（儿童型）	—	—	—	—	0.51	un	3	27	15	13.9	6	0.1	0.10	3.70	0.05	0.07	—
16-5-004	核桃乳（女性型）	—	—	—	—	0.69	un	2	31	17	17.3	6	0.1	—	1.50	0.06	0.09	—
16-5-005	核桃乳（中老年型）	—	—	—	—	—	—	2	33	16	16.2	7	0.1	0.12	1.60	0.06	0.10	—
16-5-006	核桃乳（佐餐调和型）	—	—	—	—	0.43	un	1	27	14	15.4	6	0.1	0.10	1.40	0.05	0.09	—
16-5-007	杏仁露	—	—	0.02	Tr	0.64	un	20	14	3	62.3	8	0.2	0.14	—	0.02	0.03	5.3
茶叶及茶饮料																		
16-6-111	大麦茶	—	—	3.90	75.0	—	—	270	230	960	6.0	—	10.3	—	—	—	—	—
16-6-202	大麦茶水	—	0	0	(0)	0	0	2	1	6	1.0	Tr	Tr	0.10	—	Tr	—	—
固体饮料																		
16-7-011	高乐高营养饮品	—	522.7	37.07	—	8.57	un	274	393	820	93.2	132	10.3	1.54	3.47	0.82	0.89	4.0
16-7-012	菓珍	—	—	Tr	285.0	Tr	Tr	147	84	3	196.4	4	0.2	0.38	0.25	0.01	0.07	7.2
16-7-013	桂花酸梅晶	—	1.2	Tr	30.0	Tr	Tr	6	1	7	86.1	0	0.5	—	0.18	0.04	—	Tr
16-7-014	柠檬茶	Tr	—	0.20	393.0	Tr	Tr	69	42	166	1.9	8	0.1	0.39	0.30	0.01	2.00	4.8
16-7-015	巧克力麦芽营养饮品	—	175.2	2.97	104.0	8.94	8.94	467	520	927	221.4	80	10.2	7.05	4.25	0.57	0.73	22.6
16-7-016	咖啡豆	Tr	3.2	26.32	—	11.21	un	81	204	2013	2.2	132	4.2	1.00	2.72	1.32	1.59	10.1

饮料类 Beverages

(以每100g可食部计)

编码 Code	食物名称 Food name	食部 Edible	水分 Water	能量 Energy		蛋白质 Protein	脂肪 Fat	碳水化合物 CHO	膳食纤维 (Dietary fiber)			胆固醇 Cholesterol	灰分 Ash	维生素A		硫胺素 Thiamin	核黄素 Riboflavin	维生素B_6 Vit B_6
									总 Total	可溶性 Soluble	不溶性 Insoluble			Vit A	胡萝卜素 Carotene			
		%	g	kcal	kJ	g	g	g	g	g	g	mg	g	μgRE	μg	mg	mg	mg
16-7-017	咖啡粉	100	3.1	218	911	12.2	0.5	41.1	0	—	—	0	8.8	0	—	0.01	0.07	0.03
16-7-018	咖啡伴侣	100	3.0	554	2318	2.7	34.9	57.3	—	—	—	—	2.1	33	200	0	1.00	0
冰激凌、棒冰类																		
16-8-009	冰激凌 (草莓味)	100	64.8	150	628	2.7	3.2	28.5	(0.9)	—	—	—	0.8	19	—	0.11	0.20	—
16-8-010	冰激凌 (苦咖啡味)	100	60.6	205	857	2.9	10.1	25.6	Tr	Tr	Tr	—	0.8	—	—	0.04	0.09	—
16-8-011	冰激凌 (加奶油)	100	62.4	211	884	3.5	12.8	20.5	Tr	Tr	Tr	—	0.8	—	—	0.13	0.18	—
16-8-012	冰激凌 (草莓圣代)	100	66.1	145	608	2.9	2.6	27.7	—	—	0.1	10	0.7	47	—	0.05	0.14	0.03
16-8-013	冰激凌 (巧克力圣代)	100	61.7	173	725	3.6	4.8	29.0	—	—	0.1	15	0.9	Tr	—	0.05	0.15	0.02
16-8-014	冰激凌 (脆皮甜筒)	100	66.2	158	662	3.5	5.5	23.9	—	—	0.2	16	0.9	63	—	0.04	0.11	0.02
16-8-015	冰激凌 (花心筒)	100	45.0	278	1164	4.2	13.1	36.7	0.8	—	—	—	1.0	8	—	0.06	0.16	Tr
16-8-016	冰激凌 (金百合)	100	60.7	202	847	3.3	10.5	24.5	0.8	—	—	—	1.0	Tr	—	0.12	0.19	—
16-8-017	雪糕 (百乐宝)	100	70.1	147	617	2.8	6.2	20.1	Tr	Tr	Tr	—	0.8	33	—	0.05	0.19	—
16-8-018	雪糕 (红豆缘)	100	50.7	212	888	2.7	4.8	41.2	1.7	—	—	—	0.6	—	—	0.03	0.07	—
16-8-019	棒冰 (可乐冰)	100	82.9	73	306	Tr	1.0	16.1	(0)	(0)	(0)	—	0	—	—	Tr	Tr	Tr
16-8-020	棒冰 (奇彩旋)	100	77.6	95	398	Tr	1.1	21.3	(0)	(0)	(0)	—	0	—	—	Tr	0.01	Tr
其它																		
16-9-002	纯净水 (康师傅牌)	100	100.0	0	0	(0)	(0)	0	(0)	(0)	(0)	(0)	(0)	(0)	(0)	(0)	(0)	(0)
16-9-003	纯净水 (乐百氏牌)	100	100.0	0	0	(0)	(0)	0	(0)	(0)	(0)	(0)	(0)	(0)	(0)	(0)	(0)	(0)
16-9-004	纯净水 (娃哈哈牌)	100	100.0	0	0	(0)	(0)	0	(0)	(0)	(0)	(0)	(0)	(0)	(0)	(0)	(0)	(0)
16-9-005	纯净水 (椰树牌)	100	100.0	0	0	(0)	(0)	0	(0)	(0)	(0)	(0)	(0)	(0)	(0)	(0)	(0)	(0)
16-9-006	饮用水 (农夫山泉牌)	100	100.0	0	0	(0)	(0)	0	(0)	(0)	(0)	(0)	(0)	(0)	(0)	(0)	(0)	(0)
16-9-007	饮用水 (雀巢)	100	100.0	0	0	(0)	(0)	0	(0)	(0)	(0)	(0)	(0)	(0)	(0)	(0)	(0)	(0)
16-9-008	矿泉水 (获特满牌)	100	100.0	0	0	(0)	(0)	0	(0)	(0)	(0)	(0)	(0)	(0)	(0)	(0)	(0)	(0)

（以每100g可食部计）

编码 Code	食物名称 Food name	维生素B_{12} Vit B_{12} μg	叶酸 Folate μg	烟酸 Niacin mg	维生素C Vit C mg	维生素E (Vit E) Total mg	维生素E (Vit E) α-TE mg	钙 Ca mg	磷 P mg	钾 K mg	钠 Na mg	镁 Mg mg	铁 Fe mg	锌 Zn mg	硒 Se μg	铜 Cu mg	锰 Mn mg	碘 I μg
15-7-017	咖啡粉	0	0	28.17	0	0	0	141	303	3535	37.0	327	4.4	0.35	12.60	0.14	1.71	—
15-7-018	咖啡伴侣	0	0	0	0	0	0	4	350	900	200.0	—	—	—	—	—	—	—
冰激凌、棒冰类																		
16-8-009	冰激凌(草莓味)	—	3.5	0.04	—	0.88	un	86	64	71	31.0	11	0.1	0.17	1.29	0.22	0	6.2
16-8-010	冰激凌(苦咖啡味)	—	—	0.13	—	—	—	78	42	111	56.3	7	0.3	0.27	—	0.33	0	—
16-8-011	冰激凌(加奶油)	—	3.1	0.09	—	—	—	110	86	96	41.1	10	0.1	0.33	0.90	0.12	0	3.1
16-8-012	冰激凌(草莓圣代)	1.30	10.8	Tr	—	0.04	0.04	109	76	149	45.2	7	0.1	0.23	—	0.04	0.04	—
16-8-013	冰激凌(巧克力圣代)	1.50	10.0	Tr	—	0.21	un	139	94	184	65.1	13	0.4	0.43	—	0.02	0.07	—
16-8-014	冰激凌(脆皮甜筒)	1.50	Tr	Tr	—	0.17	0.15	165	96	217	68.8	17	0.7	0.48	—	0.07	0.19	—
16-8-015	冰激凌(花心筒)	—	—	0.44	—	1.04	un	91	65	170	61.2	10	0.1	0.37	—	0.09	0	8.3
16-8-016	冰激凌(金百合)	—	Tr	0.10	—	1.62	un	98	90	93	66.3	7	0.1	0.32	2.63	0.03	0	—
16-8-017	雪糕(百乐宝)	—	4.1	0.07	—	0.11	0.11	61	54	63	50.1	—	0.1	0.11	1.72	0.14	0	—
16-8-018	雪糕(红豆缘)	—	—	Tr	—	—	—	—	47	77	44.6	—	0.5	0.10	—	0.27	0	—
16-8-019	棒冰(可乐冰)	—	Tr	Tr	—	Tr	Tr	—	—	—	—	—	0	0	—	0.31	0.02	0.1
16-8-020	棒冰(奇彩旋)	—	Tr	Tr	—	Tr	Tr	—	—	32	16.8	—	0	0	—	0.28	0.01	0.7
其它																		
16-9-002	纯净水(康师傅牌)	(0)	(0)	(0)	(0)	(0)	(0)	Tr	Tr	2	0.4	Tr	0	0.02	—	Tr	Tr	—
16-9-003	纯净水(乐百氏牌)	(0)	(0)	(0)	(0)	(0)	(0)	Tr	Tr	1	1.1	Tr	0	0.02	—	Tr	Tr	—
16-9-004	纯净水(娃哈哈牌)	(0)	(0)	(0)	(0)	(0)	(0)	Tr	Tr	2	0.6	Tr	0	0.03	—	Tr	Tr	—
16-9-005	纯净水(椰树牌)	(0)	(0)	(0)	(0)	(0)	(0)	0	Tr	4	1.2	Tr	0	0.05	—	Tr	Tr	—
16-9-006	饮用水(农夫山泉牌)	(0)	(0)	(0)	(0)	(0)	(0)	5	Tr	2	4.1	1	Tr	0.04	—	Tr	Tr	—
16-9-007	饮用水(雀巢)	(0)	(0)	(0)	(0)	(0)	(0)	3	Tr	1	8.7	2	0	0.03	—	Tr	Tr	—
16-9-008	矿泉水(获特满牌)	(0)	(0)	(0)	(0)	(0)	(0)	2	Tr	3	9.9	0	0	0.02	—	Tr	Tr	—

饮料类 Beverages

(以每100g可食部计)

编码 Code	食物名称 Food name	食部 Edible %	水分 Water g	能量 Energy kcal	能量 Energy kJ	蛋白质 Protein g	脂肪 Fat g	碳水化合物 CHO g	膳食纤维 (Dietary fiber) 总 Total g	可溶性 Soluble g	不溶性 Insoluble g	胆固醇 Cholesterol mg	灰分 Ash g	维生素A Vit A μgRE	胡萝卜素 Carotene μg	硫胺素 Thiamin mg	核黄素 Riboflavin mg	维生素B_6 Vit B_6 mg
16-9-009	矿泉水(康师傅牌)	100	100.0	0	0	(0)	(0)	0	(0)	(0)	(0)	(0)	(0)	(0)	(0)	(0)	(0)	(0)
16-9-010	矿泉水(蓝涧牌)	100	100.0	0	0	(0)	(0)	0	(0)	(0)	(0)	(0)	(0)	(0)	(0)	(0)	(0)	(0)
16-9-011	矿泉水(乐百氏牌)	100	100.0	0	0	(0)	(0)	0	(0)	(0)	(0)	(0)	(0)	(0)	(0)	(0)	(0)	(0)
16-9-012	矿泉水(雀巢)	100	100.0	0	0	(0)	(0)	0	(0)	(0)	(0)	(0)	(0)	(0)	(0)	(0)	(0)	(0)
16-9-013	矿泉水(椰树牌)	100	100.0	0	0	(0)	(0)	0	(0)	(0)	(0)	(0)	(0)	(0)	(0)	(0)	(0)	(0)

饮料类 Beverages

(以每100g可食部计)

编码 Code	食物名称 Food name	维生素 B_{12} Vit B_{12} μg	叶酸 Folate μg	烟酸 Niacin mg	维生素C Vit C mg	维生素E (Vit E) Total mg	α-TE mg	钙 Ca mg	磷 P mg	钾 K mg	钠 Na mg	镁 Mg mg	铁 Fe mg	锌 Zn mg	硒 Se μg	铜 Cu mg	锰 Mn mg	碘 I μg
16-9-009	矿泉水(康师傅牌)	(0)	(0)	(0)	(0)	(0)	(0)	0	Tr	8	1.2	1	0	0.03	—	Tr	Tr	—
16-9-010	矿泉水(蓝涧牌)	(0)	(0)	(0)	(0)	(0)	(0)	44	Tr	1	7.2	7	0	0.03	—	Tr	Tr	—
16-9-011	矿泉水(乐百氏牌)	(0)	(0)	(0)	(0)	(0)	(0)	4	0	Tr	6.6	1	0	0.03	—	Tr	Tr	—
16-9-012	矿泉水(雀巢)	(0)	(0)	(0)	(0)	(0)	(0)	42	Tr	2	10.5	12	0	0.02	—	Tr	Tr	—
16-9-013	矿泉水(椰树牌)	(0)	(0)	(0)	(0)	(0)	(0)	12	0	5	42.0	4	0	0.03	—	Tr	Tr	—

Notes

含酒精饮料

Liquor and Alcoholic Beverages

含酒精饮料是指酒精（乙醇）含量在0.5%～65.0%（V/V）的饮料。结合行业标准，分为3个亚类。

1.发酵酒：指以粮谷、水果、乳类等为原料，主要经酵母发酵等工艺制成的酒精含量小于24%（V/V）的饮料酒，包括啤酒、葡萄酒、果酒、黄酒及其它发酵酒。

2.蒸馏酒：指以粮谷、薯类、水果等为主要原料，经发酵、蒸馏、陈酿、勾兑制成的、酒精度在18%～60%（V/V）的饮料酒，包括白酒、白兰地、威士忌、俄得克（伏特加）、老姆酒（朗姆酒）和其它蒸馏酒。

3.露酒（配制酒）：指以发酵酒、蒸馏酒或食用酒精为酒基，加入可食用的辅料或食品添加剂，进行调配、混合或再加工制成的、已改变了其原酒基风格的饮料酒，包括植物类露酒、动物类露酒等。

含酒精饮料的能量值计算：

含酒精饮料从体积（ml）百分比转换为重量（g）百分比时，按附录1中的数据进行换算。

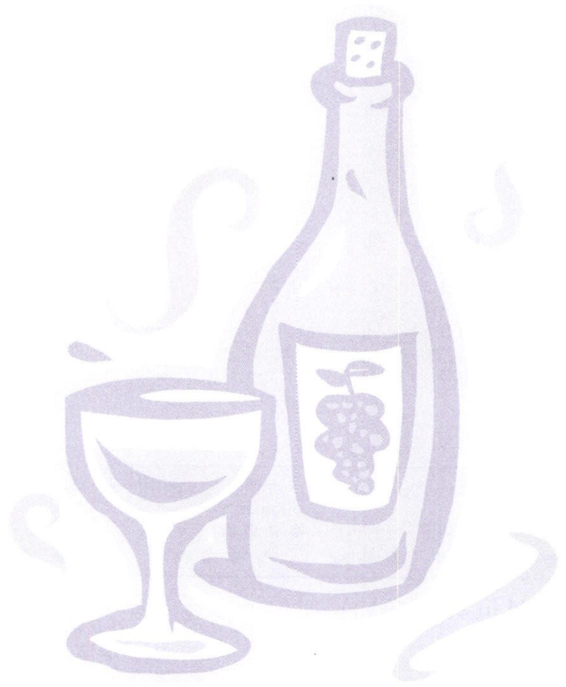

含酒精饮料 Liquor and alcoholic beverages

(以每100g可食部计)

编码 Code	食物名称 Food name	酒精度 alcohol Vol%(ml)	酒精度 alcohol Weight%(g)	食部 Edible %	水分 Water g	能量 Energy kcal	能量 Energy kJ	蛋白质 Protein g	脂肪 Fat g	碳水化合物 CHO g	灰分 Ash g	维生素A Vit A μgRE	维生素A 胡萝卜素 Carotene μg	硫胺素 Thiamin mg	核黄素 Riboflavin mg	维生素 B_6 Vit B_6 mg
发酵酒																
17-1-115	啤酒 (4.3%, 青岛牌)	4.3	3.4	100	92.9	38	159	0.4	(0)	3.1	0.2	—	—	0	0.02	—
17-1-116	啤酒 (4%, 燕京牌)	4.0	3.2	100	95.6	27	112	0.3	(0)	0.8	0.1	—	—	Tr	0.02	0.05
17-1-117	啤酒 (5.1%, 生力牌)	5.1	4.1	100	92.4	42	175	0.4	(0)	2.9	0.2	—	—	0	0.02	0.02
17-1-205	葡萄酒 (干白, 11%, 长城牌)	11.0	8.9	100	89.6	67	282	0.1	(0)	1.2	0.2	—	—	Tr	0.01	0.01
17-1-206	葡萄酒 (干白, 12%, 张裕牌)	12.0	9.7	100	88.3	75	314	0.3	(0)	1.5	0.2	—	—	Tr	Tr	0.04
17-1-207	葡萄酒 (半干白, 11.5%, 王朝牌)	11.5	9.3	100	88.6	73	304	0.3	(0)	1.6	0.2	—	—	Tr	Tr	0.04
17-1-208	葡萄酒 (干红, 11.5%, 长城牌)	11.5	9.3	100	88.7	72	300	0.2	(0)	1.5	0.3	—	—	Tr	0.01	0.02
17-1-209	葡萄酒 (干红, 11.5%, 王朝牌)	11.5	9.3	100	88.5	73	305	0.3	(0)	1.7	0.2	—	—	Tr	0.02	0.05
17-1-210	葡萄酒 (干红, 12%, 张裕牌)	12.0	9.7	100	88.2	75	314	0.3	(0)	1.5	0.3	—	—	Tr	0.02	0.04
17-1-211	黑加仑酒 (8%)	8.0	6.4	100	92.1	51	214	Tr	0.2	1.2	0.1	—	—	Tr	0.01	—
17-1-212	雪利酒	—	13.3	100	(78.8)	116	482	0.1	0	5.9	—	0	Tr	Tr	0.01	0.02
17-1-309	花雕酒 (16.5%)	16.5	13.4	100	(78.8)	124	517	(1.0)	(0)	6.5	(0.3)	—	—	Tr	Tr	—
蒸馏酒																
17-2-127	董酒 (浓香型, 46%)	46.0	38.8	100	61.2	272	1138	Tr	(0)	0	Tr	(0)	(0)	Tr	0.02	Tr
17-2-128	二锅头 (56%)	56.0	48.2	100	51.8	338	1413	Tr	(0)	0	Tr	(0)	(0)	Tr	Tr	Tr
17-2-129	汾酒 (清香型, 53%)	53.0	45.3	100	54.7	317	1327	Tr	(0)	0	Tr	(0)	(0)	Tr	0.01	Tr
17-2-130	古井贡酒 (浓香型, 38%)	38.0	31.6	100	68.2	222	929	Tr	(0)	0.2	Tr	(0)	(0)	Tr	Tr	Tr
17-2-131	剑南春 (52%)	52.0	44.4	100	55.4	312	1304	Tr	(0)	0.2	Tr	(0)	(0)	Tr	Tr	Tr
17-2-132	剑南春 (浓香型, 38%)	38.0	31.6	100	68.2	222	929	Tr	(0)	0.2	Tr	(0)	(0)	Tr	Tr	Tr
17-2-133	京酒 (浓香型, 38%)	38.0	31.6	100	68.4	221	926	Tr	(0)	0	Tr	(0)	(0)	Tr	Tr	Tr
17-2-134	茅台酒 (53%)	53.0	45.3	100	54.7	317	1327	Tr	(0)	0	Tr	(0)	(0)	Tr	Tr	Tr
17-2-135	五粮液 (52%)	52.0	44.4	100	55.6	311	1301	Tr	(0)	0	Tr	(0)	(0)	Tr	Tr	Tr

含酒精饮料 Liquor and alcoholic beverages

(以每100g可食部计)

编码 Code	食物名称 Food name	维生素 B_{12} Vit B_{12} μg	叶酸 Folate μg	烟酸 Niacin mg	维生素C Vit C mg	维生素E (Vit E) Total mg	维生素E (Vit E) α-TE mg	钙 Ca mg	磷 P mg	钾 K mg	钠 Na mg	镁 Mg mg	铁 Fe mg	锌 Zn mg	硒 Se μg	铜 Cu mg	锰 Mn mg	碘 I μg
发酵酒																		
17-1-115	啤酒 (4.3%, 青岛牌)	—	8.4	0.50	—	Tr	Tr	7	6	25	0.4	1	0.1	0.19	0.77	0.13	0.27	—
17-1-116	啤酒 (4%, 燕京牌)	0.40	—	—	—	Tr	Tr	2	14	16	3.4	6	0	0.02	—	Tr	0.13	—
17-1-117	啤酒 (5.1%, 生力牌)	—	8.2	0.49	—	Tr	Tr	6	35	44	2.3	15	0	0.01	0.33	Tr	0.02	—
17-1-205	葡萄酒 (干白, 11%, 长城牌)	0.30	Tr	—	—	Tr	Tr	6	5	83	1.7	5	0.4	0.04	0.04	0.05	0.09	—
17-1-206	葡萄酒 (干白, 12%, 张裕牌)	Tr	—	0.12	—	Tr	Tr	6	11	49	2.8	6	0.4	0.08	—	Tr	0.11	—
17-1-207	葡萄酒 (半干白, 11.5%, 王朝牌)	Tr	—	0.14	—	Tr	Tr	5	13	21	11.4	7	0.3	0.09	—	0	0.06	—
17-1-208	葡萄酒 (干红, 11.5%, 长城牌)	0.30	0.1	—	—	Tr	Tr	9	14	122	3.3	8	0.6	0.03	0.04	0.02	0.17	—
17-1-209	葡萄酒 (干红, 11.5%, 王朝牌)	0.30	—	0.11	—	Tr	Tr	5	8	72	2.1	8	0.5	0.06	—	0.01	0.17	—
17-1-210	葡萄酒 (干红, 12%, 张裕牌)	Tr	—	0.12	—	Tr	Tr	6	8	89	8.3	7	0.5	0.07	—	Tr	0.13	—
17-1-211	黑加仑酒 (8%)	Tr	Tr	0.05	—	Tr	Tr	8	2	36	2.6	2	0.5	0.45	0.26	Tr	0.08	—
17-1-212	雪利酒	Tr	Tr	0.10	0	0	0	8	24	55	27.0	5	0.4	Tr	Tr	0.04	0.01	—
17-1-309	花雕酒 (16.5%)	—	—	—	—	Tr	Tr	58	31	62	20.8	20	0.3	0.26	—	0.05	0.28	—
蒸馏酒																		
17-2-127	董酒 (浓香型, 46%)	—	—	Tr	(0)	Tr	Tr	0	—	0	0.6	Tr	—	0.03	—	Tr	Tr	—
17-2-128	二锅头 (56%)	—	—	Tr	(0)	Tr	Tr	Tr	Tr	0	0.4	0	0	0.03	—	0.01	Tr	—
17-2-129	汾酒 (清香型, 53%)	—	—	Tr	(0)	Tr	Tr	0	—	0	1.7	Tr	0	Tr	—	Tr	Tr	—
17-2-130	古井贡酒 (浓香型, 38%)	0.40	—	Tr	(0)	Tr	Tr	1	1	0	1.3	0	Tr	0.07	—	Tr	0.01	—
17-2-131	剑南春 (52%)	—	—	Tr	(0)	Tr	Tr	0	—	3	0.5	0	0	0.02	—	Tr	Tr	—
17-2-132	剑南春 (浓香型, 38%)	—	—	Tr	(0)	Tr	Tr	0	—	3	0.4	0	0	0.02	—	Tr	0.01	—
17-2-133	京酒 (浓香型, 38%)	—	—	Tr	(0)	Tr	Tr	1	Tr	0	1.1	0	0.1	0.03	—	0.01	0.01	—
17-2-134	茅台酒 (53%)	Tr	—	Tr	(0)	Tr	Tr	1	Tr	1	0.4	0	0.2	0.04	—	Tr	Tr	—
17-2-135	五粮液 (52%)	—	—	Tr	(0)	Tr	Tr	Tr	Tr	0	0.4	Tr	0	0.03	—	0.01	Tr	—

含酒精饮料 Liquor and alcoholic beverages

(以每100g可食部计)

编码 Code	食物名称 Food name	酒精度 alcohol Vol%(ml)	酒精度 alcohol Weight%(g)	食部 Edible %	水分 Water g	能量 Energy kcal	能量 Energy kJ	蛋白质 Protein g	脂肪 Fat g	碳水化合物 CHO g	灰分 Ash g	维生素A Vit A μgRE	维生素A 胡萝卜素 Carotene μg	硫胺素 Thiamin mg	核黄素 Riboflavin mg	维生素B_6 Vit B_6 mg
17-2-136	竹叶青酒 (45%)	45.0	37.9	100	51.7	307	1284	Tr	(0)	10.4	Tr	(0)	(0)	Tr	0.01	Tr
17-2-137	金奖白兰地 (38%)	38.0	31.6	100	67.3	226	944	Tr	(0)	1.1	Tr	(0)	(0)	Tr	Tr	Tr
17-2-138	伏特加	—	33.4	100	66.6	234	978	0	0	0	0	0	—	0.01	0.01	0
17-2-139	威士忌	—	36.0	100	63.9	252	1056	0	0	0.1	0	0	—	0.01	0	0
露酒																
17-3-105	苹果酒 (干型)	—	3.8	100	(92.5)	36	152	Tr	0	2.6	—	0	Tr	Tr	Tr	0.01
17-3-106	苹果酒 (甜)	—	3.7	100	(91.2)	42	176	Tr	0	4.3	—	0	Tr	Tr	Tr	0.01
17-3-107	果汁朗姆酒 (9.9%)	—	—	100	65.1	201	841[c]	0.4	1.9	28.3	0.1	—	—	0.03	0.01	—
17-3-108	鸡尾酒	—	—	100	86.9	105	439[c]	0	0	0	0.1	0	—	0	0	—
17-3-109	马提尼酒 (32%)	—	33.9	100	64.0	243	1017[c]	0	0	2.0	0.1	0	0	0	0	0
17-3-110	曼哈顿酒 (30.6%)	—	—	100	66.1	225	941[c]	0.1	0	3.2	0.1	—	—	0.01	0.01	—
17-3-111	酸味威士忌 (16.8%)	—	9.5	100	76.9	119	498[c]	0	0	13.4	0.1	1	—	0.01	0.01	0

含酒精饮料 Liquor and alcoholic beverages

(以每100g可食部计)

编码 Code	食物名称 Food name	维生素 B_{12} Vit B_{12} μg	叶酸 Folate μg	烟酸 Niacin mg	维生素C Vit C mg	维生素E (Vit E) Total mg	α-TE mg	钙 Ca mg	磷 P mg	钾 K mg	钠 Na mg	镁 Mg mg	铁 Fe mg	锌 Zn mg	硒 Se μg	铜 Cu mg	锰 Mn mg	碘 I μg
17-2-136	竹叶青酒 (45%)	0.40	—	Tr	(0)	Tr	Tr	1	—	3	5.4	1	0	0.06	—	Tr	0.01	—
17-2-137	金奖白兰地 (38%)	—	—	Tr	(0)	Tr	Tr	0	0	9	7.9	0	0	0.04	Tr	0.04	Tr	—
17-2-138	伏特加	0	0	0	0	—	—	0	5	1	1.0	0	0	0	0	0.01	0	—
17-2-139	威士忌	0	0	0.05	0	—	—	0	3	1	0	0	0	0.02	0	0.01	0.01	—
露酒																		
17-3-105	苹果酒 (干型)	Tr	—	0	0	—	—	8	3	72	7.0	3	0.5	Tr	Tr	0.04	Tr	—
17-3-106	苹果酒 (甜)	Tr	—	0	0	—	—	8	3	72	7.0	3	0.5	Tr	Tr	0.04	Tr	—
17-3-107	果汁朗姆酒 (9.9%)	—	—	0.10	5.0	—	—	8	7	71	6.0	—	0.2	—	—	—	—	—
17-3-108	鸡尾酒	—	—	0	0	—	—	4	2	2	16.0	—	0	—	—	—	—	—
17-3-109	马提尼酒 (32%)	0	0	0.04	0	0	0	1	2	16	3.0	2	0	0.01	0.10	0.01	0.02	—
17-3-110	曼哈顿酒 (30.6%)	—	—	0.10	0	—	—	2	7	26	3.0	—	0.1	—	—	—	—	—
17-3-111	酸味威士忌 (16.8%)	0	0	0.02	1.6	—	—	0	6	11	44.0	1	0	0.06	0.10	0.01	0.01	—

Notes

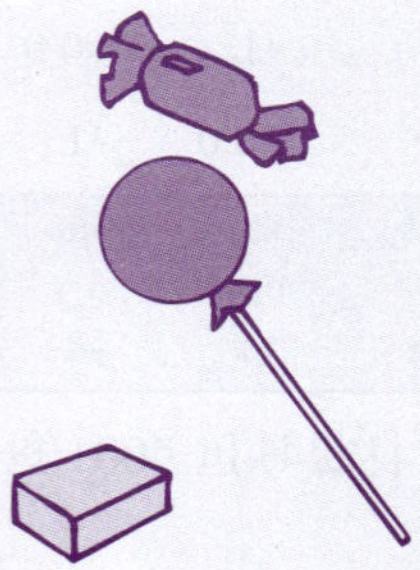

糖、果脯和蜜饯、蜂蜜

Sugars, Preserves and Honeys

该类所包括的食物均为含糖较多或经糖腌制的食品，分成糖、糖果、果脯和蜜饯、蜂蜜四个亚类。

1. 糖：主要指食用白糖、红糖、蔗糖转化糖、玉米糖浆和其它糖代用品。

2. 糖果：可分为两大类，以糖为主要成分的糖基糖果和以巧克力为主要成分的巧克力基糖果。糖基糖果包括牛轧糖、太妃糖、奶油硬糖、果汁软糖、酥糖和凝胶糖等。巧克力基糖果包括涂巧克力的糖果和巧克力条等。

3. 果脯和蜜饯：包括果脯、蜜饯等传统食品。按照制作工艺，含水但不带汁的称为果脯，如苹果脯、梨脯等。蜜饯指用浓糖浆浸渍的果品。

凉果也是我国传统食品，一般凉果保持了原果的整体形状，表面较干，有的呈盐霜状如柿饼。在本书中，将凉果归到“水果类及制品”中。

4. 蜂蜜：是以糖类为主的高浓度液体，一般含糖70%以上，主要糖分是果糖和葡萄糖。根据生产方式的不同，分为离蜜和巢蜜；根据蜜源植物种类的不同，分为油菜蜜、刺槐蜜、槐花蜜等。

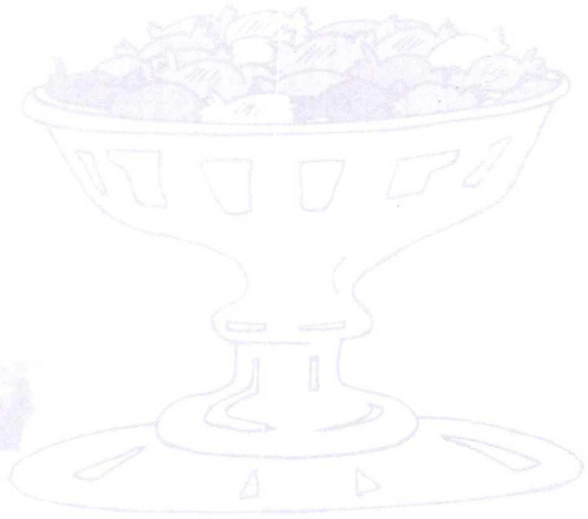

糖、果脯和蜜饯、蜂蜜 Sugars, preserves and honeys

（以每 100g 可食部计）

编码 Code	食物名称 Food name	食部 Edible %	水分 Water g	能量 Energy kcal	能量 Energy kJ	蛋白质 Protein g	脂肪 Fat g	碳水化合物 CHO g	膳食纤维 (Dietary fiber) 总 Total g	可溶性 Soluble g	不溶性 Insoluble g	胆固醇 Cholesterol mg	灰分 Ash g	维生素 A Vit A μgRE	胡萝卜素 Carotene μg	硫胺素 Thiamin mg	核黄素 Riboflavin mg	维生素 B_6 Vit B_6 mg
糖果																		
18-2-101	夹心糖	100	1.1	494	2065	2.6	20.7	74.2	Tr	Tr	Tr	—	1.4	—	—	0.04	0.11	—
18-2-102	水果味软糖	100	8.0	369	1543	6.0	0.3	85.6	(0.1)	—	—	—	0.1	—	—	0.02	0.04	—
18-2-201	牛奶糖	100	0.7	435	1822	2.2	8.2	88.2	—	—	—	—	0.7	—	—	0.07	0.10	—
18-2-202	酸奶软糖	100	1.0	404	1689	Tr	1.6	97.3	Tr	Tr	Tr	—	0.1	—	—	Tr	0.01	—
18-2-203	太妃糖	100	6.0	452	1891	3.7	16.5	72.8	—	—	0.6	—	1.0	79	—	0.02	0.14	—
18-2-301	花生牛轧糖	100	2.1	453	1896	11.7	15.5	69.5	—	—	—	—	1.2	—	—	0.05	0.09	—
18-2-302	花生芝麻糖	100	2.4	498	2082	21.3	25.3	48.7	—	—	—	—	2.3	Tr	—	0.07	0.05	—
18-2-303	四味粽子糖	100	1.0	397	1662	0.1	0.4	98.3	Tr	Tr	Tr	—	0.2	—	—	Tr	0.03	—
18-2-401	巧克力(充气)	100	1.1	543	2271	9.2	32.8	54.9	—	—	2.2	—	2.0	54	—	0.11	0.49	—
18-2-402	巧克力(果仁)	100	1.0	511	2138	9.9	33.5	53.5	—	—	11.0	—	2.1	29	—	0.10	0.37	—
18-2-403	巧克力(黑)	100	—	516	2157	4.2	30.0	63.1	5.9	—	—	0	—	2	—	0.06	0.09	0.03
18-2-404	巧克力(牛奶)	100	0.9	575	2407	8.2	39.2	49.9	—	—	2.5	—	1.8	32	—	0.11	0.24	—
果脯和蜜饯																		
18-3-012	冰糖酸角	67	27.0	257	1076	2.3	(0)	68.9	6.9	—	—	—	1.8	—	—	0.22	0.04	—
18-3-013	甘草杏	60	42.1	155	649	2.7	1.1	46.1	12.5	—	—	—	8.0	99	596	0.02	0.02	—
18-3-014	清凉杏肉	100	16.4	311	1300	2.0	0.2	79.0	—	—	3.8[a]	—	2.4	—	—	—	—	—
18-3-015	雪梅	70	17.2	260	1087	3.1	1.1	72.4	13.0	—	—	—	6.2	—	—	—	0.04	—
18-3-016	九制梅肉	100	15.0	257	1076	3.4	3.2	70.8	17.1	—	—	—	7.6	—	—	Tr	0.07	—
18-3-017	九制西梅	73	28.7	228	956	2.6	1.2	65.9	14.1	—	—	—	1.6	Tr	Tr	0.03	0.04	—
18-3-018	九制应子	83	28.7	157	655	2.3	0.6	48.6	13.1	—	—	—	19.8	Tr	Tr	0.03	0.03	—
18-3-019	梅脯	100	19.4	308	1290	0.3	1.1	78.8	4.5	—	—	—	0.4	—	—	0.02	0.01	—
18-3-020	阿胶枣	100	14.7	334	1398	2.5	0.2	82.0	—	—	1.4[a]	—	0.6	—	—	—	—	—

糖、果脯和蜜饯、蜂蜜 Sugars, preserves and honeys

（以每100g可食部计）

编码 Code	食物名称 Food name	维生素B_{12} Vit B_{12} μg	叶酸 Folate μg	烟酸 Niacin mg	维生素C Vit C mg	维生素E (Vit E) Total mg	α-TE mg	钙 Ca mg	磷 P mg	钾 K mg	钠 Na mg	镁 Mg mg	铁 Fe mg	锌 Zn mg	硒 Se μg	铜 Cu mg	锰 Mn mg	碘 I μg
糖果																		
18-2-101	夹心糖	—	7.7	Tr	—	—	—	127	67	144	246.6	26	4.0	0.86	2.43	0.50	0.22	—
18-2-102	水果味软糖	—	1.2	Tr	—	—	—	4	9	14	57.3	2	0.7	0.28	0.55	0.02	0.05	Tr
18-2-201	牛奶糖	Tr	0.7	Tr	—	—	—	65	75	200	2.7	2	0.5	1.55	0.91	0.04	0.09	14.8
18-2-202	酸奶软糖	—	0.4	Tr	—	—	—	2	1	3	8.3	1	0.1	0.07	0.44	0.01	0.03	—
18-2-203	太妃糖	—	—	Tr	—	2.74	2.15	—	—	—	—	—	—	—	—	—	—	3.5
18-2-301	花生牛轧糖	—	39.6	3.29	—	—	—	66	218	396	91.5	83	1.3	2.00	1.76	0.27	0.68	5.0
18-2-302	花生芝麻糖	—	92.1	8.68	—	13.06	—	248	599	349	63.7	164	2.1	2.69	2.55	0.63	1.25	3.8
18-2-303	四味粽子糖	—	2.4	Tr	—	—	—	4	7	145	44.6	2	0.5	0.26	Tr	Tr	2.37	—
18-2-401	巧克力(充气)	—	20.9	0.35	—	9.12	1.36	—	—	—	—	—	—	—	2.34	—	—	1.1
18-2-402	巧克力(果仁)	—	28.0	0.67	—	11.32	un	—	—	—	—	—	—	—	2.51	—	—	—
18-2-403	巧克力(黑)	0	3.0	0.43	0	—	—	32	132	365	11.0	115	—	1.62	3.10	0.70	0.80	—
18-2-404	巧克力(牛奶)	—	22.8	0.53	—	9.15	1.38	—	—	—	—	—	—	—	2.54	—	—	1.8
果脯和蜜饯																		
18-3-012	冰糖酸角	—	2.9	0.23	—	—	—	61	68	1330	120.7	61	4.3	0.34	0.70	0.28	0.28	—
18-3-013	甘草杏	—	5.4	0.80	—	—	—	378	67	1523	2574.2	51	7.2	0.61	—	0.31	0.41	3.1
18-3-014	清凉杏肉	—	—	—	0.9	—	—	22	—	—	846.4	—	2.4	—	—	—	—	—
18-3-015	雪梅	—	Tr	0.65	—	—	—	205	151	1653	895.6	100	24.7	1.06	—	0.40	0.58	—
18-3-016	九制梅肉	—	0.6	—	—	—	—	219	79	1317	958.0	184	39.0	0.65	0.56	0.36	1.26	—
18-3-017	九制西梅	—	8.7	0.77	—	—	—	100	57	1437	4.3	25	1.8	0.48	6.08	0.17	0.47	—
18-3-018	九制应子	—	4.6	Tr	—	—	—	49	23	258	8322.8	23	5.4	0.55	1.06	0.21	0.32	—
18-3-019	梅脯	—	1.2	Tr	—	0.14	0.14	52	231	179	85.5	7	2.1	1.26	—	0.03	—	—
18-3-020	阿胶枣	—	—	—	Tr	—	—	24	—	—	492.9	—	1.4	—	—	—	—	—

糖、果脯和蜜饯、蜂蜜 Sugars, preserves and honeys

(以每100g可食部计)

编码 Code	食物名称 Food name	食部 Edible %	水分 Water g	能量 Energy kcal	能量 Energy kJ	蛋白质 Protein g	脂肪 Fat g	碳水化合物 CHO g	膳食纤维 (Dietary fiber) 总 Total g	可溶性 Soluble g	不溶性 Insoluble g	胆固醇 Cholesterol mg	灰分 Ash g	维生素A Vit A μgRE	胡萝卜素 Carotene μg	硫胺素 Thiamin mg	核黄素 Riboflavin mg	维生素B₆ Vit B_6 mg
18-3-021	黑贡枣	100	17.3	305	1277	2.7	0.9	78.0	6.4	—	—	—	1.1	Tr	Tr	0.06	0.12	0.07
18-3-022	野酸枣	—	16.3	326	1362	2.7	0.5	79.6	—	—	2.1[a]	—	0.9	—	—	—	—	—
18-3-023	多味山楂	89	30.9	249	1040	1.8	1.9	61.8	—	—	5.7[a]	—	3.6	—	—	—	—	—
18-3-024	山楂脯	100	35.6	255	1065	0.5	0.6	62.9	—	—	1.1[a]	—	0.4	—	—	—	—	—
18-3-025	地瓜干	100	12.1	338	1414	2.4	0.1	83.9	—	—	2.0[a]	—	1.5	—	—	—	—	—
蜂蜜																		
18-4-001	蜂蜜	100	22.0	321	1343	0.4	1.9	75.6	—	—	—	—	0.1	—	—	Tr	0.05	—
18-4-002	蜂蜜(槐花)	100	10.0	361	1512	0.2	0.3	89.5	—	—	—	—	Tr	—	—	0.01	0.01	—
18-4-003	蜂蜜(天麻)	100	18.2	326	1364	5.2	0.3	75.7	—	—	—	—	0.6	38	228	0.11	0.14	—
18-4-004	蜂蜜(硬蜜)	100	18.5	328	1372	0.3	0.5	80.5	—	—	—	—	0.2	Tr	Tr	Tr	0.02	—
18-4-005	蜂蜜(油菜花)	100	15.8	338	1414	0.2	0.3	83.7	—	—	—	—	Tr	Tr	Tr	0.01	Tr	—

糖、果脯和蜜饯、蜂蜜 Sugars, preserves and honeys

(以每100g可食部计)

编码 Code	食物名称 Food name	维生素B_{12} Vit B_{12} μg	叶酸 Folate μg	烟酸 Niacin mg	维生素C Vit C mg	维生素E (Vit E) Total mg	α-TE mg	钙 Ca mg	磷 P mg	钾 K mg	钠 Na mg	镁 Mg mg	铁 Fe mg	锌 Zn mg	硒 Se μg	铜 Cu mg	锰 Mn mg	碘 I μg
18-3-021	黑贡枣	(0)	29.1	Tr	14.0	Tr	Tr	52	25	548	7.9	24	5.0	0.52	0.34	0.15	0.09	—
18-3-022	野酸枣	—	—	—	Tr	—	—	22	—	—	169.0	—	3.0	—	—	—	—	—
18-3-023	多味山楂	—	—	—	51.0	—	—	22	—	—	4247.5	—	2.0	—	—	—	—	—
18-3-024	山楂脯	—	—	—	6.3	—	—	21	—	—	619.3	—	1.3	—	—	—	—	—
18-3-025	地瓜干	—	—	—	23.8	—	—	10	—	—	1287.4	—	1.9	—	—	—	—	—
蜂蜜																		
18-4-001	蜂蜜	—	—	0.10	3.0	—	—	4	3	28	0.3	2	1.0	0.37	0.15	0.03	0.07	—
18-4-002	蜂蜜(槐花)	Tr	1.3	0.09	—	Tr	Tr	2	—	174	2.0	0	0.3	0.82	—	0.02	0.08	4.2
18-4-003	蜂蜜(天麻)	—	—	1.80	6.0	—	—	20	9	143	11.1	20	8.5	1.19	6.89	0.41	1.72	—
18-4-004	蜂蜜(硬蜜)	—	—	0.10	3.0	0.03	Tr	10	0	116	15.4	32	15.9	0.67	1.54	0.47	2.25	—
18-4-005	蜂蜜(油菜花)	—	—	0.10	9.0	Tr	Tr	5	3	13	4.0	1	1.3	0.11	0.41	0.90	Tr	—

Notes

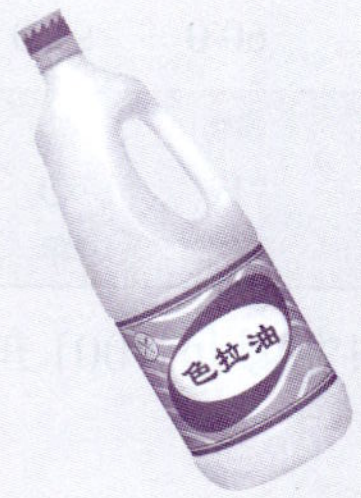

油脂类

Fats and Oils

术语油（Oil）和脂（Fat）分别指室温下的状态是液态还是固态。根据来源不同，本书将油脂类食物分为动物油脂和植物油两类。

1.动物油脂：动物脂肪包括猪脂和牛、羊等动物体脂、乳脂，以及海洋鱼类的脂肪。乳脂，又称奶油，一般指牛乳脂，因与乳类有密切的联系，在食物分类上，归入到“乳类及制品”中。动物脂肪由于脂肪酸饱和度较高，在常温下一般呈固态或半固态。

2.植物油：包括豆油、菜籽油、花生油、棉籽油、芝麻油、核桃油、棕榈油等。植物油的主要原料为大豆、玉米、菜籽、葵花子等或坚果。植物油由于含不饱和脂肪酸较多，大部分在常温下为液态。

居民消费的油脂类食物一般有：

(1)以植物原料提取的食用油脂：可分为二级油、一级油、高级烹调油和色拉油；

(2)经过深加工制得的专用油脂，如氢化油、起酥油、人造奶油、煎炸油、焙烤专用油、可可脂及其代用品等；

(3)富含功能性成分的油脂和特种油：如小麦胚芽油、沙棘油、米糠油、鱼油等；

(4)突出调味功能的芝麻香油和蛋黄酱等。

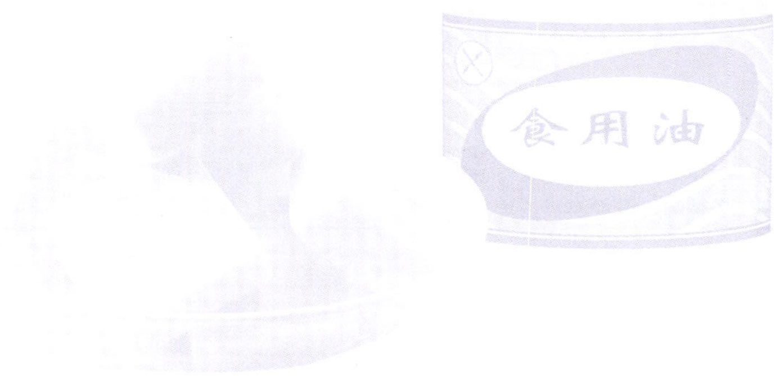

油脂类 Fats and oils

(以每100g可食部计)

编码 Code	食物名称 Food name	食部 Edible	水分 Water	能量 Energy		蛋白质 Protein	脂肪 Fat	碳水化合物 CHO	膳食纤维 (Dietary fiber) 总 Total	可溶性 Soluble	不溶性 Insoluble	胆固醇 Cholesterol	灰分 Ash	维生素A Vit A	胡萝卜素 Carotene	硫胺素 Thiamin	核黄素 Riboflavin	维生素B_6 Vit B_6
		%	g	kcal	kJ	g	g	g	g	g	g	mg	g	μgRE	μg	mg	mg	mg
植物油																		
19-2-020	核桃油	100	0.1	895	3745	(0)	99.1	0.8	(0)	(0)	(0)	—	(0)	Tr	(0)	Tr	0.01	(0)
19-2-021	花生油	100	(0)	900	3764	(0)	99.9	0.1	(0)	(0)	(0)	—	(0)	Tr	(0)	—	—	(0)
19-2-022	葵花子油	100	(0)	900	3764	(0)	99.9	0.1	(0)	(0)	(0)	—	(0)	Tr	(0)	—	—	(0)
19-2-023	粟米油 [玉米胚芽油]	100	(0)	900	3766	(0)	100.0	0	(0)	(0)	(0)	—	(0)	Tr	(0)	Tr	Tr	(0)
19-2-024	米糠油	100	(Tr)	894	3738	(0)	98.7	1.3	(0)	(0)	(0)	—	(0)	Tr	(0)	—	—	(0)
19-2-025	油茶籽油	100	0.2	898	3758	(0)	99.8	0	(0)	(0)	(0)	—	(0)	Tr	(0)	Tr	Tr	(0)
19-2-026	芝麻油 [香油]	100	0.1	898	3758	(0)	99.7	0.2	(0)	(0)	(0)	—	(0)	Tr	(0)	—	—	(0)
19-2-027	大豆色拉油	100	0	900	3764	(0)	99.9	0.1	(0)	(0)	(0)	—	(0)	Tr	(0)	—	—	(0)
19-2-028	色拉油	100	(Tr)	899	3759	(0)	99.7	0.3	(0)	(0)	(0)	—	(0)	Tr	(0)	—	—	(0)

油脂类 Fats and oils

（以每100g可食部计）

编码 Code	食物名称 Food name	维生素B12 Vit B_{12} μg	叶酸 Folate μg	烟酸 Niacin mg	维生素C Vit C mg	维生素E (Vit E) Total mg	维生素E (Vit E) α-TE mg	钙 Ca mg	磷 P mg	钾 K mg	钠 Na mg	镁 Mg mg	铁 Fe mg	锌 Zn mg	硒 Se μg	铜 Cu mg	锰 Mn mg	碘 I μg
植物油																		
19-2-020	核桃油	(0)	(0)	—	(0)	40.47	un	2	1	2	1.8	1	0.6	0.03	—	Tr	0.39	—
19-2-021	花生油	(0)	(0)	—	(0)	51.88	29.84	4	—	0	2.8	1	0.5	1.49	1.13	—	0.06	—
19-2-022	葵花子油	(0)	(0)	—	(0)	83.72	76.96	2	—	0	2.1	1	1.5	0.22	—	0.01	0.01	—
19-2-023	粟米油 [玉米胚芽油]	(0)	(0)	—	(0)	56.58	17.70	0	—	0	4.1	—	0.3	0.22	—	0.06	—	—
19-2-024	米糠油	(0)	(0)	—	(0)	35.75	un	2	—	47	1.8	1	0.4	0.57	—	—	0.05	—
19-2-025	油茶籽油	(0)	(0)	Tr	(0)	13.82	13.82	—	—	0	1.4	—	—	0.07	—	0.06	0.12	—
19-2-026	芝麻油 [香油]	(0)	(0)	—	(0)	69.79	67.39	0	—	—	0.3	—	0.2	0.14	—	—	0.02	—
19-2-027	大豆色拉油	(0)	(0)	—	(0)	102.95	23.23	1	—	1	9.1	1	0.3	1.81	—	—	—	—
19-2-028	色拉油	(0)	(0)	—	(0)	71.71	un	1	—	Tr	1.9	0	0.4	1.29	—	—	Tr	—

Notes

调味品类

Condiments

传统意义上的调味品指具有咸、甜、酸、苦、辣、鲜等味道的产品。现在，调味品的范畴已大大扩展，许多改善口味、色泽、质地的产品以及小菜等都归入调味品类。

根据调味品的生产工艺和用途，一般将其分为

1. 发酵型调味品：如醋、酱油、豆瓣酱、面酱、腐乳、味精、料酒等；

2. 非发酵型调味品：如盐、琼脂、淀粉、酵母、咸菜、糖等；

3. 香辛料：包括干制品如芥末、豆蔻、大茴香、陈皮、桂皮、花椒等和鲜品如姜、葱、蒜、鲜辣椒、香菜等。

这些食品已在前面的食物类中包括的，此处不再重复。

本节根据所包含食物的品种，将该类食物分为酱油、醋、酱、腐乳、咸菜类、香辛料和盐、味精及其它等几个亚类。

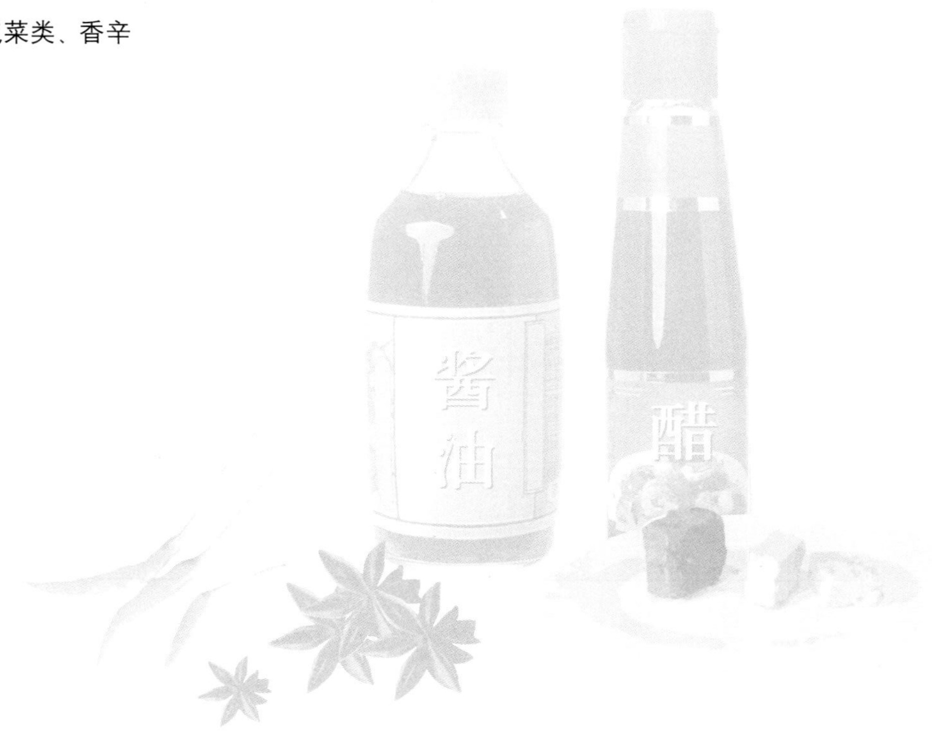

调味品类 Condiments

(以每100g可食部计)

编码 Code	食物名称 Food name	食部 Edible %	水分 Water g	能量 Energy kcal	能量 Energy kJ	蛋白质 Protein g	脂肪 Fat g	碳水化合物 CHO g	膳食纤维 (Dietary fiber) 总 Total g	可溶性 Soluble g	不溶性 Insoluble g	胆固醇 Cholesterol mg	灰分 Ash g	维生素A Vit A μgRE	胡萝卜素 Carotene μg	硫胺素 Thiamin mg	核黄素 Riboflavin mg	维生素B_6 Vit B_6 mg
酱油																		
20-1-011	黄豆酱油	100	76.2	38	159	5.1	0.2	4.3	—	—	—	—	14.3	—	—	0.02	0.15	—
20-1-012	老抽	100	51.5	129	539	7.9	0.3	23.8	—	—	—	—	16.5	—	—	0.03	0.08	—
20-1-013	生抽	100	81.2	20	83	4.8	0.1	0	Tr	Tr	Tr	—	15.5	—	—	0.02	0.11	—
酱																		
20-3-116	海鲜酱 (阿香婆)	100	14.8	492	2056	3.0	41.1	28.2	—	—	—	25	12.9	Tr	—	0.02	0.15	0.25
20-3-117	牛肉酱 (阿香婆)	100	16.8	488	2043	6.2	43.0	22.2	—	—	—	23	11.8	Tr	—	0.03	0.14	0.14
20-3-118	花生酱	100	0.4	616	2577	22.2	53.1	20.9	—	—	—	—	3.4	Tr	—	0.05	0.09	—
20-3-119	花生酱 (加巧克力)	100	0.4	633	2647	19.6	55.4	22.1	8.2	—	—	—	2.5	Tr	—	0.05	0.10	—
20-3-120	芝麻酱	100	0.4	687	2875	18.0	66.8	9.4	—	—	5.9	—	5.4	—	—	0.26	0.24	0.20
20-3-121	千岛沙拉酱	100	32.5	475	1986	2.3	43.4	19.8	1.1	—	—	15	2.0	41	—	0.03	0.06	—
20-3-122	沙拉酱	100	15.4	724	3028	2.8	78.8	1.0	—	—	—	—	2.0	87	—	0.07	0.09	—
20-3-123	奶油攀司	100	0.4	605	2530	2.9	42.0	53.8	(0)	(0)	(0)	—	0.9	130	—	0.08	0.30	—
20-3-207	草莓酱	100	29.2	284	1190	0.3	1.1	69.3	1.0	—	—	—	0.1	370	2222	Tr	0.01	—
20-3-208	番茄沙司	100	67.4	112	469	1.0	0.2	28.0	1.4	—	—	—	3.4	79	472	0.02	0.02	—
腐乳																		
20-4-006	腐乳 (香辣味)	100	67.8	158	660	13.1	11.6	0.8	—	—	0.5	—	6.8	—	—	—	—	—
20-4-007	腐乳 (白, 石宝寨牌) [酱豆腐]	100	67.4	115	479	9.5	7.7	2.7	—	—	0.9	—	12.7	18	110	0.03	0.08	—
20-4-008	腐乳 (白, 王致和牌) [酱豆腐]	100	69.2	153	642	12.3	11.6	0.6	—	—	0.6	—	6.3	—	—	—	—	—
咸菜类																		
20-5-036	剁辣椒	100	75.2	30	125	1.4	0.5	10.8	5.9	—	—	—	12.1	205	1232	Tr	0.07	—
20-5-037	酱八宝菜	100	68.9	120	501	5.6	6.1	13.8	—	—	3.3[a]	—	5.6	—	—	—	—	—

调味品类 Condiments

(以每100g可食部计)

编码 Code	食物名称 Food name	维生素 B_{12} Vit B_{12} μg	叶酸 Folate μg	烟酸 Niacin mg	维生素C Vit C mg	维生素E (Vit E) Total mg	α-TE mg	钙 Ca mg	磷 P mg	钾 K mg	钠 Na mg	镁 Mg mg	铁 Fe mg	锌 Zn mg	硒 Se μg	铜 Cu mg	锰 Mn mg	碘 I μg
酱油																		
20-1-011	黄豆酱油	Tr	15.3	1.13	—	Tr	Tr	25	78	386	5699.8	32	3.5	0.56	1.23	0.07	0.53	Tr
20-1-012	老抽	Tr	36.5	1.68	—	Tr	Tr	27	175	454	6910.4	44	6.1	0.66	1.88	0.40	0.57	2.9
20-1-013	生抽	Tr	21.0	1.08	—	Tr	Tr	16	59	342	6384.7	29	2.7	0.45	1.30	0.08	0.29	0.6
酱																		
20-3-116	海鲜酱 (阿香婆)	—	35.1	1.45	—	25.44	un	223	112	310	2107.0	44	4.3	0.90	12.42	0.23	0.37	29.1
20-3-117	牛肉酱 (阿香婆)	—	26.7	1.90	—	26.58	un	35	43	194	1260.5	18	3.8	0.54	2.48	0.15	0.39	34.5
20-3-118	花生酱	Tr	129.3	22.75	—	10.44	4.23	54	390	605	483.4	126	1.6	2.89	8.33	0.71	1.67	2.4
20-3-119	花生酱 (加巧克力)	Tr	—	10.31	—	11.36	4.99	61	224	218	214.5	131	3.8	2.30	5.78	0.58	1.04	0
20-3-120	芝麻酱	—	99.8	7.26	—	—	—	612	193	424	5.4	254	9.4	3.32	—	1.02	0.91	1.8
20-3-121	千岛沙拉酱	—	4.3	Tr	—	35.25	5.56	13	29	127	638.6	8	0.5	0.37	3.58	0.03	0.08	4.5
20-3-122	沙拉酱	—	—	Tr	—	77.75	14.60	9	71	160	733.6	4	0.6	0.47	4.34	0.02	0.05	3.2
20-3-123	奶油攀司	Tr	8.3	0.50	(Tr)	32.84	un	109	196	447	68.5	115	11.6	1.33	1.78	0.40	0.41	5.0
20-3-207	草莓酱	Tr	6.7	0.09	Tr	0.23	0.11	15	2	64	1.3	4	0.2	0.17	0.82	0.02	0.18	6.9
20-3-208	番茄沙司	Tr	1.1	0.70	8.0	1.10	0.94	10	16	324	1046.8	13	0.6	0.28	0.55	0.09	0.05	0
腐乳																		
20-4-006	腐乳 (香辣味)	—	—	—	0	—	—	91	—	—	2020.0	—	4.0	—	—	—	—	—
20-4-007	腐乳 (白, 石宝寨牌) [酱豆腐]	1.98	12.2	Tr	—	8.81	un	222	202	146	5008.2	20	5.9	4.78	14.03	0.26	1.37	13.3
20-4-008	腐乳 (白, 王致和牌) [酱豆腐]	—	—	—	0	—	—	100	—	—	2080.0	—	5.1	—	—	—	—	—
咸菜类																		
20-5-036	剁辣椒	—	8.3	1.01	—	2.21	un	9	34	211	2443.2	9	1.7	1.29	0.19	0.08	0.28	15.8
20-5-037	酱八宝菜	—	—	—	Tr	—	—	68	—	—	2620.0	—	2.4	—	—	—	—	—

调味品类 Condiments

(以每100g可食部计)

编码 Code	食物名称 Food name	食部 Edible	水分 Water	能量 Energy		蛋白质 Protein	脂肪 Fat	碳水化合物 CHO	膳食纤维 (Dietary fiber)			胆固醇 Cholesterol	灰分 Ash	维生素A		硫胺素 Thiamin	核黄素 Riboflavin	维生素B_6 Vit B_6
									总 Total	可溶性 Soluble	不溶性 Insoluble			Vit A	胡萝卜素 Carotene			
		%	g	kcal	kJ	g	g	g	g	g	g	mg	g	μgRE	μg	mg	mg	mg
20-5-038	酱甘露	100	77.4	68	285	3.0	0.4	14.0	—	—	0.9[a]	—	5.2	—	—	—	—	—
20-5-039	酱花生米	100	36.6	367	1535	17.2	31.9	11.3	—	—	8.6[a]	—	2.9	—	—	—	—	—
20-5-040	酱籽萝	100	77.3	57	237	2.9	0.4	11.2	—	—	0.7[a]	—	8.3	—	—	—	—	—
20-5-041	麻仁金丝	100	76.1	63	264	3.1	0.6	12.7	—	—	1.4[a]	—	7.5	—	—	—	—	—
20-5-042	雪菜	100	82.2	22	92	1.5	1.6	8.7	8.3	—	—	—	6.0	97	584	0.03	0.03	0.06
20-5-043	腌大头菜	100	59.4	58	243	7.0	0.2	11.3	4.2	—	—	—	22.1	—	—	0.04	0.20	0.14
20-5-044	腌芥菜头	100	68.7	20	83	2.4	0.1	5.6	3.3	—	—	—	23.2	—	—	0.02	0.03	0.03
20-5-045	腌韭菜花	100	80.0	27	112	2.8	0.6	3.8	—	—	1.1[a]	—	12.9	—	—	—	—	—
20-5-046	腌萝卜条	100	78.7	44	183	0.6	0.3	15.3	5.7	—	—	—	5.1	—	—	Tr	0.01	0.04
20-5-047	榨菜(鱼泉牌)	100	85.2	34	141	1.8	2.0	4.8	—	—	2.7	—	6.2	10	63	0.01	0.03	—
20-5-048	榨菜(正林牌)	100	87.2	10	42	1.5	0.1	4.1	3.3	—	—	—	7.1	—	—	0.01	0.02	—
香辛料																		
20-6-011	咖喱粉	100	5.7	415	1736	13.0	12.2	63.3	36.9	6.5	30.4	—	5.8	110	690	0.41	0.25	0.59
盐、味精及其它																		
20-7-202	鸡粉	100	1.6	224	937	13.2	5.1	32.4	1.1	—	—	9	47.7	Tr	—	—	0.07	—
20-7-203	鸡精	100	2.4	195	817	10.7	2.8	32.5	0.7	—	—	5	51.6	Tr	—	0.09	0.05	—
20-7-401	料酒	100	99.1	1	5	0.3	Tr	0	(0)	(0)	(0)	—	0.7	—	—	—	—	—

调味品类 Condiments

(以每100g可食部计)

编码 Code	食物名称 Food name	维生素B_{12} Vit B_{12} μg	叶酸 Folate μg	烟酸 Niacin mg	维生素C Vit C mg	维生素E (Vit E) Total mg	维生素E (Vit E) α-TE mg	钙 Ca mg	磷 P mg	钾 K mg	钠 Na mg	镁 Mg mg	铁 Fe mg	锌 Zn mg	硒 Se μg	铜 Cu mg	锰 Mn mg	碘 I μg
20-5-038	酱甘露	—	—	—	Tr	—	—	49	—	—	2470.0	—	2.2	—	—	—	—	—
20-5-039	酱花生米	—	—	—	Tr	—	—	86	—	—	970.0	—	2.2	—	—	—	—	—
20-5-040	酱籽萝	—	—	—	—	—	—	37	—	—	3020.0	—	4.4	—	—	—	—	—
20-5-041	麻仁金丝	—	—	—	Tr	—	—	63	—	—	3280.0	—	3.5	—	—	—	—	—
20-5-042	雪菜	—	4.8	Tr	—	2.16	un	74	8	31	1708.4	3	4.8	1.54	0.41	0.16	0.37	59.5
20-5-043	腌大头菜	—	24.9	1.65	Tr	Tr	Tr	—	171	11	—	7	1.1	0.14	0.33	0.01	0.07	Tr
20-5-044	腌芥菜头	—	3.9	0.43	Tr	Tr	Tr	—	43	—	—	4	2.3	0.63	0.65	0.01	0.04	Tr
20-5-045	腌韭菜花	—	—	—	Tr	—	—	75	—	—	4600.0	—	6.6	—	—	—	—	—
20-5-046	腌萝卜条	—	2.1	0.12	—	Tr	Tr	—	—	—	—	—	2.0	0.60	Tr	0.01	0.02	Tr
20-5-047	榨菜 (鱼泉牌)	—	7.7	0.21	—	Tr	Tr	46	26	49	1677.7	6	2.1	—	0.69	0.10	0.13	—
20-5-048	榨菜 (正林牌)	—	8.1	0.15	—	Tr	Tr	47	22	82	2461.7	5	2.1	0.39	0.74	0.03	0.22	—
香辛料																		
20-6-011	咖喱粉	0.10	60.0	7.00	2.0	un	4.90	540	400	1700	40.0	220	28.5	2.90	—	0.80	—	—
盐、味精及其它																		
20-7-202	鸡粉	Tr	19.2	0.84	—	Tr	Tr	22	93	147	19041.8	7	4.0	0.83	5.06	0.13	0.27	3.9
20-7-203	鸡精	Tr	11.1	0.56	—	Tr	Tr	8	66	88	18864.4	2	1.0	0.61	1.74	0.14	0.16	766.5
20-7-401	料酒	—	—	—	Tr	—	—	14	—	—	270.0	—	0.1	—	—	—	—	—

Notes

其它

Others

将难以归入到前面任何一个类别中的食物列入本节中。这里可能包括了在某地有食用习惯或有特殊利用价值的食物。

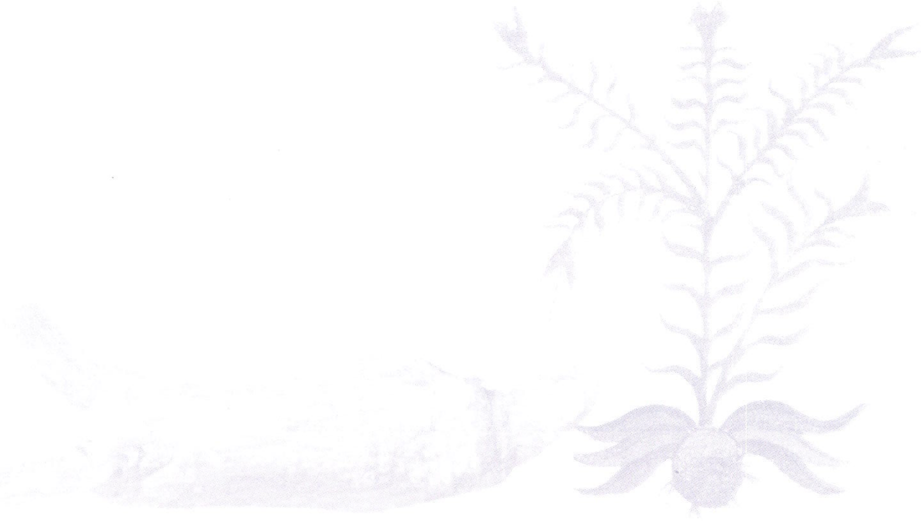

其它 Others

(以每100g可食部计)

编码 Code	食物名称 Food name	食部 Edible	水分 Water	能量 Energy		蛋白质 Protein	脂肪 Fat	碳水化合物 CHO	膳食纤维 (Dietary fiber) 总 Total	可溶性 Soluble	不溶性 Insoluble	胆固醇 Cholesterol	灰分 Ash	维生素A Vit A	胡萝卜素 Carotene	硫胺素 Thiamin	核黄素 Riboflavin	维生素B_6 Vit B_6
		%	g	kcal	kJ	g	g	g	g	g	g	mg	g	μgRE	μg	mg	mg	mg
其它																		
21-9-014	蜂蛹 [蜂胚、蜂仔]	100	80.8	100	418	10.6	5.4	2.3	—	—	—	19	0.9	—	—	0.28	0.24	—
21-9-015	蜂蛹 (油蜂)	100	7.7	669	2797	20.0	61.4	9.0	—	—	—	236	1.9	—	—	0.07	0.31	—
21-9-016	蜂蛹 (大黄蜂)	100	76.7	109	456	12.1	3.8	6.6	—	—	—	—	0.8	—	—	0.11	0.37	—
21-9-017	葛根	91	51.3	181	759	1.5	0.2	45.6	—	—	2.2	—	1.4	Tr	Tr	0.04	0.01	—
21-9-018	花椒叶 (干)	100	12.3	236	987	16.7	0.7	61.0	—	—	20.4	—	9.3	1033	6200	0.24	0.36	—
21-9-019	花粉 (油菜)	100	8.4	397	1661	24.6	11.1	52.7	—	—	3.1[a]	—	3.2	—	—	0.22	0.70	—
21-9-020	花粉 (油松) [松花粉]	100	6.4	251	1050	9.6	7.7	72.5	—	—	36.7[a]	—	3.8	—	—	0.10	0.47	—
21-9-021	花粉 (荞麦)	100	8.3	353	1477	14.9	4.2	67.3	—	—	3.4[a]	—	5.3	—	—	0.39	0.62	—
21-9-022	牛蛙	30	79.4	81	338	15.7	0.5	3.4	—	—	—	19	1.0	—	—	0.13	0.01	—
21-9-023	仙人掌 (食用)	82	92.7	9	37	0.5	Tr	4.6	2.9	1.4	1.5	—	2.2	13	79	Tr	0.01	0.07
21-9-024	仙人掌果 [仙桃]	80	90.8	17	72	1.1	0.1	6.8	3.8	1.9	1.9	—	1.2	7	44	0.01	0.01	0.12
21-9-025	仙人掌籽	100	3.5	96	401	7.4	5.1	81.7	76.6	1.6	74.9	—	2.3	Tr	—	0.04	0.05	0.08

其它 Others

(以每100g可食部计)

编码 Code	食物名称 Food name	维生素B_{12} Vit B_{12} μg	叶酸 Folate μg	烟酸 Niacin mg	维生素C Vit C mg	维生素E (Vit E) Total mg	维生素E (Vit E) α-TE mg	钙 Ca mg	磷 P mg	钾 K mg	钠 Na mg	镁 Mg mg	铁 Fe mg	锌 Zn mg	硒 Se μg	铜 Cu mg	锰 Mn mg	碘 I μg
其它																		
21-9-014	蜂蛹 [蜂胚、蜂仔]	—	—	2.60	—	—	—	1	165	249	12.0	20	2.0	2.36	4.00	0.39	0.12	—
21-9-015	蜂蛹 (油蜂)	—	—	4.80	(Tr)	2.37	un	38	281	331	299.3	35	9.3	5.09	17.65	1.89	5.08	—
21-9-016	蜂蛹 (大黄蜂)	—	—	2.80	20.0	—	—	27	157	256	15.8	22	3.8	2.21	6.10	0.08	3.61	—
21-9-017	葛根	—	—	0.40	19.0	—	—	133	44	572	3.3	76	1.6	0.56	11.45	0.33	0.19	—
21-9-018	花椒叶 (干)	(0)	—	1.00	—	—	—	—	—	—	—	—	—	—	—	—	—	—
21-9-019	花粉 (油菜)	—	—	5.90	27.0	6.36	un	345	572	555	5.7	137	22.2	2.53	8.65	0.82	2.03	—
21-9-020	花粉 (油松) [松花粉]	—	—	7.50	21.0	—	—	81	253	980	55.4	99	41.7	2.94	5.61	0.39	11.74	—
21-9-021	花粉 (荞麦)	—	—	2.50	Tr	0.26	Tr	235	92	1192	—	466	12.3	2.00	11.74	0.68	2.19	—
21-9-022	牛蛙	—	—	5.40	Tr	—	—	15	162	329	34.5	22	0.6	0.98	Tr	0.02	Tr	—
21-9-023	仙人掌 (食用)	—	2.3	0.22	4.8	0.26	0.26	534	20	70	2.8	185	0.4	0.87	0.60	0.04	2.05	1.5
21-9-024	仙人掌果 [仙桃]	—	2.5	0.24	10.7	0.50	0.50	137	5	292	14.4	62	0.4	0.40	0.40	0.06	40.89	9.5
21-9-025	仙人掌籽	—	11.3	0.58	—	2.70	un	494	207	109	15.9	92	18.7	3.26	5.10	2.36	9.04	5.9

Notes

表二 食物氨基酸含量

Table 2 Amino Acid Content of Foods

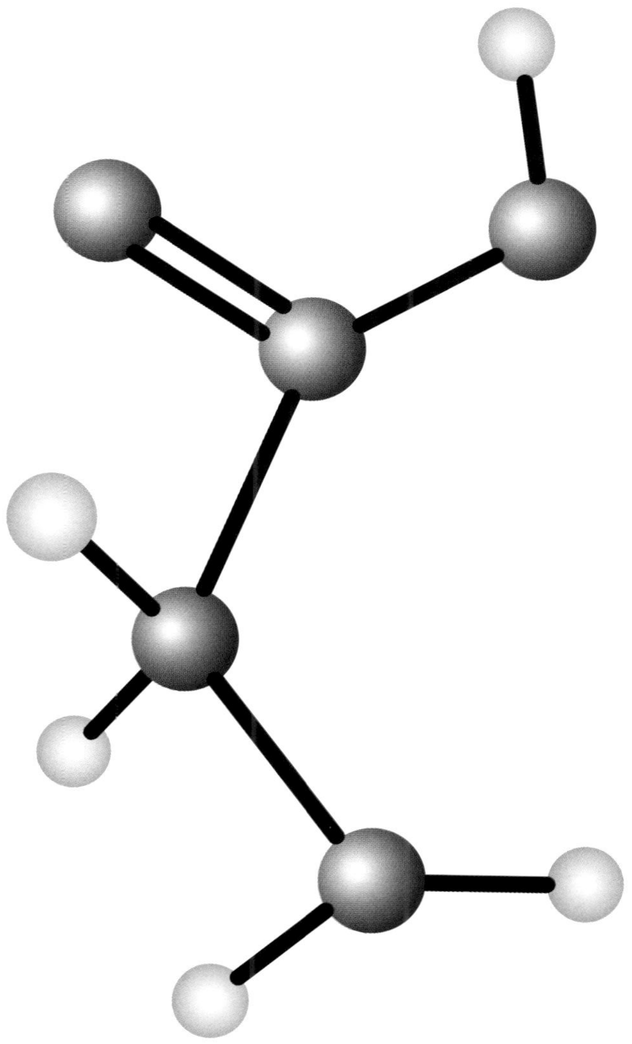

氨基酸

氨基酸是组成一切蛋白质的最基本的单位，目前已知道的有 20 多种，一般具有相同的基础结构，即

$$\begin{array}{c} R—CH—COOH \\ \quad | \\ \quad NH_2 \end{array}$$

一、氨基酸的命名

氨基酸可看作是羧酸烃基上的氢原子被氨基取代而形成的取代酸，称为氨基某酸。氨基的位置常采用希腊字母 α、β、γ 等标示在氨基酸名称前面。另外，氨基酸的俗名还是比较常用的。俗名一般多按其来源或某些性质来命名。例如氨基乙酸，因其具有甜味，故命名为甘氨酸。

二、氨基酸的分类

氨基酸存在两种异构体：L 型和 D 型。人体蛋白质中的氨基酸均为 L 型，只有微生物体内才有 D 型存在。常见的有三种分类方法。

1. 根据氨基酸侧链的极性及所带电荷分类

(1) 非极性、疏水性氨基酸　包括丙氨酸、缬氨酸、亮氨酸、异亮氨酸、脯氨酸、苯丙氨酸、色氨酸、蛋氨酸等。

(2) 极性、中性氨基酸　包括甘氨酸、丝氨酸、苏氨酸、半胱氨酸、酪氨酸、天冬酰胺和谷氨酰胺等。

(3) 碱性氨基酸　包括组氨酸、赖氨酸和精氨酸。

(4) 酸性氨基酸　包括天冬氨酸、谷氨酸。

2. 根据氨基酸侧链的化学结构分类

(1) 脂肪族氨基酸　这类氨基酸又可按其分子中含有的氨基或羧基的数目以及是否含有某些特殊元素或基团分成以下各类。

- 一氨基一羧基酸　包括甘氨酸、丙氨酸、缬氨酸、亮氨酸、异亮氨酸、丝氨酸、苏氨酸、半胱氨酸、蛋氨酸、天冬酰胺和谷氨酰胺。
- 一氨基二羧基酸　包括天冬氨酸、谷氨酸。
- 二氨基一羧基酸　包括赖氨酸和精氨酸。

(2) 芳香族氨基酸：如苯丙氨酸、酪氨酸等。

(3) 杂环类氨基酸：如脯氨酸等。

3. 根据其营养 / 生理作用分类

(1) 必需氨基酸 (essential amino acid, EAA)：即不能在体内合成或合成的速度远不能适应机体需要的氨基酸，必须由食物供给。一般来说，人体必需的氨基酸有赖氨基、亮氨基、异亮氨酸、蛋氨酸、苯丙氨酸、苏氨酸、色氨酸、缬氨酸、组氨酸 (婴幼儿必需) 。

(2) 非必需氨基酸 (nonessential amino acid)：能在体内合成的氨基酸均称为非必需氨基酸。如甘氨酸、丙氨酸、丝氨酸、半胱氨酸、酪氨酸、天冬酰胺、谷氨酰胺、天冬氨酸和谷氨酸等。

(3) 条件必需氨基酸 (conditionally essential amino acid)：这组氨基酸有两个特点：a. 在合成氨基酸中用其他氨基酸作为碳的前体，并且只限于某些特定器官；b. 合成最高速度可能是有限的，并可能受机体发育和病理生理因素所限制。包括半胱氨酸、酪氨酸、精氨酸、脯氨酸、甘氨酸。

三、食物中的氨基酸模式和限制性氨基酸

人体蛋白质与食物蛋白质在必需氨基酸的种类和含量上存在着差异。氨基酸模式是指某种食物蛋白质中必需氨基酸的构成比例。如以含量最少的色氨酸为 1，几种食物的其他氨基酸的相应比值见表 1。

表 1　几种食物蛋白质和人体蛋白质氨基酸模式

氨基酸	全鸡蛋	牛奶	牛肉	大豆	面粉	大米	人体
异亮氨酸	3.2	3.4	4.4	4.3	3.8	4.0	4.0
亮氨酸	5.1	6.8	6.8	5.7	6.4	6.3	7.0
赖氨酸	4.1	5.6	7.2	4.9	1.8	2.3	5.5
蛋氨酸 + 半胱氨酸	3.4	2.4	3.2	1.2	2.8	2.8	2.3
苯丙氨酸 + 酪氨酸	5.5	7.3	6.2	3.2	7.2	7.2	3.8
苏氨酸	2.8	3.1	3.6	2.8	2.5	2.5	2.9
缬氨酸	3.9	4.6	4.6	3.2	3.8	3.8	4.8
色氨酸	1.0	1.0	1.0	1.0	1.0	1.0	1.0

当食物蛋白质中一种或几种必需氨基酸含量较低时，其它必需氨基酸在体内则不能被充分利用，导致蛋白质营养价值降低。这些含量相对较低的氨基酸称为限制氨基酸，其中相对含量最低的氨基酸称为第一限制氨基酸。植物蛋白质中，赖氨酸、蛋氨酸、苏氨酸和色氨酸含量一般较低，其蛋白质的营养价值也相对较低。

附：常见氨基酸的表达形式和 R 结构

常见氨基酸表达形式和 R 结构

	名称	英文名称	常见缩写形式	R 部分结构
1	甘氨酸	Glycine	Gly	H—
2	丙氨酸	Alanine	Ala	CH_3—
3	缬氨酸	Valine	Val	CH_3 >CH— CH_3
4	亮氨酸	Leucine	Leu	CH_3 >CH—CH_2— CH_3
5	异亮氨酸	Isoleucine	Ile	CH_3—CH_2 >CH— CH_3
6	丝氨酸	Serine	Ser	HO—CH_2—
7	苏氨酸	Threonine	Thr	HO >CH— CH_3
8	半胱氨酸	Cysteine	Cys	HS—CH_2
9	胱氨酸	Cystine	Cys-Cys	S—CH_2— | S—CH_2—

	名称	英文名称	常见缩写形式	R 部分结构
10	蛋氨酸	Methionine	Met	$CH_3—S—CH_2—CH_2—$
11	苯丙氨酸	Phenylalanine	Phe	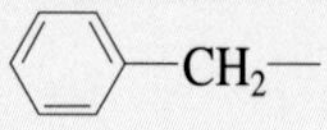
12	酪氨酸	Tyrosine	Tyr	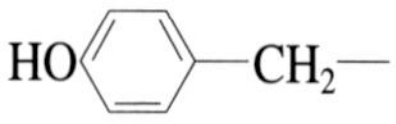
13	色氨酸	Tryptophane	Trp	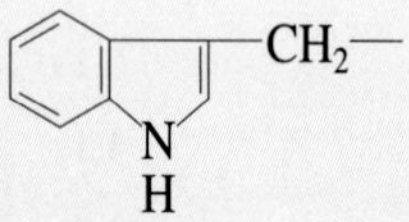
14	组氨酸	Histidine	His	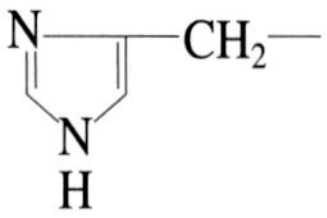
15	赖氨酸	Lysine	Lys	$NH_2—CH_2—CH_2—CH_2—CH_2—$
16	精氨酸	Arginine	Arg	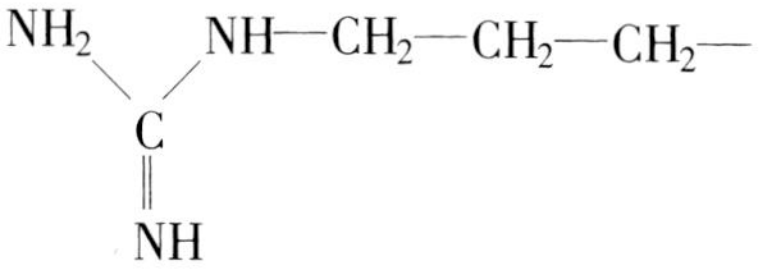
17	天冬氨酸	Aspartic acid	Asp	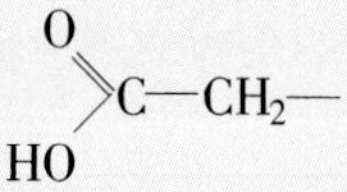
18	天冬酰胺	Asparagine	Asn	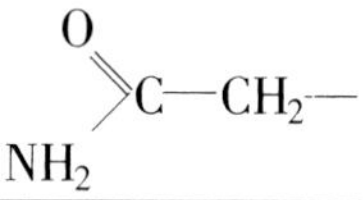
19	谷氨酸	Glutamic acid	Glu	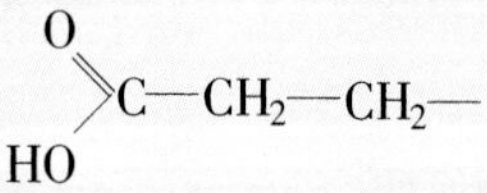
20	谷氨酰胺	Glutamine	Gln	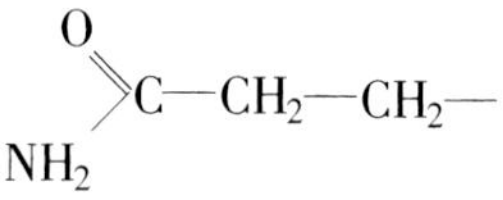
21	脯氨酸	Proline	Pro	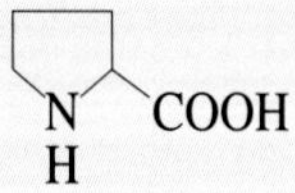
22	羟脯氨酸	Hydroxproline	Hyp	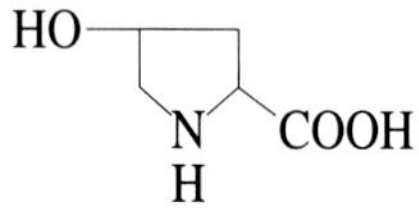
23	牛磺酸	Taurine	—	$H_2N—CH_2—CH_2—SO_3H$

注：脯氨酸、羟脯氨酸、牛磺酸为全结构

Notes

食物氨基酸含量 Amino acid content of foods

(mg/100g 可食部)

编码 Code	食物名称 Food name	水分 Water g	蛋白质 Protein g	异亮氨酸 Ile	亮氨酸 Leu	赖氨酸 Lys	含硫氨基酸 (SAA) Total	蛋氨酸 Met	胱氨酸 Cys	芳香族氨基酸 (AAA) Total	苯丙氨酸 Phe	酪氨酸 Tyr
谷类及制品												
01-1-206	小麦面粉 (标准粉)	9.9	15.7	500	1060	350	590	260	330	1170	760	410
01-1-207	小麦面粉 (富强粉、特一粉)	10.8	12.3	400	830	230	470	200	270	960	680	280
01-1-208	小麦面粉 (特制)	10.4	13.3	360	810	250	450	190	260	1000	610	390
01-1-313	挂面 (富强粉)	10.2	13.0	410	890	260	460	190	270	940	650	290
01-1-314	龙须面 (素)	10.4	10.8	360	730	200	250	80	170	910	560	350
01-1-315	龙须面 (鸡蛋)	10.2	14.0	470	900	240	550	220	330	1040	680	360
01-1-316	面条 (富强粉, 切面)	29.0	8.9	310	670	190	320	150	170	640	490	150
01-1-317	面条 (富强粉, 煮)	72.7	3.9	130	290	80	130	60	70	280	200	80
01-1-503	面筋 (肉馅)	49.2	16.2	500	1000	750	370	170	200	1070	610	460
01-2-106	粳米 (极品精米)	13.9	6.4	350	550	220	340	170	170	770	500	270
01-2-107	粳米 (西域王米)	13.3	7.5	330	640	260	360	190	170	810	550	260
01-2-108	粳米 (小站稻米)	12.9	6.9	290	510	190	330	150	180	600	400	200
01-2-215	香米	13.5	8.4	300	560	220	360	180	180	630	400	230
01-2-408	籼米饭 (蒸)	70.1	3.0	100	200	100	120	70	50	260	170	90
01-2-409	籼米粥	85.0	1.3	50	110	50	70	40	30	140	90	50
01-2-411	河粉	11.2	7.7	360	560	250	290	110	180	900	510	390
01-3-108	玉米粒 (黄, 干)	11.8	8.0	280	1150	130	340	200	140	700	410	290
01-3-109	玉米面 (黄)	11.2	8.5	280	1110	170	350	190	160	750	480	270
01-3-110	玉米糁 (黄)	12.5	7.4	270	1140	130	350	200	150	700	470	230
01-5-104	小米 (黄)	9.7	8.9	420	130	140	570	370	200	940	610	330
01-9-010	荞麦面	14.2	11.3	370	670	540	530	220	310	790	500	290
01-9-011	莜麦面	8.8	13.7	470	960	490	660	230	430	1090	690	400

食物氨基酸含量 Amino acid content of foods

(mg/100g 可食部)

编码 Code	食物名称 Food name	苏氨酸 Thr	色氨酸 Trp	缬氨酸 Val	精氨酸 Arg	组氨酸 His	丙氨酸 Ala	天冬氨酸 Asp	谷氨酸 Glu	甘氨酸 Gly	脯氨酸 Pro	丝氨酸 Ser
谷类及制品												
01-1-206	小麦面粉 (标准粉)	420	110	590	660	300	500	690	5240	570	1670	730
01-1-207	小麦面粉 (富强粉、特一粉)	300	120	550	410	220	340	470	4250	410	1320	570
01-1-208	小麦面粉 (特制)	310	130	440	450	200	400	570	4370	480	1380	590
01-1-313	挂面 (富强粉)	330	120	500	460	240	380	510	4540	440	1450	610
01-1-314	龙须面 (素)	300	130	420	400	210	320	450	3900	380	1300	520
01-1-315	龙须面 (鸡蛋)	310	120	530	500	240	380	520	4470	450	1410	600
01-1-316	面条 (富强粉, 切面)	240	90	350	300	180	300	360	1670	340	1100	460
01-1-317	面条 (富强粉, 煮)	100	30	160	90	70	110	140	1400	140	440	190
01-1-503	面筋 (肉馅)	470	120	640	770	310	780	930	3000	1010	1230	560
01-2-106	粳米 (极品精米)	190	60	340	440	130	350	540	1060	270	170	260
01-2-107	粳米 (西域王米)	240	80	380	570	150	400	650	1250	320	330	370
01-2-108	粳米 (小站稻米)	190	60	320	410	120	420	560	1030	250	250	280
01-2-215	香米	230	50	360	480	130	360	590	1200	270	250	340
01-2-408	籼米饭 (蒸)	100	30	170	210	60	160	260	520	130	120	150
01-2-409	籼米粥	50	10	90	100	30	70	120	250	60	60	70
01-2-411	河粉	270	300	370	610	160	400	680	1310	310	410	360
01-3-108	玉米粒 (黄, 干)	250	30	460	220	180	610	450	1640	210	700	390
01-3-109	玉米面 (黄)	270	40	460	260	180	660	520	1650	370	740	410
01-3-110	玉米糁 (黄)	190	20	430	230	180	610	430	1600	210	700	380
01-5-104	小米 (黄)	350	120	480	260	190	890	650	1930	250	780	470
01-9-010	荞麦面	390	110	470	930	220	430	940	2090	560	500	530
01-9-011	莜麦面	460	100	660	870	280	570	1080	2870	610	700	640

食物氨基酸含量 Amino acid content of foods

(mg/100g 可食部)

编码 Code	食物名称 Food name	水分 Water g	蛋白质 Protein g	异亮氨酸 Ile	亮氨酸 Leu	赖氨酸 Lys	含硫氨基酸 (SAA) Total	蛋氨酸 Met	胱氨酸 Cys	芳香族氨基酸 (AAA) Total	苯丙氨酸 Phe	酪氨酸 Tyr
干豆类及制品												
03-1-104	黄豆	9.2	33.1	1250	2370	1990	780	240	540	3190	1860	1330
03-1-207	豆奶粉 (多力牌)	2.6	12.3	470	830	760	270	80	190	1310	830	480
03-1-208	豆奶粉 (大磨牌)	4.3	27.4	1080	2050	1560	820	410	410	2200	1300	900
03-1-306	豆腐 (北豆腐)	78.6	9.2	340	690	520	240	120	120	780	450	330
03-1-307	豆腐 (南豆腐)	83.6	5.7	210	430	340	160	80	80	500	290	210
03-1-527	豆腐皮	9.4	51.6	2140	4020	3220	1430	750	680	4380	2440	1940
03-1-528	腐竹	7.1	54.2	2300	4200	3380	890	540	350	5780	3330	2450
03-1-529	豆腐干	30.1	19.6	1102	1320	1155	200	172	28	1582	892	690
蔬菜类及制品												
04-3-224	黄茎瓜	95.4	1.2	39	39	30	25	14	11	85	42	43
04-8-082	苜蓿 [草头、金花菜]	90.2	5.0	288	188	285	217	188	29	292	185	107
菌藻类												
05-1-031	茶树菇 (干) [柱状田头菇、茶薪菇]	12.2	23.1	2410	1720	930	600	240	360	1480	810	670
05-1-032	干巴菌	86.5	3.8	535	527	119	33	33	—	208	130	78
05-1-033	红奶浆菌 [多汁乳菇、谷熟菌]	94.0	1.5	206	149	50	16	16	—	110	75	35
05-1-034	黄蘑 (干)	11.0	24.6	1610	2490	1110	250	170	80	1870	1020	850
05-1-035	黄伞菇 (干) [多脂鳞伞、黄丝菌]	10.8	22.8	2600	1770	1070	240	190	50	1350	800	550
05-1-036	鸡腿菇 (干) [毛头鬼伞]	10.8	26.7	2530	1940	1210	480	280	200	2100	970	1130
05-1-037	鸡油菌 [黄丝菌、杏菌]	91.4	2.0	70	133	82	19	19	—	130	80	50

食物氨基酸含量 Amino acid content of foods

(mg/100g 可食部)

编码 Code	食物名称 Food name	苏氨酸 Thr	色氨酸 Trp	缬氨酸 Val	精氨酸 Arg	组氨酸 His	丙氨酸 Ala	天冬氨酸 Asp	谷氨酸 Glu	甘氨酸 Gly	脯氨酸 Pro	丝氨酸 Ser
干豆类及制品												
03-1-104	黄豆	1190	450	1140	2420	800	1360	3670	5690	1370	1510	1690
03-1-207	豆奶粉 (多力牌)	510	160	520	880	280	490	1440	2210	480	580	640
03-1-208	豆奶粉 (大磨牌)	1090	270	1010	1780	590	1020	3050	5010	990	1240	1410
03-1-306	豆腐 (北豆腐)	350	120	380	650	210	380	1040	1680	360	450	500
03-1-307	豆腐 (南豆腐)	220	50	240	420	140	240	680	1100	230	300	310
03-1-527	豆腐皮	2200	700	2440	3750	1260	2280	6080	9710	2150	2150	2790
03-1-528	腐竹	2270	400	2310	4280	1360	1950	6730	10630	2230	3220	2950
03-1-529	豆腐干	818	225	975	1252	502	900	2625	3555	938	705	945
蔬菜类及制品												
04-3-224	黄茎瓜	22	16	31	37	17	53	448	156	27	Tr	38
04-8-082	苜蓿 [草头、金花菜]	184	45	286	223	97	276	579	490	219	174	171
菌藻类												
05-1-031	茶树菇 (干) [柱状田头菇、茶薪菇]	960	210	1030	1070	340	1270	1770	3030	840	760	950
05-1-032	干巴菌	146	38	335	140	41	254	230	475	149	60	127
05-1-033	红奶浆菌 [多汁乳菇、谷熟菌]	82	15	99	88	21	100	141	255	82	24	72
05-1-034	黄蘑 (干)	1200	260	1330	1530	450	1230	2170	3020	1040	1020	1470
05-1-035	黄伞菇 (干) [多脂鳞伞、黄丝菌]	1000	210	920	1160	370	1250	1730	3240	870	910	960
05-1-036	鸡腿菇 (干) [毛头鬼伞]	1120	70	1020	1490	390	1410	2320	4290	950	1010	1140
05-1-037	鸡油菌 [黄丝菌、杏菌]	61	26	68	106	38	70	175	447	69	94	87

食物氨基酸含量 Amino acid content of foods

(mg/100g 可食部)

编码 Code	食物名称 Food name	水分 Water g	蛋白质 Protein g	异亮氨酸 Ile	亮氨酸 Leu	赖氨酸 Lys	含硫氨基酸 (SAA) Total	蛋氨酸 Met	胱氨酸 Cys	芳香族氨基酸 (AAA) Total	苯丙氨酸 Phe	酪氨酸 Tyr
05-1-039	鸡枞(干)	13.6	32.8	1940	2980	1230	280	180	100	2230	1080	1150
05-1-040	鸡枞(油炸)[油鸡枞]	16.5	4.8	200	389	235	55	55	—	390	230	160
05-1-041	鸡枞花	95.0	2.3	279	232	24	19	19	—	191	117	74
05-1-043	白牛肝菌(干)[美味牛肝菌]	11.6	27.8	1960	2840	990	690	630	60	2050	1070	980
05-1-044	黑牛肝菌[铜色牛肝菌]	90.6	3.6	310	235	104	44	44	—	199	129	70
05-1-046	乳牛肝菌(干)[粘盖牛肝菌、松树菌]	10.5	15.3	2210	1160	510	260	140	120	880	510	370
05-1-047	牛眼睛菌[马勃菌]	86.6	5.1	420	445	135	48	48	—	383	203	180
05-1-050	松蘑(干)[松茸、松口蘑]	10.6	12.5	1230	1590	290	130	70	60	530	280	250
05-1-051	杏鲍菇	89.6	1.3	122	100	40	26	10	16	112	70	42
05-1-052	血红菇(干)	7.8	22.4	2690	1790	590	190	120	70	860	460	400
05-1-053	元蘑(干)[亚侧耳、冬蘑、黄蘑]	7.8	12.3	880	1310	500	70	—	70	900	540	360
05-1-055	榛蘑(干)[小蜜环菌]	8.0	17.7	1240	1900	620	120	70	50	780	370	410
05-2-009	螺旋藻(干)	6.5	64.7	2775	4580	2308	1253	748	(505)	4041	2295	1746
05-2-010	裙带菜(干)[海芥菜、海木耳]	9.2	25.0	1050	1870	1100	800	530	270	1910	1110	800
水果类及制品												
06-2-313	小枣(干)	28.3	2.7	50	70	50	60	10	50	100	60	40
06-3-912	无花果(干)	11.5	3.6	100	171	125	104	25	79	190	111	79
06-5-027	木瓜[番木瓜]	91.7	0.6	23	32	15	2	2	—	27	21	6
坚果、种子类												
07-1-026	山核桃(熟)	2.8	8.3	510	650	220	90	90	Tr	1080	690	390

(mg/100g 可食部)

编码 Code	食物名称 Food name	苏氨酸 Thr	色氨酸 Trp	缬氨酸 Val	精氨酸 Arg	组氨酸 His	丙氨酸 Ala	天冬氨酸 Asp	谷氨酸 Glu	甘氨酸 Gly	脯氨酸 Pro	丝氨酸 Ser
05-1-039	鸡纵 (干)	1320	270	1380	1150	620	1640	1970	2830	1250	1060	1310
05-1-040	鸡纵 (油炸) [油鸡纵]	178	—	195	305	110	205	500	1280	200	270	250
05-1-041	鸡纵花	97	—	135	54	32	176	143	339	111	34	78
05-1-043	白牛肝菌 (干) [美味牛肝菌]	1230	280	890	1220	460	1400	2100	3140	1050	1210	1220
05-1-044	黑牛肝菌 [铜色牛肝菌]	167	—	256	170	44	357	332	761	223	78	184
05-1-046	乳牛肝菌 (干) [粘盖牛肝菌、松树菌]	610	90	580	630	220	680	1080	1740	540	1040	610
05-1-047	牛眼睛菌 [马勃菌]	224	—	268	199	83	296	574	1183	297	40	257
05-1-050	松蘑 (干) [松茸、松口蘑]	380	50	330	360	120	400	670	1140	330	370	380
05-1-051	杏鲍菇	43	6	55	28	18	67	36	91	42	35	21
05-1-052	血红菇 (干)	700	120	680	660	260	790	1250	2100	620	660	680
05-1-053	元蘑 (干) [亚侧耳、冬蘑、黄蘑]	570	120	490	490	190	650	940	1630	460	520	540
05-1-055	榛蘑 (干) [小蜜环菌]	680	30	590	660	230	800	1250	2030	610	440	730
05-2-009	螺旋藻 (干)	2785	1100	3434	3692	754	4388	5448	(6118)	2688	1448	2870
05-2-010	裙带菜 (干) [海芥菜、海木耳]	1080	330	1200	1100	330	1580	2190	2430	1280	900	1030
水果类及制品												
06-2-313	小枣 (干)	50	10	50	60	20	50	280	100	60	(130)	60
06-3-912	无花果 (干)	103	0	133	211	67	148	320	395	131	233	134
06-5-027	木瓜 [番木瓜]	21	10	36	18	9	38	174	57	29	21	21
坚果、种子类												
07-1-026	山核桃 (熟)	250	130	400	850	190	390	800	1510	380	430	370

食物氨基酸含量 Amino acid content of foods

(mg/100g 可食部)

编码 Code	食物名称 Food name	水分 Water g	蛋白质 Protein g	异亮氨酸 Ile	亮氨酸 Leu	赖氨酸 Lys	含硫氨基酸 (SAA) Total	蛋氨酸 Met	胱氨酸 Cys	芳香族氨基酸 (AAA) Total	苯丙氨酸 Phe	酪氨酸 Tyr
07-1-032	栗子仁 (熟)	47.3	4.5	290	390	180	120	40	80	270	160	110
07-1-033	松子 (熟)	3.4	12.9	440	740	350	180	140	40	1030	530	500
07-1-034	杏仁 (熟, 带壳)	1.7	25.1	910	1800	640	170	120	50	2220	1410	810
07-1-035	杏仁 (熟, 去壳)	3.1	28.0	900	1710	720	440	190	250	2080	1310	770
07-1-036	腰果 (熟)	2.1	24.0	940	1740	1050	760	410	350	1870	1130	740
07-1-037	榛子 (熟)	2.2	12.5	290	500	250	300	100	200	950	630	320
07-1-038	榛子仁 (熟)	2.2	15.6	560	1050	380	200	140	60	1270	760	510
07-1-040	香榧 (熟)	1.1	12.4	660	830	670	450	200	250	1170	630	540
07-2-020	花生 (烤, 勤俭牌)	2.5	26.4	940	1810	910	630	300	330	2480	1490	990
07-2-024	葵花子 (熟)	2.7	28.5	1170	1800	860	880	520	360	2120	1360	760
07-2-025	南瓜子 (熟) [白瓜子]	3.2	26.6	750	1230	600	980	410	570	1700	1000	700
07-2-026	西瓜子 (熟) [黑瓜子]	10.7	29.0	1130	2010	950	1170	770	400	2630	1620	1010
畜肉类及制品												
08-1-121	猪肉 (前臀尖, 杜长大猪)	58.6	15.3	530	1160	1210	520	360	160	1150	580	570
08-1-122	猪肉 (前臀尖, 良杂猪)	53.7	14.2	510	1030	1080	470	350	120	1090	550	540
08-1-123	猪肉 (后臀尖, 杜长大猪)	71.2	20.8	820	1750	1840	910	680	230	1780	880	900
08-1-124	猪肉 (后臀尖, 良杂猪)	68.8	20.0	700	1470	1560	670	480	190	1510	750	760
08-1-125	猪肉 (硬肋, 杜长大猪)	36.5	10.8	400	800	830	360	240	120	830	430	400
08-1-126	猪肉 (硬肋, 良杂猪)	38.4	11.6	480	950	1000	320	210	110	960	500	460
08-1-127	猪肉 (通脊, 杜长大猪)	70.7	22.3	840	1810	1920	880	660	220	1830	890	940
08-1-128	猪肉 (通脊, 良杂猪)	73.2	20.7	700	1470	1580	620	430	190	1540	770	770
08-1-129	猪肉 (里脊)	74.7	19.6	700	1590	1690	500	290	210	1660	830	830
08-1-131	猪小排 (杜长大猪)	60.0	16.8	600	1250	1310	490	330	160	1300	660	640

(mg/100g 可食部)

编码 Code	食物名称 Food name	苏氨酸 Thr	色氨酸 Trp	缬氨酸 Val	精氨酸 Arg	组氨酸 His	丙氨酸 Ala	天冬氨酸 Asp	谷氨酸 Glu	甘氨酸 Gly	脯氨酸 Pro	丝氨酸 Ser
07-1-032	栗子仁(熟)	280	60	280	170	140	300	590	620	290	270	270
07-1-033	松子(熟)	380	90	450	1470	220	560	1000	1840	530	570	600
07-1-034	杏仁(熟, 带壳)	760	—	990	2860	610	1190	2810	6860	1760	1040	1050
07-1-035	杏仁(熟, 去壳)	740	120	1060	2730	570	1160	3800	6730	1650	1440	1000
07-1-036	腰果(熟)	830	270	1270	2590	470	1200	2270	5160	1020	840	1220
07-1-037	榛子(熟)	210	150	300	830	130	620	700	1370	290	530	270
07-1-038	榛子仁(熟)	480	190	670	370	360	740	1190	3830	720	560	670
07-1-040	香榧(熟)	520	100	840	850	250	580	1250	1510	530	580	720
07-2-020	花生(烤, 勤俭牌)	750	210	1100	3220	590	1070	3310	5700	1370	1110	1410
07-2-024	葵花子(熟)	980	500	1390	2750	640	1230	2690	6750	1530	1150	1260
07-2-025	南瓜子(熟)[白瓜子]	480	610	740	2570	370	760	1540	3150	930	470	860
07-2-026	西瓜子(熟)[黑瓜子]	970	570	1280	2190	740	1420	3320	5930	1710	970	1520
畜肉类及制品												
08-1-121	猪肉(前臀尖, 杜长大猪)	600	70	620	970	460	880	1240	1970	770	630	540
08-1-122	猪肉(前臀尖, 良杂猪)	560	70	550	910	390	790	1160	1960	710	630	520
08-1-123	猪肉(后臀尖, 杜长大猪)	1020	60	940	1430	800	1290	2050	3380	950	850	920
08-1-124	猪肉(后臀尖, 良杂猪)	810	60	790	1220	650	1050	1680	2700	820	710	720
08-1-125	猪肉(硬肋, 杜长大猪)	390	70	430	650	350	580	820	1200	500	450	350
08-1-126	猪肉(硬肋, 良杂猪)	500	70	500	820	390	740	1060	1790	730	590	460
08-1-127	猪肉(通脊, 杜长大猪)	1030	60	970	1440	890	1280	2120	3440	950	830	920
08-1-128	猪肉(通脊, 良杂猪)	840	60	800	1220	760	1130	1750	2910	980	790	750
08-1-129	猪肉(里脊)	920	60	750	1280	650	1150	1890	3120	840	780	820
08-1-131	猪小排(杜长大猪)	710	70	740	1120	540	1060	1450	2380	1090	820	660

食物氨基酸含量 Amino acid content of foods

(mg/100g 可食部)

编码 Code	食物名称 Food name	水分 Water g	蛋白质 Protein g	异亮氨酸 Ile	亮氨酸 Leu	赖氨酸 Lys	含硫氨基酸 (SAA) Total	蛋氨酸 Met	胱氨酸 Cys	芳香族氨基酸 (AAA) Total	苯丙氨酸 Phe	酪氨酸 Tyr
08-1-132	猪小排 (良杂猪)	55.4	14.1	510	1030	1090	420	290	130	1060	530	530
08-1-213	猪肚	79.3	14.1	550	1090	920	490	320	170	1070	530	540
08-1-214	猪肝	72.6	19.2	640	1560	1290	680	390	290	1540	840	700
08-1-215	猪舌 [口条]	70.2	18.1	640	1340	1340	400	210	190	1340	700	640
08-1-216	猪肾 [猪腰子]	80.6	15.8	560	1270	1020	340	200	140	1280	680	600
08-1-318	火腿心全精肉	35.2	37.0	1290	2820	2900	790	520	270	2780	1410	1370
08-1-319	火腿心肉	25.6	22.2	860	1560	1700	460	390	70	1570	840	730
08-1-321	叉烧肉	60.4	20.9	890	1680	1770	730	540	190	1580	800	780
08-1-322	酱排骨	39.0	21.7	800	1630	1610	600	400	200	1570	860	710
08-1-324	熏烤小里脊	63.2	17.7	710	1530	1570	480	280	200	1390	730	660
08-1-325	猪肉脯	11.2	28.0	990	1910	1930	860	720	140	1960	1110	850
08-1-326	肉酥	2.4	30.7	1410	2510	2380	1090	880	210	2740	1610	1130
08-1-327	猪肉松	14.0	41.8	1920	3470	3500	1380	920	460	3770	1970	1800
08-1-329	酱肘子	58.9	29.6	1358	2511	2678	1153	818	335	2483	1358	1125
08-1-424	热狗肠	51.3	13.2	390	860	860	310	190	120	890	500	390
08-1-425	火腿肠	61.5	12.1	530	910	850	300	200	100	1150	640	510
08-1-426	火腿	76.6	15.5	620	1210	1190	550	430	120	1260	660	600
08-1-427	火腿 (云南)	22.1	11.4	481	898	931	289	289	—	857	487	370
08-1-429	午餐肉	55.2	9.0	410	700	670	320	240	80	810	460	350
08-2-111	牛肉 (背部肉) [上脑]	66.4	17.4	690	1330	1430	490	280	210	1330	700	630
08-2-112	牛肉 (里脊肉) [牛柳]	72.0	22.3	970	1900	2070	490	270	220	1760	950	810
08-2-113	牛肉 (臀部肉) [紫盖、白板]	72.8	22.6	885	1730	1875	725	515	210	1595	860	735
08-2-114	牛肉 (肩部肉) [肩肉]	53.3	14.1	610	1090	1170	480	320	160	1000	540	460
08-2-115	牛肉 (胸部肉) [牛胸]	58.8	16.6	670	1310	1420	550	380	170	1190	640	550

食物氨基酸含量 Amino acid content of foods

(mg/100g 可食部)

编码 Code	食物名称 Food name	苏氨酸 Thr	色氨酸 Trp	缬氨酸 Val	精氨酸 Arg	组氨酸 His	丙氨酸 Ala	天冬氨酸 Asp	谷氨酸 Glu	甘氨酸 Gly	脯氨酸 Pro	丝氨酸 Ser
08-1-132	猪小排(良杂猪)	460	60	570	900	400	780	1190	1980	680	580	520
08-1-213	猪肚	650	90	660	1070	280	1050	1320	2100	1550	1000	730
08-1-214	猪肝	800	80	910	1060	460	1160	1640	2330	1150	880	870
08-1-215	猪舌 [口条]	750	80	750	1120	420	1070	1520	2540	1150	840	740
08-1-216	猪肾 [猪腰子]	660	80	740	950	370	930	1350	1830	940	720	720
08-1-318	火腿心全精肉	1540	330	1570	2030	1120	1930	3080	4990	1430	1330	1250
08-1-319	火腿心肉	980	150	960	1240	640	1130	1950	3170	1030	800	820
08-1-321	叉烧肉	1010	190	1010	1240	560	1180	1990	3230	930	780	860
08-1-322	酱排骨	940	200	1020	1390	480	1480	1980	3130	1830	1370	840
08-1-324	熏烤小里脊	860	220	880	1170	590	1150	1710	2820	960	800	740
08-1-325	猪肉脯	1030	100	1070	1420	730	1310	2180	4330	980	1010	860
08-1-326	肉酥	1420	270	1540	1920	930	1690	2990	6550	1340	1240	1300
08-1-327	猪肉松	2030	370	2050	2790	1250	2290	3990	7040	1740	1460	1730
08-1-329	酱肘子	1395	316	1414	2223	781	1795	2799	4799	1395	1256	1228
08-1-424	热狗肠	470	130	500	790	320	740	1060	1890	1020	770	500
08-1-425	火腿肠	570	60	550	920	360	690	1150	1920	710	610	570
08-1-426	火腿	670	120	700	970	510	1020	1420	2240	1050	920	640
08-1-427	火腿(云南)	510	—	503	685	426	595	1006	2158	543	138	449
08-1-429	午餐肉	390	70	420	540	300	510	850	1380	500	520	380
08-2-111	牛肉(青部肉)[上脑]	670	60	740	1040	500	920	1440	2450	730	630	600
08-2-112	牛肉(里脊肉)[牛柳]	1110	130	1080	1430	880	1300	2310	3650	920	780	950
08-2-113	牛肉(臀部肉)[紫盖、白板]	985	200	1020	1315	810	1185	2010	3260	865	690	835
08-2-114	牛肉(肩部肉)[肩肉]	590	40	630	850	450	750	1220	1990	600	480	500
08-2-115	牛肉(胸部肉)[牛胸]	700	50	760	1050	550	950	1460	2460	810	630	620

食物氨基酸含量 Amino acid content of foods

(mg/100g 可食部)

编码 Code	食物名称 Food name	水分 Water g	蛋白质 Protein g	异亮氨酸 Ile	亮氨酸 Leu	赖氨酸 Lys	含硫氨基酸 (SAA) Total	蛋氨酸 Met	胱氨酸 Cys	芳香族氨基酸 (AAA) Total	苯丙氨酸 Phe	酪氨酸 Tyr
08-2-116	牛肉(腹部肉)[牛腩]	57.6	17.1	770	1410	1520	300	160	140	1280	690	590
08-2-117	牛肉(膝圆肉)[和尚头]	74.6	22.4	850	1630	1790	340	140	200	1460	770	690
08-2-118	牛肉(股内肉)[针扒、米龙、黄瓜条]	72.5	22.8	890	1710	1860	640	430	210	1530	810	720
08-2-119	牛肉(小腿肉)[牛展、牛腱子]	73.4	23.0	800	1530	1650	620	400	220	1470	770	700
08-2-210	牛百叶(黑)	85.6	13.2	360	700	580	280	170	110	660	340	320
08-2-307	牛肉(酱,五香)	55.5	33.2	1410	2757	2876	1237	937	300	2493	1274	1219
08-2-308	牛肉(清香)	63.6	25.8	1058	2116	2226	911	653	258	1941	984	957
08-2-309	牛腱子(香叶)	53.9	35.6	1230	2460	2550	1080	710	370	2240	1230	1010
08-2-310	牛肉干(长富牌)	14.6	41.8	1463	2627	2627	1344	896	448	2597	1582	1015
08-3-113	羊肉(上脑)	78.0	19.0	820	1530	1630	730	530	200	1550	790	760
08-3-114	羊肉(腰窝)	73.5	18.9	810	1510	1610	710	520	190	1490	790	700
08-3-115	羊肉(前腿)	77.1	19.8	880	1660	1760	870	650	220	1610	840	770
08-3-116	羊肉(后腿)	75.1	20.6	820	1560	1660	790	600	190	1530	790	740
08-3-309	烧羊肉(五香)	59.4	33.6	1370	2700	2820	910	590	320	2530	1370	1160
08-3-310	羊肉串(生)	74.5	13.0	530	1000	130	470	320	150	980	520	460
08-4-304	驴肉(五香)	64.9	28.2	1170	2320	2250	730	660	70	2280	1240	1040
禽肉类及制品												
09-1-112	鸡胸脯肉	71.7	24.6	930	1900	2020	980	730	250	1620	870	750
09-1-113	鸡腿	71.7	20.2	610	1320	1430	670	490	180	1120	580	540
09-1-114	鸡翅	63.3	19.0	710	1340	1400	690	510	180	1280	690	590
09-1-115	鸡块(带浆粉)	58.2	12.2	420	800	750	420	250	170	750	430	320
09-1-116	野山鸡	70.3	20.4	890	1620	1760	840	600	240	1590	800	790

食物氨基酸含量 Amino acid content of foods

(mg/100g 可食部)

编码 Code	食物名称 Food name	苏氨酸 Thr	色氨酸 Trp	缬氨酸 Val	精氨酸 Arg	组氨酸 His	丙氨酸 Ala	天冬氨酸 Asp	谷氨酸 Glu	甘氨酸 Gly	脯氨酸 Pro	丝氨酸 Ser
08-2-116	牛肉(腹部肉)[牛腩]	800	120	830	1140	590	1020	1710	2690	870	680	700
08-2-117	牛肉(膝圆肉)[和尚头]	950	220	930	1260	710	1130	2000	3190	830	670	810
08-2-118	牛肉(股内肉)[针扒、米龙、黄瓜条]	1000	140	1000	1330	810	1230	2060	3300	950	720	860
08-2-119	牛肉(小腿肉)[牛展、牛腱子]	840	170	890	1230	590	1120	1750	2960	940	720	740
08-2-210	牛百叶(黑)	390	40	420	630	170	570	870	1240	820	500	440
08-2-307	牛肉(酱,五香)	1620	300	1638	2266	937	2038	3194	5214	1747	1356	1392
08-2-308	牛肉(清香)	1242	230	1214	1656	773	1647	2512	4076	1509	1104	1021
08-2-309	牛腱子(香叶)	1370	260	1500	2390	840	2380	2940	4860	3150	2040	1350
08-2-310	牛肉干(长富牌)	1463	597	1463	1970	776	1910	2896	5194	1463	1253	1254
08-3-113	羊肉(上脑)	880	90	940	1230	540	1070	1750	3000	810	660	760
08-3-114	羊肉(腰窝)	870	90	1030	1350	540	1350	1780	3020	1250	890	790
08-3-115	羊肉(前腿)	950	(154)	1140	1350	570	1210	1880	3190	850	720	800
08-3-116	羊肉(后腿)	890	140	1070	1250	550	1160	1800	2950	850	690	770
08-3-309	烧羊肉(五香)	1510	350	1640	2540	800	2410	3160	5070	2950	1930	1320
08-3-310	羊肉串(生)	580	110	610	800	350	700	1220	2290	540	470	550
08-4-304	驴肉(五香)	1340	210	1330	1840	850	1780	2620	4430	1860	1460	1250
禽肉类及制品												
09-1-112	鸡胸脯肉	1080	300	1120	1560	870	1360	2260	3570	990	780	960
09-1-113	鸡腿	740	140	710	1150	420	1020	1580	2780	900	670	710
09-1-114	鸡翅	740	130	760	1190	460	1100	1580	2640	1090	760	680
09-1-115	鸡块(带浆粉)	420	90	490	620	330	560	900	1680	460	490	430
09-1-116	野山鸡	960	160	1030	1350	650	1180	1940	3080	800	670	850

食物氨基酸含量 Amino acid content of foods

(mg/100g 可食部)

编码 Code	食物名称 Food name	水分 Water g	蛋白质 Protein g	异亮氨酸 Ile	亮氨酸 Leu	赖氨酸 Lys	含硫氨基酸 (SAA) Total	蛋氨酸 Met	胱氨酸 Cys	芳香族氨基酸 (AAA) Total	苯丙氨酸 Phe	酪氨酸 Tyr
09-1-308	扒鸡 (五香脱骨)	59.7	23.4	820	1710	1760	570	350	220	1620	800	820
09-1-310	童子鸡 (熟)	66.8	15.8	690	1240	1330	650	460	190	1270	640	630
09-2-307	烤鸭 (老唐牌)	57.0	20.3	830	1720	1750	530	300	230	1650	830	820
09-3-302	腊鹅	15.8	24.6	880	1680	1710	890	640	250	1500	810	690
09-4-301	火鸡腿	72.5	16.7	760	1430	1410	690	500	190	1440	770	670
09-9-003	乳鸽	57.5	11.3	510	990	1020	440	330	110	1010	530	480
09-9-004	乳鸽 (红烧)	59.0	16.9	631	1287	1230	451	385	66	1279	672	607
乳类及制品												
10-1-105	牛乳 (光明牌)	88.0	3.1	133	271	217	106	83	23	280	151	129
10-1-106	牛乳 (乐百氏牌)	87.4	3.3	140	287	230	109	76	33	284	148	136
10-1-107	牛乳 (帕玛拉特牌)	87.9	3.0	124	241	195	101	75	26	245	135	110
10-1-108	牛乳 (三元牌)	86.9	3.4	133	275	225	116	86	30	274	146	128
10-1-110	牛乳 (龙丹牌)	87.5	2.9	128	262	209	106	80	26	257	137	120
10-1-111	牛乳 (蒙牛牌)	87.2	3.1	143	288	241	123	88	35	290	152	138
10-1-112	牛乳 (新南洋牌)	87.4	3.1	142	267	223	117	79	38	274	146	128
10-9-004	全脂甜炼乳 (雀巢)	15.9	7.5	310	680	520	220	150	70	470	330	140
蛋类及制品												
11-1-109	鸡蛋 (红皮)	77.1	12.2	720	1080	840	490	440	50	1190	680	510
11-1-110	藏鸡蛋	72.7	12.6	570	1030	780	720	400	320	1090	600	490
11-1-111	乌鸡蛋 (绿皮)	69.7	12.6	640	1200	910	500	290	210	1210	670	540
11-2-203	咸鸭蛋 (煮)	70.0	13.8	700	1050	830	710	530	180	1340	760	580
鱼虾蟹贝类												
12-1-131	草鱼 [白鲩、草包鱼]	78.2	17.7	600	1190	1350	610	460	150	1140	640	500

食物氨基酸含量 Amino acid content of foods

(mg/100g 可食部)

编码 Code	食物名称 Food name	苏氨酸 Thr	色氨酸 Trp	缬氨酸 Val	精氨酸 Arg	组氨酸 His	丙氨酸 Ala	天冬氨酸 Asp	谷氨酸 Glu	甘氨酸 Gly	脯氨酸 Pro	丝氨酸 Ser
09-1-308	扒鸡 (五香脱骨)	970	230	1000	1670	650	1480	2070	3100	1830	1230	830
09-1-310	童子鸡 (熟)	700	110	770	990	440	880	1460	2380	640	590	630
09-2-307	烤鸭 (老詰牌)	1020	180	1040	1590	550	1420	2080	3250	1580	1130	920
09-3-302	腊鹅	970	360	1100	1560	530	1760	2000	3340	2220	1410	910
09-4-301	火鸡腿	800	180	740	1200	420	1000	1750	3020	850	810	820
09-9-003	乳鸽	550	60	600	810	280	740	1100	1970	610	480	490
09-9-004	乳鸽 (红烧)	722	148	935	1197	377	1279	1448	2337	1550	1050	681
乳类及制品												
10-1-105	牛乳 (光明牌)	110	53	171	96	75	89	196	566	51	266	144
10-1-106	牛乳 (乐百氏牌)	119	65	191	102	78	102	211	622	57	284	160
10-1-107	牛乳 (帕玛拉特牌)	95	49	145	85	60	84	173	486	48	227	127
10-1-108	牛乳 (三元牌)	121	64	167	96	72	92	216	621	53	271	165
10-1-110	牛乳 (龙丹牌)	104	53	160	92	68	88	183	527	51	246	137
10-1-111	牛乳 (蒙牛牌)	117	64	187	104	77	98	209	588	57	276	153
10-1-112	牛乳 (新南洋牌)	110	60	168	96	73	94	196	559	63	264	146
10-9-004	全脂甜炼乳 (雀巢)	280	60	390	200	170	220	510	1520	130	640	380
蛋类及制品												
11-1-109	鸡蛋 (红皮)	600	200	700	740	250	670	1290	1640	400	450	950
11-1-110	藏鸡蛋	590	180	570	740	260	630	1220	1480	400	440	930
11-1-111	乌鸡蛋 (绿皮)	640	240	740	810	280	690	1290	1570	420	490	960
11-2-203	咸鸭蛋 (煮)	710	200	730	680	270	590	1150	1600	390	460	970
鱼虾蟹贝类												
12-1-131	草鱼 [白鲩、草包鱼]	660	150	710	900	550	900	1550	2180	720	540	620

食物氨基酸含量 Amino acid content of foods

(mg/100g 可食部)

编码 Code	食物名称 Food name	水分 Water g	蛋白质 Protein g	异亮氨酸 Ile	亮氨酸 Leu	赖氨酸 Lys	含硫氨基酸 (SAA) Total	蛋氨酸 Met	胱氨酸 Cys	芳香族氨基酸 (AAA) Total	苯丙氨酸 Phe	酪氨酸 Tyr
12-1-132	鲢鱼 [白鲢、胖子、连子鱼]	82.8	16.3	620	1310	1460	680	530	150	1260	670	590
12-1-133	鲫鱼 [喜头鱼、海附鱼]	78.6	18.0	660	1450	1670	740	570	170	1380	760	620
12-1-241	带鱼 (切段)	78.8	17.6	660	1220	1380	710	530	180	1140	580	560
12-1-242	黄鱼 (小黄花鱼)	79.4	17.0	700	1320	1500	730	540	190	1320	680	640
12-1-244	鲭鱼	45.2	14.4	627	1096	1237	711	418	293	1068	557	511
12-1-245	双髻鲨	73.6	27.4	1071	1666	1795	923	446	477	1589	864	725
12-1-303	金鲨鱼翅 (干)	12.0	84.1	2010	2550	2990	1930	1280	650	7010	1810	5200
12-1-304	鱼排	61.2	10.1	390	730	700	410	300	110	810	450	360
12-1-305	鱼丸	72.5	11.1	440	830	930	460	350	110	810	460	350
12-1-306	鱼子酱	55.9	9.6	490	840	520	320	240	80	650	330	320
12-1-401	草鱼 (熏)	45.6	24.0	880	1720	1780	800	660	140	1660	890	770
12-1-402	丁香鱼 (香辣味)	30.3	19.0	800	1540	1300	700	540	160	1570	920	650
12-1-403	凤尾鱼 (熟)	19.5	23.5	920	1850	1930	870	710	160	1660	910	750
12-1-404	箭鱼 (炸)	47.8	20.8	930	1780	1830	950	700	250	1560	870	690
12-1-407	鲮鱼 (豆豉, 熟)	18.8	25.5	690	1240	1120	570	450	120	1360	760	600
12-1-408	鳗鱼 (红烧)	55.4	21.3	830	1550	1620	740	590	150	1560	880	680
12-1-409	鲭鱼 (烤, 150℃, 10分)	45.8	16.5	753	1329	1455	914	514	400	1286	672	614
12-1-410	鲭鱼 (烤, 150℃, 20分)	45.7	19.1	817	1416	1578	948	551	397	1378	729	649
12-1-411	鲭鱼 (烤, 150℃, 30分)	32.0	19.9	881	1551	1681	1024	599	425	1502	787	715
12-1-412	鲭鱼 (烤, 180℃, 10分)	47.3	20.2	865	1534	1653	1064	588	476	1490	786	704
12-1-413	鲭鱼 (烤, 210℃, 10分)	39.0	19.0	860	1508	1629	1008	569	439	1464	769	695
12-1-414	鲭鱼 (炸)	28.3	17.2	884	1564	1768	942	579	363	1465	779	686
12-1-415	鲭鱼 (蒸)	47.0	14.6	720	1268	1410	719	397	322	1227	646	581
12-1-416	鲭鱼 (煮)	49.3	14.9	665	1171	1294	759	442	317	1141	598	543

食物氨基酸含量 Amino acid content of foods

(mg/100g 可食部)

编码 Code	食物名称 Food name	苏氨酸 Thr	色氨酸 Trp	缬氨酸 Val	精氨酸 Arg	组氨酸 His	丙氨酸 Ala	天冬氨酸 Asp	谷氨酸 Glu	甘氨酸 Gly	脯氨酸 Pro	丝氨酸 Ser
12-1-132	鲢鱼 [白鲢、胖子、连子鱼]	730	110	760	1020	440	960	1680	2530	750	490	740
12-1-133	鲫鱼 [喜头鱼、海附鱼]	830	190	810	1060	520	1060	1880	2840	780	540	770
12-1-241	带鱼 (切段)	730	100	760	920	300	1020	1580	2360	800	570	650
12-1-242	黄鱼 (小黄花鱼)	790	110	830	1020	300	1000	1730	2670	750	540	740
12-1-244	鲭鱼	619	206	735	886	734	801	1334	1898	645	466	534
12-1-245	双髻鲨	911	263	1026	1282	529	1147	1975	2926	873	655	706
12-1-303	金鲨鱼翅 (干)	2050	670	2720	7170	1200	8670	6060	8510	17190	9480	2960
12-1-304	鱼排	390	70	430	510	170	510	850	2390	400	450	410
12-1-305	鱼丸	510	80	500	700	200	650	1100	2290	590	410	480
12-1-306	鱼子酱	460	70	540	420	160	670	710	2430	280	450	400
12-1-401	草鱼 (熏)	1050	180	1090	1390	560	1540	2310	3460	1630	1150	960
12-1-402	丁香鱼 (香辣味)	910	150	1020	1220	410	1090	2060	3430	950	700	920
12-1-403	凤尾鱼 (熟)	1090	190	1140	1420	410	1570	2390	3790	1370	1040	1010
12-1-404	箭鱼 (炸)	930	140	1090	1330	450	1390	2130	3690	1180	940	890
12-1-407	鲮鱼 (豆豉, 熟)	680	180	810	1170	380	1390	1780	2450	1940	1410	770
12-1-408	鳗鱼 (红烧)	870	160	900	1220	430	1340	1940	4490	1360	980	820
12-1-409	鲭鱼 (烤, 150℃, 10 分)	748	245	889	1072	801	986	1630	2323	830	591	657
12-1-410	鲭鱼 (烤, 150℃, 20 分)	800	237	956	1142	864	1091	1737	2490	963	669	707
12-1-411	鲭鱼 (烤, 150℃, 30 分)	869	250	1030	1238	872	1155	1887	2705	985	700	765
12-1-412	鲭鱼 (烤, 180℃, 10 分)	859	234	1012	1197	893	1164	1870	2661	1024	716	768
12-1-413	鲭鱼 (烤, 210℃, 10 分)	848	259	1007	1208	898	1118	1836	2620	950	672	750
12-1-414	鲭鱼 (炸)	843	260	933	1260	454	1150	1930	2872	883	645	726
12-1-415	鲭鱼 (蒸)	716	140	837	1017	761	945	1560	2211	833	587	630
12-1-416	鲭鱼 (煮)	658	187	770	937	625	859	1429	2025	722	523	580

食物氨基酸含量 Amino acid content of foods

(mg/100g 可食部)

编码 Code	食物名称 Food name	水分 Water g	蛋白质 Protein g	异亮氨酸 Ile	亮氨酸 Leu	赖氨酸 Lys	含硫氨基酸 (SAA) Total	蛋氨酸 Met	胱氨酸 Cys	芳香族氨基酸 (AAA) Total	苯丙氨酸 Phe	酪氨酸 Tyr
12-1-417	沙丁鱼 (茄汁, 熟)	70.4	13.8	610	1070	1100	550	440	110	1100	580	520
12-1-420	午餐鱼 (香辣味)	37.5	24.4	810	1730	1850	720	550	170	1690	890	800
12-2-203	虾酱	72.3	10.8	660	740	580	400	280	120	930	480	450
12-2-204	虾仁 (红)	87.8	10.4	340	670	750	410	290	120	680	360	320
12-2-301	虾仁肉丸	70.0	4.6	167	302	314	137	85	52	299	167	132
12-3-006	海蟹 (小)	79.2	14.2	520	920	950	510	350	160	980	480	500
12-3-301	蟹足棒	67.4	9.0	370	670	760	380	290	90	740	410	330
12-4-117	海蚌 [西施舌]	87.7	9.5	349	631	691	302	302	Tr	649	266	383
12-9-014	甲鱼蛋	75.2	12.5	580	980	Tr	290	290	Tr	1030	510	520
12-9-301	墨鱼圈	84.8	13.0	400	750	760	440	310	130	650	330	320
12-9-302	墨鱼丸	71.0	13.4	500	930	1010	530	380	150	910	480	430
婴幼儿食品												
13-2-002	鸡肝蔬菜泥 (亨氏)	82.5	4.0	170	310	240	110	60	50	390	200	190
13-3-011	米粉 (高蛋白, 亨氏)	3.1	15.7	680	1190	820	500	250	250	1450	860	590
小吃、甜饼												
14-1-039	黑芝麻汤圆	37.2	4.4	170	330	140	220	120	100	420	270	150
14-2-212	月饼 (奶油莲芸)	20.5	5.5	128	240	121	131	41	90	299	184	115
速食食品												
15-1-011	比萨饼 (夹奶酪)	47.8	12.2	504	995	868	397	276	121	1134	582	552
15-1-012	比萨饼 (夹奶酪、肉和蔬菜)	47.7	16.5	689	1344	1218	540	376	164	1457	757	700
15-1-015	三明治 (夹鸡肉片, 无调料酱)	47.3	13.3	666	978	958	517	334	183	972	554	418
15-1-016	三明治 (夹烤牛肉片)	48.6	15.5	679	1191	1111	557	366	191	1123	634	489

食物氨基酸含量 Amino acid content of foods

(mg/100g 可食部)

编码 Code	食物名称 Food name	苏氨酸 Thr	色氨酸 Trp	缬氨酸 Val	精氨酸 Arg	组氨酸 His	丙氨酸 Ala	天冬氨酸 Asp	谷氨酸 Glu	甘氨酸 Gly	脯氨酸 Pro	丝氨酸 Ser
12-1-417	沙丁鱼(茄汁,熟)	650	120	710	750	510	830	1390	2130	710	580	580
12-1-420	午餐鱼(香辣味)	990	200	1020	1330	570	1420	2200	2740	1290	900	850
12-2-203	虾酱	390	10	510	320	160	540	930	2100	620	490	390
12-2-204	虾仁(红)	360	10	370	820	160	530	960	1470	650	270	340
12-2-301	虾仁肉丸	168	0	186	290	129	237	371	139	213	170	158
12-3-006	海蟹(小)	560	60	550	1210	240	740	1200	1930	640	460	500
12-3-301	蟹足棒	390	60	420	510	150	530	860	1950	380	270	370
12-4-117	海蚌[西施舌]	308	125	501	918	163	632	793	1314	644	379	370
12-9-014	甲鱼蛋	590	Tr	550	870	340	710	1090	1480	370	640	480
12-9-301	墨鱼圈	430	60	430	710	190	600	980	1440	550	480	420
12-9-302	墨鱼丸	560	90	540	710	250	660	1210	2510	450	430	520
婴幼儿食品												
13-2-002	鸡肝蔬菜泥(亨氏)	170	—	210	190	90	180	370	530	140	220	180
13-3-011	米粉(高蛋白,亨氏)	650	190	790	1130	380	730	1670	2920	630	780	850
小吃、甜饼												
14-1-039	黑芝麻汤圆	160	30	240	410	100	230	400	840	200	220	230
14-2-212	月饼(奶油莲芸)	104	66	174	183	76	137	256	839	134	206	186
速食食品												
15-1-011	比萨饼(夹奶酪)	397	145	635	478	373	361	743	3044	280	1197	625
15-1-012	比萨饼(夹奶酪、肉和蔬菜)	571	199	850	746	510	612	1111	3812	555	1462	805
15-1-015	三明治(夹鸡肉片,无调料酱)	523	155	659	743	383	670	1077	2440	622	732	504
15-1-016	三明治(夹烤牛肉片)	629	176	755	908	489	855	1291	2813	795	875	629

食物氨基酸含量 Amino acid content of foods

(mg/100g 可食部)

编码 Code	食物名称 Food name	水分 Water g	蛋白质 Protein g	异亮氨酸 Ile	亮氨酸 Leu	赖氨酸 Lys	含硫氨基酸 (SAA) Total	蛋氨酸 Met	胱氨酸 Cys	芳香族氨基酸 (AAA) Total	苯丙氨酸 Phe	酪氨酸 Tyr
15-1-018	干酪汉堡包 (夹熏肉, 加调料酱)	43.6	16.4	696	1271	1239	534	365	169	1234	683	551
15-1-019	干酪汉堡包 (普通型, 夹单层肉饼, 无调料酱)	37.3	14.5	618	1135	998	474	310	164	1118	635	483
15-1-020	干酪汉堡包 (普通型, 夹奶酪、单层肉饼, 加调料酱)	47.7	14.1	601	1103	971	465	303	162	1086	617	469
15-1-021	干酪汉堡包 (普通型, 夹奶酪、单层肉饼, 加调料酱和蔬菜)	55.2	11.6	493	901	794	377	246	131	889	506	383
15-1-022	干酪汉堡包 (普通型, 夹奶酪、双层肉饼、双层面包, 加调料酱和蔬菜)	46.6	13.0	558	1023	949	425	286	139	998	558	440
15-1-023	汉堡包 (普通型, 夹肉饼, 加调料酱和蔬菜)	49.4	11.7	495	892	726	388	240	148	832	499	333
15-1-024	热狗 (原味)	54.0	10.6	453	769	641	346	199	147	699	417	282
15-2-105	早餐奶	86.3	2.3	115	213	169	91	69	22	194	106	88
15-2-112	黑芝麻糊粉	2.3	6.9	280	450	150	270	130	140	700	440	260
15-2-115	燕麦片	9.0	14.4	490	1060	540	300	270	30	1300	820	480
15-2-116	燕麦片 (果仁, 甜)	5.4	8.9	320	580	290	260	190	70	870	550	320
15-2-202	鸡汁味干脆面 (面饼+调味料)	2.3	11.4	360	680	220	340	190	150	880	540	340
15-2-203	海鲜味方便面 (面饼+调味料+油料)	6.2	10.4	350	650	210	330	180	150	880	550	330
15-2-209	鳕鱼方便面 (面饼+调味料+珍料+调味油+蔬菜)	5.0	10.2	350	640	430	320	210	110	770	440	330
15-2-210	鳕鱼方便面 (面饼+调味料+蔬菜)	2.4	10.2	320	600	180	290	160	130	810	490	320
15-2-211	油酱料 (珍料+调味油料, 鳕鱼方便面)	77.6	10.2	380	700	790	340	290	50	700	350	350
15-2-218	海鲜鸡汁味米线 (米线+调味料+蔬菜+肉酱)	58.1	4.5	220	390	160	200	110	90	540	390	150

食物氨基酸含量 Amino acid content of foods

(mg/100g 可食部)

编码 Code	食物名称 Food name	苏氨酸 Thr	色氨酸 Trp	缬氨酸 Val	精氨酸 Arg	组氨酸 His	丙氨酸 Ala	天冬氨酸 Asp	谷氨酸 Glu	甘氨酸 Gly	脯氨酸 Pro	丝氨酸 Ser
15-1-018	干酪汉堡包 (夹熏肉, 加调料酱)	617	199	826	948	508	852	1292	3034	956	1112	630
15-1-019	干酪汉堡包 (普通型, 夹单层肉饼, 无调料酱)	524	182	739	787	438	701	1064	3102	756	1128	592
15-1-020	干酪汉堡包 (普通型, 夹奶酪、单层肉饼, 加调料酱)	511	178	719	765	425	682	1040	3033	735	1096	576
15-1-021	干酪汉堡包 (普通型, 夹奶酪、单层肉饼, 加调料酱和蔬菜)	419	146	588	626	349	557	863	2503	601	891	472
15-1-022	干酪汉堡包 (普通型, 夹奶酪、双层肉饼、双层面包, 加调料酱和蔬菜)	482	164	661	728	402	652	989	2615	705	949	511
15-1-023	汉堡包 (普通型, 夹肉饼, 加调料酱和蔬菜)	438	142	576	672	325	633	917	2579	711	841	510
15-1-024	热狗 (原味)	360	98	483	666	295	598	872	2385	646	765	481
15-2-105	早餐奶	72	34	124	78	49	73	165	436	43	208	106
15-2-112	黑芝麻糊粉	200	70	270	440	130	250	370	1920	270	540	290
15-2-115	燕麦片	520	380	720	970	280	680	1200	3170	690	700	740
15-2-116	燕麦片 (果仁, 甜)	280	190	400	620	160	350	700	1650	370	430	410
15-2-202	鸡汁味干脆面 (面饼+调味料)	270	120	450	460	200	320	450	4910	390	1080	480
15-2-203	海鲜味方便面 (面饼 + 调味料 + 油料)	240	150	390	370	180	290	400	4170	340	1090	440
15-2-209	鳕鱼方便面 (面饼+调味料+珍料+调味油+蔬菜)	330	130	410	450	180	370	630	3740	360	750	440
15-2-210	鳕鱼方便面 (面饼+调味料+蔬菜)	260	80	380	370	180	270	420	4430	330	1040	450
15-2-211	油酱料 (珍料 + 调味油料, 鳕鱼方便面)	440	190	460	570	180	520	950	2720	390	320	420
15-2-218	海鲜鸡汁味米线 (米线+调味料+蔬菜+肉酱)	140	60	220	280	90	220	350	910	170	210	190

食物氨基酸含量 Amino acid content of foods

(mg/100g 可食部)

编码 Code	食物名称 Food name	水分 Water g	蛋白质 Protein g	异亮氨酸 Ile	亮氨酸 Leu	赖氨酸 Lys	含硫氨基酸 (SAA) Total	蛋氨酸 Met	胱氨酸 Cys	芳香族氨基酸 (AAA) Total	苯丙氨酸 Phe	酪氨酸 Tyr
15-2-219	海鲜鸡汁味米线 (米线 + 调味料 + 蔬菜)	58.8	3.9	220	390	160	200	110	90	550	400	150
15-2-220	肉酱 (海鲜鸡汁味米线)	7.9	7.2	140	220	200	150	90	60	280	180	100
15-2-221	冬菜虾仁馄饨	58.9	9.1	312	623	454	402	188	214	662	386	276
15-2-222	韭菜合子	59.7	7.5	314	580	419	262	0	262	636	373	263
15-2-223	糯米饭团	37.0	5.9	212	424	182	265	27	238	495	282	213
15-2-224	什锦炒饭	58.7	5.0	216	400	259	207	75	132	458	243	215
15-2-225	虾仁炒饭	64.8	4.7	162	317	197	154	55	99	360	187	173
15-2-507	饺子 (猪肉香菇馅)	59.7	12.3	498	898	940	337	258	79	831	468	363
15-2-508	饺子 (猪肉虾仁馅)	50.4	10.0	567	1032	993	404	273	131	980	563	417
15-2-509	饺子 (鸡肉蘑菇馅)	61.0	7.4	267	518	389	269	98	171	533	325	208
15-2-510	饺子 (海鳗猪肉馅)	55.9	14.3	606	1080	1193	690	371	319	1013	543	470
15-2-511	饺子 (海鳗虾仁馅)	54.7	12.3	574	1009	1132	453	331	122	962	510	452
15-3-103	蛋酥卷	2.1	8.1	330	400	180	300	130	170	620	370	250
15-3-105	法式卷饼	2.0	7.6	300	570	300	260	160	100	660	380	280
15-3-202	锅巴 (豆香)	0.9	7.6	320	580	310	220	100	120	770	480	290
15-3-301	怪味胡豆	2.5	12.6	530	930	730	150	80	70	1190	760	430
15-3-308	鱼肉粒	6.3	27.1	1060	2000	1820	990	860	130	2150	1230	920
饮料类												
16-4-003	AD 钙奶	86.0	1.1	52	108	84	23	17	6	80	53	27
16-7-017	咖啡粉	3.1	12.2	172	478	96	225	23	202	427	262	165
含酒精饮料												
17-1-117	啤酒 (5.1%, 生力牌)	92.4	0.4	10	16	10	9	2	7	26	14	12

食物氨基酸含量 Amino acid content of foods

(mg/100g 可食部)

编码 Code	食物名称 Food name	苏氨酸 Thr	色氨酸 Trp	缬氨酸 Val	精氨酸 Arg	组氨酸 His	丙氨酸 Ala	天冬氨酸 Asp	谷氨酸 Glu	甘氨酸 Gly	脯氨酸 Pro	丝氨酸 Ser
15-2-219	海鲜鸡汁味米线 (米线+调味料+蔬菜)	140	60	220	280	90	220	360	170	170	210	190
15-2-220	肉酱 (海鲜鸡汁味米线)	100	—	130	200	60	170	240	4650	150	110	100
15-2-221	冬菜虾仁馄饨	289	0	343	485	226	397	616	2245	416	670	375
15-2-222	韭菜合子	296	262	352	457	181	399	723	2274	324	563	406
15-2-223	糯米饭团	186	70	266	332	148	249	377	1657	230	555	282
15-2-224	什锦炒饭	191	0	289	381	126	274	469	858	206	223	261
15-2-225	虾仁炒饭	138	0	209	331	103	216	379	836	170	181	181
15-2-507	饺子 (猪肉香菇馅)	484	126	534	737	336	633	1080	2046	490	466	461
15-2-508	饺子 (猪肉虾仁馅)	506	107	611	795	342	751	1101	2714	793	707	487
15-2-509	饺子 (鸡肉蘑菇馅)	253	24	317	399	192	412	511	2083	588	749	318
15-2-510	饺子 (海鳗猪肉馅)	571	48	668	1048	365	893	1327	2111	974	734	531
15-2-511	饺子 (海鳗虾仁馅)	526	30	624	909	344	770	1225	2101	630	526	475
15-3-103	蛋酥卷	180	160	230	250	90	200	370	990	150	390	300
15-3-105	法式卷饼	260	260	350	260	140	260	440	1650	250	670	360
15-3-202	锅巴 (豆香)	240	80	330	510	150	350	720	1310	300	400	350
15-3-301	怪味胡豆	470	100	590	1120	290	540	1370	2070	510	560	620
15-3-308	鱼肉粒	1150	90	1220	1420	530	1420	2460	5420	1180	1230	1080
饮料类												
16-4-003	AD 钙奶	48	12	67	34	30	39	84	252	22	106	62
16-7-017	咖啡粉	142	30	276	53	165	335	478	2030	441	351	126
含酒精饮料												
17-1-117	啤酒 (5.1%, 生力牌)	8	5	18	16	8	21	20	69	19	53	12

食物氨基酸含量 Amino acid content of foods

(mg/100g 可食部)

编码 Code	食物名称 Food name	水分 Water g	蛋白质 Protein g	异亮氨酸 Ile	亮氨酸 Leu	赖氨酸 Lys	含硫氨基酸 (SAA) Total	蛋氨酸 Met	胱氨酸 Cys	芳香族氨基酸 (AAA) Total	苯丙氨酸 Phe	酪氨酸 Tyr
糖、果脯和蜜饯、蜂蜜												
18-4-002	蜂蜜 (槐花)	10.0	0.2	9	9	6	6	2	4	25	17	7
调味品类												
20-1-012	老抽	51.5	7.9	310	460	350	90	90	—	390	250	140
20-3-117	牛肉酱 (阿香婆)	16.8	6.2	270	350	180	100	70	30	440	260	180
20-3-121	千岛沙拉酱	32.5	2.3	123	145	117	53	43	10	264	146	118
20-3-122	沙拉酱	15.4	2.8	144	208	172	88	78	10	309	165	144
20-4-007	腐乳 (白,石宝寨牌) [酱豆腐]	67.4	9.5	550	770	460	200	120	80	810	510	300
其它												
21-9-014	蜂蛹 [蜂胚、蜂仔]	80.8	10.6	606	1032	411	318	318	—	993	450	543
21-9-016	蜂蛹 (大黄蜂)	76.7	12.1	786	1104	378	192	192	—	726	417	309
21-9-018	花椒叶 (干)	12.3	16.7	920	2080	—	260	260	—	1920	1200	720
21-9-020	花粉 (油松) [松花粉]	6.4	9.6	447	751	745	88	88	—	837	548	289
21-9-021	花粉 (荞麦)	8.3	14.9	540	880	560	140	140	—	980	600	380
21-9-022	牛蛙	79.4	15.7	662	1334	1258	393	393	—	1297	651	646
21-9-023	仙人掌 (食用)	92.7	0.5	16	29	21	13	7	6	39	22	17
21-9-024	仙人掌果 [仙桃]	90.8	1.1	39	79	32	52	22	30	106	60	46
21-9-025	仙人掌籽	3.5	7.4	300	470	150	490	190	300	1110	620	490

食物氨基酸含量 Amino acid content of foods

(mg/100g 可食部)

编码 Code	食物名称 Food name	苏氨酸 Thr	色氨酸 Trp	缬氨酸 Val	精氨酸 Arg	组氨酸 His	丙氨酸 Ala	天冬氨酸 Asp	谷氨酸 Glu	甘氨酸 Gly	脯氨酸 Pro	丝氨酸 Ser
糖、果脯和蜜饯、蜂蜜												
18-4-002	蜂蜜 (槐花)	5	2	7	8	3	6	19	13	6	35	7
调味品类												
20-1-012	老抽	250	50	360	170	110	320	810	1490	260	380	330
20-3-117	牛肉酱 (阿香婆)	180	40	220	320	110	270	610	1890	250	250	210
20-3-121	千岛沙拉酱	68	30	93	88	36	93	213	675	54	92	91
20-3-122	沙拉酱	99	30	138	149	52	122	210	519	95	123	164
20-4-007	腐乳 (白, 石宝寨牌) [酱豆腐]	230	10	440	350	130	640	750	1450	370	310	300
其它												
21-9-014	蜂蛹 [蜂胚、蜂仔]	399	81	636	411	204	304	735	1962	522	693	411
21-9-016	蜂蛹 (大黄蜂)	543	92	1080	285	309	1293	780	1611	1164	1017	450
21-9-018	花椒叶 (干)	1080	—	1820	900	320	940	520	520	1120	2000	440
21-9-020	花粉 (油松) [松花粉]	384	—	654	666	217	604	886	1384	515	522	422
21-9-021	花粉 (荞麦)	560	150	680	560	220	340	1220	3000	580	2180	720
21-9-022	牛蛙	580	276	778	492	336	437	964	3876	205	1357	483
21-9-023	仙人掌 (食用)	16	5	27	15	6	20	40	70	17	14	22
21-9-024	仙人掌果 [仙桃]	37	19	55	126	24	50	90	210	75	51	46
21-9-025	仙人掌籽	180	80	670	740	130	260	470	1180	440	380	220

Notes

表三 食物脂肪酸含量

Table 3 Fatty Acid Content of Foods

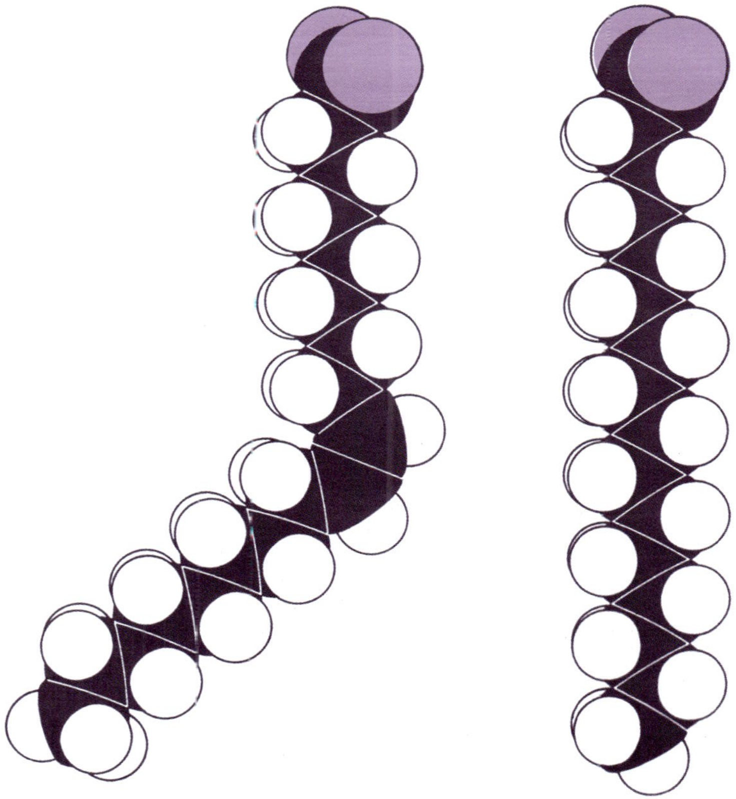

脂肪酸

脂肪酸 (fatty acid, FA) 的化学形式为 R-COOH，式中的 R 为由碳原子所组成的烷基链。自然界中的脂肪酸主要是含双数碳原子的脂肪酸。

一、脂肪酸的命名和表达

脂肪酸分子上的碳原子用阿拉伯数字编号定位，通常有两种顺序相反的系统，即从羧基 (—COOH) 碳原子算起的“Δ 编号系统”和从甲基 (CH_3—) 的碳原子算起的“n 或 ω 编号系统”。

如：	CH_3 —	CH_2 —	CH_2 —	CH_2 —	CH_2 —	COOH
Δ 编号系统	6	5	4	3	2	1
n 或 ω 编号系统	1	2	3	4	5	6

与上述排序方式相对应，对脂肪酸的表达也存在两种形式。以棕榈油酸为例，如果以“Δ编号系统”定位，则表示为 Δ^9 16：1；如果以“*n* 或 ω 编号系统”定位，表示为 16：1，*n*-7。目前通常使用的是后一种表达方法。

脂肪酸的表达方式也常常简化为只包括碳原子与不饱和键的数目，如棕榈酸为 16 个碳的脂肪酸，其中没有不饱和键，故以 16：0 表示；而油酸含有 18 个碳和一个不饱和键 (即一个烯)，以 18：1 表示。在本书的食物脂肪酸含量表中即是采用这种方式。

二、脂肪酸的分类

常见的有三种分类方法。

1. 按碳链的长短分类

(1) 短链脂肪酸：碳原子数为 2 ~ 6 个

(2) 中链脂肪酸：碳原子数为 8 ~ 12 个

(3) 长链脂肪酸：碳原子数为 14 ~ 28 个

2. 按脂肪酸的饱和程度分类

(1) 饱和脂肪酸 (saturated fatty acid, SFA)：碳原子链中不含有不饱和键。

(2) 单不饱和脂肪酸 (monounsaturated fatty acids, MUFA)：碳原子链中含有一个不饱和键。

(3) 多不饱和脂肪酸 (polyunsaturated fatty acid, PUFA)：碳原子链中含两个及两个以上不饱和键。在多不饱和脂肪酸中，有重要生物学意义的是 n-3 和 n-6 系列。

脂肪酸的不饱和键能与氢结合变成饱和键，随着饱和程度的增加，油脂可由液态变为固态，这一过程称为氢化。氢化可以使大部分不饱和脂肪酸变为饱和，并呈顺式与反式两类。

3.根据其营养、生理作用分类

(1) 必需脂肪酸 (essential fatty acid, EFA)：包括亚油酸和α-亚麻酸，它们在体内不能被合成，必须通过食物供给。

(2) 非必需脂肪酸：除两种必需脂肪酸以外，其它脂肪酸均属此类。

三、食物中的脂肪酸

动物性脂肪如猪油、奶油、牛油等含饱和脂肪酸 40% ~ 60%。植物性油脂则含丰富的不饱和脂肪酸，饱和脂肪酸仅占 10% ~ 20%，但椰子油含饱和脂肪酸较高。

附：常见脂肪酸的结构和表达形式

常见脂肪酸的结构和表达形式

系统名 (化学名称) (Systematic name)	通俗名 (Common name)	简写符号 (Shorthand nomenclature)	常用缩写形式
1. 饱和脂肪酸 (Saturated)			
短链的 (Short-chain)			
丁酸 (Butanoic)	酪酸 (Butyric)	4:0	
己酸 (Hexanoic)	羊油酸 (Caproic)	6:0	
中链的 (Medium-chain)			
辛酸 (Octanoic)	羊脂酸 (Caprylic)	8:0	
葵酸 (Decanoic)	羊蜡酸 (Capric)	10:0	
十一酸 (Henedecanoic)	(Undecylic)	11:0	
十二酸 (Dodecanoic)	月桂酸 (Lauric)	12:0	
十三酸 (Tridecanoic)	(Tridecylic)	13:0	
长链的 (Long-chain)			
十四酸 (Tetradecanoic)	[肉] 豆蔻酸 (Myristic)	14:0	
十五酸 (Pentadecanoic)	(Pentadecylic)	15:0	
十六酸 (Hexadecanoic)	棕榈酸 (软脂酸) (Palmitic)	16:0	PA
十七酸 (Heptadecanoic)	珠光脂酸或真珠酸 (Margaric)	17:0	
十八酸 (Octadecanoic)	硬脂酸 (Stearic)	18:0	SA
十九酸 (Nonadecanoic)	(Nondecylic)	19:0	
二十酸 (Eicosanoic)	花生酸 (Arachidic)	20:0	
二十二酸 (Docosanoic)	山萮酸 (Behenic)	22:0	

续表

系统名（化学名称） (Systematic name)	通俗名 (Common name)	简写符号 (Shorthand nomenclature)	常用缩写形式
2. **单不饱和脂肪酸** (Monounsaturated)			
十四碳-9-烯酸（顺） (cis-9-Tetradecenoic)	肉豆蔻油酸 (Myristoleic)	14:1 (n-5)	
十五碳-10-烯酸 (10-Pentadecenoic)		15:1 (n-5)	
十六碳-9-烯酸（顺） (cis-9-Hexadecenoic)	棕榈油酸 (Palmitoleic)	16:1 (n-7)	POA
十七碳-10-烯酸 (10-Heptadecenoic)		17:1 (n-7)	
十八碳-9-烯酸（顺） (cis-9-Octadecenoic)	油酸 (Oleic)	18:1 (n-9)	OA
十八碳-9-烯酸（反） (trans-9-Octadecenoic)	反油酸 (Elaidic)	18:1 (n-9) trans	
二十碳-9-烯酸（顺） (cis-9-Eicosenoic)	鳕油酸 (Gadoleic)	20:1 (n-11)	
二十二碳-13-烯酸（顺） (cis-13-Docosenoic)	芥子酸 (Erucic)	22:1 (n-9)	
二十二碳-13-烯酸（反） (trans-13-Docosenoic)	蔓菁酸 (Brassidic)	22:1 (n-9) trans	
3. **多不饱和脂肪酸** (Polyunsaturated)			
十八碳-9, 12-二烯酸（顺, 顺） (cis, cis-9, 12-Octadecadienoic)	亚油酸 (Linoleic)	18:2 (n-6)	LA
十八碳-9, 12, 15-三烯酸（全顺） (all cis-9, 12, 15- Octadecatrienoic)	α-亚麻酸 (α-Linolenic)	18:3 (n-3)	ALA
十八碳-6, 9, 12-三烯酸（全顺） (all cis-6, 9, 12- Octadecatrienoic)	γ-亚麻酸 (γ-Linolenic)	18:3 (n-6)	GLA
十八碳-6, 9, 9-三烯酸（顺, 顺, 反） (cis6, cis9, 13trans- Octadecatrienoic)	哥伦比酸 (Columbinic)	18:3 (n-9)	
二十碳-11, 14-二烯酸（全顺） (cis, cis-11, 14-Eicosadienoic)		20:2 (n-6)	
二十碳-5, 8, 11-三烯酸（全顺） (all cis-5, 8, 11-Eicosatrienoic)	“蜜”酸 (“Mead”)	20:3 (n-9)	MA
二十碳-8, 11, 14-三烯酸（全顺） (all cis-8, 11, 14-Eicosatrienoic)	二高-γ-亚麻酸 (Dihomo-γ-linolenic)	20:3 (n-6)	DGLA
二十碳-5, 8, 11, 14-四烯酸（全顺） (all cis-5, 8, 11, 14-Eicosatetraenoic)	花生四烯酸 (Arachidonic)	20:4 (n-6)	AA
二十碳-5, 8, 11, 14, 17-五烯酸（全顺） (all cis-5, 8, 11, 14, 17-Eicosapentaenoic)		20:5 (n-3)	EPA
二十二碳-13, 16, 19-三烯酸（全顺） (all cis-13, 16, 19-Docosatrienoic)		22:3 (n-3)	

续表

系统名 (化学名称) (Systematic name)	通俗名 (Common name)	简写符号 (Shorthand nomenclature)	常用缩写形式
二十二碳-7, 10, 13, 16-四烯酸 (全顺) (all cis-7, 10, 13, 16-Docosatetraenoic)		22:4 (n-6)	
二十二碳-7, 10, 13, 16, 19-五烯酸 (全顺) (all cis-7, 10, 13, 16, 19-Docosapentaenoic)		22:5 (n-3)	DPA
二十二碳-4, 7, 10, 13, 16, 19-六烯酸 (全顺) (all cis-4, 7, 10, 13, 16, 19-Docosahexaenoic)		22:6 (n-3)	DHA
二十四碳-15-烯酸 (顺) (cis-15-Tetracosenoic)	神经酸 (Nervonic) 或鲨油酸 (Selacholeic)	24:1 (n-9)	

cis: 顺式; trans: 反式

食物脂肪酸含量 Fatty acid content of foods

编码 Code	食物名称 Food name	脂肪 Fat g	脂肪酸 Fatty acid (g/100g 可食部) Total	饱和 SFA	单不饱和 MUFA	多不饱和 PUFA	未知 UN.K	饱和脂肪酸/总脂肪酸(%) Total	6:0	8:0	10:0	11:0	12:0	13:0	14:0	15:0	16:0	17:0	18:0	19:0	20:0	22:0	24:0
谷类及制品																							
01-1-206	小麦面粉(标准粉)	2.5	1.7	0.9	0.5	0.2	0	54.6	Tr	Tr	Tr	Tr	1.2	Tr	0.3	0.7	49.6	Tr	2.8	Tr	Tr	Tr	Tr
01-1-207	小麦面粉(富强粉、特一粉)	1.5	1.0	0.3	0.1	0.6	0	29.1	Tr	Tr	Tr	Tr	0.7	Tr	0.3	0.1	25.3	Tr	2.7	Tr	Tr	Tr	Tr
01-1-313	挂面(富强粉)	1.5	1.0	0.7	0.2	0.1	0	64.8	Tr	Tr	Tr	Tr	1.8	Tr	0.6	0.6	58.3	Tr	3.5	Tr	Tr	Tr	Tr
01-1-314	龙须面(素)	1.8	1.2	0.8	0	0.3	0	69.4	Tr	Tr	2.4	Tr	1.5	Tr	0.3	Tr	65.2	Tr	Tr	Tr	Tr	Tr	Tr
01-1-315	龙须面(鸡蛋)	1.8	1.2	0.6	0.3	0.2	0	51.4	Tr	Tr	1.0	Tr	0.6	Tr	0.6	Tr	46.3	Tr	2.9	Tr	Tr	Tr	Tr
01-1-316	面条(富强粉,切面)	0.4	0.3	0.1	0.1	0.1	0	53.4	Tr	Tr	Tr	Tr	1.2	Tr	1.1	Tr	44.6	Tr	6.5	Tr	Tr	Tr	Tr
01-1-317	面条(富强粉,煮)	0.4	0.3	0.1	0	0.2	0	28.3	Tr	Tr	Tr	Tr	1.7	Tr	0.2	Tr	25.1	Tr	1.3	Tr	Tr	Tr	Tr
01-1-410	花卷(加牛奶)	3.2	2.1	0.8	0.7	0.6	0	36.8	Tr	Tr	Tr	Tr	1.4	Tr	1.6	Tr	31.2	Tr	2.6	Tr	Tr	Tr	Tr
01-1-411	馒头(富强粉)	1.3	0.9	0.7	0.2	0	0	75.3	Tr	Tr	Tr	Tr	1.6	Tr	0.5	Tr	66.8	Tr	6.4	Tr	Tr	Tr	Tr
01-1-503	面筋(肉馅)	33.2	un	un	un	un	un	26.3	Tr	Tr	Tr	Tr	Tr	Tr	1.2	Tr	25.1	Tr	Tr	Tr	Tr	Tr	Tr
01-2-214	籼米	1.1	0.9	0.3	0.2	0.4	0	36.2	Tr	Tr	Tr	Tr	0.6	Tr	1.2	Tr	32.0	Tr	2.4	Tr	Tr	Tr	Tr
01-2-408	籼米饭(蒸)	0.4	0.3	0.1	0.1	0.1	0	36.9	Tr	Tr	Tr	Tr	1.6	Tr	0.9	Tr	32.2	Tr	2.2	Tr	Tr	Tr	Tr
01-2-409	籼米粥	0.2	0.2	0.1	0	0.1	0	39.3	Tr	Tr	Tr	Tr	2.3	Tr	0.8	Tr	33.2	Tr	3.0	Tr	Tr	Tr	Tr
01-2-410	米粉	0.8	0.7	0.3	0.1	0.3	0	48.7	Tr	Tr	Tr	Tr	9.6	Tr	2.3	Tr	36.8	Tr	Tr	Tr	Tr	Tr	Tr
01-3-108	玉米粒(黄，干)	0.8	0.7	0.2	0.1	0.4	0	24.2	Tr	Tr	Tr	Tr	1.1	Tr	Tr	Tr	21.5	Tr	1.6	Tr	Tr	Tr	Tr
01-3-109	玉米面(黄)	1.5	1.3	0.3	0.3	0.7	0	22.2	Tr	Tr	Tr	Tr	0.6	Tr	Tr	Tr	19.1	Tr	2.5	Tr	Tr	Tr	Tr
01-3-110	玉米糁(黄)	1.2	1.0	0.2	0.2	0.6	0	22.7	Tr	Tr	Tr	Tr	0.9	Tr	Tr	Tr	20.2	Tr	1.6	Tr	Tr	Tr	Tr
01-5-104	小米(黄)	3.0	2.6	1.2	0.8	0.5	0	49.0	Tr	Tr	0.4	Tr	0.3	Tr	0.2	Tr	44.6	Tr	3.5	Tr	Tr	Tr	Tr
01-9-010	荞麦面	2.8	1.9	0.3	0.6	0.9	0	16.1	Tr	Tr	0.2	Tr	0.1	Tr	0.1	Tr	15.0	Tr	0.7	Tr	Tr	Tr	Tr
01-9-011	莜麦面	8.6	5.8	1.7	3.1	0.9	0	30.1	Tr	Tr	Tr	Tr	Tr	Tr	0.4	Tr	27.8	Tr	1.9	Tr	Tr	Tr	Tr
干豆类及制品																							
03-1-207	豆奶粉(多力牌)	6.5	4.3	2.5	1.2	0.6	0	58.0	Tr	Tr	0.6	Tr	0.4	Tr	0.4	Tr	44.5	Tr	12.1	Tr	Tr	Tr	Tr

编码 Code	食物名称 Food name	单不饱和/总脂肪酸(%) Total	14:1	16:1	17:1	18:1	20:1	22:1	24:1	多不饱和/总脂肪酸(%) Total	16:2	18:2	18:3	18:4	20:2	20:3	20:4	20:5	22:3	22:4	22:5	22:6	未知 %
谷类及制品																							
01-1-206	小麦面粉(标准粉)	30.3	Tr	0.3	Tr	30.0	Tr	Tr	Tr	14.5	Tr	13.2	1.3	Tr	Tr	Tr	Tr	Tr	Tr	Tr	Tr	Tr	0.6
01-1-207	小麦面粉(富强粉、特一粉)	11.6	Tr	Tr	Tr	11.6	Tr	Tr	Tr	59.3	Tr	56.1	3.2	Tr	Tr	Tr	Tr	Tr	Tr	Tr	Tr	Tr	0
01-1-313	挂面(富强粉)	24.8	Tr	0.3	Tr	24.5	Tr	Tr	Tr	10.4	Tr	9.3	1.1	Tr	Tr	Tr	Tr	Tr	Tr	Tr	Tr	Tr	0
01-1-314	龙须面(素)	2.7	Tr	Tr	Tr	2.7	Tr	Tr	Tr	27.9	Tr	20.7	7.2	Tr	Tr	Tr	Tr	Tr	Tr	Tr	Tr	Tr	0
01-1-315	龙须面(鸡蛋)	28.8	Tr	2.3	Tr	26.5	Tr	Tr	Tr	19.7	Tr	19.7	Tr	Tr	Tr	Tr	Tr	Tr	Tr	Tr	Tr	Tr	0.1
01-1-316	面条(富强粉,切面)	24.6	Tr	0.8	Tr	23.8	Tr	Tr	Tr	21.6	Tr	21.6	Tr	Tr	Tr	Tr	Tr	Tr	Tr	Tr	Tr	Tr	0.4
01-1-317	面条(富强粉,煮)	10.7	Tr	Tr	Tr	10.7	Tr	Tr	Tr	61.0	Tr	56.5	4.5	Tr	Tr	Tr	Tr	Tr	Tr	Tr	Tr	Tr	0
01-1-410	花卷(加牛奶)	33.4	Tr	Tr	Tr	33.4	Tr	Tr	Tr	29.9	Tr	28.9	1.0	Tr	Tr	Tr	Tr	Tr	Tr	Tr	Tr	Tr	0
01-1-411	馒头(富强粉)	21.3	Tr	0.8	Tr	20.5	Tr	Tr	Tr	3.3	Tr	3.3	Tr	Tr	Tr	Tr	Tr	Tr	Tr	Tr	Tr	Tr	0.1
01-1-503	面筋(肉馅)	53.7	Tr	Tr	Tr	53.7	Tr	Tr	Tr	19.3	Tr	14.4	4.9	Tr	Tr	Tr	Tr	Tr	Tr	Tr	Tr	Tr	0.7
01-2-214	籼米	22.6	Tr	Tr	Tr	22.6	Tr	Tr	Tr	39.6	Tr	39.6	Tr	Tr	Tr	Tr	Tr	Tr	Tr	Tr	Tr	Tr	1.6
01-2-408	籼米饭(蒸)	20.6	Tr	0.5	Tr	20.1	Tr	Tr	Tr	42.6	Tr	39.4	3.2	Tr	Tr	Tr	Tr	Tr	Tr	Tr	Tr	Tr	0
01-2-409	籼米粥	21.7	Tr	Tr	Tr	21.7	Tr	Tr	Tr	38.9	Tr	38.9	Tr	Tr	Tr	Tr	Tr	Tr	Tr	Tr	Tr	Tr	0.1
01-2-410	米粉	7.6	Tr	Tr	Tr	7.6	Tr	Tr	Tr	43.3	Tr	30.9	12.4	Tr	Tr	Tr	Tr	Tr	Tr	Tr	Tr	Tr	0.4
01-3-108	玉米粒(黄，干)	20.1	Tr	Tr	Tr	20.1	Tr	Tr	Tr	55.0	Tr	51.7	3.3	Tr	Tr	Tr	Tr	Tr	Tr	Tr	Tr	Tr	0.7
01-3-109	玉米面(黄)	25.6	Tr	1.5	Tr	24.1	Tr	Tr	Tr	52.8	Tr	52.2	0.6	Tr	Tr	Tr	Tr	Tr	Tr	Tr	Tr	Tr	0
01-3-110	玉米糁(黄)	19.7	Tr	Tr	Tr	19.7	Tr	Tr	Tr	57.5	Tr	54.6	2.9	Tr	Tr	Tr	Tr	Tr	Tr	Tr	Tr	Tr	0.1
01-5-104	小米(黄)	33.3	Tr	2.8	Tr	30.5	Tr	Tr	Tr	17.7	Tr	17.7	Tr	Tr	Tr	Tr	Tr	Tr	Tr	Tr	Tr	Tr	0
01-9-010	荞麦面	34.4	Tr	Tr	Tr	34.4	Tr	Tr	Tr	49.5	Tr	44.1	5.4	Tr	Tr	Tr	Tr	Tr	Tr	Tr	Tr	Tr	0
01-9-011	莜麦面	53.8	Tr	1.5	Tr	52.3	Tr	Tr	Tr	15.9	Tr	15.2	0.7	Tr	Tr	Tr	Tr	Tr	Tr	Tr	Tr	Tr	0.2
干豆类及制品																							
03-1-207	豆奶粉(多力牌)	28.2	Tr	1.2	Tr	27.0	Tr	Tr	Tr	13.9	Tr	2.4	11.5	Tr	Tr	Tr	Tr	Tr	Tr	Tr	Tr	Tr	0

食物脂肪酸含量 Fatty acid content of foods

编码 Code	食物名称 Food name	脂肪 Fat g	脂肪酸 Fatty acid (g/100g 可食部) Total	饱和 SFA	单不饱和 MUFA	多不饱和 PUFA	未知 UN.K	饱和脂肪酸/总脂肪酸 (%) Total	6:0	8:0	10:0	11:0	12:0	13:0	14:0	15:0	16:0	17:0	18:0	19:0	20:0	22:0	24:0
03-1-208	豆奶粉 (大磨牌)	13.0	8.6	2.7	1.8	4.1	0	31.4	Tr	Tr	Tr	Tr	6.3	Tr	2.6	0.8	18.8	Tr	2.9	Tr	Tr	Tr	Tr
03-1-306	豆腐 (北豆腐)	8.1	7.5	3.8	2.9	0.6	0.3	50.6	Tr	Tr	Tr	Tr	Tr	Tr	0.4	Tr	37.8	Tr	12.4	Tr	Tr	Tr	Tr
03-1-307	豆腐 (南豆腐)	5.8	5.4	1.9	2.0	1.6	0	34.3	Tr	Tr	Tr	Tr	Tr	Tr	0.4	Tr	26.0	Tr	7.9	Tr	Tr	Tr	Tr
03-1-405	豆浆	1.6	1.5	0.8	0.5	0.2	0	51.3	Tr	Tr	0.2	Tr	0.2	Tr	0.2	Tr	40.3	Tr	10.4	Tr	Tr	Tr	Tr
03-1-527	豆腐皮	23.0	21.4	5.6	6.5	9.2	0	26.1	Tr	Tr	Tr	Tr	Tr	Tr	0.3	Tr	21.1	Tr	4.7	Tr	Tr	Tr	Tr
03-1-528	腐竹	27.2	25.3	10.3	12.1	2.9	0	40.7	Tr	Tr	0.1	Tr	0.1	Tr	0.1	0.1	33.0	Tr	7.3	Tr	Tr	Tr	Tr
03-1-529	豆腐干	35.2	32.7	11.1	12.5	9.2	0	33.8	Tr	Tr	2.3	Tr	Tr	Tr	2.7	Tr	23.4	Tr	5.4	Tr	Tr	Tr	Tr
菌藻类																							
05-1-031	茶树菇 (干) [柱状田头菇、茶薪菇]	2.6	1.5	0.5	0.1	0.9	0	31.8	Tr	Tr	0.9	Tr	0.6	Tr	0.4	0.6	27.2	Tr	2.1	Tr	Tr	Tr	Tr
05-1-034	黄蘑 (干)	6.4	3.6	0.7	1.5	1.4	0	18.4	Tr	Tr	0.2	Tr	0.5	Tr	0.6	Tr	16.4	Tr	0.7	Tr	Tr	Tr	Tr
05-1-035	黄伞菇 (干) [多脂鳞伞、黄丝菌]	3.2	1.8	0.3	0.1	1.4	0	15.3	Tr	Tr	0.3	Tr	0.2	Tr	0.1	0.3	13.0	Tr	1.4	Tr	Tr	Tr	Tr
05-1-039	鸡坳 (干)	3.7	2.1	1.5	0.6	Tr	0	72.2	Tr	Tr	1.2	Tr	0.8	Tr	1.1	0.3	53.2	Tr	15.6	Tr	Tr	Tr	Tr
05-1-043	白牛肝菌 (干) [美味牛肝菌]	1.6	0.9	0.2	0.4	0.3	0	17.0	Tr	Tr	Tr	Tr	1.0	Tr	0.5	Tr	13.4	Tr	2.1	Tr	Tr	Tr	Tr
05-1-046	乳牛肝菌 (干) [粘盖牛肝菌、松树菌]	2.8	1.6	0.2	0.6	0.7	0	15.1	Tr	Tr	0.7	Tr	0.5	Tr	Tr	0.4	10.8	Tr	2.7	Tr	Tr	Tr	Tr
05-1-050	松蘑 (干) [松茸、松口蘑]	3.0	1.7	0.2	0.8	0.7	0	12.9	Tr	Tr	0.3	Tr	0.2	Tr	0.1	0.6	11.7	Tr	Tr	Tr	Tr	Tr	Tr
05-1-052	血红菇 (干)	6.7	3.8	0.8	1.9	1.3	0	21.8	Tr	Tr	Tr	Tr	Tr	Tr	0.2	6.3	13.5	Tr	1.8	Tr	Tr	Tr	Tr
05-1-053	元蘑 (干) [亚侧耳、冬蘑、黄蘑]	1.5	0.8	0.4	0.3	0.2	0	47.5	Tr	Tr	1.8	Tr	1.5	Tr	0.8	0.8	39.3	Tr	3.3	Tr	Tr	Tr	Tr
05-1-055	榛蘑 (干) [小蜜环菌]	10.8	6.1	1.0	4.2	0.9	0	15.8	Tr	Tr	0.1	Tr	1.8	Tr	0.6	0.4	11.7	Tr	1.2	Tr	Tr	Tr	Tr
05-2-010	裙带菜 (干) [海芥菜、海木耳]	1.7	1.4	1.0	0.3	0.1	0.1	72.0	Tr	Tr	Tr	Tr	7.3	Tr	10.3	9.0	40.6	Tr	4.8	Tr	Tr	Tr	Tr

编码 Code	食物名称 Food name	单不饱和/总脂肪酸(%)								多不饱和/总脂肪酸(%)														未知 %
		Total	14:1	15:1	17:1	18:1	20:1	22:1	24:1	Total	16:2	18:2	18:3	18:4	20:2	20:3	20:4	20:5	22:3	22:4	22:5	22:6	
03-1-208	豆奶粉(大磨牌)	20.5	Tr	Tr	Tr	20.5	Tr	Tr	Tr	48.0	Tr	41.9	6.1	Tr	Tr	Tr	Tr	Tr	Tr	Tr	Tr	Tr	0.1
03-1-306	豆腐(北豆腐)	38.5	Tr	0.8	Tr	35.4	Tr	2.3	Tr	7.4	Tr	7.3	0.1	Tr	Tr	Tr	Tr	Tr	Tr	Tr	Tr	Tr	3.5
03-1-307	豆腐(南豆腐)	36.6	Tr	0.4	Tr	31.9	Tr	4.3	Tr	28.9	Tr	28.4	0.5	Tr	Tr	Tr	Tr	Tr	Tr	Tr	Tr	Tr	0.2
03-1-405	豆浆	36.6	Tr	Tr	Tr	36.6	Tr	Tr	Tr	10.2	Tr	10.2	Tr	Tr	Tr	Tr	Tr	Tr	Tr	Tr	Tr	Tr	1.9
03-1-527	豆腐皮	30.6	Tr	2.0	Tr	28.6	Tr	Tr	Tr	43.2	Tr	39.4	3.8	Tr	Tr	Tr	Tr	Tr	Tr	Tr	Tr	Tr	0.1
03-1-528	腐竹	48.0	Tr	2.1	Tr	45.9	Tr	Tr	Tr	11.3	Tr	11.3	Tr	Tr	Tr	Tr	Tr	Tr	Tr	Tr	Tr	Tr	0
03-1-529	豆腐干	38.1	Tr	0.6	Tr	37.5	Tr	Tr	Tr	28.0	Tr	25.9	2.1	Tr	Tr	Tr	Tr	Tr	Tr	Tr	Tr	Tr	0.1
菌藻类																							
05-1-031	茶树菇(干)[柱状田头菇、茶薪菇]	9.7	Tr	0.3	Tr	9.4	Tr	Tr	Tr	58.4	Tr	58.4	Tr	Tr	Tr	Tr	Tr	Tr	Tr	Tr	Tr	Tr	0.1
05-1-034	黄蘑(干)	42.5	Tr	0.2	Tr	42.3	Tr	Tr	Tr	39.0	Tr	37.0	2.0	Tr	Tr	Tr	Tr	Tr	Tr	Tr	Tr	Tr	0.1
05-1-035	黄伞菇[多脂鳞伞、黄丝菌]	5.0	Tr	Tr	Tr	5.0	Tr	Tr	Tr	79.4	Tr	79.4	Tr	Tr	Tr	Tr	Tr	Tr	Tr	Tr	Tr	Tr	0.3
05-1-039	鸡枞(干)	27.9	Tr	0.9	Tr	27.0	Tr	Tr	Tr	Tr	Tr	Tr	Tr	Tr	Tr	Tr	Tr	Tr	Tr	Tr	Tr	Tr	0
05-1-043	白牛肝菌(干)[美味牛肝菌]	47.2	Tr	Tr	Tr	47.2	Tr	Tr	Tr	35.4	Tr	35.4	Tr	Tr	Tr	Tr	Tr	Tr	Tr	Tr	Tr	Tr	0.4
05-1-046	乳牛肝菌(干)[粘盖牛肝菌、松树菌]	39.2	Tr	1.3	Tr	37.9	Tr	Tr	Tr	45.7	Tr	45.7	Tr	Tr	Tr	Tr	Tr	Tr	Tr	Tr	Tr	Tr	0
05-1-050	松蘑(干)[松茸、松口蘑]	44.8	Tr	3.0	Tr	41.8	Tr	Tr	Tr	42.3	Tr	42.3	Tr	Tr	Tr	Tr	Tr	Tr	Tr	Tr	Tr	Tr	0
05-1-052	血红菇(干)	50.7	Tr	Tr	Tr	50.7	Tr	Tr	Tr	33.2	Tr	33.2	Tr	Tr	Tr	Tr	Tr	Tr	Tr	Tr	Tr	Tr	0
05-1-053	元蘑(干)[亚侧耳、冬蘑、黄蘑]	30.0	Tr	Tr	Tr	30.0	Tr	Tr	Tr	22.5	Tr	22.5	Tr	Tr	Tr	Tr	Tr	Tr	Tr	Tr	Tr	Tr	0
05-1-055	榛蘑(干)[小蜜环菌]	68.8	Tr	20.7	Tr	48.1	Tr	Tr	Tr	15.3	Tr	15.3	Tr	Tr	Tr	Tr	Tr	Tr	Tr	Tr	Tr	Tr	0.1
05-2-010	裙带菜(干)[海芥菜、海木耳]	18.4	Tr	6.6	Tr	11.8	Tr	Tr	Tr	4.7	Tr	4.7	Tr	Tr	Tr	Tr	Tr	Tr	Tr	Tr	Tr	Tr	4.9

食物脂肪酸含量 Fatty acid content of foods

编码 Code	食物名称 Food name	脂肪 Fat g	脂肪酸 Fatty acid (g/100g 可食部) Total	饱和 SFA	单不饱和 MUFA	多不饱和 PUFA	未知 UN.K	饱和脂肪酸/总脂肪酸(%) Total	6:0	8:0	10:0	11:0	12:0	13:0	14:0	15:0	16:0	17:0	18:0	19:0	20:0	22:0	24:0
05-2-011	海带菜	7.5	6.0	2.5	2.6	0.7	0.2	41.8	Tr	Tr	Tr	Tr	0.4	Tr	0.8	Tr	33.3	Tr	7.3	Tr	Tr	Tr	Tr
水果类及制品																							
06-3-912	无花果(干)	4.3	3.4	0.4	0.6	2.4	0	11.7	Tr	Tr	Tr	Tr	Tr	Tr	Tr	Tr	7.8	Tr	3.4	Tr	0.5	Tr	Tr
坚果、种子类																							
07-1-026	山核桃(熟)	64.5	61.7	4.0	44.8	12.9	0	6.5	Tr	Tr	0.1	Tr	Tr	Tr	Tr	Tr	5.4	Tr	1.0	Tr	Tr	Tr	Tr
07-1-032	栗子仁(熟)	1.5	1.4	0.3	0.4	0.7	0	24.4	Tr	Tr	1.4	Tr	0.9	Tr	Tr	1.8	17.1	Tr	3.2	Tr	Tr	Tr	Tr
07-1-033	松子(熟)	40.4	38.6	4.4	20.8	13.5	0	11.3	Tr	Tr	Tr	Tr	Tr	Tr	0.1	Tr	9.4	Tr	1.8	Tr	Tr	Tr	Tr
07-1-034	杏仁(熟，带壳)	58.4	55.8	6.6	36.2	13.2	0	11.9	Tr	Tr	Tr	Tr	Tr	Tr	0.2	Tr	10.8	Tr	0.9	Tr	Tr	Tr	Tr
07-1-035	杏仁(熟，去壳)	54.4	52.0	4.8	36.0	11.2	0	9.2	Tr	Tr	Tr	Tr	Tr	Tr	Tr	Tr	8.5	Tr	0.7	Tr	Tr	Tr	Tr
07-1-036	腰果(熟)	50.9	48.7	10.6	28.1	9.9	0	21.8	Tr	Tr	Tr	Tr	Tr	Tr	0.1	Tr	14.8	Tr	6.9	Tr	Tr	Tr	Tr
07-1-037	榛子(熟)	57.3	54.8	4.3	41.7	8.8	0	7.8	Tr	Tr	0.1	Tr	Tr	Tr	0.1	Tr	6.6	Tr	1.0	Tr	Tr	Tr	Tr
07-1-038	榛子仁(熟)	52.9	50.6	3.0	37.6	10.0	0	6.0	Tr	Tr	Tr	Tr	Tr	Tr	Tr	Tr	6.0	Tr	Tr	Tr	Tr	Tr	Tr
07-1-039	开心果(熟)	53.0	50.7	8.0	33.8	8.9	0	15.8	Tr	Tr	0.2	Tr	0.1	Tr	0.1	Tr	14.1	Tr	1.3	Tr	Tr	Tr	Tr
07-1-040	香榧(熟)	57.0	54.5	4.9	18.1	26.9	4.5	9.0	Tr	Tr	Tr	Tr	Tr	Tr	Tr	Tr	9.0	Tr	Tr	Tr	Tr	Tr	Tr
07-2-020	花生(烤，勤俭牌)	46.3	44.0	8.5	25.1	10.6	0	19.4	Tr	Tr	0.2	Tr	Tr	Tr	Tr	Tr	15.7	Tr	3.5	Tr	Tr	Tr	Tr
07-2-021	花生(烤，密日兴牌)	22.3	21.2	6.1	12.5	2.6	0	28.7	Tr	Tr	Tr	Tr	Tr	Tr	0.4	Tr	21.7	Tr	6.6	Tr	Tr	Tr	Tr
07-2-023	葵花子(奶油香瓜子)	54.1	51.7	9.2	12.5	30.5	0	17.7	Tr	Tr	0.2	Tr	0.1	Tr	Tr	Tr	11.3	Tr	6.1	Tr	Tr	Tr	Tr
07-2-024	葵花子(熟)	49.0	46.8	9.3	18.8	18.6	0	19.9	Tr	Tr	Tr	Tr	0.3	Tr	0.1	Tr	13.0	Tr	6.5	Tr	Tr	Tr	Tr
07-2-025	南瓜子(熟)[白瓜子]	52.8	50.5	15.7	16.5	18.2	0.1	31.2	Tr	Tr	0.2	Tr	0.3	Tr	Tr	Tr	23.6	Tr	7.1	Tr	Tr	Tr	Tr
07-2-026	西瓜子(熟)[黑瓜子]	46.0	44.0	15.0	7.7	20.5	0.7	34.2	Tr	Tr	Tr	Tr	0.4	Tr	0.1	Tr	23.2	Tr	10.5	Tr	Tr	Tr	Tr
畜肉类及制品																							
08-1-121	猪肉(前臀尖，杜长大猪)	25.3	23.0	11.8	10.7	0.4	0.1	51.4	Tr	Tr	Tr	Tr	0.1	Tr	1.7	Tr	31.4	Tr	18.2	Tr	Tr	Tr	Tr

食物脂肪酸含量 Fatty acid content of foods

编码 Code	食物名称 Food name	单不饱和/总脂肪酸(%) Total	14:1	16:1	17:1	18:1	20:1	22:1	24:1	多不饱和/总脂肪酸(%) Total	16:2	18:2	18:3	18:4	20:2	20:3	20:4	20:5	22:3	22:4	22:5	22:6	未知 %
05-2-011	海带菜	43.3	Tr	3.1	Tr	40.2	Tr	Tr	Tr	11.6	Tr	11.6	Tr	Tr	Tr	Tr	Tr	Tr	Tr	Tr	Tr	Tr	3.3
水果类及制品																							
06-3-912	无花果(干)	18.1	Tr	Tr	Tr	17.9	0.2	Tr	Tr	70.2	Tr	35.3	34.9	Tr	Tr	Tr	Tr	Tr	Tr	Tr	Tr	Tr	0
坚果、种子类																							
07-1-026	山核桃(熟)	72.6	Tr	Tr	Tr	72.6	Tr	Tr	Tr	20.9	Tr	18.1	2.8	Tr	Tr	Tr	Tr	Tr	Tr	Tr	Tr	Tr	0
07-1-032	栗子仁(熟)	27.9	Tr	Tr	Tr	27.9	Tr	Tr	Tr	47.7	Tr	45.5	2.2	Tr	Tr	Tr	Tr	Tr	Tr	Tr	Tr	Tr	0
07-1-033	松子(熟)	53.9	Tr	0.8	Tr	53.1	Tr	Tr	Tr	34.9	Tr	34.6	0.3	Tr	Tr	Tr	Tr	Tr	Tr	Tr	Tr	Tr	0
07-1-034	杏仁(熟，带壳)	64.8	Tr	1.1	Tr	63.7	Tr	Tr	Tr	23.6	Tr	23.6	Tr	Tr	Tr	Tr	Tr	Tr	Tr	Tr	Tr	Tr	0
07-1-035	杏仁(熟，去壳)	69.2	Tr	Tr	Tr	69.2	Tr	Tr	Tr	21.6	Tr	21.6	Tr	Tr	Tr	Tr	Tr	Tr	Tr	Tr	Tr	Tr	0
07-1-036	腰果(熟)	57.8	Tr	Tr	Tr	57.8	Tr	Tr	Tr	20.4	Tr	20.4	Tr	Tr	Tr	Tr	Tr	Tr	Tr	Tr	Tr	Tr	0
07-1-037	榛子(熟)	76.2	Tr	Tr	Tr	76.2	Tr	Tr	Tr	16.0	Tr	16.0	Tr	Tr	Tr	Tr	Tr	Tr	Tr	Tr	Tr	Tr	0
07-1-038	榛子仁(熟)	74.3	Tr	Tr	Tr	74.3	Tr	Tr	Tr	19.7	Tr	19.7	Tr	Tr	Tr	Tr	Tr	Tr	Tr	Tr	Tr	Tr	0
07-1-039	开心果(熟)	66.7	Tr	Tr	Tr	66.7	Tr	Tr	Tr	17.5	Tr	17.1	0.4	Tr	Tr	Tr	Tr	Tr	Tr	Tr	Tr	Tr	0
07-1-040	香榧(熟)	33.3	Tr	Tr	Tr	33.3	Tr	Tr	Tr	49.4	Tr	49.3	0.1	Tr	Tr	Tr	Tr	Tr	Tr	Tr	Tr	Tr	8.3
07-2-020	花生(烤，勤俭牌)	57.0	Tr	0.6	Tr	56.4	Tr	Tr	Tr	24.1	Tr	22.5	1.6	Tr	Tr	Tr	Tr	Tr	Tr	Tr	Tr	Tr	0
07-2-021	花生(烤，密日兴牌)	59.0	Tr	3.8	Tr	55.2	Tr	Tr	Tr	12.4	Tr	12.4	Tr	Tr	Tr	Tr	Tr	Tr	Tr	Tr	Tr	Tr	0
07-2-023	葵花子(奶油香瓜子)	24.2	Tr	Tr	Tr	24.2	Tr	Tr	Tr	59.0	Tr	59.0	Tr	Tr	Tr	Tr	Tr	Tr	Tr	Tr	Tr	Tr	0
07-2-024	葵花子(熟)	40.2	Tr	Tr	Tr	40.2	Tr	Tr	Tr	39.8	Tr	39.8	Tr	Tr	Tr	Tr	Tr	Tr	Tr	Tr	Tr	Tr	0.1
07-2-025	南瓜子(熟)[白瓜子]	32.6	Tr	Tr	Tr	32.6	Tr	Tr	Tr	36.1	Tr	36.1	Tr	Tr	Tr	Tr	Tr	Tr	Tr	Tr	Tr	Tr	0.1
07-2-026	西瓜子(熟)[黑瓜子]	17.6	Tr	Tr	Tr	17.6	Tr	Tr	Tr	46.7	Tr	46.7	Tr	Tr	Tr	Tr	Tr	Tr	Tr	Tr	Tr	Tr	1.5
畜肉类及制品																							
08-1-121	猪肉(前臀尖，杜长大猪)	46.6	Tr	2.5	Tr	44.1	Tr	Tr	Tr	1.6	Tr	0.5	1.1	Tr	Tr	Tr	Tr	Tr	Tr	Tr	Tr	Tr	0.4

编码 Code	食物名称 Food name	脂肪 Fat g	脂肪酸 Fatty acid (g/100g 可食部) Total	饱和 SFA	单不饱和 MUFA	多不饱和 PUFA	未知 UN.K	饱和脂肪酸/总脂肪酸 (%) Total	6:0	8:0	10:0	11:0	12:0	13:0	14:0	15:0	16:0	17:0	18:0	19:0	20:0	22:0	24:0
08-1-122	猪肉(前臀尖，良杂猪)	30.4	27.7	12.8	13.7	1.0	0.1	46.4	Tr	Tr	Tr	Tr	0.1	Tr	1.7	Tr	28.6	Tr	16.0	Tr	Tr	Tr	Tr
08-1-123	猪肉(后臀尖，杜长大猪)	9.1	8.3	3.4	4.5	0.3	0	41.3	Tr	Tr	Tr	Tr	0.2	Tr	1.4	Tr	26.5	Tr	13.2	Tr	Tr	Tr	Tr
08-1-124	猪肉(后臀尖，良杂猪)	10.5	9.6	3.9	5.0	0.6	0	41.0	Tr	Tr	Tr	Tr	0.1	Tr	1.5	Tr	26.5	Tr	12.9	Tr	Tr	Tr	Tr
08-1-125	猪肉(硬肋，杜长大猪)	57.1	52.0	23.2	26.1	2.5	0.2	44.7	Tr	Tr	Tr	Tr	0.1	Tr	1.7	Tr	27.2	Tr	15.7	Tr	Tr	Tr	Tr
08-1-126	猪肉(硬肋，良杂猪)	54.4	49.5	27.0	21.7	2.7	0	54.5	Tr	Tr	Tr	Tr	0.2	Tr	1.8	0.3	34.2	Tr	18.0	Tr	Tr	Tr	Tr
08-1-127	猪肉(通脊，杜长大猪)	7.8	7.1	3.2	3.6	0.3	0	45.0	Tr	Tr	Tr	Tr	0.1	Tr	1.5	Tr	28.5	Tr	14.9	Tr	Tr	Tr	Tr
08-1-128	猪肉(通脊，良杂猪)	6.4	5.8	2.6	2.9	0.3	0	45.2	Tr	Tr	Tr	Tr	Tr	Tr	1.7	Tr	28.8	Tr	14.7	Tr	Tr	Tr	Tr
08-1-130	猪皮	28.1	26.8	10.7	15.2	0.9	0.1	39.8	Tr	Tr	Tr	Tr	0.1	Tr	1.9	Tr	27.6	Tr	10.2	Tr	Tr	Tr	Tr
08-1-131	猪小排(杜长大猪)	25.3	23.0	10.7	11.3	1.1	0	46.3	Tr	Tr	Tr	Tr	0.1	Tr	1.7	Tr	28.0	Tr	16.5	Tr	Tr	Tr	Tr
08-1-132	猪小排(良杂猪)	32.7	29.8	14.1	14.2	1.3	0.1	47.4	Tr	Tr	Tr	Tr	0.1	Tr	1.8	Tr	29.0	Tr	16.5	Tr	Tr	Tr	Tr
08-1-213	猪肚	3.5	2.8	1.8	0.9	0.1	0	63.5	Tr	Tr	Tr	Tr	0.3	Tr	2.0	Tr	35.9	Tr	25.3	Tr	Tr	Tr	Tr
08-1-214	猪肝	4.7	3.5	2.0	1.3	0.1	0	58.7	Tr	Tr	Tr	Tr	0.5	Tr	1.8	Tr	34.0	Tr	22.4	Tr	Tr	Tr	Tr
08-1-215	猪舌[口条]	12.4	11.3	5.3	5.3	0.6	0	46.8	Tr	Tr	Tr	Tr	0.1	Tr	1.6	Tr	30.7	Tr	14.4	Tr	Tr	Tr	Tr
08-1-216	猪肾[猪腰子]	1.8	1.3	1.0	0.3	Tr	0	74.9	Tr	Tr	Tr	Tr	2.0	Tr	2.3	0.4	47.2	Tr	23.0	Tr	Tr	Tr	Tr
08-1-318	火腿心全精肉	19.3	17.6	6.2	8.9	2.4	0	35.1	Tr	Tr	Tr	Tr	Tr	Tr	1.4	Tr	31.7	Tr	2.0	Tr	Tr	Tr	Tr
08-1-319	火腿心肉	48.8	44.4	17.8	24.8	1.7	0.1	40.1	Tr	Tr	1.2	Tr	Tr	Tr	1.7	Tr	27.0	Tr	10.2	Tr	Tr	Tr	Tr
08-1-321	叉烧肉	9.8	8.7	2.1	5.2	1.4	0	24.0	Tr	Tr	Tr	Tr	0.1	Tr	0.9	Tr	18.4	Tr	4.6	Tr	Tr	Tr	Tr
08-1-322	酱排骨	26.7	25.2	9.3	11.7	4.2	0	36.9	Tr	Tr	Tr	Tr	Tr	Tr	1.2	Tr	32.4	Tr	3.3	Tr	Tr	Tr	Tr
08-1-323	香糟块肉	53.3	50.4	16.9	24.4	9.0	0.1	33.6	Tr	Tr	Tr	Tr	Tr	Tr	1.4	Tr	26.8	Tr	5.4	Tr	Tr	Tr	Tr
08-1-324	熏烤小里脊	3.9	3.5	2.2	0.9	0.4	0	62.3	Tr	Tr	12.9	Tr	20.4	Tr	Tr	Tr	22.0	Tr	7.0	Tr	Tr	Tr	Tr
08-1-325	猪肉脯	8.8	7.8	3.4	3.6	0.8	0	43.4	Tr	Tr	Tr	Tr	Tr	Tr	3.2	Tr	32.6	Tr	7.6	Tr	Tr	Tr	Tr
08-1-326	肉酥	27.1	24.0	7.7	11.7	4.5	0	32.3	Tr	Tr	Tr	Tr	Tr	Tr	1.2	Tr	25.4	Tr	5.7	Tr	Tr	Tr	Tr
08-1-327	猪肉松	10.2	9.0	3.9	4.4	0.7	0	43.2	Tr	Tr	Tr	Tr	Tr	Tr	2.4	Tr	31.0	Tr	9.8	Tr	Tr	Tr	Tr
08-1-328	扒猪脸	29.6	28.0	10.2	13.8	2.3	1.6	36.6	Tr	Tr	Tr	Tr	Tr	Tr	0.7	Tr	26.1	1.1	8.7	Tr	Tr	Tr	Tr

食物脂肪酸含量 Fatty acid content of foods

编码 Code	食物名称 Food name	单不饱和/总脂肪酸(%) Total	14:1	16:1	17:1	18:1	20:1	22:1	24:1	多不饱和/总脂肪酸(%) Total	16:2	18:2	18:3	18:4	20:2	20:3	20:4	20:5	22:3	22:4	22:5	22:6	未知 %
08-1-122	猪肉(前臀尖，良杂猪)	49.7	Tr	2.9	Tr	46.8	Tr	Tr	Tr	3.6	Tr	2.4	1.2	Tr	Tr	Tr	Tr	Tr	Tr	Tr	Tr	Tr	0.3
08-1-123	猪肉(后臀尖，杜长大猪)	54.3	Tr	3.2	Tr	51.1	Tr	Tr	Tr	4.2	Tr	2.3	1.9	Tr	Tr	Tr	Tr	Tr	Tr	Tr	Tr	Tr	0.2
08-1-124	猪肉(后臀尖，良杂猪)	52.7	Tr	3.4	Tr	49.3	Tr	Tr	Tr	6.0	Tr	4.8	1.2	Tr	Tr	Tr	Tr	Tr	Tr	Tr	Tr	Tr	0.3
08-1-125	猪肉(硬肋，杜长大猪)	50.2	Tr	2.8	Tr	47.4	Tr	Tr	Tr	4.8	Tr	3.5	1.3	Tr	Tr	Tr	Tr	Tr	Tr	Tr	Tr	Tr	0.3
08-1-126	猪肉(硬肋，良杂猪)	43.8	Tr	2.9	Tr	40.9	Tr	Tr	Tr	5.4	Tr	0.4	5.0	Tr	Tr	Tr	Tr	Tr	Tr	Tr	Tr	Tr	0
08-1-127	猪肉(通脊，杜长大猪)	50.4	Tr	4.8	Tr	45.6	Tr	Tr	Tr	4.5	Tr	3.3	1.2	Tr	Tr	Tr	Tr	Tr	Tr	Tr	Tr	Tr	0.1
08-1-128	猪肉(通脊，良杂猪)	49.4	Tr	3.2	Tr	46.2	Tr	Tr	Tr	5.0	Tr	1.4	3.6	Tr	Tr	Tr	Tr	Tr	Tr	Tr	Tr	Tr	0.4
08-1-130	猪皮	56.6	Tr	4.3	Tr	52.3	Tr	Tr	Tr	3.2	Tr	2.2	1.0	Tr	Tr	Tr	Tr	Tr	Tr	Tr	Tr	Tr	0.4
08-1-131	猪小排(杜长大猪)	48.9	Tr	2.7	Tr	46.2	Tr	Tr	Tr	4.6	Tr	2.0	2.6	Tr	Tr	Tr	Tr	Tr	Tr	Tr	Tr	Tr	0.2
08-1-132	猪小排(良杂猪)	47.8	Tr	3.0	Tr	44.8	Tr	Tr	Tr	4.3	Tr	2.6	1.7	Tr	Tr	Tr	Tr	Tr	Tr	Tr	Tr	Tr	0.5
08-1-213	猪肚	32.5	Tr	2.0	Tr	30.5	Tr	Tr	Tr	3.9	Tr	0.7	3.2	Tr	Tr	Tr	Tr	Tr	Tr	Tr	Tr	Tr	0.1
08-1-214	猪肝	37.9	Tr	4.8	Tr	33.1	Tr	Tr	Tr	3.2	Tr	2.8	0.4	Tr	Tr	Tr	Tr	Tr	Tr	Tr	Tr	Tr	0.2
08-1-215	猪舌[口条]	47.3	Tr	3.6	Tr	43.7	Tr	Tr	Tr	5.6	Tr	4.0	1.6	Tr	Tr	Tr	Tr	Tr	Tr	Tr	Tr	Tr	0.3
08-1-216	猪肾[猪腰子]	24.6	Tr	1.2	Tr	23.4	Tr	Tr	Tr	Tr	Tr	Tr	Tr	Tr	Tr	Tr	Tr	Tr	Tr	Tr	Tr	Tr	0.5
08-1-318	火腿心全精肉	50.8	Tr	Tr	Tr	50.8	Tr	Tr	Tr	13.9	Tr	10.9	3.0	Tr	Tr	Tr	Tr	Tr	Tr	Tr	Tr	Tr	0.2
08-1-319	火腿心肉	55.9	Tr	5.6	Tr	50.3	Tr	Tr	Tr	3.8	Tr	2.9	0.9	Tr	Tr	Tr	Tr	Tr	Tr	Tr	Tr	Tr	0.2
08-1-321	叉烧肉	59.5	Tr	6.0	Tr	53.5	Tr	Tr	Tr	16.3	Tr	14.6	1.7	Tr	Tr	Tr	Tr	Tr	Tr	Tr	Tr	Tr	0.2
08-1-322	酱排骨	46.4	Tr	Tr	Tr	46.0	Tr	0.4	Tr	16.7	Tr	14.6	2.1	Tr	Tr	Tr	Tr	Tr	Tr	Tr	Tr	Tr	0
08-1-323	香糟块肉	48.4	Tr	Tr	Tr	48.4	Tr	Tr	Tr	17.9	Tr	15.2	2.7	Tr	Tr	Tr	Tr	Tr	Tr	Tr	Tr	Tr	0.1
08-1-324	熏烤小里脊	26.0	Tr	Tr	Tr	26.0	Tr	Tr	Tr	11.5	Tr	11.5	Tr	Tr	Tr	Tr	Tr	Tr	Tr	Tr	Tr	Tr	0.2
08-1-325	猪肉脯	46.2	Tr	3.3	Tr	42.9	Tr	Tr	Tr	10.5	Tr	10.5	Tr	Tr	Tr	Tr	Tr	Tr	Tr	Tr	Tr	Tr	0
08-1-326	肉酥	48.7	Tr	Tr	Tr	48.7	Tr	Tr	Tr	18.8	Tr	16.4	2.4	Tr	Tr	Tr	Tr	Tr	Tr	Tr	Tr	Tr	0.2
08-1-327	猪肉松	48.8	Tr	4.2	Tr	44.6	Tr	Tr	Tr	7.9	Tr	7.9	Tr	Tr	Tr	Tr	Tr	Tr	Tr	Tr	Tr	Tr	0.1
08-1-328	扒猪脸	49.5	Tr	Tr	1.2	48.3	Tr	Tr	Tr	8.1	Tr	8.1	Tr	Tr	Tr	Tr	Tr	Tr	Tr	Tr	Tr	Tr	5.8

食物脂肪酸含量 Fatty acid content of foods

编码 Code	食物名称 Food name	脂肪 Fat g	脂肪酸 Fatty acid (g/100g 可食部) Total	饱和 SFA	单不饱和 MUFA	多不饱和 PUFA	未知 UN.K	饱和脂肪酸/总脂肪酸(%) Total	6:0	8:0	10:0	11:0	12:0	13:0	14:0	15:0	16:0	17:0	18:0	19:0	20:0	22:0	24:0
08-1-423	脆皮肠	24.0	21.4	8.6	10.7	2.1	0	40.1	Tr	Tr	0.9	Tr	0.6	Tr	2.0	0.1	26.6	Tr	9.9	Tr	Tr	Tr	Tr
08-1-424	热狗肠	25.2	22.4	17.2	4.8	0.4	0	76.8	Tr	Tr	2.0	Tr	15.9	Tr	20.8	2.6	28.2	Tr	7.3	Tr	Tr	Tr	Tr
08-1-425	火腿肠	14.6	13.0	7.4	5.2	0.3	0	57.0	Tr	Tr	Tr	Tr	Tr	Tr	3.7	Tr	44.1	Tr	9.2	Tr	Tr	Tr	Tr
08-1-426	火腿	3.4	3.0	0.9	1.7	0.4	0	30.3	Tr	Tr	0.1	Tr	0.1	Tr	1.2	Tr	22.0	Tr	6.9	Tr	Tr	Tr	Tr
08-1-428	三明治火腿	4.5	4.0	2.4	1.6	Tr	0	60.2	Tr	Tr	Tr	Tr	Tr	20.2	Tr	Tr	37.0	Tr	3.0	Tr	Tr	Tr	Tr
08-1-429	午餐肉	30.1	28.4	10.5	14.0	3.8	0.1	36.9	Tr	Tr	Tr	Tr	Tr	Tr	1.2	Tr	27.9	Tr	7.8	Tr	Tr	Tr	Tr
08-2-111	牛肉(背部肉)[上脑]	12.4	11.4	6.0	5.1	0.2	0	52.9	Tr	Tr	Tr	Tr	Tr	Tr	3.5	0.4	26.9	Tr	22.1	Tr	Tr	Tr	Tr
08-2-112	牛肉(里脊肉)[牛柳]	5.0	4.6	2.3	2.0	0.2	0	50.8	Tr	Tr	Tr	Tr	Tr	Tr	2.8	0.3	26.3	Tr	21.4	Tr	Tr	Tr	Tr
08-2-113	牛肉(臀部肉)[紫盖、白板]	2.6	2.4	1.1	1.2	0.1	0	45.7	Tr	Tr	Tr	Tr	Tr	Tr	2.9	1.3	25.9	Tr	15.6	Tr	Tr	Tr	Tr
08-2-114	牛肉(肩部肉)[肩肉]	31.7	29.0	16.5	11.9	0.5	0.1	56.8	Tr	Tr	Tr	Tr	Tr	Tr	4.5	1.7	28.6	Tr	22.0	Tr	Tr	Tr	Tr
08-2-115	牛肉(胸部肉)[牛胸]	28.8	26.4	14.4	11.4	0.5	0.1	54.7	Tr	Tr	Tr	Tr	Tr	Tr	4.1	1.6	26.6	Tr	22.4	Tr	Tr	Tr	Tr
08-2-116	牛肉(腹部肉)[牛腩]	29.3	27.9	14.7	13.3	0.3	0	52.7	Tr	Tr	Tr	Tr	0.4	Tr	4.8	2.0	28.7	Tr	16.8	Tr	Tr	Tr	Tr
08-2-117	牛肉(膝圆肉)[和尚头]	1.8	1.6	0.7	0.8	0.1	0	44.6	Tr	Tr	Tr	Tr	Tr	Tr	2.2	0.7	25.2	Tr	16.5	Tr	Tr	Tr	Tr
08-2-118	牛肉(股内肉)[针扒、米龙、黄瓜条]	2.9	2.7	1.5	1.2	0	0	55.2	Tr	Tr	Tr	Tr	0.2	Tr	3.9	1.5	30.7	Tr	18.9	Tr	Tr	Tr	Tr
08-2-119	牛肉(小腿肉)[牛展、牛腱子]	3.3	3.0	1.6	1.4	0.1	0	52.0	Tr	Tr	Tr	Tr	Tr	Tr	3.3	1.2	28.3	Tr	19.2	Tr	Tr	Tr	Tr
08-2-210	牛百叶(黑)	1.9	1.5	0.8	0.6	0.2	0	49.9	Tr	Tr	Tr	Tr	0.2	Tr	2.4	0.9	25.6	Tr	20.8	Tr	Tr	Tr	Tr
08-2-307	牛肉(酱,五香)	10.7	9.5	5.2	3.6	0.6	0	55.0	Tr	Tr	Tr	Tr	Tr	Tr	2.9	Tr	33.0	Tr	19.1	Tr	Tr	Tr	Tr
08-2-308	牛肉(清香)	10.7	9.5	4.0	4.9	0.6	0	42.3	Tr	Tr	Tr	Tr	Tr	Tr	1.4	0.4	28.1	Tr	12.4	Tr	Tr	Tr	Tr
08-2-309	牛腱子(香叶)	5.5	5.0	2.2	2.6	0.3	0	42.8	Tr	Tr	0.1	Tr	0.3	Tr	6.1	0.7	24.6	Tr	11.0	Tr	Tr	Tr	Tr
08-2-310	牛肉干(长富牌)	5.1	4.9	2.5	2.1	0.2	0	52.4	Tr	Tr	0.2	Tr	0.2	Tr	3.9	1.1	28.8	Tr	18.2	Tr	Tr	Tr	Tr
08-3-309	烧羊肉(五香)	5.4	4.8	1.5	2.6	0.7	0	30.5	Tr	Tr	0.2	Tr	0.2	Tr	1.6	Tr	21.0	Tr	7.5	Tr	Tr	Tr	Tr
08-3-310	羊肉串(生)	4.8	4.3	1.9	1.9	0.4	0	44.8	Tr	Tr	Tr	Tr	0.1	Tr	2.8	0.6	26.3	Tr	15.0	Tr	Tr	Tr	Tr

编码 Code	食物名称 Food name	单不饱和/总脂肪酸(%)								多不饱和/总脂肪酸(%)													未知 %
		Total	14:1	16:1	17:1	18:1	20:1	22:1	24:1	Total	16:2	18:2	18:3	18:4	20:2	20:3	20:4	20:5	22:3	22:4	22:5	22:6	
08-1-423	脆皮肠	50.2	Tr	4.6	Tr	45.6	Tr	Tr	Tr	9.7	Tr	8.7	1.0	Tr	Tr	Tr	Tr	Tr	Tr	Tr	Tr	Tr	0
08-1-424	热狗肠	21.2	Tr	Tr	Tr	21.2	Tr	Tr	Tr	1.9	Tr	1.9	Tr	Tr	Tr	Tr	Tr	Tr	Tr	Tr	Tr	Tr	0.1
08-1-425	火腿肠	40.4	Tr	1.1	Tr	39.3	Tr	Tr	Tr	2.6	Tr	2.6	Tr	Tr	Tr	Tr	Tr	Tr	Tr	Tr	Tr	Tr	0
08-1-426	火腿	56.8	Tr	5.6	Tr	51.2	Tr	Tr	Tr	13.9	Tr	12.7	1.2	Tr	Tr	Tr	Tr	Tr	Tr	Tr	Tr	Tr	0
08-1-428	三明治火腿	39.7	Tr	Tr	Tr	39.7	Tr	Tr	Tr	Tr	Tr	Tr	Tr	Tr	Tr	Tr	Tr	Tr	Tr	Tr	Tr	Tr	0.1
08-1-429	午餐肉	49.3	Tr	Tr	Tr	49.3	Tr	Tr	Tr	13.3	Tr	11.6	1.7	Tr	Tr	Tr	Tr	Tr	Tr	Tr	Tr	Tr	0.5
08-2-111	牛肉(背部肉)[上脑]	45.3	Tr	4.2	Tr	41.1	Tr	Tr	Tr	1.5	Tr	1.4	0.1	Tr	Tr	Tr	Tr	Tr	Tr	Tr	Tr	Tr	0.3
08-2-112	牛肉(里脊肉)[牛柳]	44.5	Tr	3.7	Tr	40.8	Tr	Tr	Tr	4.6	Tr	3.9	0.7	Tr	Tr	Tr	Tr	Tr	Tr	Tr	Tr	Tr	0.1
08-2-113	牛肉(臀部肉)[紫盖、白板]	49.3	Tr	5.9	Tr	43.4	Tr	Tr	Tr	5.1	Tr	4.4	0.7	Tr	Tr	Tr	Tr	Tr	Tr	Tr	Tr	Tr	0
08-2-114	牛肉(肩部肉)[肩肉]	41.1	Tr	4.6	Tr	36.5	Tr	Tr	Tr	1.8	Tr	1.6	0.2	Tr	Tr	Tr	Tr	Tr	Tr	Tr	Tr	Tr	0.3
08-2-115	牛肉(胸部肉)[牛胸]	43.2	Tr	4.8	Tr	38.4	Tr	Tr	Tr	1.9	Tr	1.7	0.2	Tr	Tr	Tr	Tr	Tr	Tr	Tr	Tr	Tr	0.2
08-2-116	牛肉(腹部肉)[牛腩]	47.5	Tr	7.2	Tr	40.3	Tr	Tr	Tr	1.0	Tr	0.9	0.1	Tr	Tr	Tr	Tr	Tr	Tr	Tr	Tr	Tr	0
08-2-117	牛肉(膝圆肉)[和尚头]	48.6	Tr	5.6	Tr	43.0	Tr	Tr	Tr	6.3	Tr	5.6	0.7	Tr	Tr	Tr	Tr	Tr	Tr	Tr	Tr	Tr	0.5
08-2-118	牛肉(股内肉)[针扒、米龙、黄瓜条]	43.6	Tr	5.3	Tr	38.3	Tr	Tr	Tr	1.0	Tr	1.0	Tr	Tr	Tr	Tr	Tr	Tr	Tr	Tr	Tr	Tr	0.2
08-2-119	牛肉(小腿肉)[牛展、牛腱子]	45.7	Tr	4.7	Tr	41.0	Tr	Tr	Tr	2.1	Tr	1.8	0.3	Tr	Tr	Tr	Tr	Tr	Tr	Tr	Tr	Tr	0.2
08-2-210	牛百叶(黑)	39.1	Tr	3.4	Tr	35.7	Tr	Tr	Tr	10.7	Tr	10.7	Tr	Tr	Tr	Tr	Tr	Tr	Tr	Tr	Tr	Tr	0.3
08-2-307	牛肉(酱,五香)	38.0	Tr	Tr	Tr	38.0	Tr	Tr	Tr	6.6	Tr	5.3	1.3	Tr	Tr	Tr	Tr	Tr	Tr	Tr	Tr	Tr	0.4
08-2-308	牛肉(清香)	51.2	Tr	Tr	Tr	51.2	Tr	Tr	Tr	6.3	Tr	4.9	1.4	Tr	Tr	Tr	Tr	Tr	Tr	Tr	Tr	Tr	0.2
08-2-309	牛腱子(香叶)	50.8	Tr	7.6	Tr	43.2	Tr	Tr	Tr	6.4	Tr	4.8	1.6	Tr	Tr	Tr	Tr	Tr	Tr	Tr	Tr	Tr	0
08-2-310	牛肉干(长富牌)	44.2	Tr	6.0	Tr	38.2	Tr	Tr	Tr	3.4	Tr	2.8	0.6	Tr	Tr	Tr	Tr	Tr	Tr	Tr	Tr	Tr	0
08-3-309	烧羊肉(五香)	54.1	Tr	6.1	Tr	48.0	Tr	Tr	Tr	14.9	Tr	13.6	1.3	Tr	Tr	Tr	Tr	Tr	Tr	Tr	Tr	Tr	0.5
08-3-310	羊肉串(生)	44.6	Tr	Tr	Tr	44.6	Tr	Tr	Tr	10.5	Tr	8.2	2.3	Tr	Tr	Tr	Tr	Tr	Tr	Tr	Tr	Tr	0.1

食物脂肪酸含量 Fatty acid content of foods

编码 Code	食物名称 Food name	脂肪 Fat g	脂肪酸 Fatty acid (g/100g 可食部) Total	饱和 SFA	单不饱和 MUFA	多不饱和 PUFA	未知 UN.K	饱和脂肪酸/总脂肪酸(%) Total	6:0	8:0	10:0	11:0	12:0	13:0	14:0	15:0	16:0	17:0	18:0	19:0	20:0	22:0	24:0
08-4-304	驴肉(五香)	6.0	5.3	2.3	2.6	0.5	0	42.5	Tr	Tr	0.1	Tr	0.2	Tr	4.3	0.7	30.6	Tr	6.6	Tr	Tr	Tr	Tr
08-9-006	鹿肉(梅花鹿)	1.3	1.2	0.5	0.4	0.2	0	39.9	Tr	Tr	0.7	Tr	0.7	Tr	1.7	Tr	30.1	Tr	6.7	Tr	Tr	Tr	Tr
禽肉类及制品																							
09-1-112	鸡胸脯肉	1.9	1.8	1.0	0.7	0.1	0	53.2	Tr	Tr	Tr	Tr	0.4	Tr	0.8	0.2	37.3	Tr	14.5	Tr	Tr	Tr	Tr
09-1-113	鸡腿	7.2	6.8	2.4	3.8	0.6	0	35.1	Tr	Tr	Tr	Tr	Tr	Tr	0.8	0.3	27.8	Tr	6.2	Tr	Tr	Tr	Tr
09-1-114	鸡翅	11.5	10.9	5.6	5.1	0.1	0	51.7	Tr	Tr	Tr	Tr	Tr	Tr	1.0	0.3	40.7	Tr	9.7	Tr	Tr	Tr	Tr
09-1-115	鸡块(带浆粉)	9.1	8.6	3.1	4.4	1.1	0	35.5	Tr	Tr	Tr	Tr	Tr	Tr	1.8	0.8	24.4	Tr	8.5	Tr	Tr	Tr	Tr
09-1-116	野山鸡	2.0	1.9	0.7	0.8	0.4	0	36.8	Tr	Tr	0.2	Tr	0.2	Tr	0.9	0.2	33.7	Tr	1.6	Tr	Tr	Tr	Tr
09-1-308	扒鸡(五香脱骨)	10.8	10.2	2.4	5.0	1.9	0.9	23.3	Tr	Tr	Tr	Tr	Tr	Tr	0.7	Tr	19.0	Tr	3.6	Tr	Tr	Tr	Tr
09-1-309	烤鸡	16.9	16.0	4.1	8.6	3.2	0	25.7	Tr	Tr	Tr	Tr	Tr	Tr	0.7	Tr	21.7	Tr	3.3	Tr	Tr	Tr	Tr
09-1-310	童子鸡(熟)	18.1	17.1	5.4	7.4	4.3	0	31.7	Tr	Tr	Tr	Tr	1.9	Tr	2.6	Tr	27.2	Tr	Tr	Tr	Tr	Tr	Tr
09-2-307	烤鸭(老唐牌)	25.3	23.9	8.9	10.9	4.1	0	37.1	Tr	Tr	Tr	Tr	0.7	Tr	1.2	Tr	30.7	Tr	4.5	Tr	Tr	Tr	Tr
09-3-302	腊鹅	21.5	20.3	7.2	9.7	2.7	0.6	35.6	Tr	Tr	Tr	Tr	Tr	Tr	0.5	0.2	33.1	Tr	1.8	Tr	Tr	Tr	Tr
09-9-003	乳鸽	34.1	32.2	5.3	19.4	7.5	0	16.3	Tr	Tr	Tr	Tr	Tr	Tr	0.4	0.3	15.6	Tr	Tr	Tr	Tr	Tr	Tr
09-9-004	乳鸽(红烧)	20.8	19.7	4.4	12.4	2.8	0.1	22.3	Tr	Tr	Tr	Tr	Tr	Tr	0.5	Tr	18.6	Tr	3.2	Tr	Tr	Tr	Tr
乳类及制品																							
10-1-105	牛乳(光明牌)	3.2	3.0	2.0	0.8	0.1	0.1	66.6	Tr	Tr	2.6	Tr	(3.5)	0.1	17.0	3.4	32.1	Tr	7.9	Tr	Tr	Tr	Tr
10-1-106	牛乳(乐百氏牌)	3.8	3.6	2.3	1.1	0.1	0.1	64.9	Tr	Tr	2.2	Tr	(3.5)	0.1	15.4	3.2	29.9	Tr	10.6	Tr	Tr	Tr	Tr
10-1-107	牛乳(帕玛拉特牌)	3.1	2.9	1.9	0.9	0.1	0.1	65.5	Tr	Tr	2.8	Tr	(3.5)	0.2	16.3	3.7	30.1	Tr	8.9	Tr	Tr	Tr	Tr
10-1-108	牛乳(三元牌)	3.9	3.7	2.4	1.1	0.1	0.1	66.0	Tr	Tr	2.0	Tr	(3.5)	0.1	15.1	1.9	32.8	Tr	10.6	Tr	Tr	Tr	Tr
10-1-109	牛乳(完达山牌)	3.2	3.0	2.4	0.5	0.1	0	79.9	Tr	Tr	3.3	Tr	13.6	Tr	21.9	3.3	31.5	Tr	6.3	Tr	Tr	Tr	Tr
10-1-110	牛乳(龙丹牌)	3.8	3.6	2.3	1.0	0.1	0.1	64.9	Tr	Tr	1.5	Tr	(3.5)	Tr	16.8	3.6	30.2	Tr	9.3	Tr	Tr	Tr	Tr
10-1-111	牛乳(蒙牛牌)	3.7	3.5	2.2	1.2	0.1	0.1	62.8	Tr	Tr	1.9	Tr	(3.5)	0.1	14.7	3.0	28.4	Tr	11.2	Tr	Tr	Tr	Tr

编码 Code	食物名称 Food name	单不饱和/总脂肪酸(%) Total	14:1	16:1	17:1	18:1	20:1	22:1	24:1	多不饱和/总脂肪酸(%) Total	16:2	18:2	18:3	18:4	20:2	20:3	20:4	20:5	22:3	22:4	22:5	22:6	未知 %
08-4-304	驴肉(五香)	48.8	Tr	9.6	Tr	39.2	Tr	Tr	Tr	8.7	Tr	6.4	2.3	Tr	Tr	Tr	Tr	Tr	Tr	Tr	Tr	Tr	0
08-9-006	鹿肉(梅花鹿)	38.6	Tr	Tr	Tr	38.6	Tr	Tr	Tr	21.3	Tr	20.2	1.1	Tr	Tr	Tr	Tr	Tr	Tr	Tr	Tr	Tr	0.2
禽肉类及制品																							
09-1-112	鸡胸脯肉	41.0	Tr	4.0	Tr	37.0	Tr	Tr	Tr	5.8	Tr	5.4	0.4	Tr	Tr	Tr	Tr	Tr	Tr	Tr	Tr	Tr	0
09-1-113	鸡腿	56.4	Tr	10.0	Tr	46.4	Tr	Tr	Tr	9.5	Tr	8.7	0.8	Tr	Tr	Tr	Tr	Tr	Tr	Tr	Tr	Tr	0
09-1-114	鸡翅	46.9	Tr	7.6	Tr	39.3	Tr	Tr	Tr	1.2	Tr	1.2	Tr	Tr	Tr	Tr	Tr	Tr	Tr	Tr	Tr	Tr	0.2
09-1-115	鸡块(带浆粉)	51.4	Tr	9.4	Tr	42.0	Tr	Tr	Tr	12.8	Tr	12.5	0.3	Tr	Tr	Tr	Tr	Tr	Tr	Tr	Tr	Tr	0.3
09-1-116	野山鸡	43.3	Tr	Tr	Tr	43.3	Tr	Tr	Tr	18.8	Tr	18.8	Tr	Tr	Tr	Tr	Tr	Tr	Tr	Tr	Tr	Tr	1.1
09-1-308	扒鸡(五香脱骨)	48.6	Tr	8.4	Tr	40.2	Tr	Tr	Tr	18.9	Tr	18.0	0.9	Tr	Tr	Tr	Tr	Tr	Tr	Tr	Tr	Tr	9.2
09-1-309	烤鸡	53.9	Tr	7.3	Tr	46.6	Tr	Tr	Tr	20.1	Tr	19.9	0.2	Tr	Tr	Tr	Tr	Tr	Tr	Tr	Tr	Tr	0.3
09-1-310	童子鸡(熟)	43.4	Tr	Tr	Tr	43.4	Tr	Tr	Tr	24.9	Tr	22.7	2.2	Tr	Tr	Tr	Tr	Tr	Tr	Tr	Tr	Tr	0
09-2-307	烤鸭(老唐牌)	45.6	Tr	Tr	Tr	45.3	Tr	0.3	Tr	17.1	Tr	15.9	1.2	Tr	Tr	Tr	Tr	Tr	Tr	Tr	Tr	Tr	0.2
09-3-302	腊鹅	47.8	Tr	Tr	Tr	47.8	Tr	Tr	Tr	13.5	Tr	12.1	1.4	Tr	Tr	Tr	Tr	Tr	Tr	Tr	Tr	Tr	3.1
09-9-003	乳鸽	60.2	Tr	16.9	Tr	43.3	Tr	Tr	Tr	23.4	Tr	21.7	1.7	Tr	Tr	Tr	Tr	Tr	Tr	Tr	Tr	Tr	0.1
09-9-004	乳鸽(红烧)	62.9	Tr	17.5	Tr	45.4	Tr	Tr	Tr	14.4	Tr	13.7	0.7	Tr	Tr	Tr	Tr	Tr	Tr	Tr	Tr	Tr	0.4
乳类及制品																							
10-1-105	牛乳(光明牌)	26.8	Tr	3.2	Tr	23.6	Tr	Tr	Tr	3.1	Tr	3.1	Tr	Tr	Tr	Tr	Tr	Tr	Tr	Tr	Tr	Tr	3.5
10-1-106	牛乳(乐百氏牌)	29.9	Tr	2.9	Tr	27.0	Tr	Tr	Tr	1.9	Tr	1.9	Tr	Tr	Tr	Tr	Tr	Tr	Tr	Tr	Tr	Tr	3.3
10-1-107	牛乳(帕玛拉特牌)	29.1	Tr	3.3	Tr	25.8	Tr	Tr	Tr	2.0	Tr	2.0	Tr	Tr	Tr	Tr	Tr	Tr	Tr	Tr	Tr	Tr	3.4
10-1-108	牛乳(三元牌)	29.2	Tr	3.2	Tr	26.0	Tr	Tr	Tr	2.4	Tr	2.4	Tr	Tr	Tr	Tr	Tr	Tr	Tr	Tr	Tr	Tr	2.4
10-1-109	牛乳(完达山牌)	18.1	Tr	Tr	Tr	18.1	Tr	Tr	Tr	2.0	Tr	2.0	Tr	Tr	Tr	Tr	Tr	Tr	Tr	Tr	Tr	Tr	0
10-1-110	牛乳(龙丹牌)	28.2	Tr	2.5	Tr	25.7	Tr	Tr	Tr	2.9	Tr	2.9	Tr	Tr	Tr	Tr	Tr	Tr	Tr	Tr	Tr	Tr	4.0
10-1-111	牛乳(蒙牛牌)	33.0	Tr	3.0	Tr	30.0	Tr	Tr	Tr	2.1	Tr	2.1	Tr	Tr	Tr	Tr	Tr	Tr	Tr	Tr	Tr	Tr	2.1

食物脂肪酸含量 Fatty acid content of foods

编码 Code	食物名称 Food name	脂肪 Fat g	脂肪酸 Fatty acid (g/100g 可食部) Total	饱和 SFA	单不饱和 MUFA	多不饱和 PUFA	未知 UN.K	饱和脂肪酸/总脂肪酸(%) Total	6:0	8:0	10:0	11:0	12:0	13:0	14:0	15:0	16:0	17:0	18:0	19:0	20:0	22:0	24:0
10-1-112	牛乳(新南洋牌)	3.8	3.6	2.3	1.1	0.1	0.1	64.4	Tr	Tr	1.1	Tr	(3.5)	0.1	13.9	3.0	31.4	Tr	11.4	Tr	Tr	Tr	Tr
10-1-113	牛乳(帕玛拉特)	3.2	3.0	1.9	0.9	0.1	0.1	64.5	Tr	Tr	2.7	Tr	(3.5)	0.1	15.3	3.4	29.7	Tr	9.8	Tr	Tr	Tr	Tr
10-1-114	牛乳(伊利牌)	3.7	3.5	2.3	1.1	0.1	0	67.0	Tr	Tr	1.9	Tr	7.1	Tr	14.8	2.6	31.0	Tr	9.6	Tr	Tr	Tr	Tr
10-1-115	牛乳(部分脱脂, 帕玛拉特)	1.3	1.2	0.9	0.3	Tr	0	76.7	Tr	Tr	4.0	Tr	13.7	Tr	18.2	2.6	30.4	Tr	7.8	Tr	Tr	Tr	Tr
10-1-116	牛乳(脱脂, 帕玛拉特)	0.2	0.2	0.1	0.1	Tr	0	49.4	Tr	Tr	15.9	Tr	20.4	Tr	13.1	Tr	Tr	Tr	Tr	Tr	Tr	Tr	Tr
10-1-117	牛乳(强化锌、钙, 帕玛拉特)	3.1	2.9	1.9	0.8	0.1	0.1	66.1	Tr	Tr	2.9	Tr	(3.5)	0.1	16.2	3.6	30.5	Tr	9.3	Tr	Tr	Tr	Tr
10-1-118	牛奶(草莓味, 卡夫牌)	3.0	2.8	1.8	0.7	0.1	0.2	65.7	Tr	Tr	2.9	Tr	(3.5)	Tr	16.6	Tr	33.4	Tr	9.3	Tr	Tr	Tr	Tr
10-1-119	牛奶(巧克力味, 卡夫牌)	3.2	3.0	1.9	1.0	0.1	0.1	62.7	Tr	Tr	2.8	Tr	(3.5)	0.1	15.5	3.3	32.8	Tr	4.7	Tr	Tr	Tr	Tr
10-1-120	牛奶(巧克力味, 三元牌)	2.8	2.6	1.8	0.7	0	0.1	68.4	Tr	Tr	2.9	Tr	(3.5)	0.1	17.4	3.7	31.6	Tr	9.2	Tr	Tr	Tr	Tr
10-1-121	学生奶	2.6	2.5	1.8	0.7	0	0	72.0	Tr	Tr	1.5	Tr	13.4	Tr	16.8	2.4	28.9	Tr	9.0	Tr	Tr	Tr	Tr
10-2-106	全脂奶粉(三鹿牌)	29.6	28.0	16.6	9.2	0.9	1.3	59.2	Tr	Tr	0.9	Tr	Tr	0.1	12.8	2.5	29.8	Tr	13.1	Tr	Tr	Tr	Tr
10-2-107	全脂奶粉(伊利牌)	26.0	24.6	15.2	8.3	1.0	0	62.0	Tr	Tr	1.1	Tr	5.2	0.1	13.5	3.0	28.4	Tr	10.7	Tr	Tr	Tr	Tr
10-2-108	全脂甜奶粉(三鹿牌)	21.1	19.9	12.2	6.3	0.4	1.1	61.1	Tr	Tr	1.7	Tr	Tr	0.1	15.2	1.2	31.6	Tr	11.3	Tr	Tr	Tr	Tr
10-2-109	全脂甜奶粉(伊利牌)	21.0	19.8	15.2	4.2	0.4	0	76.5	Tr	Tr	2.3	Tr	16.2	Tr	20.9	2.5	27.2	Tr	7.4	Tr	Tr	Tr	Tr
10-2-111	低脂奶粉(高钙高铁, 伊利牌)	11.0	10.4	7.5	2.6	0.2	0	72.5	Tr	Tr	1.8	Tr	15.5	Tr	17.6	2.0	26.7	Tr	8.9	Tr	Tr	Tr	Tr
10-2-117	儿童奶粉(三鹿牌)	17.5	16.5	8.5	5.2	2.2	0.6	51.5	Tr	Tr	3.0	Tr	Tr	Tr	8.3	0.4	31.7	Tr	8.1	Tr	Tr	Tr	Tr
10-2-118	儿童奶粉(完达山牌)	18.0	17.0	9.2	5.3	2.6	0	53.9	Tr	Tr	2.4	Tr	3.7	Tr	9.9	2.1	27.1	Tr	8.7	Tr	Tr	Tr	Tr
10-2-123	中老年奶粉(三鹿牌)	5.8	5.5	3.4	1.2	Tr	0.8	62.1	Tr	Tr	Tr	Tr	Tr	Tr	22.5	Tr	33.4	Tr	6.2	Tr	Tr	Tr	Tr
10-3-007	酸奶(调味)	3.2	3.0	2.5	0.5	Tr	0	83.6	Tr	Tr	Tr	Tr	20.9	Tr	23.3	Tr	35.1	Tr	4.3	Tr	Tr	Tr	Tr
10-3-008	酸奶(果粒)	2.9	2.7	2.2	0.5	Tr	0	80.3	Tr	Tr	Tr	Tr	14.2	Tr	21.4	3.8	34.5	Tr	6.4	Tr	Tr	Tr	Tr
10-4-012	奶酪(光明牌)	28.4	26.8	19.6	6.4	0.7	0.1	73.2	Tr	Tr	1.6	Tr	6.6	Tr	17.0	3.9	37.4	Tr	6.7	Tr	Tr	Tr	Tr
10-4-014	低脂奶酪	11.6	11.0	9.5	1.4	Tr	0	86.5	Tr	Tr	Tr	Tr	15.3	Tr	24.4	2.5	39.4	Tr	4.9	Tr	Tr	Tr	Tr

编码 Code	食物名称 Food name	单不饱和/总脂肪酸 (%)								多不饱和/总脂肪酸 (%)													未知 %
		Total	14:1	16:1	17:1	18:1	20:1	22:1	24:1	Total	16:2	18:2	18:3	18:4	20:2	20:3	20:4	20:5	22:3	22:4	22:5	22:6	
10-1-112	牛乳 (新南洋牌)	31.4	Tr	2.9	Tr	28.5	Tr	Tr	Tr	2.4	Tr	2.4	Tr	Tr	Tr	Tr	Tr	Tr	Tr	Tr	Tr	Tr	1.8
10-1-113	牛乳 (帕玛拉特)	30.5	Tr	3.3	Tr	27.2	Tr	Tr	Tr	2.1	Tr	2.1	Tr	Tr	Tr	Tr	Tr	Tr	Tr	Tr	Tr	Tr	2.9
10-1-114	牛乳 (伊利牌)	30.3	Tr	Tr	Tr	30.3	Tr	Tr	Tr	2.8	Tr	2.3	0.5	Tr	Tr	Tr	Tr	Tr	Tr	Tr	Tr	Tr	0
10-1-115	牛乳 (部分脱脂, 帕玛拉特)	23.3	Tr	Tr	Tr	23.3	Tr	Tr	Tr	Tr	Tr	Tr	Tr	Tr	Tr	Tr	Tr	Tr	Tr	Tr	Tr	Tr	0
10-1-116	牛乳 (脱脂, 帕玛拉特)	32.7	Tr	Tr	Tr	32.7	Tr	Tr	Tr	Tr	Tr	Tr	Tr	Tr	Tr	Tr	Tr	Tr	Tr	Tr	Tr	Tr	17.9
10-1-117	牛乳 (强化锌、钙, 帕玛拉特)	27.9	Tr	3.2	Tr	24.7	Tr	Tr	Tr	2.1	Tr	2.1	Tr	Tr	Tr	Tr	Tr	Tr	Tr	Tr	Tr	Tr	3.9
10-1-118	牛奶 (草莓味, 卡夫牌)	24.1	Tr	1.0	Tr	23.1	Tr	Tr	Tr	1.8	Tr	1.8	Tr	Tr	Tr	Tr	Tr	Tr	Tr	Tr	Tr	Tr	8.4
10-1-119	牛奶 (巧克力味, 卡夫牌)	32.7	Tr	3.0	Tr	29.7	Tr	Tr	Tr	2.4	Tr	2.4	Tr	Tr	Tr	Tr	Tr	Tr	Tr	Tr	Tr	Tr	2.2
10-1-120	牛奶 (巧克力味, 三元牌)	26.1	Tr	2.2	Tr	23.9	Tr	Tr	Tr	1.5	Tr	1.5	Tr	Tr	Tr	Tr	Tr	Tr	Tr	Tr	Tr	Tr	4.0
10-1-121	学生奶	26.5	Tr	1.0	Tr	25.5	Tr	Tr	Tr	1.4	Tr	1.4	Tr	Tr	Tr	Tr	Tr	Tr	Tr	Tr	Tr	Tr	0.1
10-2-106	全脂奶粉 (三鹿牌)	33.0	Tr	2.8	Tr	30.2	Tr	Tr	Tr	3.1	Tr	2.4	0.7	Tr	Tr	Tr	Tr	Tr	Tr	Tr	Tr	Tr	4.7
10-2-107	全脂奶粉 (伊利牌)	33.8	Tr	3.7	Tr	30.1	Tr	Tr	Tr	4.0	Tr	3.0	1.0	Tr	Tr	Tr	Tr	Tr	Tr	Tr	Tr	Tr	0.2
10-2-108	全脂甜奶粉 (三鹿牌)	31.8	Tr	3.0	Tr	28.8	Tr	Tr	Tr	1.8	Tr	1.8	Tr	Tr	Tr	Tr	Tr	Tr	Tr	Tr	Tr	Tr	5.3
10-2-109	全脂甜奶粉 (伊利牌)	21.4	Tr	Tr	Tr	21.4	Tr	Tr	Tr	2.0	Tr	2.0	Tr	Tr	Tr	Tr	Tr	Tr	Tr	Tr	Tr	Tr	0.1
10-2-111	低脂奶粉 (高钙高铁, 伊利牌)	25.4	Tr	Tr	Tr	24.8	Tr	0.6	Tr	2.1	Tr	2.1	Tr	Tr	Tr	Tr	Tr	Tr	Tr	Tr	Tr	Tr	0
10-2-117	儿童奶粉 (三鹿牌)	31.6	Tr	1.2	Tr	30.4	Tr	Tr	Tr	13.3	Tr	13.3	Tr	Tr	Tr	Tr	Tr	Tr	Tr	Tr	Tr	Tr	3.6
10-2-118	儿童奶粉 (完达山牌)	31.1	Tr	2.3	Tr	28.8	Tr	Tr	Tr	15.1	Tr	13.2	1.9	Tr	Tr	Tr	Tr	Tr	Tr	Tr	Tr	Tr	0
10-2-123	中老年奶粉 (三鹿牌)	22.5	Tr	Tr	Tr	22.5	Tr	Tr	Tr	Tr	Tr	Tr	Tr	Tr	Tr	Tr	Tr	Tr	Tr	Tr	Tr	Tr	15.4
10-3-007	酸奶 (调味)	16.2	Tr	Tr	Tr	16.2	Tr	Tr	Tr	Tr	Tr	Tr	Tr	Tr	Tr	Tr	Tr	Tr	Tr	Tr	Tr	Tr	0.2
10-3-008	酸奶 (果粒)	19.7	Tr	1.3	Tr	18.4	Tr	Tr	Tr	Tr	Tr	Tr	Tr	Tr	Tr	Tr	Tr	Tr	Tr	Tr	Tr	Tr	0
10-4-012	奶酪 (光明牌)	23.9	Tr	Tr	Tr	23.9	Tr	Tr	Tr	2.6	Tr	1.4	1.2	Tr	Tr	Tr	Tr	Tr	Tr	Tr	Tr	Tr	0.3
10-4-014	低脂奶酪	13.1	Tr	Tr	Tr	13.1	Tr	Tr	Tr	Tr	Tr	Tr	Tr	Tr	Tr	Tr	Tr	Tr	Tr	Tr	Tr	Tr	0.4

食物脂肪酸含量 Fatty acid content of foods

编码 Code	食物名称 Food name	脂肪 Fat g	脂肪酸 Fatty acid (g/100g 可食部) Total	饱和 SFA	单不饱和 MUFA	多不饱和 PUFA	未知 UN.K	饱和脂肪酸/总脂肪酸(%) Total	6:0	8:0	10:0	11:0	12:0	13:0	14:0	15:0	16:0	17:0	18:0	19:0	20:0	22:0	24:0
10-5-008	奶油	86.0	81.3	62.1	17.6	1.5	0	76.4	Tr	Tr	1.0	Tr	6.3	Tr	17.6	4.0	39.6	Tr	7.9	Tr	Tr	Tr	Tr
10-9-004	全脂甜炼乳(雀巢)	10.0	9.5	5.9	3.2	0.4	0	62.1	Tr	Tr	Tr	Tr	3.4	Tr	11.0	3.5	40.4	Tr	3.8	Tr	Tr	Tr	Tr
10-9-005	全脂甜炼乳(燕山牌)	10.0	9.5	5.1	3.7	0.6	0	54.0	Tr	Tr	Tr	Tr	1.9	Tr	11.1	Tr	32.7	Tr	8.3	Tr	Tr	Tr	Tr
蛋类及制品																							
11-1-109	鸡蛋(红皮)	10.5	8.7	6.8	1.8	0.1	0	78.5	Tr	Tr	Tr	Tr	Tr	Tr	0.2	27.6	4.3	Tr	46.4	Tr	Tr	Tr	Tr
11-1-111	乌鸡蛋(绿皮)	10.6	8.8	3.2	5.2	0.4	0	36.1	Tr	Tr	0.1	Tr	Tr	0.1	0.6	0.2	29.1	Tr	6.0	Tr	Tr	Tr	Tr
11-2-104	海鸭蛋	13.8	11.5	3.9	7.3	0.2	0	34.2	Tr	Tr	Tr	Tr	Tr	Tr	0.5	Tr	33.0	Tr	0.7	Tr	Tr	Tr	Tr
11-2-203	咸鸭蛋(煮)	13.5	11.2	4.2	7.0	Tr	0	37.3	Tr	Tr	Tr	Tr	Tr	Tr	0.4	Tr	36.1	Tr	0.8	Tr	Tr	Tr	Tr
鱼虾蟹贝类																							
12-1-131	草鱼[白鲩、草包鱼]	2.6	1.8	0.7	0.9	0.3	0	36.7	Tr	Tr	Tr	Tr	4.3	Tr	1.3	Tr	23.6	Tr	7.5	Tr	Tr	Tr	Tr
12-1-132	鲢鱼[白鲢、胖子、连子鱼]	2.1	1.5	0.8	0.7	0	0	52.1	Tr	Tr	Tr	Tr	0.9	Tr	7.0	1.7	31.3	Tr	11.2	Tr	Tr	Tr	Tr
12-1-133	鲫鱼[喜头鱼、海附鱼]	1.6	1.1	0.4	0.5	0.2	0	37.5	Tr	Tr	Tr	Tr	0.6	Tr	2.2	0.4	26.7	Tr	7.6	Tr	Tr	Tr	Tr
12-1-241	带鱼(切段)	4.2	2.9	1.5	1.4	0	0	50.5	Tr	Tr	0.1	Tr	0.2	Tr	8.5	1.1	33.6	Tr	7.0	Tr	Tr	Tr	Tr
12-1-242	黄鱼(小黄花鱼)	5.1	3.6	1.5	2.0	0.1	0	41.7	Tr	Tr	Tr	Tr	0.2	Tr	6.2	Tr	30.4	Tr	4.9	Tr	Tr	Tr	Tr
12-1-244	鲭鱼	39.4	27.6	6.4	12.5	8.7	0	23.1	Tr	Tr	Tr	Tr	Tr	Tr	9.1	Tr	12.5	Tr	1.5	Tr	Tr	Tr	Tr
12-1-245	双髻鲨	0.1	0.1	0	0	0	0	39.0	Tr	Tr	Tr	Tr	Tr	Tr	Tr	Tr	25.1	Tr	13.9	Tr	Tr	Tr	Tr
12-1-304	鱼排	2.4	2.2	1.3	0.7	0.1	0	62.4	Tr	Tr	0.4	Tr	0.4	Tr	2.2	Tr	50.4	Tr	9.0	Tr	Tr	Tr	Tr
12-1-305	鱼丸	1.3	1.2	0.7	0.4	0.1	0	59.4	Tr	Tr	1.3	Tr	0.8	Tr	2.0	Tr	47.5	Tr	7.8	Tr	Tr	Tr	Tr
12-1-306	鱼子酱	7.1	6.4	1.1	1.5	3.8	0	16.8	Tr	Tr	Tr	Tr	Tr	Tr	0.4	Tr	15.8	Tr	0.6	Tr	Tr	Tr	Tr
12-1-401	草鱼(熏)	16.5	15.3	1.8	6.2	7.3	0	12.0	Tr	Tr	Tr	Tr	Tr	Tr	0.6	Tr	9.8	Tr	1.6	Tr	Tr	Tr	Tr
12-1-402	丁香鱼(香辣味)	28.2	25.4	3.8	6.1	15.1	0.4	14.9	Tr	Tr	Tr	Tr	0.2	Tr	0.2	Tr	14.1	Tr	0.4	Tr	Tr	Tr	Tr
12-1-404	箭鱼(炸)	16.1	11.3	2.6	4.5	4.2	0	23.3	Tr	Tr	Tr	Tr	0.4	Tr	0.6	Tr	18.8	Tr	3.5	Tr	Tr	Tr	Tr

食物脂肪酸含量 Fatty acid content of foods

编码 Code	食物名称 Food name	单不饱和/总脂肪酸(%) Total	14:1	16:1	17:1	18:1	20:1	22:1	24:1	多不饱和/总脂肪酸(%) Total	16:2	18:2	18:3	18:4	20:2	20:3	20:4	20:5	22:3	22:4	22:5	22:6	未知 %
10-5-008	奶油	21.7	Tr	Tr	Tr	21.7	Tr	Tr	Tr	1.9	Tr	1.4	0.5	Tr	Tr	Tr	Tr	Tr	Tr	Tr	Tr	Tr	0
10-9-004	全脂甜炼乳(雀巢)	33.9	Tr	Tr	Tr	33.9	Tr	Tr	Tr	4.0	Tr	3.7	0.3	Tr	Tr	Tr	Tr	Tr	Tr	Tr	Tr	Tr	0
10-9-005	全脂甜炼乳(燕山牌)	39.3	Tr	Tr	Tr	39.3	Tr	Tr	Tr	6.7	Tr	5.9	0.8	Tr	Tr	Tr	Tr	Tr	Tr	Tr	Tr	Tr	0
蛋类及制品																							
11-1-109	鸡蛋(红皮)	20.2	Tr	8.4	Tr	11.8	Tr	Tr	Tr	1.0	Tr	1.0	Tr	Tr	Tr	Tr	Tr	Tr	Tr	Tr	Tr	Tr	0.3
11-1-111	乌鸡蛋(绿皮)	58.8	Tr	6.2	Tr	52.6	Tr	Tr	Tr	5.1	Tr	4.9	0.2	Tr	Tr	Tr	Tr	Tr	Tr	Tr	Tr	Tr	0
11-2-104	海鸭蛋	64.1	Tr	Tr	Tr	64.1	Tr	Tr	Tr	1.4	Tr	Tr	Tr	Tr	Tr	Tr	1.4	Tr	Tr	Tr	Tr	Tr	0.3
11-2-203	咸鸭蛋(煮)	62.6	Tr	Tr	Tr	62.6	Tr	Tr	Tr	Tr	Tr	Tr	Tr	Tr	Tr	Tr	Tr	Tr	Tr	Tr	Tr	Tr	0.1
鱼虾蟹贝类																							
12-1-131	草鱼[白鲩、草包鱼]	47.9	Tr	5.7	Tr	42.2	Tr	Tr	Tr	14.9	Tr	14.9	Tr	Tr	Tr	Tr	Tr	Tr	Tr	Tr	Tr	Tr	0.5
12-1-132	鲢鱼[白鲢、胖子、连子鱼]	45.4	Tr	13.6	Tr	31.8	Tr	Tr	Tr	2.5	Tr	2.5	Tr	Tr	Tr	Tr	Tr	Tr	Tr	Tr	Tr	Tr	0
12-1-133	鲫鱼[喜头鱼、海附鱼]	44.1	Tr	7.8	Tr	36.3	Tr	Tr	Tr	18.1	Tr	14.2	3.9	Tr	Tr	Tr	Tr	Tr	Tr	Tr	Tr	Tr	0.3
12-1-241	带鱼(切段)	48.0	Tr	15.7	Tr	32.3	Tr	Tr	Tr	1.3	Tr	1.0	0.3	Tr	Tr	Tr	Tr	Tr	Tr	Tr	Tr	Tr	0.2
12-1-242	黄鱼(小黄花鱼)	55.6	Tr	24.8	Tr	30.8	Tr	Tr	Tr	2.6	Tr	2.2	0.4	Tr	Tr	Tr	Tr	Tr	Tr	Tr	Tr	Tr	0.1
12-1-244	鲭鱼	45.3	Tr	4.2	Tr	10.7	11.5	18.9	Tr	31.6	Tr	1.5	1.9	7.0	Tr	Tr	1.5	7.2	Tr	Tr	1.1	11.4	0
12-1-245	双髻鲨	25.6	Tr	2.4	Tr	16.8	1.2	5.2	Tr	35.5	Tr	Tr	Tr	Tr	Tr	Tr	6.0	4.9	Tr	Tr	24.6	Tr	0
12-1-304	鱼排	31.7	Tr	Tr	Tr	31.7	Tr	Tr	Tr	6.0	Tr	6.0	Tr	Tr	Tr	Tr	Tr	Tr	Tr	Tr	Tr	Tr	0
12-1-305	鱼丸	32.4	Tr	Tr	Tr	32.4	Tr	Tr	Tr	8.2	Tr	6.8	1.4	Tr	Tr	Tr	Tr	Tr	Tr	Tr	Tr	Tr	0
12-1-306	鱼子酱	23.7	Tr	Tr	Tr	23.7	Tr	Tr	Tr	59.8	Tr	49.6	10.2	Tr	Tr	Tr	Tr	Tr	Tr	Tr	Tr	Tr	0
12-1-401	草鱼(熏)	40.5	Tr	5.4	Tr	35.1	Tr	Tr	Tr	47.3	Tr	17.8	12.1	Tr	Tr	Tr	17.4	Tr	Tr	Tr	Tr	Tr	0.2
12-1-402	丁香鱼(香辣味)	24.1	Tr	Tr	Tr	24.1	Tr	Tr	Tr	59.5	Tr	41.8	11.7	Tr	Tr	Tr	6.0	Tr	Tr	Tr	Tr	Tr	1.5
12-1-404	箭鱼(炸)	39.7	Tr	1.4	Tr	38.3	Tr	Tr	Tr	37.0	Tr	33.7	3.3	Tr	Tr	Tr	Tr	Tr	Tr	Tr	Tr	Tr	0

食物脂肪酸含量 Fatty acid content of foods

编码 Code	食物名称 Food name	脂肪 Fat g	脂肪酸 Fatty acid (g/100g 可食部) Total	饱和 SFA	单不饱和 MUFA	多不饱和 PUFA	未知 UN.K	饱和脂肪酸/总脂肪酸(%) Total	6:0	8:0	10:0	11:0	12:0	13:0	14:0	15:0	16:0	17:0	18:0	19:0	20:0	22:0	24:0
12-1-407	鲮鱼 (豆豉, 熟)	33.1	29.8	8.5	10.3	11.4	0	28.4	Tr	Tr	Tr	Tr	Tr	Tr	0.7	0.2	26.1	Tr	1.4	Tr	Tr	Tr	Tr
12-1-408	鳗鱼 (红烧)	9.8	6.9	1.2	1.9	3.8	0	16.8	Tr	Tr	Tr	Tr	Tr	Tr	0.4	Tr	15.7	Tr	0.7	Tr	Tr	Tr	Tr
12-1-409	鲭鱼 (烤, 150℃, 10 分)	37.8	26.5	5.8	11.8	8.9	0	22.1	Tr	Tr	Tr	Tr	Tr	Tr	7.9	Tr	12.2	Tr	2.0	Tr	Tr	Tr	Tr
12-1-410	鲭鱼 (烤, 150℃, 20 分)	34.8	24.4	5.7	10.8	7.9	0	23.3	Tr	Tr	Tr	Tr	Tr	Tr	8.3	Tr	13.0	Tr	2.0	Tr	Tr	Tr	Tr
12-1-411	鲭鱼 (烤, 150℃, 30 分)	50.0	35.0	8.1	15.8	11.2	0	23.0	Tr	Tr	Tr	Tr	Tr	Tr	8.1	Tr	12.8	Tr	2.1	Tr	Tr	Tr	Tr
12-1-412	鲭鱼 (烤, 180℃, 10 分)	31.8	22.3	5.1	10.2	6.9	0	23.1	Tr	Tr	Tr	Tr	Tr	Tr	8.4	Tr	12.8	Tr	1.9	Tr	Tr	Tr	Tr
12-1-413	鲭鱼 (烤, 210℃, 10 分)	43.4	30.4	7.0	13.7	9.7	0	23.1	Tr	Tr	Tr	Tr	Tr	Tr	7.9	Tr	13.0	Tr	2.2	Tr	Tr	Tr	Tr
12-1-414	鲭鱼 (炸)	53.4	48.1	10.7	16.9	20.6	0	22.2	Tr	Tr	Tr	Tr	Tr	Tr	6.2	Tr	13.4	Tr	2.6	Tr	Tr	Tr	Tr
12-1-415	鲭鱼 (蒸)	36.5	25.6	6.2	11.2	8.2	0	24.1	Tr	Tr	Tr	Tr	Tr	Tr	9.1	Tr	13.1	Tr	1.9	Tr	Tr	Tr	Tr
12-1-416	鲭鱼 (煮)	34.5	24.2	6.0	10.3	7.9	0	24.7	Tr	Tr	Tr	Tr	Tr	Tr	8.8	Tr	13.9	Tr	2.0	Tr	Tr	Tr	Tr
12-1-417	沙丁鱼 (茄汁, 熟)	9.8	6.9	2.5	1.8	2.5	0	36.3	Tr	Tr	Tr	Tr	Tr	Tr	3.1	0.9	30.8	Tr	1.5	Tr	Tr	Tr	Tr
12-1-420	午餐鱼 (香辣味)	30.2	27.2	3.9	7.0	16.2	0.1	14.5	Tr	Tr	Tr	Tr	Tr	Tr	0.2	Tr	13.9	Tr	0.4	Tr	Tr	Tr	Tr
12-2-203	虾酱	7.6	5.3	1.6	2.2	1.5	0	30.9	Tr	Tr	Tr	Tr	Tr	Tr	0.5	Tr	25.8	Tr	4.6	Tr	Tr	Tr	Tr
12-2-301	虾仁肉丸	7.4	un	un	un	un	un	38.8	Tr	Tr	0.1	Tr	0.1	Tr	1.3	Tr	23.6	0.2	13.2	Tr	0.3	Tr	Tr
12-3-006	海蟹 (小)	1.1	0.6	0.2	0.3	0.1	0	29.3	Tr	Tr	1.0	Tr	1.0	Tr	1.2	Tr	20.6	Tr	5.5	Tr	Tr	Tr	Tr
12-3-301	蟹足棒	0.6	0.3	0.1	0.1	0.1	0	35.4	Tr	Tr	1.2	Tr	0.9	Tr	2.0	Tr	26.8	Tr	4.5	Tr	Tr	Tr	Tr
12-4-601	文蛤丸	9.2	8.3	3.1	3.6	1.7	0	37.1	Tr	Tr	Tr	Tr	0.5	Tr	1.4	Tr	23.4	0.3	11.2	Tr	0.3	Tr	Tr
12-9-014	甲鱼蛋	7.3	6.1	1.2	4.1	0.8	0	19.4	Tr	Tr	Tr	Tr	Tr	Tr	1.3	Tr	14.7	Tr	2.5	Tr	0.9	Tr	Tr
12-9-301	墨鱼圈	2.2	2.0	1.2	0.5	0.3	0	62.8	Tr	Tr	0.6	Tr	Tr	Tr	2.9	0.2	53.5	Tr	5.6	Tr	Tr	Tr	Tr
12-9-302	墨鱼丸	4.7	4.2	1.9	1.8	0.4	0	45.8	Tr	Tr	0.1	Tr	0.1	Tr	2.1	0.2	39.2	Tr	4.1	Tr	Tr	Tr	Tr
婴幼儿食品																							
13-1-114	婴儿配方奶粉 (完达山牌)	27.5	26.0	12.3	8.0	5.6	0.1	47.3	Tr	Tr	2.0	Tr	2.8	Tr	5.8	0.5	30.4	Tr	5.8	Tr	Tr	Tr	Tr
13-1-214	较大婴幼儿配方奶粉 (完达山牌)	18.0	17.0	11.0	4.4	1.5	0	64.8	Tr	Tr	5.3	Tr	6.4	Tr	14.1	3.0	29.1	Tr	6.9	Tr	Tr	Tr	Tr

编码 Code	食物名称 Food name	单不饱和/总脂肪酸(%)								多不饱和/总脂肪酸(%)													未知 %
		Total	14:1	16:1	17:1	18:1	20:1	22:1	24:1	Total	16:2	18:2	18:3	18:4	20:2	20:3	20:4	20:5	22:3	22:4	22:5	22:6	
12-1-407	鲮鱼(豆豉,熟)	34.5	Tr	Tr	Tr	34.5	Tr	Tr	Tr	38.3	Tr	33.0	5.3	Tr	Tr	Tr	Tr	Tr	Tr	Tr	Tr	Tr	0
12-1-408	鳗鱼(红烧)	27.6	Tr	Tr	Tr	27.6	Tr	Tr	Tr	55.4	Tr	51.9	3.5	Tr	Tr	Tr	Tr	Tr	Tr	Tr	Tr	Tr	0.2
12-1-409	鲭鱼(烤,150℃,10分)	44.5	Tr	4.0	Tr	11.8	12.1	16.6	Tr	33.5	Tr	1.7	2.1	7.0	Tr	Tr	1.8	7.9	Tr	Tr	1.3	11.7	0
12-1-410	鲭鱼(烤,150℃,20分)	44.3	Tr	4.2	Tr	11.8	11.6	16.7	Tr	32.4	Tr	1.7	1.9	6.4	Tr	Tr	1.8	7.5	Tr	Tr	1.3	11.8	0
12-1-411	鲭鱼(烤,150℃,30分)	45.2	Tr	4.2	Tr	12.3	12.0	16.7	Tr	32.1	Tr	1.7	1.9	6.2	Tr	Tr	1.8	7.8	Tr	Tr	1.3	11.4	0
12-1-412	鲭鱼(烤,180℃,10分)	45.8	Tr	4.1	Tr	10.7	12.6	18.4	Tr	31.0	Tr	1.7	2.0	6.3	Tr	Tr	1.7	7.1	Tr	Tr	1.1	11.1	0.1
12-1-413	鲭鱼(烤,210℃,10分)	45.1	Tr	4.4	Tr	12.6	11.7	16.4	Tr	31.8	Tr	1.7	1.9	6.2	Tr	Tr	1.8	7.6	Tr	Tr	1.2	11.4	0
12-1-414	鲭鱼(炸)	35.1	Tr	3.0	Tr	15.4	6.4	10.3	Tr	42.9	Tr	20.3	3.8	4.0	Tr	Tr	1.0	5.1	Tr	Tr	0.7	8.0	0
12-1-415	鲭鱼(蒸)	43.8	Tr	4.2	Tr	11.3	11.6	16.7	Tr	32.2	Tr	1.7	1.9	6.7	Tr	Tr	1.7	7.4	Tr	Tr	1.2	11.6	0
12-1-416	鲭鱼(煮)	42.7	Tr	4.2	Tr	13.2	10.0	15.3	Tr	32.6	Tr	1.7	1.8	6.4	Tr	Tr	1.6	7.8	Tr	Tr	1.2	12.1	0
12-1-417	沙丁鱼(茄汁,熟)	26.7	Tr	Tr	Tr	26.7	Tr	Tr	Tr	36.8	Tr	30.1	6.7	Tr	Tr	Tr	Tr	Tr	Tr	Tr	Tr	Tr	0.2
12-1-420	午餐鱼(香辣味)	25.8	Tr	Tr	Tr	25.8	Tr	Tr	Tr	59.5	Tr	34.1	12.0	Tr	Tr	Tr	13.4	Tr	Tr	Tr	Tr	Tr	0.2
12-2-203	虾酱	40.6	Tr	3.0	Tr	37.6	Tr	Tr	Tr	28.3	Tr	26.1	2.2	Tr	Tr	Tr	Tr	Tr	Tr	Tr	Tr	Tr	0.2
12-2-301	虾仁肉丸	45.1	Tr	2.1	Tr	42.1	0.9	Tr	Tr	16.2	Tr	14.2	0.8	Tr	Tr	Tr	0.3	0.1	Tr	Tr	0.4	0.4	0
12-3-006	海蟹(小)	54.9	Tr	9.0	Tr	45.9	Tr	Tr	Tr	15.8	Tr	14.6	1.2	Tr	Tr	Tr	Tr	Tr	Tr	Tr	Tr	Tr	0
12-3-301	蟹足棒	29.0	Tr	Tr	Tr	29.0	Tr	Tr	Tr	35.6	Tr	Tr	35.6	Tr	Tr	Tr	Tr	Tr	Tr	Tr	Tr	Tr	0
12-4-601	文蛤丸	42.9	Tr	2.2	Tr	39.5	1.2	Tr	Tr	20.0	Tr	17.8	1.2	Tr	Tr	Tr	Tr	0.2	Tr	Tr	0.3	0.5	0
12-9-014	甲鱼蛋	67.4	Tr	15.0	0.5	51.9	Tr	Tr	Tr	12.8	Tr	8.2	0.8	Tr	0.7	Tr	1.3	Tr	Tr	Tr	1.8	Tr	0.4
12-9-301	墨鱼圈	23.2	Tr	Tr	Tr	23.2	Tr	Tr	Tr	14.0	Tr	6.7	7.3	Tr	Tr	Tr	Tr	Tr	Tr	Tr	Tr	Tr	0
12-9-302	墨鱼丸	43.7	Tr	Tr	Tr	43.7	Tr	Tr	Tr	10.6	Tr	10.6	Tr	Tr	Tr	Tr	Tr	Tr	Tr	Tr	Tr	Tr	0
婴幼儿食品																							
13-1-114	婴儿配方奶粉(完达山牌)	30.9	Tr	0.9	Tr	30.0	Tr	Tr	Tr	21.6	Tr	19.2	2.4	Tr	Tr	Tr	Tr	Tr	Tr	Tr	Tr	Tr	0.2
13-1-214	较大婴幼儿配方奶粉(完达山牌)	26.0	Tr	1.9	Tr	24.1	Tr	Tr	Tr	9.1	Tr	7.8	1.3	Tr	Tr	Tr	Tr	Tr	Tr	Tr	Tr	Tr	0.1

食物脂肪酸含量 Fatty acid content of foods

编码 Code	食物名称 Food name	脂肪 Fat g	脂肪酸 Fatty acid (g/100g 可食部) Total	饱和 SFA	单不饱和 MUFA	多不饱和 PUFA	未知 UN.K	饱和脂肪酸/总脂肪酸(%) Total	6:0	8:0	10:0	11:0	12:0	13:0	14:0	15:0	16:0	17:0	18:0	19:0	20:0	22:0	24:0
13-2-002	鸡肝蔬菜泥 (亨氏)	2.2	1.6	1.0	0.5	0	0	63.8	Tr	Tr	Tr	Tr	2.8	Tr	9.1	2.8	36.0	Tr	13.1	Tr	Tr	Tr	Tr
13-3-011	米粉 (高蛋白, 亨氏)	2.0	1.7	1.2	0.3	0.2	0	68.7	Tr	Tr	1.5	Tr	1.1	Tr	1.5	Tr	56.6	Tr	8.0	Tr	Tr	Tr	Tr
小吃、甜饼																							
14-1-038	春卷 (素馅)	4.6	un	un	un	un	un	32.6	Tr	Tr	0.2	Tr	0.1	Tr	0.4	Tr	26.0	Tr	5.9	Tr	Tr	Tr	Tr
14-1-039	黑芝麻汤圆	13.8	un	un	un	un	un	43.2	Tr	Tr	Tr	Tr	0.9	Tr	1.3	Tr	35.3	Tr	5.7	Tr	Tr	Tr	Tr
14-1-040	醪糟	0.2	un	un	un	un	un	47.3	Tr	Tr	4.1	Tr	2.4	Tr	1.8	Tr	35.7	Tr	3.3	Tr	Tr	Tr	Tr
14-1-041	煎饼	3.5	un	un	un	un	un	19.0	Tr	Tr	0.2	Tr	0.1	Tr	0.1	Tr	17.0	Tr	1.6	Tr	Tr	Tr	Tr
14-2-209	月饼 (蛋黄)	20.0	un	un	un	un	un	45.6	Tr	Tr	Tr	Tr	0.9	Tr	0.8	Tr	38.4	Tr	5.5	Tr	Tr	Tr	Tr
14-2-210	月饼 (豆沙)	6.9	un	un	un	un	un	40.3	Tr	Tr	Tr	Tr	1.2	Tr	0.8	Tr	34.1	Tr	4.2	Tr	Tr	Tr	Tr
14-2-211	月饼 (桂花板栗)	6.6	un	un	un	un	un	68.0	Tr	Tr	Tr	Tr	5.1	Tr	Tr	5.7	52.2	Tr	5.0	Tr	Tr	Tr	Tr
14-2-212	月饼 (奶油莲芸)	13.0	un	un	un	un	un	29.2	Tr	Tr	0.5	Tr	0.7	Tr	2.2	Tr	15.4	Tr	6.6	Tr	1.2	2.6	2.6
14-2-332	沙琪玛蛋酥	30.4	28.8	16.6	10.3	1.3	0.5	57.8	Tr	Tr	Tr	Tr	0.6	Tr	1.8	Tr	52.7	Tr	2.7	Tr	Tr	Tr	Tr
速食食品																							
15-1-011	比萨饼 (夹奶酪)	5.1	4.8	2.4	1.6	0.8	0	un	un	un	un	un	un	un	un	un	un	un	un	un	un	un	un
15-1-012	比萨饼 (夹奶酪、肉和蔬菜)	6.8	6.3	1.9	3.2	1.2	0	un	un	un	un	un	un	un	un	un	un	un	un	un	un	un	un
15-1-015	三明治 (夹鸡肉片, 无调料酱)	16.2	14.9	4.6	5.7	4.6	0	un	un	un	un	un	un	un	un	un	un	un	un	un	un	un	un
15-1-016	三明治 (夹烤牛肉片)	9.9	8.7	2.6	4.9	1.2	0	un	un	un	un	un	un	un	un	un	un	un	un	un	un	un	un
15-1-020	干酪汉堡包 (普通型, 夹奶酪、单层肉饼, 加调料酱)	12.5	10.9	5.3	4.6	1.0	0	un	un	un	un	un	un	un	un	un	un	un	un	un	un	un	un
15-1-021	干酪汉堡包 (普通型, 夹奶酪、单层肉饼, 加调料酱和蔬菜)	12.9	11.3	5.6	4.7	1.0	0	un	un	un	un	un	un	un	un	un	un	un	un	un	un	un	un
15-1-022	干酪汉堡包 (普通型, 夹奶酪、双层肉饼、双层面包, 加调料酱和蔬菜)	15.5	13.6	5.4	5.4	2.8	0	un	un	un	un	un	un	un	un	un	un	un	un	un	un	un	un
15-1-024	热狗 (原味)	14.8	13.7	5.0	7.0	1.7	0	un	un	un	un	un	un	un	un	un	un	un	un	un	un	un	un

编码 Code	食物名称 Food name	单不饱和/总脂肪酸(%)								多不饱和/总脂肪酸(%)													未知 %
		Total	14:1	16:1	17:1	18:1	20:1	22:1	24:1	Total	16:2	18:2	18:3	18:4	20:2	20:3	20:4	20:5	22:3	22:4	22:5	22:6	
13-2-002	鸡肝蔬菜泥(亨氏)	32.6	Tr	Tr	Tr	32.6	Tr	Tr	Tr	2.8	Tr	2.8	Tr	Tr	Tr	Tr	Tr	Tr	Tr	Tr	Tr	Tr	0.8
13-3-011	米粉(高蛋白,亨氏)	19.5	Tr	0.3	Tr	19.2	Tr	Tr	Tr	11.8	Tr	9.4	2.4	Tr	Tr	Tr	Tr	Tr	Tr	Tr	Tr	Tr	0
小吃、甜饼																							
14-1-038	春卷(素馅)	36.5	Tr	1.2	Tr	35.3	Tr	Tr	Tr	31.0	Tr	28.9	2.1	Tr	Tr	Tr	Tr	Tr	Tr	Tr	Tr	Tr	0
14-1-039	黑芝麻汤圆	41.2	Tr	Tr	Tr	41.2	Tr	Tr	Tr	15.6	Tr	15.6	Tr	Tr	Tr	Tr	Tr	Tr	Tr	Tr	Tr	Tr	0
14-1-040	醪糟	28.9	Tr	Tr	Tr	28.9	Tr	Tr	Tr	23.7	Tr	23.7	Tr	Tr	Tr	Tr	Tr	Tr	Tr	Tr	Tr	Tr	0.1
14-1-041	煎饼	40.7	Tr	0.4	Tr	40.3	Tr	Tr	Tr	40.3	Tr	40.3	Tr	Tr	Tr	Tr	Tr	Tr	Tr	Tr	Tr	Tr	0
14-2-209	月饼(蛋黄)	45.9	Tr	Tr	Tr	45.9	Tr	Tr	Tr	7.9	Tr	7.9	Tr	Tr	Tr	Tr	Tr	Tr	Tr	Tr	Tr	Tr	0.6
14-2-210	月饼(豆沙)	43.9	Tr	Tr	Tr	43.9	Tr	Tr	Tr	14.3	Tr	14.3	Tr	Tr	Tr	Tr	Tr	Tr	Tr	Tr	Tr	Tr	1.5
14-2-211	月饼(桂花板栗)	31.6	Tr	Tr	Tr	31.6	Tr	Tr	Tr	Tr	Tr	Tr	Tr	Tr	Tr	Tr	Tr	Tr	Tr	Tr	Tr	Tr	0.4
14-2-212	月饼(奶油莲芸)	39.5	Tr	1.3	Tr	38.2	Tr	Tr	Tr	31.2	Tr	29.1	2.1	Tr	Tr	Tr	Tr	Tr	Tr	Tr	Tr	Tr	0.1
14-2-332	沙琪玛蛋酥	35.9	Tr	Tr	Tr	35.9	Tr	Tr	Tr	4.4	Tr	4.4	Tr	Tr	Tr	Tr	Tr	Tr	Tr	Tr	Tr	Tr	1.9
速食食品																							
15-1-011	比萨饼(夹奶酪)	un	un	un	un	un	un	un	un	un	un	un	un	un	un	un	un	un	un	un	un	un	un
15-1-012	比萨饼(夹奶酪、肉和蔬菜)	un	un	un	un	un	un	un	un	un	un	un	un	un	un	un	un	un	un	un	un	un	un
15-1-015	三明治(夹鸡肉片,无调料酱)	un	un	un	un	un	un	un	un	un	un	un	un	un	un	un	un	un	un	un	un	un	un
15-1-016	三明治(夹烤牛肉片)	un	un	un	un	un	un	un	un	un	un	un	un	un	un	un	un	un	un	un	un	un	un
15-1-020	干酪汉堡包(普通型,夹奶酪、单层肉饼,加调料酱)	un	un	un	un	un	un	un	un	un	un	un	un	un	un	un	un	un	un	un	un	un	un
15-1-021	干酪汉堡包(普通型,夹奶酪、单层肉饼,加调料酱和蔬菜)	un	un	un	un	un	un	un	un	un	un	un	un	un	un	un	un	un	un	un	un	un	un
15-1-022	干酪汉堡包(普通型,夹奶酪,双层肉饼、双层面包,加调料酱和蔬菜)	un	un	un	un	un	un	un	un	un	un	un	un	un	un	un	un	un	un	un	un	un	un
15-1-024	热狗(原味)	un	un	un	un	un	un	un	un	un	un	un	un	un	un	un	un	un	un	un	un	un	un

食物脂肪酸含量 Fatty acid content of foods

编码 Code	食物名称 Food name	脂肪 Fat g	脂肪酸 Fatty acid (g/100g 可食部) Total	饱和 SFA	单不饱和 MUFA	多不饱和 PUFA	未知 UN.K	饱和脂肪酸/总脂肪酸 (%) Total	6:0	8:0	10:0	11:0	12:0	13:0	14:0	15:0	16:0	17:0	18:0	19:0	20:0	22:0	24:0
15-2-105	早餐奶	3.1	2.9	1.8	0.8	0.1	0.2	61.7	Tr	Tr	2.4	Tr	Tr	0.1	16.4	3.5	31.6	Tr	7.7	Tr	Tr	Tr	Tr
15-2-106	八宝粥 (康师傅牌)	4.4	un	un	un	un	un	28.3	Tr	Tr	2.6	Tr	0.6	Tr	0.2	Tr	19.5	Tr	5.4	Tr	Tr	Tr	Tr
15-2-107	八宝粥 (亲亲牌)	4.0	un	un	un	un	un	38.1	Tr	Tr	3.4	Tr	1.1	Tr	0.2	Tr	26.4	Tr	7.0	Tr	Tr	Tr	Tr
15-2-109	八宝粥 (娃哈哈牌)	0.9	un	un	un	un	un	100.0	Tr	Tr	28.1	Tr	Tr	Tr	Tr	Tr	71.9	Tr	Tr	Tr	Tr	Tr	Tr
15-2-110	八宝粥 (无糖, 娃哈哈牌)	0.8	un	un	un	un	un	40.8	Tr	Tr	Tr	Tr	Tr	Tr	Tr	Tr	40.8	Tr	Tr	Tr	Tr	Tr	Tr
15-2-112	黑芝麻糊粉	7.5	un	un	un	un	un	19.4	Tr	Tr	0.1	Tr	Tr	Tr	Tr	Tr	14.3	Tr	5.0	Tr	Tr	Tr	Tr
15-2-113	麦片	9.7	9.1	5.4	1.5	2.2	0	59.2	Tr	Tr	Tr	Tr	29.0	Tr	9.8	Tr	20.4	Tr	Tr	Tr	Tr	Tr	Tr
15-2-114	麦片 (原味香奶)	9.0	8.5	1.8	5.6	1.0	0	21.4	Tr	Tr	Tr	Tr	0.5	Tr	0.6	Tr	12.6	Tr	7.7	Tr	Tr	Tr	Tr
15-2-115	燕麦片	9.7	9.1	2.0	5.0	2.1	0	22.1	Tr	Tr	Tr	Tr	0.3	Tr	0.3	Tr	20.4	Tr	1.1	Tr	Tr	Tr	Tr
15-2-116	燕麦片 (果仁、甜)	11.1	10.4	3.7	3.3	3.5	0	35.5	Tr	Tr	Tr	Tr	Tr	Tr	0.6	Tr	34.2	Tr	0.7	Tr	Tr	Tr	Tr
15-2-202	鸡汁味干脆面 (面饼 + 调味料)	27.0	23.8	12.7	8.9	2.2	0	53.4	Tr	Tr	0.7	Tr	0.9	Tr	1.1	Tr	47.3	Tr	3.4	Tr	Tr	Tr	Tr
15-2-203	海鲜味方便面 (面饼 + 调味料 + 油料)	19.2	17.0	2.3	10.3	4.3	0	13.7	Tr	Tr	0.6	Tr	0.3	Tr	0.1	Tr	11.6	Tr	1.1	Tr	Tr	Tr	Tr
15-2-206	红烧牛肉方便面 (面饼+调味料+蔬菜+肉酱)	17.9	15.8	9.9	5.1	0.8	0	62.4	Tr	Tr	2.2	Tr	2.9	Tr	0.7	Tr	53.8	Tr	2.8	Tr	Tr	Tr	Tr
15-2-209	鳕鱼方便面 (面饼+调味料+珍料+调味油+蔬菜)	24.2	21.4	13.5	7.0	0.9	0	63.4	Tr	Tr	0.7	Tr	0.8	Tr	1.6	Tr	57.1	Tr	3.2	Tr	Tr	Tr	Tr
15-2-212	铁板牛肉炒面 (面饼+汤料+蔬菜+调味酱)	18.8	16.6	10.1	5.7	0.9	0	60.6	Tr	Tr	1.7	Tr	1.8	Tr	1.4	Tr	52.4	Tr	3.3	Tr	Tr	Tr	Tr
15-2-215	玉米红烧牛肉味方便面 (面饼+调味料+蔬菜+肉酱)	4.1	3.6	1.6	1.5	0.6	0	43.4	Tr	Tr	0.2	Tr	0.1	Tr	0.1	Tr	38.8	Tr	4.2	Tr	Tr	Tr	Tr
15-2-221	冬菜虾仁馄饨	4.3	un	un	un	un	un	35.7	Tr	Tr	Tr	Tr	Tr	Tr	1.3	Tr	23.4	0.3	10.4	Tr	0.3	Tr	Tr
15-2-222	韭菜合子	11.3	un	un	un	un	un	24.0	Tr	Tr	Tr	Tr	Tr	Tr	0.4	Tr	18.4	Tr	4.7	Tr	0.2	0.2	0.2
15-2-223	糯米饭团	17.6	un	un	un	un	un	22.0	Tr	Tr	Tr	Tr	Tr	Tr	0.3	Tr	17.2	0.2	4.1	Tr	0.2	Tr	Tr
15-2-224	什锦炒饭	5.6	un	un	un	un	un	19.4	Tr	Tr	Tr	Tr	Tr	Tr	Tr	Tr	13.7	Tr	5.1	Tr	0.3	0.3	0.3

食物脂肪酸含量 Fatty acid content of foods

编码 Code	食物名称 Food name	单不饱和/总脂肪酸 (%)								多不饱和/总脂肪酸 (%)													未知 %
		Total	14:1	16:1	17:1	18:1	20:1	22:1	24:1	Total	16:2	18:2	18:3	18:4	20:2	20:3	20:4	20:5	22:3	22:4	22:5	22:6	
15-2-105	早餐奶	28.3	Tr	3.5	Tr	24.8	Tr	Tr	Tr	3.2	Tr	3.2	Tr	Tr	Tr	Tr	Tr	Tr	Tr	Tr	Tr	Tr	6.8
15-2-106	八宝粥 (康师傅牌)	55.9	Tr	Tr	Tr	55.9	Tr	Tr	Tr	15.7	Tr	15.3	0.4	Tr	Tr	Tr	Tr	Tr	Tr	Tr	Tr	Tr	0.1
15-2-107	八宝粥 (亲亲牌)	57.3	Tr	Tr	Tr	57.3	Tr	Tr	Tr	4.7	Tr	3.5	1.2	Tr	Tr	Tr	Tr	Tr	Tr	Tr	Tr	Tr	0
15-2-109	八宝粥 (娃哈哈牌)	Tr	Tr	Tr	Tr	Tr	Tr	Tr	Tr	Tr	Tr	Tr	Tr	Tr	Tr	Tr	Tr	Tr	Tr	Tr	Tr	Tr	0
15-2-110	八宝粥 (无糖, 娃哈哈牌)	59.2	Tr	Tr	Tr	59.2	Tr	Tr	Tr	Tr	Tr	Tr	Tr	Tr	Tr	Tr	Tr	Tr	Tr	Tr	Tr	Tr	0
15-2-112	黑芝麻糊粉	45.8	Tr	0.7	Tr	45.1	Tr	Tr	Tr	34.6	Tr	34.6	Tr	Tr	Tr	Tr	Tr	Tr	Tr	Tr	Tr	Tr	0.2
15-2-113	麦片	16.5	Tr	Tr	Tr	16.5	Tr	Tr	Tr	24.1	Tr	18.8	5.3	Tr	Tr	Tr	Tr	Tr	Tr	Tr	Tr	Tr	0.2
15-2-114	麦片 (原味香奶)	66.7	Tr	Tr	Tr	66.7	Tr	Tr	Tr	11.9	Tr	11.9	Tr	Tr	Tr	Tr	Tr	Tr	Tr	Tr	Tr	Tr	0
15-2-115	燕麦片	55.2	Tr	1.6	Tr	53.6	Tr	Tr	Tr	23.0	Tr	23.0	Tr	Tr	Tr	Tr	Tr	Tr	Tr	Tr	Tr	Tr	0
15-2-116	燕麦片 (果仁、甜)	31.2	Tr	Tr	Tr	31.2	Tr	Tr	Tr	33.3	Tr	29.7	3.6	Tr	Tr	Tr	Tr	Tr	Tr	Tr	Tr	Tr	0
15-2-202	鸡汁味干脆面 (面饼 + 调味料)	37.3	Tr	Tr	Tr	37.3	Tr	Tr	Tr	9.1	Tr	8.9	0.2	Tr	Tr	Tr	Tr	Tr	Tr	Tr	Tr	Tr	0.2
15-2-203	海鲜味方便面 (面饼 + 调味料 + 油料)	60.7	Tr	2.0	Tr	58.7	Tr	Tr	Tr	25.6	Tr	25.1	0.5	Tr	Tr	Tr	Tr	Tr	Tr	Tr	Tr	Tr	0
15-2-206	红烧牛肉方便面 (面饼+调味料+蔬菜+肉酱)	32.4	Tr	Tr	Tr	32.4	Tr	Tr	Tr	5.1	Tr	5.1	Tr	Tr	Tr	Tr	Tr	Tr	Tr	Tr	Tr	Tr	0.1
15-2-209	鳕鱼方便面 (面饼 + 调味料 + 珍料 + 凋味油 + 蔬菜)	32.7	Tr	Tr	Tr	32.7	Tr	Tr	Tr	4.0	Tr	3.9	0.1	Tr	Tr	Tr	Tr	Tr	Tr	Tr	Tr	Tr	0
15-2-212	铁板牛肉炒面 (面饼+汤料+蔬菜+调味酱)	34.1	Tr	Tr	Tr	34.1	Tr	Tr	Tr	5.2	Tr	5.2	Tr	Tr	Tr	Tr	Tr	Tr	Tr	Tr	Tr	Tr	0.1
15-2-215	玉米红烧牛肉味方便面 (面饼+调味料+蔬菜+肉酱)	41.3	Tr	1.2	Tr	40.1	Tr	Tr	Tr	15.2	Tr	15.2	Tr	Tr	Tr	Tr	Tr	Tr	Tr	Tr	Tr	Tr	0.1
15-2-221	冬菜虾仁馄饨	40.5	Tr	1.9	Tr	38.0	0.6	Tr	Tr	23.8	Tr	21.4	1.4	Tr	Tr	Tr	0.4	0.2	Tr	Tr	Tr	0.4	0
15-2-222	韭菜合子	24.7	Tr	0.6	Tr	23.9	0.2	Tr	Tr	51.3	Tr	45.0	5.5	Tr	Tr	Tr	0.8	Tr	Tr	Tr	Tr	Tr	0
15-2-223	糯米饭团	22.5	Tr	0.2	Tr	22.0	0.2	0.1	Tr	55.5	Tr	49.8	5.4	Tr	Tr	Tr	0.2	0.1	Tr	Tr	Tr	Tr	0
15-2-224	什锦炒饭	25.3	Tr	0.4	Tr	24.9	Tr	Tr	Tr	55.0	Tr	48.1	6.4	Tr	Tr	Tr	0.5	Tr	Tr	Tr	Tr	Tr	0.3

食物脂肪酸含量 Fatty acid content of foods

编码 Code	食物名称 Food name	脂肪 Fat g	脂肪酸 Fatty acid (g/100g 可食部) Total	饱和 SFA	单不饱和 MUFA	多不饱和 PUFA	未知 UN-K	饱和脂肪酸/总脂肪酸(%) Total	6:0	8:0	10:0	11:0	12:0	13:0	14:0	15:0	16:0	17:0	18:0	19:0	20:0	22:0	24:0
15-2-225	虾仁炒饭	1.7	un	un	un	un	un	16.3	Tr	Tr	Tr	Tr	Tr	Tr	Tr	Tr	11.6	Tr	4.0	Tr	0.3	0.4	0.4
15-2-415	饼干(三明治)	30.4	28.8	11.0	6.0	11.7	0	38.3	Tr	Tr	Tr	Tr	4.0	Tr	2.2	Tr	32.1	Tr	Tr	Tr	Tr	Tr	Tr
15-2-416	饼干(夹心)	15.9	15.0	7.4	5.7	1.9	0	49.4	Tr	Tr	Tr	Tr	0.2	Tr	1.0	Tr	47.1	Tr	1.1	Tr	Tr	Tr	Tr
15-2-417	饼干(甜酥夹心)	35.1	33.2	23.6	8.0	1.6	0	71.1	Tr	Tr	0.4	Tr	33.7	Tr	13.0	Tr	20.5	Tr	3.5	Tr	Tr	Tr	Tr
15-2-418	饼干(苏打夹心)	19.3	18.3	13.8	4.1	0.3	0	75.8	Tr	Tr	Tr	Tr	38.2	Tr	9.6	Tr	24.5	Tr	3.5	Tr	Tr	Tr	Tr
15-2-419	饼干(咸)	25.6	24.2	11.9	9.8	2.5	0	49.2	Tr	Tr	Tr	Tr	0.3	Tr	1.1	Tr	46.8	Tr	1.0	Tr	Tr	Tr	Tr
15-2-501	饺子(素馅)	5.6	un	un	un	un	un	18.2	Tr	Tr	Tr	Tr	Tr	Tr	0.2	Tr	16.4	Tr	1.6	Tr	Tr	Tr	Tr
15-2-502	饺子(三鲜馅)	12.3	un	un	un	un	un	34.9	Tr	Tr	Tr	Tr	Tr	Tr	1.3	Tr	31.4	Tr	2.2	Tr	Tr	Tr	Tr
15-2-503	饺子(猪肉白菜馅)	10.8	un	un	un	un	un	36.2	Tr	Tr	Tr	Tr	Tr	Tr	1.2	Tr	31.8	Tr	3.2	Tr	Tr	Tr	Tr
15-2-504	饺子(猪肉韭菜馅)	14.4	un	un	un	un	un	35.0	Tr	Tr	Tr	Tr	Tr	Tr	1.3	Tr	31.8	Tr	1.9	Tr	Tr	Tr	Tr
15-2-505	饺子(猪肉芹菜馅)	16.8	un	un	un	un	un	37.7	Tr	Tr	Tr	Tr	Tr	Tr	1.6	Tr	34.3	Tr	1.8	Tr	Tr	Tr	Tr
15-2-506	饺子(猪肉茴香馅)	9.1	un	un	un	un	un	38.3	Tr	Tr	Tr	Tr	Tr	Tr	1.4	Tr	34.8	Tr	2.1	Tr	Tr	Tr	Tr
15-2-507	饺子(猪肉香菇馅)	15.3	un	un	un	un	un	37.4	Tr	Tr	0.1	Tr	0.1	Tr	1.3	0.1	23.6	0.3	10.9	0.2	0.8	Tr	Tr
15-2-508	饺子(猪肉虾仁馅)	15.4	un	un	un	un	un	37.5	Tr	Tr	Tr	Tr	Tr	Tr	1.3	Tr	23.4	Tr	11.7	0.2	0.9	Tr	Tr
15-2-509	饺子(鸡肉蘑菇馅)	7.4	un	un	un	un	un	35.5	Tr	Tr	0.1	Tr	0.1	Tr	1.2	Tr	22.6	Tr	11.2	Tr	0.3	Tr	Tr
15-2-510	饺子(海鳗猪肉馅)	17.7	un	un	un	un	un	38.4	Tr	Tr	Tr	Tr	Tr	Tr	1.5	Tr	24.3	Tr	12.2	Tr	0.3	0.1	0.1
15-2-511	饺子(海鳗虾仁馅)	20.0	un	un	un	un	un	37.4	Tr	Tr	Tr	Tr	Tr	Tr	1.3	Tr	24.1	Tr	11.6	Tr	0.3	0.1	0.1
15-2-513	包子(猪肉馅)	10.0	un	un	un	un	un	32.6	Tr	Tr	Tr	Tr	Tr	Tr	1.0	Tr	29.0	Tr	2.6	Tr	Tr	Tr	Tr
15-3-101	米饼(鸡蛋牛奶味)	29.9	28.3	15.8	5.9	4.6	2.0	55.8	Tr	Tr	1.2	Tr	1.4	Tr	5.3	Tr	31.7	Tr	16.2	Tr	Tr	Tr	Tr
15-3-102	雪米饼	17.6	16.6	9.4	6.0	1.2	0	56.5	Tr	Tr	Tr	Tr	1.2	Tr	Tr	Tr	52.1	Tr	3.2	Tr	Tr	Tr	Tr
15-3-103	蛋酥卷	35.3	33.4	16.1	13.3	3.9	0.1	48.2	Tr	Tr	0.3	Tr	0.4	Tr	1.4	Tr	41.7	Tr	4.4	Tr	Tr	Tr	Tr
15-3-104	巧克力派	17.7	13.0	8.8	4.2	Tr	0	67.8	Tr	Tr	Tr	Tr	22.1	Tr	4.0	Tr	35.0	Tr	6.7	Tr	Tr	Tr	Tr
15-3-105	法式卷饼	34.0	32.2	14.5	12.6	5.1	0	45.2	Tr	Tr	Tr	Tr	0.4	Tr	2.6	1.8	30.9	Tr	9.5	Tr	Tr	Tr	Tr
15-3-106	立体脆	24.7	23.4	11.7	9.3	2.0	0.4	50.0	Tr	Tr	0.5	Tr	Tr	Tr	0.7	Tr	45.8	Tr	3.0	Tr	Tr	Tr	Tr

食物脂肪酸含量 Fatty acid content of foods

编码 Code	食物名称 Food name	单不饱和/总脂肪酸(%) Total	14:1	16:1	17:1	18:1	20:1	22:1	24:1	多不饱和/总脂肪酸(%) Total	16:2	18:2	18:3	18:4	20:2	20:3	20:4	20:5	22:3	22:4	22:5	22:6	未知 %
15-2-225	虾仁炒饭	23.1	Tr	Tr	Tr	22.9	0.2	Tr	Tr	60.6	Tr	51.8	7.8	Tr	Tr	Tr	Tr	0.8	Tr	Tr	Tr	0.2	0
15-2-415	饼干(三明治)	21.0	Tr	Tr	Tr	21.0	Tr	Tr	Tr	40.6	Tr	32.5	8.1	Tr	Tr	Tr	Tr	Tr	Tr	Tr	Tr	Tr	0.1
15-2-416	饼干(夹心)	37.9	Tr	Tr	Tr	37.9	Tr	Tr	Tr	12.7	Tr	12.7	Tr	Tr	Tr	Tr	Tr	Tr	Tr	Tr	Tr	Tr	0
15-2-417	饼干(甜酥夹心)	24.0	Tr	Tr	Tr	24.0	Tr	Tr	Tr	4.8	Tr	4.7	0.1	Tr	Tr	Tr	Tr	Tr	Tr	Tr	Tr	Tr	0.1
15-2-418	饼干(苏打夹心)	22.7	Tr	Tr	Tr	22.7	Tr	Tr	Tr	1.9	Tr	1.9	Tr	Tr	Tr	Tr	Tr	Tr	Tr	Tr	Tr	Tr	0
15-2-419	饼干(咸)	40.3	Tr	Tr	Tr	40.3	Tr	Tr	Tr	10.4	Tr	10.4	Tr	Tr	Tr	Tr	Tr	Tr	Tr	Tr	Tr	Tr	0.1
15-2-501	饺子(素馅)	28.9	Tr	Tr	Tr	28.9	Tr	Tr	Tr	52.8	Tr	36.2	16.6	Tr	Tr	Tr	Tr	Tr	Tr	Tr	Tr	Tr	0.1
15-2-502	饺子(三鲜馅)	44.7	Tr	Tr	Tr	44.7	Tr	Tr	Tr	20.3	Tr	20.3	Tr	Tr	Tr	Tr	Tr	Tr	Tr	Tr	Tr	Tr	0.1
15-2-503	饺子(猪肉白菜馅)	46.0	Tr	Tr	Tr	46.0	Tr	Tr	Tr	17.7	Tr	16.3	1.4	Tr	Tr	Tr	Tr	Tr	Tr	Tr	Tr	Tr	0.1
15-2-504	饺子(猪肉韭菜馅)	44.0	Tr	Tr	Tr	44.0	Tr	Tr	Tr	21.0	Tr	19.1	1.9	Tr	Tr	Tr	Tr	Tr	Tr	Tr	Tr	Tr	0
15-2-505	饺子(猪肉芹菜馅)	48.9	Tr	Tr	Tr	48.9	Tr	Tr	Tr	13.3	Tr	13.3	Tr	Tr	Tr	Tr	Tr	Tr	Tr	Tr	Tr	Tr	0.1
15-2-506	饺子(猪肉茴香馅)	48.0	Tr	Tr	Tr	48.0	Tr	Tr	Tr	13.6	Tr	13.3	0.3	Tr	Tr	Tr	Tr	Tr	Tr	Tr	Tr	Tr	0.1
15-2-507	饺子(猪肉香菇馅)	47.5	Tr	2.5	Tr	44.8	0.2	Tr	Tr	15.1	Tr	13.7	0.8	Tr	Tr	Tr	0.1	Tr	Tr	Tr	0.3	0.2	0
15-2-508	饺子(猪肉虾仁馅)	43.4	Tr	2.2	Tr	41.0	0.2	Tr	Tr	19.0	Tr	15.8	1.0	Tr	Tr	Tr	Tr	Tr	Tr	Tr	0.3	1.9	0.1
15-2-509	饺子(鸡肉蘑菇馅)	39.8	Tr	0.2	Tr	38.8	0.8	Tr	Tr	24.9	Tr	22.4	2.1	Tr	Tr	Tr	Tr	Tr	Tr	Tr	0.2	0.2	0
15-2-510	饺子(海鳗猪肉馅)	47.4	Tr	2.4	Tr	43.6	1.1	0.3	Tr	14.5	Tr	13.1	0.8	Tr	Tr	Tr	Tr	Tr	Tr	Tr	0.2	0.4	0
15-2-511	饺子(海鳗虾仁馅)	45.2	Tr	2.2	Tr	41.7	1.0	0.3	Tr	18.6	Tr	17.0	1.2	Tr	Tr	Tr	Tr	Tr	Tr	Tr	0.2	0.2	0
15-2-513	包子(猪肉馅)	45.4	Tr	Tr	Tr	45.4	Tr	Tr	Tr	21.9	Tr	20.3	1.6	Tr	Tr	Tr	Tr	Tr	Tr	Tr	Tr	Tr	0.1
15-3-101	米饼(鸡蛋牛奶味)	21.0	Tr	Tr	Tr	21.0	Tr	Tr	Tr	16.2	Tr	16.2	Tr	Tr	Tr	Tr	Tr	Tr	Tr	Tr	Tr	Tr	7.0
15-3-102	雪米饼	36.0	Tr	Tr	Tr	36.0	Tr	Tr	Tr	7.5	Tr	7.5	Tr	Tr	Tr	Tr	Tr	Tr	Tr	Tr	Tr	Tr	0
15-3-103	蛋酥卷	39.8	Tr	Tr	Tr	39.8	Tr	Tr	Tr	11.8	Tr	11.7	0.1	Tr	Tr	Tr	Tr	Tr	Tr	Tr	Tr	Tr	0.2
15-3-104	巧克力派	32.4	Tr	Tr	Tr	32.4	Tr	Tr	Tr	Tr	Tr	Tr	Tr	Tr	Tr	Tr	Tr	Tr	Tr	Tr	Tr	Tr	0
15-3-105	法式卷饼	39.1	Tr	Tr	Tr	39.1	Tr	Tr	Tr	15.8	Tr	14.1	1.7	Tr	Tr	Tr	Tr	Tr	Tr	Tr	Tr	Tr	0
15-3-106	立体脆	39.8	Tr	Tr	Tr	39.8	Tr	Tr	Tr	8.7	Tr	8.7	Tr	Tr	Tr	Tr	Tr	Tr	Tr	Tr	Tr	Tr	1.5

食物脂肪酸含量 Fatty acid content of foods

编码 Code	食物名称 Food name	脂肪 Fat g	脂肪酸 Fatty acid (g/100g 可食部) Total	饱和 SFA	单不饱和 MUFA	多不饱和 PUFA	未知 UN.K	饱和脂肪酸/总脂肪酸(%) Total	6:0	8:0	10:0	11:0	12:0	13:0	14:0	15:0	16:0	17:0	18:0	19:0	20:0	22:0	24:0
15-3-107	粟米脆	34.7	32.8	14.9	13.0	4.9	0	45.3	Tr	Tr	Tr	Tr	0.2	Tr	1.0	Tr	43.5	Tr	0.6	Tr	Tr	Tr	Tr
15-3-108	通心脆	29.6	28.0	16.9	10.1	1.0	0.1	60.2	Tr	Tr	Tr	Tr	1.6	Tr	1.7	Tr	53.1	Tr	3.8	Tr	Tr	Tr	Tr
15-3-109	洋葱圈	21.3	20.1	12.0	7.2	1.0	0	59.8	Tr	Tr	1.3	Tr	4.6	Tr	2.1	0.4	48.2	Tr	3.2	Tr	Tr	Tr	Tr
15-3-202	锅巴(豆香)	30.6	28.9	14.0	11.9	3.0	0	48.4	Tr	Tr	Tr	Tr	0.4	Tr	1.1	Tr	46.2	Tr	0.7	Tr	Tr	Tr	Tr
15-3-203	锅巴(小米)	36.9	34.9	16.9	9.4	8.6	0	48.4	Tr	Tr	Tr	Tr	1.7	Tr	1.5	Tr	43.8	Tr	1.4	Tr	Tr	Tr	Tr
15-3-204	海苔	4.8	2.7	2.7	Tr	Tr	0	100.8	Tr	Tr	6.0	Tr	25.5	Tr	2.0	3.7	63.6	Tr	Tr	Tr	Tr	Tr	Tr
15-3-205	香菇片	12.4	7.0	3.1	2.8	1.0	0	45.1	Tr	Tr	Tr	Tr	0.3	Tr	1.1	Tr	43.0	Tr	0.7	Tr	Tr	Tr	Tr
15-3-206	薯片(烧烤味)	37.6	35.4	15.8	14.7	4.9	0.1	44.7	Tr	Tr	0.5	Tr	Tr	Tr	1.1	Tr	40.4	Tr	2.7	Tr	Tr	Tr	Tr
15-3-207	薯片(香辣味)	40.0	37.7	20.2	15.0	2.4	0.1	53.5	Tr	Tr	1.2	Tr	1.8	Tr	1.7	0.2	44.4	Tr	4.2	Tr	Tr	Tr	Tr
15-3-208	薯圈	42.6	40.1	23.4	14.6	2.0	0.2	58.3	Tr	Tr	1.3	Tr	1.2	Tr	2.0	Tr	51.2	Tr	2.6	Tr	Tr	Tr	Tr
15-3-301	怪味胡豆	12.1	9.4	4.2	3.9	1.2	0.1	45.0	Tr	Tr	Tr	Tr	0.2	Tr	0.9	Tr	42.8	Tr	1.1	Tr	Tr	Tr	Tr
15-3-303	夹心米果	41.9	39.6	23.7	13.4	2.5	0	59.9	Tr	Tr	Tr	Tr	3.9	Tr	2.7	Tr	51.2	Tr	2.1	Tr	Tr	Tr	Tr
15-3-304	乐芙球	45.0	42.6	19.7	18.4	4.6	0	46.3	Tr	Tr	0.2	Tr	0.5	Tr	1.6	0.2	39.5	Tr	4.3	Tr	Tr	Tr	Tr
15-3-305	玉米花	13.4	11.4	5.9	4.2	1.3	0	51.9	Tr	Tr	6.8	Tr	Tr	Tr	Tr	Tr	38.2	Tr	6.9	Tr	Tr	Tr	Tr
15-3-308	鱼肉粒	3.3	2.3	1.0	1.0	0.3	0	43.8	Tr	Tr	0.7	Tr	0.6	Tr	9.3	0.3	28.1	Tr	4.8	Tr	Tr	Tr	Tr
饮料类																							
16-2-013	菠萝汁饮料(大湖牌)	0.2	0.2	0.1	Tr	0.1	0	48.4	Tr	Tr	Tr	Tr	5.1	Tr	6.5	Tr	36.8	Tr	Tr	Tr	Tr	Tr	Tr
16-2-026	西柚汁饮料	0.4	0.3	0.1	0	0.2	0	31.2	Tr	Tr	Tr	Tr	2.6	Tr	1.7	Tr	26.9	Tr	Tr	Tr	Tr	Tr	Tr
16-2-027	椰子汁饮料	2.4	1.9	1.7	0.2	0	0	90.1	Tr	Tr	Tr	Tr	48.9	Tr	21.9	Tr	16.9	Tr	2.4	Tr	Tr	Tr	Tr
16-4-004	健康快车奶饮料	0.6	0.6	0.6	Tr	Tr	0	100.0	Tr	Tr	Tr	Tr	31.9	Tr	28.1	Tr	40.0	Tr	Tr	Tr	Tr	Tr	Tr
16-4-005	粒粒果奶饮料	0.6	0.6	0.5	0.1	Tr	0	86.5	Tr	Tr	Tr	Tr	24.6	Tr	23.5	Tr	38.4	Tr	Tr	Tr	Tr	Tr	Tr
16-4-006	酸乳饮料	1.3	1.2	0.8	0.3	Tr	0.2	65.7	Tr	Tr	Tr	Tr	Tr	Tr	21.9	0.7	31.7	Tr	11.4	Tr	Tr	Tr	Tr
16-7-011	高乐高营养饮品	2.4	un	un	un	un	un	100.0	Tr	Tr	33.9	Tr	Tr	Tr	Tr	Tr	66.1	Tr	Tr	Tr	Tr	Tr	Tr

编码 Code	食物名称 Food name	单不饱和/总脂肪酸(%) Total	14:1	16:1	17:1	18:1	20:1	22:1	24:1	多不饱和/总脂肪酸(%) Total	16:2	18:2	18:3	18:4	20:2	20:3	20:4	20:5	22:3	22:4	22:5	22:6	未知 %
15-3-107	粟米脆	39.7	Tr	Tr	Tr	39.7	Tr	Tr	Tr	14.9	Tr	14.9	Tr	Tr	Tr	Tr	Tr	Tr	Tr	Tr	Tr	Tr	0.1
15-3-108	通心脆	35.9	Tr	Tr	Tr	35.9	Tr	Tr	Tr	3.6	Tr	3.6	Tr	Tr	Tr	Tr	Tr	Tr	Tr	Tr	Tr	Tr	0.3
15-3-109	洋葱圈	35.6	Tr	Tr	Tr	35.6	Tr	Tr	Tr	4.8	Tr	4.8	Tr	Tr	Tr	Tr	Tr	Tr	Tr	Tr	Tr	Tr	0
15-3-202	锅巴(豆香)	41.2	Tr	Tr	Tr	41.2	Tr	Tr	Tr	10.3	Tr	10.3	Tr	Tr	Tr	Tr	Tr	Tr	Tr	Tr	Tr	Tr	0.1
15-3-203	锅巴(小米)	26.9	Tr	Tr	Tr	26.9	Tr	Tr	Tr	24.7	Tr	3.6	21.1	Tr	Tr	Tr	Tr	Tr	Tr	Tr	Tr	Tr	0
15-3-204	海苔	Tr	Tr	Tr	Tr	Tr	Tr	Tr	Tr	Tr	Tr	Tr	Tr	Tr	Tr	Tr	Tr	Tr	Tr	Tr	Tr	Tr	0
15-3-205	香菇片	39.8	Tr	Tr	Tr	39.8	Tr	Tr	Tr	15.0	Tr	15.0	Tr	Tr	Tr	Tr	Tr	Tr	Tr	Tr	Tr	Tr	0.1
15-3-206	薯片(烧烤味)	41.4	Tr	Tr	Tr	41.4	Tr	Tr	Tr	13.7	Tr	12.5	1.2	Tr	Tr	Tr	Tr	Tr	Tr	Tr	Tr	Tr	0.2
15-3-207	薯片(香辣味)	39.8	Tr	Tr	Tr	39.8	Tr	Tr	Tr	6.4	Tr	6.4	Tr	Tr	Tr	Tr	Tr	Tr	Tr	Tr	Tr	Tr	0.3
15-3-208	薯圈	36.3	Tr	Tr	Tr	36.3	Tr	Tr	Tr	4.9	Tr	4.9	Tr	Tr	Tr	Tr	Tr	Tr	Tr	Tr	Tr	Tr	0.5
15-3-301	怪味胡豆	41.3	Tr	Tr	Tr	41.3	Tr	Tr	Tr	12.9	Tr	11.9	0.1	Tr	Tr	Tr	0.9	Tr	Tr	Tr	Tr	Tr	0.8
15-3-303	夹心米果	33.7	Tr	Tr	Tr	33.7	Tr	Tr	Tr	6.4	Tr	6.4	Tr	Tr	Tr	Tr	Tr	Tr	Tr	Tr	Tr	Tr	0
15-3-304	乐芙球	43.2	Tr	Tr	Tr	43.2	Tr	Tr	Tr	10.7	Tr	10.4	0.3	Tr	Tr	Tr	Tr	Tr	Tr	Tr	Tr	Tr	0
15-3-305	玉米花	36.7	Tr	Tr	Tr	36.7	Tr	Tr	Tr	11.2	Tr	11.2	Tr	Tr	Tr	Tr	Tr	Tr	Tr	Tr	Tr	Tr	0.2
15-3-308	鱼肉粒	42.5	Tr	Tr	Tr	42.5	Tr	Tr	Tr	13.7	Tr	7.5	6.2	Tr	Tr	Tr	Tr	Tr	Tr	Tr	Tr	Tr	0
饮料类																							
16-2-013	菠萝汁饮料(大湖牌)	Tr	Tr	Tr	Tr	Tr	Tr	Tr	Tr	51.4	Tr	31.3	20.1	Tr	Tr	Tr	Tr	Tr	Tr	Tr	Tr	Tr	0.2
16-2-026	西柚汁饮料	14.6	Tr	3.6	Tr	11.0	Tr	Tr	Tr	56.5	Tr	20.6	35.9	Tr	Tr	Tr	Tr	Tr	Tr	Tr	Tr	Tr	0
16-2-027	椰子汁饮料	8.7	Tr	Tr	Tr	8.7	Tr	Tr	Tr	1.1	Tr	1.1	Tr	Tr	Tr	Tr	Tr	Tr	Tr	Tr	Tr	Tr	0.1
16-4-004	健康快车奶饮料	Tr	Tr	Tr	Tr	Tr	Tr	Tr	Tr	Tr	Tr	Tr	Tr	Tr	Tr	Tr	Tr	Tr	Tr	Tr	Tr	Tr	0
16-4-005	粒粒果奶饮料	13.3	Tr	Tr	Tr	13.3	Tr	Tr	Tr	Tr	Tr	Tr	Tr	Tr	Tr	Tr	Tr	Tr	Tr	Tr	Tr	Tr	0.2
16-4-006	酸乳饮料	21.3	Tr	Tr	Tr	21.3	Tr	Tr	Tr	Tr	Tr	Tr	Tr	Tr	Tr	Tr	Tr	Tr	Tr	Tr	Tr	Tr	13.0
16-7-011	高乐高营养饮品	Tr	Tr	Tr	Tr	Tr	Tr	Tr	Tr	Tr	Tr	Tr	Tr	Tr	Tr	Tr	Tr	Tr	Tr	Tr	Tr	Tr	0

食物脂肪酸含量 Fatty acid content of foods

编码 Code	食物名称 Food name	脂肪 Fat g	脂肪酸 Fatty acid (g/100g 可食部) Total	饱和 SFA	单不饱和 MUFA	多不饱和 PUFA	未知 UN.K	饱和脂肪酸/总脂肪酸(%) Total	6:0	8:0	10:0	11:0	12:0	13:0	14:0	15:0	16:0	17:0	18:0	19:0	20:0	22:0	24:0
16-7-012	菓珍	2.2	1.8	0.7	0.8	0.3	0	37.6	Tr	Tr	1.0	Tr	1.4	0.2	1.5	Tr	24.6	Tr	8.9	Tr	Tr	Tr	Tr
16-7-014	柠檬茶	1.7	1.4	0.4	0.4	0.5	0	33.0	Tr	Tr	2.4	Tr	1.7	Tr	1.1	Tr	23.6	Tr	4.2	Tr	Tr	Tr	Tr
16-7-015	巧克力麦芽营养饮品	4.0	2.9	2.9	Tr	Tr	0	100.0	Tr	Tr	Tr	Tr	26.4	Tr	29.0	Tr	44.6	Tr	Tr	Tr	Tr	Tr	Tr
16-7-016	咖啡豆	8.8	8.3	3.4	0.8	4.1	0	41.4	Tr	Tr	Tr	Tr	Tr	Tr	Tr	Tr	37.2	Tr	4.2	Tr	Tr	Tr	Tr
16-7-017	咖啡粉	0.5	0.4	0.2	0	0.2	0	un	un	un	un	un	un	un	un	un	un	un	un	un	un	un	un
16-8-009	冰激凌(草莓味)	3.2	3.0	1.9	1.0	0.1	0	63.6	Tr	Tr	3.1	Tr	1.3	Tr	16.2	Tr	28.8	Tr	14.2	Tr	Tr	Tr	Tr
16-8-010	冰激凌(苦咖啡味)	10.1	9.5	8.7	0.6	0.2	0	90.9	Tr	6.9	7.9	Tr	43.1	Tr	20.8	Tr	9.2	Tr	3.0	Tr	Tr	Tr	Tr
16-8-011	冰激凌(加奶油)	12.8	12.1	7.6	4.1	Tr	0.4	62.6	Tr	Tr	2.1	Tr	0.7	Tr	15.9	Tr	29.3	Tr	14.6	Tr	Tr	Tr	Tr
16-8-015	冰激凌(花心筒)	13.1	12.4	·7.5	3.7	1.2	0	60.5	Tr	1.8	1.5	Tr	16.4	Tr	8.1	Tr	26.5	Tr	6.2	Tr	Tr	Tr	Tr
16-8-016	冰激凌(金百合)	10.5	9.9	9.0	0.7	0.2	0	91.1	Tr	7.0	8.0	Tr	43.4	Tr	20.9	Tr	9.0	Tr	2.8	Tr	Tr	Tr	Tr
16-8-017	雪糕(百乐宝)	6.2	5.9	5.0	0.8	0.1	0	85.0	Tr	5.7	6.5	Tr	38.3	Tr	18.5	Tr	12.6	Tr	3.4	Tr	Tr	Tr	Tr
16-8-018	雪糕(红豆缘)	4.8	4.5	3.8	0.7	Tr	0	84.1	Tr	5.9	Tr	Tr	44.6	Tr	16.0	Tr	15.3	Tr	2.3	Tr	Tr	Tr	Tr
16-8-019	棒冰(可乐冰)	1.0	0.9	0.5	0.4	0.1	0	49.0	Tr	Tr	Tr	Tr	Tr	Tr	1.8	Tr	37.6	Tr	9.6	Tr	Tr	Tr	Tr
16-8-020	棒冰(奇彩旋)	1.1	1.0	0.5	0.1	0.4	0.1	44.1	Tr	Tr	1.6	Tr	Tr	Tr	5.7	Tr	36.6	Tr	0.2	Tr	Tr	Tr	Tr
糖、果脯和蜜饯、蜂蜜																							
18-2-101	夹心糖	20.7	un	un	un	un	un	64.7	Tr	Tr	Tr	Tr	22.4	Tr	6.1	Tr	33.5	Tr	2.7	Tr	Tr	Tr	Tr
18-2-201	牛奶糖	8.2	un	un	un	un	un	62.8	Tr	Tr	Tr	Tr	10.7	Tr	8.9	1.8	36.1	Tr	5.3	Tr	Tr	Tr	Tr
18-2-301	花生牛轧糖	15.5	un	un	un	un	un	15.0	Tr	Tr	Tr	Tr	Tr	Tr	Tr	Tr	15.0	Tr	Tr	Tr	Tr	Tr	Tr
18-2-302	花生芝麻糖	25.3	un	un	un	un	un	14.9	Tr	Tr	Tr	Tr	Tr	Tr	Tr	Tr	14.9	Tr	Tr	Tr	Tr	Tr	Tr
18-3-015	雪梅	1.1	0.8	0.5	0.1	0.2	0	62.7	Tr	Tr	4.2	Tr	3.1	Tr	1.4	Tr	47.9	Tr	6.1	Tr	Tr	Tr	Tr
18-3-016	九制梅肉	3.2	2.2	0.2	0.7	1.3	0	10.1	Tr	Tr	0.6	Tr	0.3	Tr	Tr	Tr	6.5	Tr	2.7	Tr	Tr	Tr	Tr
18-3-017	九制西梅	1.2	0.8	0.5	Tr	0.4	0	56.9	Tr	Tr	Tr	Tr	2.7	Tr	5.5	Tr	44.6	Tr	4.1	Tr	Tr	Tr	Tr
18-3-018	九制应子	0.6	0.4	0.2	0	0.2	0	58.6	Tr	Tr	Tr	Tr	1.9	Tr	2.0	Tr	54.7	Tr	Tr	Tr	Tr	Tr	Tr

编码 Code	食物名称 Food name	单不饱和/总脂肪酸(%) Total	14:1	16:1	17:1	18:1	20:1	22:1	24:1	多不饱和/总脂肪酸(%) Total	16:2	18:2	18:3	18:4	20:2	20:3	20:4	20:5	22:3	22:4	22:5	22:6	未知 %
16-7-012	菓珍	44.3	Tr	Tr	Tr	44.3	Tr	Tr	Tr	17.8	Tr	15.9	1.9	Tr	Tr	Tr	Tr	Tr	Tr	Tr	Tr	Tr	0.3
16-7-014	柠檬茶	29.6	Tr	Tr	Tr	29.6	Tr	Tr	Tr	37.3	Tr	18.9	18.4	Tr	Tr	Tr	Tr	Tr	Tr	Tr	Tr	Tr	0.1
16-7-015	巧克力麦芽营养饮品	Tr	Tr	Tr	Tr	Tr	Tr	Tr	Tr	Tr	Tr	Tr	Tr	Tr	Tr	Tr	Tr	Tr	Tr	Tr	Tr	Tr	0
16-7-016	咖啡豆	9.1	Tr	Tr	Tr	9.1	Tr	Tr	Tr	49.2	Tr	45.6	3.6	Tr	Tr	Tr	Tr	Tr	Tr	Tr	Tr	Tr	0.3
16-7-017	咖啡粉	un	un	un	un	un	un	un	un	un	un	un	un	un	un	un	un	un	un	un	un	un	un
16-8-009	冰激凌	32.8	Tr	0.5	Tr	32.3	Tr	Tr	Tr	3.5	Tr	3.5	Tr	Tr	Tr	Tr	Tr	Tr	Tr	Tr	Tr	Tr	0.1
16-8-010	冰激凌(苦咖啡味)	6.8	Tr	Tr	Tr	6.8	Tr	Tr	Tr	2.2	Tr	2.2	Tr	Tr	Tr	Tr	Tr	Tr	Tr	Tr	Tr	Tr	0.1
16-8-011	冰激凌(加奶油)	33.8	Tr	0.4	Tr	33.4	Tr	Tr	Tr	Tr	Tr	Tr	Tr	Tr	Tr	Tr	Tr	Tr	Tr	Tr	Tr	Tr	3.6
16-8-015	冰激凌(花心筒)	30.1	Tr	Tr	Tr	30.1	Tr	Tr	Tr	9.3	Tr	8.7	0.6	Tr	Tr	Tr	Tr	Tr	Tr	Tr	Tr	Tr	0.1
16-8-016	冰激凌(金百合)	6.6	Tr	Tr	Tr	6.6	Tr	Tr	Tr	2.2	Tr	2.2	Tr	Tr	Tr	Tr	Tr	Tr	Tr	Tr	Tr	Tr	0.1
16-8-017	雪糕(百乐宝)	13.6	Tr	Tr	Tr	13.6	Tr	Tr	Tr	1.4	Tr	1.4	Tr	Tr	Tr	Tr	Tr	Tr	Tr	Tr	Tr	Tr	0
16-8-018	雪糕(红豆缘)	15.9	Tr	Tr	Tr	15.9	Tr	Tr	Tr	Tr	Tr	Tr	Tr	Tr	Tr	Tr	Tr	Tr	Tr	Tr	Tr	Tr	0
16-8-019	棒冰(可乐冰)	41.6	Tr	Tr	Tr	41.6	Tr	Tr	Tr	9.3	Tr	9.3	Tr	Tr	Tr	Tr	Tr	Tr	Tr	Tr	Tr	Tr	0.1
16-8-020	棒冰(奇彩旋)	8.4	Tr	Tr	Tr	8.4	Tr	Tr	Tr	38.8	Tr	38.8	Tr	Tr	Tr	Tr	Tr	Tr	Tr	Tr	Tr	Tr	8.7
糖、果脯和蜜饯、蜂蜜																							
18-2-101	夹心糖	25.6	Tr	Tr	Tr	25.6	Tr	Tr	Tr	9.7	Tr	9.7	Tr	Tr	Tr	Tr	Tr	Tr	Tr	Tr	Tr	Tr	0
18-2-201	牛奶糖	30.3	Tr	Tr	Tr	30.3	Tr	Tr	Tr	6.9	Tr	6.0	0.9	Tr	Tr	Tr	Tr	Tr	Tr	Tr	Tr	Tr	0
18-2-301	花生牛轧糖	4.3	Tr	Tr	Tr	4.3	Tr	Tr	Tr	80.3	Tr	53.3	27.0	Tr	Tr	Tr	Tr	Tr	Tr	Tr	Tr	Tr	0.4
18-2-302	花生芝麻糖	0.4	Tr	Tr	Tr	0.4	Tr	Tr	Tr	84.5	Tr	45.7	38.8	Tr	Tr	Tr	Tr	Tr	Tr	Tr	Tr	Tr	0.2
18-3-015	雪梅	12.7	Tr	Tr	Tr	12.7	Tr	Tr	Tr	24.6	Tr	17.9	6.7	Tr	Tr	Tr	Tr	Tr	Tr	Tr	Tr	Tr	0
18-3-016	九制梅肉	32.8	Tr	Tr	Tr	32.8	Tr	Tr	Tr	57.0	Tr	35.7	21.3	Tr	Tr	Tr	Tr	Tr	Tr	Tr	Tr	Tr	0.1
18-3-017	九制西梅	Tr	Tr	Tr	Tr	Tr	Tr	Tr	Tr	43.2	Tr	33.3	9.9	Tr	Tr	Tr	Tr	Tr	Tr	Tr	Tr	Tr	0
18-3-018	九制应子	1.5	Tr	Tr	Tr	1.5	Tr	Tr	Tr	39.8	Tr	26.3	13.5	Tr	Tr	Tr	Tr	Tr	Tr	Tr	Tr	Tr	0.1

食物脂肪酸含量 Fatty acid content of foods

编码 Code	食物名称 Food name	脂肪 Fat g	脂肪酸 Fatty acid (g/100g 可食部) Total	饱和 SFA	单不饱和 MUFA	多不饱和 PUFA	未知 UN.K	饱和脂肪酸/总脂肪酸(%) Total	6:0	8:0	10:0	11:0	12:0	13:0	14:0	15:0	16:0	17:0	18:0	19:0	20:0	22:0	24:0
18-3-019	梅脯	1.1	0.8	0.4	0.2	0.1	0	57.2	Tr	Tr	1.1	Tr	1.2	Tr	0.6	Tr	50.3	Tr	4.0	Tr	Tr	Tr	Tr
油脂类																								
19-2-020	核桃油	99.1	94.7	7.2	18.6	68.8	0.2	7.6	Tr	Tr	Tr	Tr	Tr	Tr	Tr	Tr	6.4	Tr	1.2	Tr	Tr	Tr	Tr
19-2-021	花生油	99.9	95.5	12.9	43.1	39.4	0.1	13.5	Tr	Tr	Tr	Tr	Tr	Tr	0.1	Tr	13.4	Tr	Tr	Tr	Tr	Tr	Tr
19-2-022	葵花子油	99.9	95.5	9.6	20.5	65.3	0.1	10.0	Tr	Tr	Tr	Tr	Tr	Tr	Tr	Tr	8.8	Tr	1.2	Tr	Tr	Tr	Tr
19-2-023	粟米油 [玉米胚芽油]	100.0	95.6	13.3	27.2	55.3	0	13.9	Tr	Tr	Tr	Tr	Tr	Tr	Tr	Tr	13.4	Tr	0.5	Tr	Tr	Tr	Tr
19-2-024	米糠油	98.7	94.4	14.0	35.0	45.0	0.4	14.8	Tr	Tr	Tr	Tr	Tr	Tr	Tr	Tr	12.5	Tr	2.3	Tr	Tr	Tr	Tr
19-2-025	油茶籽油	99.8	95.4	9.8	72.9	12.6	0.1	10.3	Tr	Tr	Tr	Tr	Tr	Tr	Tr	Tr	9.3	Tr	1.0	Tr	Tr	Tr	Tr
19-2-026	芝麻油 [香油]	99.7	95.3	11.7	35.6	47.9	0.1	12.3	Tr	Tr	Tr	Tr	Tr	Tr	Tr	Tr	9.3	Tr	3.0	Tr	Tr	Tr	Tr
19-2-027	大豆色拉油	99.9	95.5	13.5	29.6	52.4	0	14.1	Tr	Tr	Tr	Tr	Tr	Tr	0.3	Tr	13.8	Tr	Tr	Tr	Tr	Tr	Tr
19-2-028	色拉油	99.7	95.3	13.9	20.3	61.9	0	14.6	Tr	Tr	Tr	Tr	0.9	Tr	Tr	Tr	11.2	Tr	2.5	Tr	Tr	Tr	Tr
调味品类																								
20-1-012	老抽	0.3	0.3	0.1	0.1	0.1	0	41.8	Tr	Tr	Tr	Tr	0.6	Tr	1.2	Tr	38.6	Tr	1.4	Tr	Tr	Tr	Tr
20-3-116	海鲜酱 (阿香婆)	41.1	un	un	un	un	un	4.6	Tr	Tr	Tr	Tr	Tr	Tr	Tr	Tr	Tr	4.6	Tr	Tr	Tr	Tr	Tr
20-3-117	牛肉酱 (阿香婆)	43.0	un	un	un	un	un	7.3	Tr	Tr	Tr	Tr	Tr	Tr	Tr	Tr	Tr	6.0	Tr	1.3	Tr	Tr	Tr
20-3-118	花生酱	53.1	50.5	8.3	24.4	17.8	0	16.4	Tr	Tr	Tr	Tr	Tr	Tr	Tr	Tr	15.5	Tr	0.9	Tr	Tr	Tr	Tr
20-3-119	花生酱 (加巧克力)	55.4	52.7	9.5	25.6	17.4	0.1	18.1	Tr	Tr	Tr	Tr	Tr	Tr	0.3	Tr	17.4	Tr	0.4	Tr	Tr	Tr	Tr
20-3-120	芝麻酱	66.8	63.9	5.9	24.1	33.9	0	9.2	Tr	Tr	Tr	Tr	Tr	Tr	Tr	Tr	9.2	Tr	Tr	Tr	Tr	Tr	Tr
20-3-121	千岛沙拉酱	43.4	41.1	5.7	9.4	26.1	0	13.8	Tr	Tr	Tr	Tr	Tr	Tr	0.1	Tr	11.8	Tr	1.9	Tr	Tr	Tr	Tr
20-3-122	沙拉酱	78.8	74.7	10.6	18.5	45.6	0.1	14.2	Tr	Tr	Tr	Tr	Tr	Tr	0.1	Tr	12.2	Tr	1.9	Tr	Tr	Tr	Tr
20-3-123	奶油攀司	42.0	39.7	5.3	12.1	22.1	0.1	13.4	Tr	Tr	Tr	Tr	Tr	Tr	0.7	Tr	12.7	Tr	Tr	Tr	Tr	Tr	Tr
20-3-207	草莓酱	1.1	0.8	0.3	0.2	0.2	0	44.4	Tr	Tr	1.8	Tr	1.2	Tr	Tr	Tr	39.0	Tr	2.4	Tr	Tr	Tr	Tr
20-3-208	番茄沙司	0.2	0.1	0	0	0.1	0	29.7	Tr	Tr	1.8	Tr	1.4	Tr	1.4	Tr	22.2	Tr	2.9	Tr	Tr	Tr	Tr

编码 Code	食物名称 Food name	单不饱和/总脂肪酸(%)								多不饱和/总脂肪酸(%)													未知 %
		Total	14:1	16:1	17:1	18:1	20:1	22:1	24:1	Total	16:2	18:2	18:3	18:4	20:2	20:3	20:4	20:5	22:3	22:4	22:5	22:6	
18-3-019	梅脯	25.7	Tr	Tr	Tr	25.7	Tr	Tr	Tr	17.0	Tr	14.0	3.0	Tr	Tr	Tr	Tr	Tr	Tr	Tr	Tr	Tr	0.1
油脂类																							
19-2-020	核桃油	19.6	Tr	Tr	Tr	19.6	Tr	Tr	Tr	72.6	Tr	64.9	7.7	Tr	Tr	Tr	Tr	Tr	Tr	Tr	Tr	Tr	0.2
19-2-021	花生油	45.1	Tr	Tr	Tr	45.1	Tr	Tr	Tr	41.3	Tr	41.3	Tr	Tr	Tr	Tr	Tr	Tr	Tr	Tr	Tr	Tr	0.1
19-2-022	葵花子油	21.5	Tr	Tr	Tr	21.5	Tr	Tr	Tr	68.4	Tr	68.4	Tr	Tr	Tr	Tr	Tr	Tr	Tr	Tr	Tr	Tr	0.1
19-2-023	粟米油[玉米胚芽油]	28.4	Tr	Tr	Tr	28.4	Tr	Tr	Tr	57.8	Tr	56.2	1.6	Tr	Tr	Tr	Tr	Tr	Tr	Tr	Tr	Tr	0
19-2-024	米糠油	37.1	Tr	Tr	Tr	34.6	Tr	2.5	Tr	47.7	Tr	47.7	Tr	Tr	Tr	Tr	Tr	Tr	Tr	Tr	Tr	Tr	0.4
19-2-025	油茶籽油	76.4	Tr	Tr	Tr	76.4	Tr	Tr	Tr	13.2	Tr	12.2	1.0	Tr	Tr	Tr	Tr	Tr	Tr	Tr	Tr	Tr	0.1
19-2-026	芝麻油[香油]	37.3	Tr	Tr	Tr	37.3	Tr	Tr	Tr	50.3	Tr	50.3	Tr	Tr	Tr	Tr	Tr	Tr	Tr	Tr	Tr	Tr	0.1
19-2-027	大豆色拉油	31.0	Tr	1.2	Tr	29.8	Tr	Tr	Tr	54.9	Tr	49.3	5.6	Tr	Tr	Tr	Tr	Tr	Tr	Tr	Tr	Tr	0
19-2-028	色拉油	21.3	Tr	Tr	Tr	21.3	Tr	Tr	Tr	64.9	Tr	55.7	9.2	Tr	Tr	Tr	Tr	Tr	Tr	Tr	Tr	Tr	0
调味品类																							
20-1-012	老抽	38.8	Tr	Tr	Tr	38.8	Tr	Tr	Tr	19.3	Tr	19.3	Tr	Tr	Tr	Tr	Tr	Tr	Tr	Tr	Tr	Tr	0.1
20-3-116	海鲜酱(阿香婆)	28.3	Tr	Tr	Tr	Tr	28.3	Tr	Tr	67.1	Tr	Tr	21.1	17.8	Tr	Tr	Tr	28.2	Tr	Tr	Tr	Tr	0
20-3-117	牛肉酱(阿香婆)	32.0	Tr	Tr	Tr	Tr	32.0	Tr	Tr	60.4	Tr	Tr	19.6	15.7	Tr	Tr	Tr	25.1	Tr	Tr	Tr	Tr	0.3
20-3-118	花生酱	48.4	Tr	Tr	Tr	48.4	Tr	Tr	Tr	35.2	Tr	35.2	Tr	Tr	Tr	Tr	Tr	Tr	Tr	Tr	Tr	Tr	0
20-3-119	花生酱(加巧克力)	48.6	Tr	Tr	Tr	48.6	Tr	Tr	Tr	33.1	Tr	32.2	0.9	Tr	Tr	Tr	Tr	Tr	Tr	Tr	Tr	Tr	0.2
20-3-120	芝麻酱	37.7	Tr	Tr	Tr	37.7	Tr	Tr	Tr	53.1	Tr	53.1	Tr	Tr	Tr	Tr	Tr	Tr	Tr	Tr	Tr	Tr	0
20-3-121	千岛沙拉酱	22.8	Tr	Tr	Tr	22.8	Tr	Tr	Tr	63.4	Tr	53.1	10.3	Tr	Tr	Tr	Tr	Tr	Tr	Tr	Tr	Tr	0
20-3-122	沙拉酱	24.7	Tr	Tr	Tr	24.7	Tr	Tr	Tr	61.0	Tr	52.2	8.8	Tr	Tr	Tr	Tr	Tr	Tr	Tr	Tr	Tr	0.1
20-3-123	奶油攀司	30.5	Tr	Tr	Tr	30.5	Tr	Tr	Tr	55.8	Tr	45.4	10.4	Tr	Tr	Tr	Tr	Tr	Tr	Tr	Tr	Tr	0.3
20-3-207	草莓酱	23.3	Tr	Tr	Tr	23.3	Tr	Tr	Tr	32.2	Tr	26.5	5.7	Tr	Tr	Tr	Tr	Tr	Tr	Tr	Tr	Tr	0.1
20-3-208	番茄沙司	20.8	Tr	Tr	Tr	20.8	Tr	Tr	Tr	49.5	Tr	42.8	6.7	Tr	Tr	Tr	Tr	Tr	Tr	Tr	Tr	Tr	0

食物脂肪酸含量 Fatty acid content of foods

编码 Code	食物名称 Food name	脂肪 Fat g	脂肪酸 Fatty acid (g/100g 可食部) Total	饱和 SFA	单不饱和 MUFA	多不饱和 PUFA	未知 UN.K	饱和脂肪酸/总脂肪酸 (%) Total	6:0	8:0	10:0	11:0	12:0	13:0	14:0	15:0	16:0	17:0	18:0	19:0	20:0	22:0	24:0
20-4-007	腐乳 (白, 石宝寨牌) [酱豆腐]	7.7	7.2	2.6	2.7	1.9	0	36.2	Tr	Tr	0.3	Tr	Tr	Tr	Tr	Tr	31.6	Tr	4.3	Tr	Tr	Tr	Tr
20-5-036	剁辣椒	0.5	0.4	0.1	0	0.3	0	26.9	Tr	Tr	Tr	Tr	1.0	Tr	0.6	Tr	23.2	Tr	2.1	Tr	Tr	Tr	Tr
20-5-042	雪菜	1.6	1.3	0.7	0.5	0.1	0	52.3	Tr	Tr	Tr	Tr	1.7	Tr	0.2	Tr	42.2	Tr	8.2	Tr	Tr	Tr	Tr
20-7-202	鸡粉	5.1	4.8	1.1	2.4	1.2	0.2	23.0	Tr	Tr	Tr	Tr	0.1	Tr	0.6	Tr	18.8	Tr	3.5	Tr	Tr	Tr	Tr
20-7-203	鸡精	2.8	2.6	0.9	1.3	0.5	0	33.3	Tr	Tr	0.1	Tr	0.1	Tr	0.8	Tr	28.2	Tr	4.1	Tr	Tr	Tr	Tr
其它																							
21-9-015	蜂蛹 (油蜂)	61.4	un	un	un	un	un	11.0	Tr	Tr	Tr	Tr	Tr	Tr	0.6	Tr	6.5	Tr	2.6	Tr	1.3	Tr	Tr

编码 Code	食物名称 Food name	单不饱和/总脂肪酸 (%)								多不饱和/总脂肪酸 (%)													未知 %
		Total	14:1	16:1	17:1	18:1	20:1	22:1	24:1	Total	16:2	18:2	18:3	18:4	20:2	20:3	20:4	20:5	22:3	22:4	22:5	22:6	
20-4-007	腐乳 (白, 石宝寨牌) [酱豆腐]	37.5	Tr	2.2	Tr	35.3	Tr	Tr	Tr	26.2	Tr	Tr	26.2	Tr	Tr	Tr	Tr	Tr	Tr	Tr	Tr	Tr	0.1
20-5-036	剁辣椒	10.5	Tr	Tr	Tr	10.5	Tr	Tr	Tr	62.8	Tr	54.6	8.2	Tr	Tr	Tr	Tr	Tr	Tr	Tr	Tr	Tr	0
20-5-042	雪菜	42.8	Tr	4.2	Tr	38.6	Tr	Tr	Tr	4.9	Tr	4.9	Tr	Tr	Tr	Tr	Tr	Tr	Tr	Tr	Tr	Tr	0
20-7-202	鸡粉	48.8	Tr	10.3	Tr	38.5	Tr	Tr	Tr	24.5	Tr	23.2	1.3	Tr	Tr	Tr	Tr	Tr	Tr	Tr	Tr	Tr	3.7
20-7-203	鸡精	49.3	Tr	8.5	Tr	40.8	Tr	Tr	Tr	18.1	Tr	18.1	Tr	Tr	Tr	Tr	Tr	Tr	Tr	Tr	Tr	Tr	0
其它																							
21-9-015	蜂蛹 (油蜂)	65.8	Tr	Tr	Tr	33.7	6.4	25.7	Tr	22.5	Tr	13.6	8.9	Tr	Tr	Tr	Tr	Tr	Tr	Tr	Tr	Tr	0.7

Notes

表四 食物胆碱、生物素、泛酸、维生素K、维生素D含量

Table 4 Choline, Biotin, Pantothenic Acid, Vitamin K and Vitamin D Content of Foods

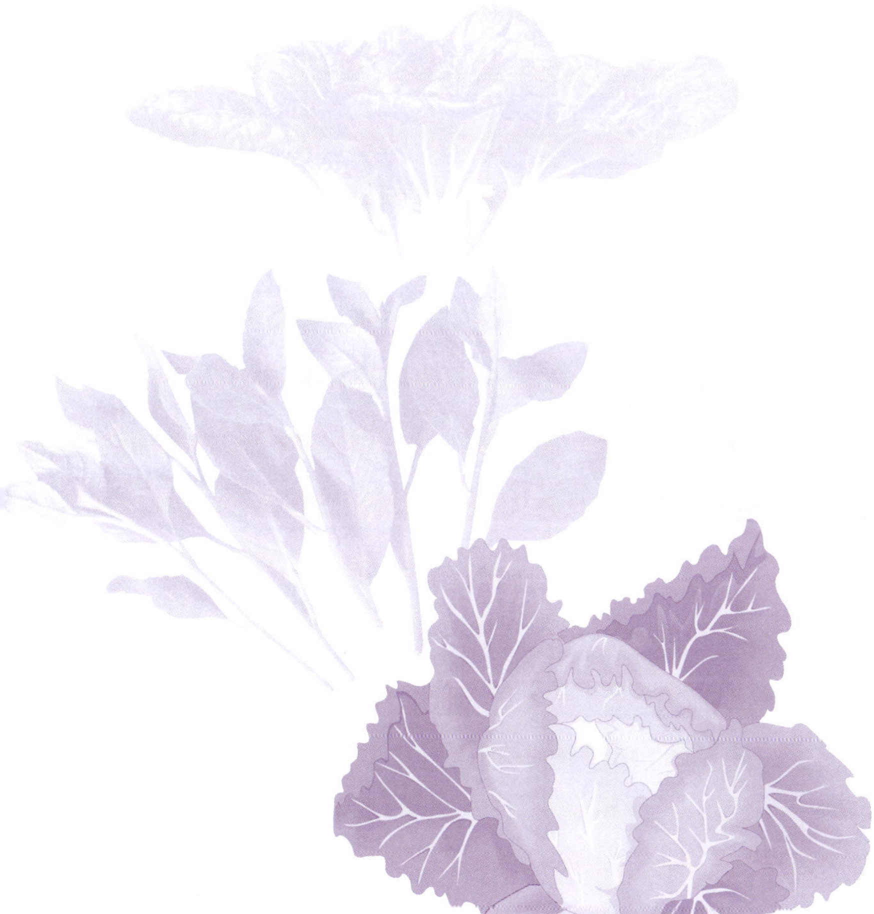

Notes

表四 食物胆碱、生物素、泛酸、维生素K、维生素D含量

Table 4 Choline, Biotin, Pantothenic Acid, Vitamin K and Vitamin D Content of Foods

(以每100g可食部计)

编码 Code	食物名称 Food name	胆碱 Cholin mg	生物素 Biotin μg	泛酸 Pantothenic acid mg	维生素K Vit K μg	维生素D Vit D IU
谷类及制品						
01-1-206	小麦面粉(标准粉)	41.8	7.6	—	—	—
01-1-207	小麦面粉(富强粉、特一粉)	46.9	3.8	—	—	—
01-1-208	小麦面粉(特制)	45.6	2.3	—	—	—
01-1-313	挂面(富强粉)	37.3	4.4	—	—	—
01-1-314	龙须面(素)	30.8	1.7	—	—	—
01-1-316	面条(富强粉, 切面)	16.8	3.3	—	—	—
01-1-317	面条(富强粉, 煮)	14.6	1.6	—	—	—
01-1-410	花卷(加牛奶)	20.7	—	—	—	—
01-1-411	馒头(富强粉)	38.9	4.6	—	—	—
01-2-106	粳米(极品精米)	29.4	1.3	—	—	—
01-2-107	粳米(西域王米)	58.6	4.3	—	—	—
01-2-108	粳米(小站稻米)	38.7	1.5	—	—	—
01-2-214	籼米	22.2	3.1	—	—	—
01-2-215	香米	19.8	1.1	—	—	—
01-2-408	籼米饭(蒸)	12.3	0.4	—	—	—
01-2-409	籼米粥	—	1.2	—	—	—
01-2-410	米粉	14.2	Tr	—	—	—
01-2-411	河粉	16.6	1.3	—	—	—
01-3-108	玉米粒(黄、干)	22.8	4.5	—	—	—
01-3-109	玉米面(黄)	35.6	5.8	—	—	—
01-3-110	玉米糁(黄)	23.6	5.4	—	—	—
01-5-104	小米(黄)	50.6	6.9	—	—	—
01-9-010	荞麦面	—	11.5	—	—	—
01-9-011	莜麦面	—	11.9	—	—	—
薯类、淀粉及制品						
02-1-104	马铃薯[土豆、洋芋]	—	4.2	—	—	—
02-1-205	甘薯(红心)[山芋、红薯]		2.0	—	—	—

食物胆碱、生物素、泛酸、维生素K、维生素D含量

Choline, biotin, pantothenic acid, vitamin K and vitamin D content of foods

(以每100g可食部计)

编码 Code	食物名称 Food name	胆碱 Cholin mg	生物素 Biotin μg	泛酸 Pantothenic acid mg	维生素K Vit K μg	维生素D Vit D IU
干豆类及制品						
03-1-207	豆奶粉(多力牌)	18.4	8.0	—	—	—
03-1-208	豆奶粉(大磨牌)	123.5	16.3	—	—	—
03-1-306	豆腐(北豆腐)	26.5	7.2	—	—	—
03-1-307	豆腐(南豆腐)	18.3	6.4	—	—	—
03-1-405	豆浆	6.4	3.2	—	—	—
03-1-527	豆腐皮	137.0	37.1	—	—	—
03-1-528	腐竹	34.1	39.4	—	—	—
03-1-529	豆腐干	12.2	6.6	—	—	—
蔬菜类及制品						
04-1-111	白萝卜[莱菔]	—	0.8	—	—	—
04-1-112	白萝卜(圆)	—	0.4	—	—	—
04-1-113	青萝卜	—	0.7	—	—	—
04-1-114	变萝卜[红皮萝卜]	—	0.5	—	—	—
04-1-115	樱桃萝卜	—	1.5	—	—	—
04-1-204	胡萝卜	—	3.1	—	—	—
04-1-402	根芹[根洋芹、球根塘蒿]	—	6.9	—	—	—
04-1-403	紫菜头	—	0.5	—	—	—
04-2-118	扁豆	—	2.5	—	—	—
04-2-119	豇豆	—	9.9	—	—	—
04-2-120	四季豆[菜豆、芸豆]	—	2.6	—	—	—
04-2-121	四棱豆[杨桃豆、翅豆]	—	1.8	—	—	—
04-2-122	甜脆荷兰豆[甜豆]	—	4.1	—	—	—
04-2-205	黄豆芽	—	4.1	—	—	—
04-2-206	绿豆芽	—	1.0	—	—	—
04-2-207	黑豆苗	—	1.2	—	—	—
04-2-208	豌豆苗	—	8.7	—	—	—
04-3-115	茄子(白皮，长)	—	1.4	—	—	—
04-3-116	茄子(紫皮，长)	—	1.2	—	—	—
04-3-117	茄子(紫皮，圆)	—	1.2	—	—	—
04-3-118	香瓜茄	—	1.1	—	—	—
04-3-119	番茄[西红柿]	—	2.3	—	—	—

食物胆碱、生物素、泛酸、维生素K、维生素D含量

Choline, biotin, pantothenic acid, vitamin K and vitamin D content of foods

(以每100g可食部计)

编码 Code	食物名称 Food name	胆碱 Cholin mg	生物素 Biotin μg	泛酸 Pantothenic acid mg	维生素K Vit K μg	维生素D Vit D IU
04-3-120	樱桃番茄[小西红柿]	—	2.4	—	—	—
04-3-122	辣椒(小红尖辣椒，干)	—	41.1	—	—	—
04-3-123	辣椒(青，尖)	—	1.6	—	—	—
04-3-124	甜椒[灯笼椒、柿子椒]	—	1.2	—	—	—
04-3-125	彩椒	—	2.1	—	—	—
04-3-126	秋葵[黄秋葵、羊角豆]	—	2.8	—	—	—
04-3-221	冬瓜	—	0.2	—	—	—
04-3-222	飞碟瓜	—	1.3	—	—	—
04-3-223	黄金西葫芦	—	2.2	—	—	—
04-3-225	迷你黄瓜[荷兰乳黄瓜]	—	0.8	—	—	—
04-3-226	秋黄瓜[旱黄瓜]	—	1.0	—	—	—
04-3-227	南瓜(栗面)	—	1.2	—	—	—
04-3-228	丝瓜	—	1.4	—	—	—
04-4-206	大葱	—	0.8	—	—	—
04-4-207	细香葱[香葱、四季葱]	—	1.5	—	—	—
04-4-404	韭菜	—	2.3	—	—	—
04-5-117	大白菜(白口)	—	1.2	—	—	—
04-5-118	大白菜(青口)	—	1.2	—	—	—
04-5-119	酸白菜[酸菜]	—	1.8	—	—	—
04-5-120	小白菜[青菜]	—	1.3	—	—	—
04-5-122	鸡毛菜	—	1.7	—	—	—
04-5-123	娃娃菜	—	2.0	—	—	—
04-5-125	油菜	—	Tr	—	—	—
04-5-126	油菜心	—	6.7	—	—	—
04-5-210	结球甘蓝(绿)[圆白菜]	—	1.2	—	—	—
04-5-211	结球甘蓝(紫)	—	2.9	—	—	—
04-5-212	抱子甘蓝	—	6.4	—	—	—
04-5-213	羽衣甘蓝	—	9.8	—	—	—
04-5-214	盖菜	—	0.8	—	—	—
04-5-215	芥蓝[甘蓝菜、盖蓝菜]	—	8.7	—	—	—
04-5-216	菜花[花椰菜]	—	3.7	—	—	—
04-5-217	西兰花[绿菜花]	—	4.6	—	—	—
04-5-327	番杏[新西兰菠菜、夏菠菜]	—	2.4	—	—	—

食物胆碱、生物素、泛酸、维生素K、维生素D含量

Choline, biotin, pantothenic acid, vitamin K and vitamin D content of foods

(以每100g可食部计)

编码 Code	食物名称 Food name	胆碱 Cholin mg	生物素 Biotin μg	泛酸 Pantothenic acid mg	维生素K Vit K μg	维生素D Vit D IU
04-5-328	樱桃萝卜缨	—	2.6	—	—	—
04-5-329	白凤菜	—	0.8	—	—	—
04-5-330	紫背天葵 [红风菜、血皮菜]	—	4.1	—	—	—
04-5-331	芹菜 (茎)	—	1.1	—	—	—
04-5-332	西芹 [西洋芹菜、美芹]	—	1.7	—	—	—
04-5-333	生菜	—	0.8	—	—	—
04-5-334	油麦菜	—	6.2	—	—	—
04-5-335	叶甜菜 (白梗)	—	1.0	—	—	—
04-5-336	莴笋叶 [莴苣菜]	—	0.7	—	—	—
04-5-337	蕹菜 [空心菜、藤藤菜]	—	4.6	—	—	—
04-5-339	球茎茴香 [甜茴香、意大利茴香]	—	1.4	—	—	—
04-5-415	芦笋 (绿) [石刁柏、龙须菜]	—	3.0	—	—	—
04-5-416	芦笋 (紫)	—	1.3	—	—	—
04-5-417	结球菊苣	—	2.9	—	—	—
04-5-418	软化白菊苣	—	1.5	—	—	—
04-6-010	藕 [莲藕]	—	2.6	—	—	—
04-7-203	芋头 [芋艿、毛芋]	—	2.8	—	—	—
04-8-081	苦苣菜 [苦菜、天精菜]	—	7.6	—	—	—
04-8-083	鱼腥草 (叶) [蕺菜、臭菜]	—	5.7	—	—	—
04-8-084	鱼腥草 (根)	—	2.9	—	—	—
菌藻类						
05-1-030	草菇 [大黑头细花草、稻菇]	—	2.5	—	—	—
05-1-031	茶树菇 (干) [柱状田头菇、茶薪菇]	26.8	86.5	—	—	—
05-1-034	黄蘑 (干)	93.3	79.3	—	—	—
05-1-035	黄伞菇 (干) [多脂鳞伞、黄丝菌]	124.7	31.7	—	—	—
05-1-036	鸡腿菇 (干) [毛头鬼伞]	94.0	79.4	—	—	—
05-1-039	鸡坳 (干)	48.1	84.3	—	—	—
05-1-043	白牛肝菌 (干) [美味牛肝菌]	46.5	55.2	—	—	—
05-1-046	乳牛肝菌 (干) [粘盖牛肝菌、松树菌]	139.4	54.2	—	—	—
05-1-048	平菇 [糙皮侧耳、青蘑]	—	4.3	—	—	—
05-1-050	松蘑 (干) [松茸、松口蘑]	—	73.0	—	—	—
05-1-052	血红菇 (干)	140.7	31.0	—	—	—
05-1-053	元蘑 (干) [亚侧耳、冬蘑、黄蘑]	42.4	74.9	—	—	—

食物胆碱、生物素、泛酸、维生素K、维生素D含量

Choline, biotin, pantothenic acid, vitamin K and vitamin D content of foods

（以每100g可食部计）

编码 Code	食物名称 Food name	胆碱 Cholin mg	生物素 Biotin μg	泛酸 Pantothenic acid mg	维生素K Vit K μg	维生素D Vit D IU
05-1-055	榛蘑(干)[小蜜环菌]	55.5	85.1	—	—	—
05-2-010	裙带菜(干)[海芥菜、海木耳]	—	28.1	—	—	—
05-2-011	海带菜	40.4	2.3	—	—	—
水果类及制品						
06-1-907	蛇果	—	0.5	—	—	—
06-2-207	布朗	—	0.3	—	—	—
06-2-208	西梅	—	0.2	—	—	—
06-2-312	冬枣	—	2.8	—	—	—
06-3-911	红提子葡萄	—	1.0	—	—	—
06-4-304	葡萄柚(以色列)[西柚]	—	1.0	—	—	—
06-5-021	桂圆(干)	—	7.8	—	—	—
06-5-022	红毛丹	—	0.3	—	—	—
06-5-023	火龙果[仙蜜果、红龙果]	—	1.6	—	—	—
06-5-025	榴莲	—	8.5	—	—	—
06-5-030	山竹	—	0.8	—	—	—
06-5-031	香蕉(红皮,海南)	—	1.1	—	—	—
06-5-032	香蕉(红皮,泰国)	—	0.8	—	—	—
06-6-206	小西瓜[地雷瓜]	—	1.7	—	—	—
坚果、种子类						
07-1-026	山核桃(熟)	14.8	13.0	—	—	—
07 1 032	栗子仁(熟)	—	87.1	—	—	—
07-1-033	松子(熟)	69.2	8.2	—	—	—
07-1-034	杏仁(熟,带壳)	23.0	25.6	—	—	—
07-1-035	杏仁(熟,去壳)	29.3	49.0	—	—	—
07-1-036	腰果(熟)	45.6	18.9	—	—	—
07-1-037	榛子(熟)	—	90.1	—	—	—
07-1-038	榛子仁(熟)	94.8	45.8	—	—	—
07-1-039	开心果(熟)	89.7	15.9	—	—	—
07-1-040	香榧(熟)	19.8	1.1	—	—	—
07-2-020	花生(烤,勤俭牌)	36.0	107.9	—	—	—
07-2-023	葵花子(奶油香瓜子)	95.9	84.6	—	—	—
07-2-024	葵花子(熟)	103.0	104.0	—	—	—

食物胆碱、生物素、泛酸、维生素K、维生素D含量
Choline, biotin, pantothenic acid, vitamin K and vitamin D content of foods

(以每100g可食部计)

编码 Code	食物名称 Food name	胆碱 Cholin mg	生物素 Biotin μg	泛酸 Pantothenic acid mg	维生素K Vit K μg	维生素D Vit D IU
07-2-025	南瓜子(熟)[白瓜子]	70.6	12.0	—	—	—
07-2-026	西瓜子(熟)[黑瓜子]	61.5	8.7	—	—	—
畜肉类及制品						
08-1-121	猪肉(前臀尖,杜长大猪)	63.2	2.9	—	—	—
08-1-122	猪肉(前臀尖,良杂猪)	55.2	4.4	—	—	—
08-1-123	猪肉(后臀尖,杜长大猪)	70.5	5.1	—	—	—
08-1-124	猪肉(后臀尖,良杂猪)	61.4	—	—	—	—
08-1-125	猪肉(硬肋,杜长大猪)	51.6	7.1	—	—	—
08-1-126	猪肉(硬肋,良杂猪)	51.6	3.7	—	—	—
08-1-127	猪肉(通脊,杜长大猪)	59.6	2.9	—	—	—
08-1-128	猪肉(通脊,良杂猪)	53.2	1.8	—	—	—
08-1-129	猪肉(里脊)	59.9	2.4	—	—	—
08-1-130	猪皮	44.2	2.9	—	—	—
08-1-131	猪小排(杜长大猪)	45.2	5.4	—	—	—
08-1-132	猪小排(良杂猪)	42.6	3.6	—	—	—
08-1-213	猪肚	—	6.2	—	—	—
08-1-214	猪肝	359.4	61.9	—	—	—
08-1-215	猪舌[口条]	143.4	8.8	—	—	—
08-1-216	猪肾[猪腰子]	171.6	—	—	—	—
08-1-318	火腿心全精肉	32.8	1.6	—	—	—
08-1-319	火腿心肉	72.0	3.6	—	—	—
08-1-321	叉烧肉	—	0.5	—	—	—
08-1-322	酱排骨	—	2.6	—	—	—
08-1-323	香糟块肉	—	7.0	—	—	—
08-1-324	熏烤小里脊	70.0	—	—	—	—
08-1-325	猪肉脯	18.5	5.3	—	—	—
08-1-326	肉酥	—	2.0	—	—	—
08-1-327	猪肉松	86.8	3.7	—	—	—
08-1-423	脆皮肠	26.4	—	—	—	—
08-1-424	热狗肠	31.0	—	—	—	—
08-1-425	火腿肠	39.1	—	—	—	—
08-1-426	火腿	—	1.5	—	—	—

食物胆碱、生物素、泛酸、维生素K、维生素D含量
Choline, biotin, pantothenic acid, vitamin K and vitamin D content of foods

(以每100g可食部计)

编码 Code	食物名称 Food name	胆碱 Cholin mg	生物素 Biotin μg	泛酸 Pantothenic acid mg	维生素K Vit K μg	维生素D Vit D IU
08-1-428	三明治火腿	37.7	1.6	—	—	—
08-1-429	午餐肉	—	2.7	—	—	—
08-2-111	牛肉(背部肉)[上脑]	38.9	0.7	—	—	—
08-2-112	牛肉(里脊肉)[牛柳]	24.6	0.8	—	—	—
08-2-113	牛肉(臀部肉)[紫盖、白板]	27.4	0.9	—	—	—
08-2-114	牛肉(肩部肉)[肩肉]	26.2	0.7	—	—	—
08-2-115	牛肉(胸部肉)[牛胸]	26.1	0.9	—	—	—
08-2-116	牛肉(腹部肉)[牛腩]	30.6	0.6	—	—	—
08-2-117	牛肉(膝圆肉)[和尚头]	25.0	0.8	—	—	—
08-2-118	牛肉(股内肉)[针扒、米龙、黄瓜条]	24.0	0.7	—	—	—
08-2-119	牛肉(小腿肉)[牛展、牛腱子]	25.1	1.3	—	—	—
08-2-210	牛百叶(黑)	32.6	1.4	—	—	—
08-2-307	牛肉(酱,五香)	60.0	2.0	—	—	—
08-2-308	牛肉(清香)	50.6	1.5	—	—	—
08-2-309	牛腱子(香叶)	62.2	2.7	—	—	—
08-2-310	牛肉干(长富牌)	178.5	—	—	—	—
08-3-309	烧羊肉(五香)	—	1.3	—	—	—
08-3-310	羊肉串(生)	—	2.0	—	—	—
08-4-304	驴肉(五香)	138.5	2.6	—	—	—
08-9-006	鹿肉(梅花鹿)	26.6	—	—	—	—
	禽肉类及制品					
09-1-112	鸡胸脯肉	13.8	1.5	—	—	—
09-1-113	鸡腿	12.4	1.6	—	—	—
09-1-114	鸡翅	12.6	4.7	—	—	—
09-1-115	鸡块(带浆粉)	—	2.3	—	—	—
09-1-116	野山鸡	32.1	2.8	—	—	—
09-1-309	烤鸡	—	3.3	—	—	—
09-1-310	童子鸡(熟)	25.2	2.6	—	—	—
09-2-307	烤鸭(老唐牌)	—	5.8	—	—	—
09-3-302	腊鹅	63.5	5.0	—	—	—
09-4-301	火鸡腿	—	5.9	—	—	—
09-9-003	乳鸽	—	1.5	—	—	—

食物胆碱、生物素、泛酸、维生素K、维生素D含量

Choline, biotin, pantothenic acid, vitamin K and vitamin D content of foods

(以每100g可食部计)

编码 Code	食物名称 Food name	胆碱 Cholin mg	生物素 Biotin μg	泛酸 Pantothenic acid mg	维生素K Vit K μg	维生素D Vit D IU
09-9-004	乳鸽(红烧)	—	2.7	—	—	—
	乳类及制品					
10-1-105	牛乳(光明牌)	22.2	1.2	—	—	—
10-1-106	牛乳(乐百氏牌)	21.9	2.8	—	—	—
10-1-107	牛乳(帕玛拉特牌)	27.8	2.7	—	—	—
10-1-108	牛乳(三元牌)	26.6	2.4	—	—	—
10-1-109	牛乳(完达山牌)	29.0	1.4	—	—	—
10-1-110	牛乳(龙丹牌)	23.0	2.4	—	—	—
10-1-111	牛乳(蒙牛牌)	35.2	4.5	—	—	—
10-1-112	牛乳(新南洋牌)	25.9	3.3	—	—	—
10-1-113	牛乳(帕玛拉特)	15.0	2.8	—	—	—
10-1-114	牛乳(伊利牌)	—	3.2	—	—	—
10-1-115	牛乳(部分脱脂,帕玛拉特)	—	2.3	—	—	—
10-1-116	牛乳(脱脂,帕玛拉特)	—	2.2	—	—	—
10-1-117	牛乳(强化锌、钙,帕玛拉特)	15.0	2.9	—	—	—
10-1-118	牛奶(草莓味,卡夫牌)	31.5	1.8	—	—	—
10-1-119	牛奶(巧克力味,卡夫牌)	31.5	1.9	—	—	—
10-1-120	牛奶(巧克力味,三元牌)	18.3	2.0	—	—	—
10-1-121	学生奶	—	2.0	—	—	—
10-2-106	全脂奶粉(三鹿牌)	47.8	—	2.52	—	—
10-2-107	全脂奶粉(伊利牌)	—	—	—	—	300
10-2-109	全脂甜奶粉(伊利牌)	—	—	—	—	300
10-2-111	低脂奶粉(高钙高铁,伊利牌)	—	—	—	—	300
10-2-113	儿童奶粉(安儿健A+,美赞臣)	64.0	16.7	3.10	50.0	280
10-2-114	儿童奶粉(适体健,美赞臣)	32.0	10.0	2.50	16.5	165
10-2-115	儿童奶粉(惠氏)	—	5.4	1.40	—	360
10-2-116	儿童奶粉(可淇牌)	—	—	—	—	280
10-2-118	儿童奶粉(完达山牌)	—	—	—	28.0	300
10-2-119	孕妇乳母奶粉(惠氏)	—	122.0	5.30	41.0	163
10-2-120	孕妇乳母奶粉(美赞臣)	—	120.0	4.00	—	160
10-2-122	中老年奶粉(雀巢)	—	—	1.85	—	270
10-2-124	中老年奶粉(森永牌)	—	—	—	—	330
10-3-007	酸奶(调味)	—	0.9	—	—	—

食物胆碱、生物素、泛酸、维生素K、维生素D含量

Choline, biotin, pantothenic acid, vitamin K and vitamin D content of foods

(以每100g可食部计)

编码 Code	食物名称 Food name	胆碱 Cholin mg	生物素 Biotin μg	泛酸 Pantothenic acid mg	维生素K Vit K μg	维生素D Vit D IU
10-3-008	酸奶(果粒)	6.1	2.0	—	—	—
10-4-012	奶酪(光明牌)	Tr	2.3	—	—	—
10-4-014	低脂奶酪	9.4	3.8	—	—	—
10-4-015	硬质干酪	—	3.0	—	—	—
10-5-008	奶油	—	1.4	—	—	—
10-9-004	全脂甜炼乳(雀巢)	—	3.4	—	—	—
蛋类及制品						
11-1-109	鸡蛋(红皮)	124.4	9.4	—	—	—
11-1-111	乌鸡蛋(绿皮)	222.9	41.4	—	—	—
11-2-104	海鸭蛋	183.3	—	—	—	—
11-2-203	咸鸭蛋(煮)	179.3	17.1	—	—	—
鱼虾蟹贝类						
12-1-131	草鱼[白鲩、草包鱼]	16.6	0.6	—	—	—
12-1-132	鲢鱼[白鲢、胖子、连子鱼]	16.0	3.0	—	—	—
12-1-133	鲫鱼[喜头鱼、海附鱼]	14.3	1.3	—	—	—
12-1-241	带鱼(切段)	107.9	2.2	—	—	—
12-1-242	黄鱼(小黄花鱼)	110.8	1.8	—	—	—
12-1-243	金鳇鱼	31.0	—	—	—	—
12-1-303	金鲨鱼翅(干)	108.7	Tr	—	—	—
12-1-304	鱼排	33.3	—	—	—	—
12-1-305	鱼丸	19.8	—	—	—	—
12-1-306	鱼子酱	58.6	6.3	—	—	—
12-1-401	草鱼(熏)	—	0.7	—	—	—
12-1-402	丁香鱼(香辣味)	—	5.8	—	—	—
12-1-403	凤尾鱼(熟)	—	6.4	—	—	—
12-1-404	箭鱼(炸)	—	2.2	—	—	—
12-1-405	金枪鱼(盐水浸)	—	2.0	—	—	—
12-1-406	金枪鱼(油浸)	—	3.0	—	—	—
12-1-407	鲮鱼(豆豉,熟)	—	6.7	—	—	—
12-1-408	鳗鱼(红烧)	—	1.1	—	—	—
12-1-417	沙丁鱼(茄汁,熟)	—	5.7	—	—	—
12-1-418	沙丁鱼(盐水浸)	—	10.0	—	—	—

食物胆碱、生物素、泛酸、维生素K、维生素D含量

Choline, biotin, pantothenic acid, vitamin K and vitamin D content of foods

(以每100g可食部计)

编码 Code	食物名称 Food name	胆碱 Cholin mg	生物素 Biotin μg	泛酸 Pantothenic acid mg	维生素K Vit K μg	维生素D Vit D IU
12-1-419	沙丁鱼(油浸)	—	5.0	—	—	—
12-1-420	午餐鱼(香辣味)	—	1.7	—	—	—
12-1-421	鳕鱼(烤)	—	1.0	—	—	—
12-1-422	鳕鱼(炸)	—	3.0	—	—	—
12-2-203	虾酱	108.2	11.7	—	—	—
12-2-204	虾仁(红)	59.4	0.5	—	—	—
12-3-006	海蟹(小)	75.4	2.7	—	—	—
12-3-301	蟹足棒	17.6	—	—	—	—
12-9-301	墨鱼圈	53.0	5.2	—	—	—
婴幼儿食品						
13-1-101	婴儿配方奶粉(爱儿乐,惠氏)	79.0	16.0	2.36	53.0	335
13-1-102	婴儿配方奶粉(爱儿乐,惠氏,金装)	79.0	16.0	2.36	53.0	335
13-1-103	婴儿配方奶粉(爱力大1,美赞臣)	54.0	11.6	2.50	65.0	280
13-1-104	婴儿配方奶粉(安婴儿,美赞臣)	63.0	15.0	3.00	47.0	310
13-1-105	婴儿配方奶粉(安婴儿A+,美赞臣)	63.0	15.0	3.00	47.0	310
13-1-106	婴儿配方奶粉(安婴乐,美赞臣)	62.0	16.0	2.60	57.0	310
13-1-107	婴儿配方奶粉(吉利蜜1,森永牌)	—	10.0	3.00	50.0	330
13-1-108	婴儿配方奶粉(可淇牌)	38.0	11.0	1.60	22.0	300
13-1-109	婴儿配方奶粉(力多精1,雀巢)	51.0	11.0	2.30	41.0	300
13-1-110	婴儿配方奶粉(美素力1)	105.0	8.5	1.71	39.0	372
13-1-111	婴儿配方奶粉(美素力H)	60.0	8.5	1.73	39.0	372
13-1-112	婴儿配方奶粉(美素力,袋装)	60.0	8.5	1.73	39.0	372
13-1-113	婴儿配方奶粉(圣元牌)	100.0	15.0	2.60	42.0	322
13-1-114	婴儿配方奶粉(完达山牌)	47.5	10.0	2.00	27.5	300
13-1-115	婴儿奶粉(高钙,圣元牌)	60.0	15.0	2.60	42.0	322
13-1-116	婴儿配方豆粉(爱儿素,惠氏)	65.0	27.0	2.31	77.0	327
13-1-201	较大婴儿配方奶粉(爱力大2,美赞臣)	70.0	14.0	3.00	68.0	360
13-1-202	较大婴儿配方奶粉(安婴宝,美赞臣)	74.0	14.4	3.00	68.0	270
13-1-203	较大婴儿配方奶粉(安婴宝A+,美赞臣)	88.0	14.5	3.10	39.0	270
13-1-204	较大婴儿配方奶粉(健儿乐,惠氏)	70.0	14.0	2.11	47.0	300
13-1-205	较大婴儿配方奶粉(健儿乐,惠氏,金装)	70.0	14.0	2.11	47.0	300
13-1-206	较大婴儿配方奶粉(可淇牌)	—	10.4	1.95	26.0	400
13-1-207	较大婴儿配方奶粉(美素乐2)	125.0	15.0	2.50	35.0	344

食物胆碱、生物素、泛酸、维生素K、维生素D含量

Choline, biotin, pantothenic acid, vitamin K and vitamin D content of foods

(以每 100g 可食部计)

编码 Code	食物名称 Food name	胆碱 Cholin mg	生物素 Biotin μg	泛酸 Pantothenic acid mg	维生素 K Vit K μg	维生素 D Vit D IU
13-1-208	较大婴儿配方奶粉(美素乐, 全能装)	61.0	15.0	2.20	36.0	345
13-1-209	较大婴儿配方奶粉(美素乐, 袋装)	61.0	15.0	2.20	36.0	345
13-1-210	较大婴幼儿配方奶粉(吉利蜜2, 森永牌)	—	10.0	2.00	50.0	400
13-1-211	较大婴幼儿配方奶粉(力多精2, 雀巢)	46.0	16.0	3.20	21.0	420
13-1-212	较大婴儿配方奶粉(圣元牌)	—	15.0	2.60	42.0	400
13-1-213	较大婴幼儿奶粉(高钙, 圣元牌)	—	15.0	2.60	42.0	400
13-1-214	较大婴幼儿配方奶粉(完达山牌)	60.0	—	1.88	42.0	300
13-1-301	幼儿奶粉(爱力大3, 美赞臣)	81.0	12.6	3.10	71.0	320
13-1-302	幼儿奶粉(安儿宝, 美赞臣)	54.0	14.3	3.40	54.0	310
13-1-303	幼儿奶粉(安儿宝A+, 美赞臣)	54.0	14.3	3.40	54.0	310
13-1-304	幼儿奶粉(惠氏)	—	11.0	1.60	23.0	225
13-1-305	幼儿奶粉(惠氏, 金装)	—	11.0	2.30	28.0	284
13-1-306	幼儿奶粉(可淇牌)	—	10.4	2.00	30.0	450
13-1-307	幼儿奶粉(美素高)	75.0	21.0	3.10	22.0	324
13-1-308	幼儿奶粉(美素高, 全能装)	75.0	21.0	3.10	22.0	324
13-1-309	幼儿奶粉(美素高, 袋装)	75.0	21.0	3.10	22.0	324
13-1-310	幼儿奶粉(雀巢)	—	28.0	4.20	21.0	464
13-1-311	幼儿奶粉(雀巢金牌)	—	28.0	4.20	21.0	460
13-1-312	幼儿奶粉(森永牌)	—	20.0	3.00	50.0	370
13-1-313	幼儿奶粉(圣元牌)	—	16.0	2.60	42.0	400
13-2-001	胡萝卜苹果泥(亨氏)	—	1.7	—	—	—
13-2-002	鸡肝蔬菜泥(亨氏)	54.9	27.3	—	—	146
13-2-003	香甜胡萝卜泥(亨氏)	—	2.3	—	—	—
13-3-009	米粉(雀巢)	—	25.0	1.50	—	350
13-3-010	米粉(高蛋白, 雀巢)	—	20.0	1.90	—	300
13-3-011	米粉(高蛋白, 亨氏)	15.6	11.0	—	—	350
13-3-012	米粉(苹果, 雀巢)	—	25.0	1.50	—	350
13-3-013	米粉(蔬菜, 亨氏)	—	—	—	—	300
13-3-014	米粉(蔬菜, 雀巢)	—	25.0	1.50	—	350
13-3-015	米粉(胡萝卜, 亨氏)	—	—	—	—	250
13-3-016	米粉(胡萝卜, 雀巢)	—	25.0	1.50	—	350
13-3-017	米粉(番茄, 亨氏)	—	—	—	—	250
13-3-018	米粉(猪肝蔬菜, 亨氏)	—	—	—	—	300

食物胆碱、生物素、泛酸、维生素K、维生素D含量

Choline, biotin, pantothenic acid, vitamin K and vitamin D content of foods

(以每100g可食部计)

编码 Code	食物名称 Food name	胆碱 Cholin mg	生物素 Biotin μg	泛酸 Pantothenic acid mg	维生素K Vit K μg	维生素D Vit D IU
13-3-019	米粉(鱼肉蔬菜, 亨氏)	—	—	—	—	350
13-3-020	麦粉(蜂蜜, 雀巢)	—	25.0	1.50	—	350
	小吃、甜饼					
14-1-038	春卷(素馅)	22.0	—	—	—	—
14-1-039	黑芝麻汤圆	15.7	1.9	—	—	—
14-1-041	煎饼	41.2	—	—	—	—
14-2-209	月饼(蛋黄)	99.4	4.9	—	—	—
14-2-210	月饼(豆沙)	22.9	2.2	—	—	—
14-2-211	月饼(桂花板栗)	21.6	2.0	—	—	—
14-2-332	沙琪玛蛋酥	—	2.9	—	—	—
	速食食品					
15-1-002	香芋甜心(肯德基)	26.0	1.1	—	—	—
15-1-003	鸡肉汉堡(肯德基)	34.0	1.8	—	—	—
15-1-004	鸡肉卷(肯德基)	51.6	1.9	—	—	—
15-1-007	新奥尔良鸡翅(肯德基)	46.4	2.7	—	—	—
15-1-008	劲爆鸡米花(肯德基)	78.7	2.1	—	—	—
15-2-105	早餐奶	18.3	1.7	—	—	—
15-2-106	八宝粥(康师傅牌)	15.0	1.3	—	—	—
15-2-107	八宝粥(亲亲牌)	23.6	1.9	—	—	—
15-2-108	八宝粥(同茂牌)	12.5	1.5	—	—	—
15-2-109	八宝粥(娃哈哈牌)	9.4	1.2	—	—	—
15-2-110	八宝粥(无糖, 娃哈哈牌)	13.2	1.0	—	—	—
15-2-111	八宝粥(椰树牌)	—	2.4	—	—	—
15-2-112	黑芝麻糊粉	9.4	3.3	—	—	—
15-2-113	麦片	20.4	8.7	—	—	—
15-2-114	麦片(原味香奶)	35.2	3.4	—	—	—
15-2-115	燕麦片	53.5	15.2	—	—	—
15-2-116	燕麦片(果仁, 甜)	27.6	3.3	—	—	—
15-2-202	鸡汁味干脆面(面饼+调味料)	—	2.2	—	—	—
15-2-203	海鲜味方便面(面饼+调味料+油料)	—	0.9	—	—	—
15-2-204	海鲜味方便面(面饼+调味料)	—	0.9	—	—	—
15-2-205	油料(海鲜味方便面)	—	Tr	—	—	—

食物胆碱、生物素、泛酸、维生素K、维生素D含量

Choline, biotin, pantothenic acid, vitamin K and vitamin D content of foods

(以每100g可食部计)

编码 Code	食物名称 Food name	胆碱 Cholin mg	生物素 Biotin μg	泛酸 Pantothenic acid mg	维生素K Vit K μg	维生素D Vit D IU
15-2-206	红烧牛肉方便面 (面饼+调味料+蔬菜+肉酱)	—	2.0	—	—	—
15-2-207	红烧牛肉方便面(面饼+调味料+蔬菜)	—	2.1	—	—	—
15-2-208	肉酱(红烧牛肉方便面)	—	0.9	—	—	—
15-2-209	鳕鱼方便面 (面饼+调味料+珍料+调味油+蔬菜)	—	1.9	—	—	—
15-2-210	鳕鱼方便面(面饼+调味料+蔬菜)	—	1.8	—	—	—
15-2-211	油酱料(珍料+调味油料，鳕鱼方便面)	—	2.1	—	—	—
15-2-212	铁板牛肉炒面 (面饼+汤料+蔬菜+调味酱)	—	2.9	—	—	—
15-2-213	铁板牛肉炒面(面饼+汤料+蔬菜)	—	2.9	—	—	—
15-2-214	调味酱(铁板牛肉炒面)	—	2.9	—	—	—
15-2-215	玉米红烧牛肉味方便面 (面饼+调味料+蔬菜+肉酱)	—	1.2	—	—	—
15-2-216	玉米红烧牛肉味方便面 (面饼+调味料+蔬菜)	—	1.2	—	—	—
15-2-217	肉酱(玉米红烧牛肉味方便面)	—	1.5	—	—	—
15-2-218	海鲜鸡汁味米线 (米线+调味料+蔬菜+肉酱)	—	0.7	—	—	—
15-2-219	海鲜鸡汁味米线 (米线+调味料+蔬菜)	—	0.7	—	—	—
15-2-220	肉酱(海鲜鸡汁味米线)	—	1.1	—	—	—
15-2-415	饼干(三明治)	17.8	3.6	—	—	—
15-2-416	饼干(夹心)	22.4	5.8	—	—	—
15-2-418	饼干(苏打夹心)	13.4	4.9	—	—	—
15-2-419	饼干(咸)	20.4	3.1	—	—	—
15-2-421	早茶饼	22.8	2.6	—	—	—
15-2-501	饺子(素馅)	26.4	—	—	—	—
15-2-502	饺子(三鲜馅)	21.2	—	—	—	—
15-2-503	饺子(猪肉白菜馅)	17.8	—	—	—	—
15-2-504	饺子(猪肉韭菜馅)	16.6	—	—	—	—
15-2-505	饺子(猪肉芹菜馅)	16.2	—	—	—	—
15-2-506	饺子(猪肉茴香馅)	19.2	—	—	—	—
15-2-512	包子(三鲜馅)	20.5	—	—	—	—
15-2-513	包子(猪肉馅)	20.4	—	—	—	—

食物胆碱、生物素、泛酸、维生素K、维生素D含量

Choline, biotin, pantothenic acid, vitamin K and vitamin D content of foods

(以每100g可食部计)

编码 Code	食物名称 Food name	胆碱 Cholin mg	生物素 Biotin μg	泛酸 Pantothenic acid mg	维生素K Vit K μg	维生素D Vit D IU
15-3-102	雪米饼	78.0	1.6	—	—	—
15-3-103	蛋酥卷	132.0	12.6	—	—	—
15-3-104	巧克力派	42.1	2.1	—	—	—
15-3-105	法式卷饼	92.0	9.5	—	—	—
15-3-106	立体脆	6.5	7.2	—	—	—
15-3-107	粟米脆	—	2.3	—	—	—
15-3-108	通心脆	—	1.0	—	—	—
15-3-202	锅巴(豆香)	14.0	4.1	—	—	—
15-3-203	锅巴(小米)	—	5.4	—	—	—
15-3-204	海苔	46.2	—	—	—	—
15-3-205	香菇片	92.8	3.9	—	—	—
15-3-206	薯片(烧烤味)	14.0	7.0	—	—	—
15-3-208	薯圈	—	7.0	—	—	—
15-3-301	怪味胡豆	18.4	3.7	—	—	—
15-3-302	奶油五香豆	9.8	16.9	—	—	—
15-3-303	夹心米果	—	3.8	—	—	—
15-3-304	乐芙球	75.7	8.6	—	—	—
15-3-305	玉米花	—	6.9	—	—	—
15-3-308	鱼肉粒	—	5.9	—	—	—
15-3-401	果冻(草莓水果冻)	—	0.1	—	—	—
15-3-402	果冻(蒟蒻冻)	—	Tr	—	—	—
15-3-403	果冻(蒟蒻椰果冻)	—	Tr	—	—	—
	饮料类					
16-2-013	菠萝汁饮料(大湖牌)	—	0.2	—	—	—
16-2-014	苹果汁饮料(光明牌)	—	0.8	—	—	—
16-2-015	苹果汁饮料(亨氏)	—	0.3	—	—	—
16-2-016	苹果果肉饮料	—	0.3	—	—	—
16-2-017	橙汁饮料(光明牌)	—	1.0	—	—	—
16-2-023	山楂果肉饮料	—	0.6	—	—	—
16-2-024	酸枣果汁饮料	—	0.5	—	—	—
16-2-025	西番莲汁饮料	—	0.3	—	—	—
16-2-026	西柚汁饮料	—	0.4	—	—	—
16-2-027	椰子汁饮料	—	0.7	—	—	—

食物胆碱、生物素、泛酸、维生素K、维生素D含量

Choline, biotin, pantothenic acid, vitamin K and vitamin D content of foods

(以每100g可食部计)

编码 Code	食物名称 Food name	胆碱 Cholin mg	生物素 Biotin μg	泛酸 Pantothenic acid mg	维生素K Vit K μg	维生素D Vit D IU
16-3-002	胡萝卜汁饮料	—	0.3	—	—	—
16-4-004	健康快车奶饮料	—	0.6	—	—	—
16-4-005	粒粒果奶饮料	—	0.7	—	—	—
16-4-006	酸乳饮料	19.8	0.8	—	—	—
16-4-007	酸乳饮料(发酵)	—	0.4	—	—	—
16-7-013	桂花酸梅晶	—	1.5	—	—	—
16-7-016	咖啡豆	102.0	56.1	—	—	—
16-8-012	冰激凌(草莓圣代)	30.1	2.1	—	—	—
16-8-013	冰激凌(巧克力圣代)	38.5	2.8	—	—	—
16-8-014	冰激凌(脆皮甜筒)	30.5	2.0	—	—	—
含酒精饮料						
17-1-115	啤酒(4.3%, 青岛牌)	—	0.8	—	—	—
17-1-117	啤酒(5.1%, 生力牌)	—	0.9	—	—	—
17-1-205	葡萄酒(干白, 11%, 长城牌)	—	1.0	—	—	—
17-1-208	葡萄酒(干红, 11.5%, 长城牌)	—	3.0	—	—	—
17-1-211	黑加仑酒(8%)	—	0.7	—	—	—
17-1-212	雪利酒	—	1.0	—	—	—
17-2-137	金奖白兰地(38%)	—	Tr	—	—	—
17-3-105	苹果酒(干型)	—	1.0	—	—	—
17-3-106	苹果酒(甜)	—	1.0	—	—	—
糖、果脯和蜜饯、蜂蜜						
18-2-102	水果味软糖	—	Tr	—	—	—
18-2-201	牛奶糖	—	1.6	—	—	—
18-2-202	酸奶软糖	—	0.1	—	—	—
18-2-203	太妃糖	—	1.1	—	—	—
18-2-301	花生牛轧糖	23.4	14.7	—	—	—
18-2-302	花生芝麻糖	26.4	—	—	—	—
18-2-303	四味粽子糖	37.8	—	—	—	—
18-2-401	巧克力(充气)	13.2	5.4	—	—	—
18-2-402	巧克力(果仁)	16.7	5.0	—	—	—
18-2-404	巧克力(牛奶)	9.2	3.9	—	—	—
18-3-012	冰糖酸角	—	1.7	—	—	—

食物胆碱、生物素、泛酸、维生素K、维生素D含量

Choline, biotin, pantothenic acid, vitamin K and vitamin D content of foods

（以每100g可食部计）

编码 Code	食物名称 Food name	胆碱 Cholin mg	生物素 Biotin μg	泛酸 Pantothenic acid mg	维生素K Vit K μg	维生素D Vit D IU
18-3-013	甘草杏	23.1	—	—	—	—
18-3-015	雪梅	85.6	1.2	—	—	—
18-3-016	九制梅肉	82.5	1.1	—	—	—
18-3-017	九制西梅	34.5	—	—	—	—
18-3-018	九制应子	32.3	—	—	—	—
18-3-021	黑贡枣	—	1.2	—	—	—
18-4-002	蜂蜜(槐花)	58.0	Tr	—	—	—
调味品类						
20-1-011	黄豆酱油	—	3.9	—	—	—
20-1-012	老抽	—	3.7	—	—	—
20-1-013	生抽	—	3.3	—	—	—
20-3-116	海鲜酱(阿香婆)	17.0	9.4	—	—	—
20-3-117	牛肉酱(阿香婆)	14.2	11.2	—	—	—
20-3-118	花生酱	—	82.3	—	—	—
20-3-119	花生酱(加巧克力)	—	34.6	—	—	—
20-3-120	芝麻酱	—	22.3	—	—	—
20-3-122	沙拉酱	—	5.1	—	—	—
20-3-123	奶油攀司	—	4.4	—	—	—
20-3-208	番茄沙司	—	3.1	—	—	—
20-4-007	腐乳(白,石宝寨牌)[酱豆腐]	54.2	9.6	—	—	—
20-5-036	剁辣椒	28.1	4.7	—	—	—
20-5-042	雪菜	—	1.3	—	—	—
20-5-043	腌大头菜	13.1	12.9	—	—	—
20-5-044	腌芥菜头	8.1	3.0	—	—	—
20-5-046	腌萝卜条	7.8	1.9	—	—	—
20-5-047	榨菜(鱼泉牌)	9.4	Tr	—	—	—
20-5-048	榨菜(正林牌)	9.4	—	—	—	—
20-7-203	鸡精	—	0.6	—	—	—
其它						
21-9-023	仙人掌(食用)	—	0.8	—	—	—
21-9-024	仙人掌果[仙桃]	—	8.4	—	—	—
21-9-025	仙人掌籽	—	9.5	—	—	—

附录 1　Appendix 1

酒精相对密度与质量分数、体积分数关系表（15℃）

The Relative Density of Alcohol and the Concentration of Alcohol Expressed by Percentage of W/W, V/V and W/V (15℃)

相对密度	质量分数 /%	体积分数 /%	100ml 中的质量 /g	相对密度	质量分数 /%	体积分数 /%	100ml 中的质量 /g
1.000	0.00	0.00	0.00	0.969	22.10	26.96	21.40
0.999	0.53	0.67	0.53	0.968	22.87	27.87	22.12
0.998	1.06	1.34	1.06	0.967	23.63	28.76	22.82
0.997	1.61	2.02	1.60	0.966	24.37	29.64	23.52
0.996	2.17	2.72	2.16	0.965	25.09	30.49	24.19
0.995	2.73	3.42	2.72	0.964	25.81	31.32	24.85
0.994	3.31	4.14	3.29	0.963	26.51	32.14	25.50
0.993	3.90	4.88	3.87	0.962	27.19	32.93	26.13
0.992	4.51	5.63	4.47	0.961	27.86	33.71	26.75
0.991	5.13	6.40	5.08	0.960	28.52	34.47	27.36
0.990	5.76	7.18	5.70	0.959	29.17	35.22	27.95
0.989	6.41	7.99	6.34	0.958	29.81	35.95	28.53
0.988	7.08	8.81	6.99	0.957	30.43	36.67	29.10
0.987	7.77	9.66	7.66	0.956	31.05	37.37	29.66
0.986	8.48	10.52	8.35	0.955	31.66	38.06	30.21
0.985	9.20	11.41	9.06	0.954	32.25	38.74	30.74
0.984	9.94	12.32	9.78	0.953	32.84	39.40	31.27
0.983	10.71	13.25	10.52	0.952	33.42	40.60	31.79
0.982	11.48	14.20	11.27	0.951	33.99	40.70	32.30
0.981	12.28	15.16	12.03	0.950	34.56	41.33	32.80
0.980	13.08	16.14	12.81	0.949	35.11	41.95	33.30
0.979	13.90	17.14	13.60	0.948	35.66	42.57	33.78
0.978	14.73	18.14	14.39	0.947	36.21	43.17	34.26
0.977	15.56	19.14	15.19	0.946	36.75	43.77	34.73
0.976	16.40	20.15	15.99	0.945	37.28	44.35	35.20
0.975	17.23	21.16	16.79	0.944	37.80	44.93	35.66
0.974	18.07	22.16	17.58	0.943	38.32	45.50	36.11
0.973	18.89	23.14	18.37	0.942	38.84	46.07	36.56
0.972	19.71	24.12	19.14	0.941	39.35	46.63	37.00
0.971	20.52	25.08	19.91	0.940	39.86	47.18	37.44
0.970	21.32	26.03	20.66	0.939	40.37	47.72	37.87

续表

相对密度	质量分数/%	体积分数/%	100ml 中的质量/g	相对密度	质量分数/%	体积分数/%	100ml 中的质量/g
0.938	40.87	48.26	38.03	0.901	57.84	65.61	52.07
0.937	41.36	48.80	38.72	0.900	58.27	66.03	52.40
0.936	41.85	49.33	39.14	0.899	58.71	66.45	52.74
0.935	42.34	49.85	39.56	0.898	59.15	66.87	53.07
0.934	42.83	50.37	39.97	0.897	59.58	67.29	53.40
0.933	43.31	50.88	40.38	0.896	60.02	67.70	53.73
0.932	43.79	51.39	40.78	0.895	60.45	68.12	54.05
0.931	44.27	51.89	41.18	0.894	60.88	68.53	54.38
0.930	44.75	52.39	41.58	0.893	61.51	68.94	54.71
0.929	45.22	52.89	41.97	0.892	61.75	69.34	55.03
0.928	45.69	53.39	42.37	0.891	62.18	69.75	55.35
0.927	46.16	53.88	42.76	0.890	62.61	70.16	55.67
0.926	46.63	54.36	43.14	0.889	63.04	70.56	55.99
0.925	47.09	54.84	43.52	0.888	63.47	70.96	56.31
0.924	47.55	55.32	43.90	0.887	63.90	71.36	56.63
0.923	48.01	55.80	44.28	0.886	64.33	71.76	56.94
0.922	48.47	56.27	44.65	0.885	64.75	72.15	57.26
0.921	48.93	56.74	45.03	0.884	65.18	72.55	57.57
0.920	49.39	57.21	45.40	0.883	65.61	72.94	57.88
0.919	49.84	57.67	45.76	0.882	66.04	73.33	58.19
0.918	50.29	58.13	46.13	0.881	66.46	73.72	58.50
0.917	50.75	58.59	46.49	0.880	66.89	74.11	58.81
0.916	51.20	59.05	46.86	0.879	67.31	74.49	59.12
0.915	51.65	59.50	47.22	0.878	67.74	74.88	59.42
0.914	52.09	59.95	47.57	0.877	68.16	75.26	59.73
0.913	52.54	60.40	47.93	0.876	68.58	75.64	60.03
0.912	52.99	60.84	48.28	0.875	69.01	76.02	60.33
0.911	53.43	61.29	48.64	0.874	69.43	76.40	60.63
0.910	53.88	61.73	48.99	0.873	69.85	76.78	60.93
0.909	54.32	62.17	49.33	0.872	70.27	77.15	61.23
0.908	54.76	62.61	49.68	0.871	70.70	77.53	61.52
0.907	55.20	63.04	50.03	0.870	71.12	77.90	61.82
0.906	55.65	63.47	50.37	0.869	71.54	78.27	62.11
0.905	56.09	63.91	50.71	0.868	71.95	78.64	62.40
0.904	56.52	64.34	51.06	0.867	72.37	79.00	62.69
0.903	56.96	64.76	51.39	0.866	72.79	79.37	62.98
0.902	57.40	65.19	51.73	0.865	73.21	79.73	63.27

续表

相对密度	质量分数/%	体积分数/%	100ml 中的质量/g
0.864	73.63	80.09	63.56
0.863	74.04	80.45	63.85
0.862	74.46	80.81	64.13
0.861	74.87	81.17	64.41
0.860	75.29	81.52	64.69
0.859	75.70	81.87	64.97
0.858	76.12	82.23	65.25
0.857	76.53	82.57	65.53
0.856	76.94	82.92	65.81
0.855	77.35	83.27	66.08
0.854	77.76	83.61	66.36
0.853	78.17	83.96	66.63
0.852	78.58	84.30	66.90
0.851	78.99	84.64	67.16
0.850	79.40	84.97	67.43
0.849	79.81	85.31	67.70
0.848	80.21	85.64	67.96
0.847	80.62	85.97	68.23
0.846	81.02	86.30	68.49
0.845	81.43	86.63	68.75
0.844	81.83	86.95	69.00
0.843	82.23	87.28	69.26
0.842	82.63	87.60	69.52
0.841	83.03	87.92	69.77
0.840	83.43	88.23	70.02
0.839	83.83	88.55	70.27
0.838	84.22	88.86	70.52
0.837	84.62	89.18	70.77
0.836	85.01	89.48	71.01
0.835	85.41	89.79	71.26
0.834	85.80	90.09	71.50
0.833	86.19	90.40	71.74
0.832	86.58	90.70	71.97
0.831	86.97	90.99	72.21
0.830	87.35	91.29	72.44
0.829	87.74	91.58	72.67
0.828	88.12	91.87	72.90
0.827	88.50	92.15	73.13
0.826	88.88	92.44	73.66
0.825	89.26	92.72	73.58
0.824	89.64	93.00	73.80
0.823	90.02	93.28	74.02
0.822	90.39	93.55	74.24
0.821	90.76	93.82	74.45
0.820	91.13	94.09	74.66
0.819	91.50	94.35	74.87
0.818	91.87	94.61	75.08
0.817	92.23	94.87	75.29
0.816	92.59	95.13	75.49
0.815	92.96	95.38	75.69
0.814	93.31	95.63	75.89
0.813	93.67	95.88	76.09
0.812	94.03	96.13	76.29
0.811	94.38	96.37	76.48
0.810	94.73	96.61	76.67
0.809	95.08	96.85	76.86
0.808	95.43	97.08	77.04
0.807	95.77	97.31	77.22
0.806	96.11	97.54	77.40
0.805	96.46	97.76	77.58
0.804	96.79	97.99	77.76
0.803	97.13	98.20	77.93
0.802	97.47	98.42	78.10
0.801	97.80	98.63	78.27
0.800	98.13	98.84	78.44
0.799	98.46	99.05	78.61
0.798	98.79	99.26	78.77
0.797	99.11	99.46	78.93
0.796	99.44	99.66	79.08
0.795	99.76	99.86	79.24
0.79425	100.00	100.00	79.36

摘自：杨桂馥主编. 软饮料工业手册. 北京：中国轻工业出版社, 2002

附录2　Appendix 2

中国居民膳食营养素参考摄入量

Chinese Dietary Reference Intakes (Chinese DRIs)

（中国营养学会2000年4月制定）

DRIs是在RDAs基础上发展起来的一组每日平均膳食营养素摄入量的参考值，包括4项内容：平均需要量（EAR）、推荐摄入量（RNI）、适宜摄入量（AI）和可耐受最高摄入量（UL）。

一、平均需要量 (Estimated Average Requirement，EAR)

EAR是某一特定性别、年龄及生理状况群体中对某营养素需要量的平均值。摄入量达到EAR水平时可以满足群体中半数个体对该营养素的需要，而不能满足另外半数个体的需要。

EAR是RNI的基础，如果个体摄入量呈常态分布，一个人群的RNI＝EAR＋2SD。针对人群，EAR可以用于评估群体中摄入量不足的发生率。针对个体，可以检查其摄入不足的可能性。

二、推荐摄入量 (Recommended Nutrient Intake，RNI)

RNI相当于传统使用的RDA，它可以满足某一特定群体中绝大多数（97%～98%）个体的需要。长期摄入RNI水平，可以维持组织中有适当的储备。

RNI是健康个体的膳食营养素摄入量目标，个体摄入量低于RNI时并不一定表明该个体未达到适宜营养状态。如果某个体的平均摄入量达到或超过了RNI，可以认为该个体没有摄入不足的危险。

三、适宜摄入量 (Adequate Intake，AI)

AI是通过观察或实验获得的健康人群某种营养素的摄入量。AI应能满足目标人群中几乎所有个体的需要。AI的准确性远不如RNI，可能显著高于RNI。

AI主要用作个体的营养素摄入目标，同时用作限制过多摄入的标准。当健康个体摄入量达到AI时，出现营养缺乏的危险性很小。如长期摄入超过AI，则有可能产生毒副作用。

四、可耐受最高摄入量 (Tolerable Upper Intake Level，UL)

UL是平均每日可以摄入该营养素的最高量。这个量对一般人群中的几乎所有个体似不致于损害健康。

UL的主要用途是检查个体摄入量过高的可能，避免发生中毒。当摄入量超过UL时，发生毒副作用的危险性会增加。在大多数情况下，UL包括膳食、强化食物和添加剂等各种来源的营养素之和。

表1. 能量和蛋白质的RNIs及脂肪供能比

Table 1 RNIs of energy and protein and percentage of energy from fat

年龄 Age (岁 Year)	能量 Energy #				蛋白质 Protein		脂肪 Fat
	RNI/MJ		RNI/kcal		RNI/g		AI 占能量百分比
	男 M	女 F	男 M	女 F	男 M	女 F	Energy/%
0~	0.40MJ/kg		95kcal/kg *		1.5~3g/(kg·d)		45~50
0.5~							35~40
1~	4.60	4.40	1100	1050	35	35	
2~	5.02	4.81	1200	1150	40	40	30~35
3~	5.64	5.43	1350	1300	45	45	
4~	6.06	5.83	1450	1400	50	50	
5~	6.70	6.27	1600	1500	55	55	
6~	7.10	6.70	1700	1600	55	55	
7~	7.53	7.10	1800	1700	60	60	25~30
8~	7.94	7.53	1900	1800	65	65	
9~	8.36	7.94	2000	1900	65	65	
10~	8.80	8.36	2100	2000	70	65	
11~	10.04	9.20	2400	2200	75	75	
14~	12.13	10.04	2900	2400	85	80	25~30
18~							20~30
体力活动水平 PAL▲							
轻 Light	10.04	8.80	2400	2100	75	65	
中 Moderate	11.30	9.62	2700	2300	80	70	
重 Heavy	13.38	11.30	3200	2700	90	80	
孕妇 Pregnant women		+0.84		+200		+5, +15, +20	
乳母 Lactating mothers		+2.09		+500		+20	
50~							20~30
体力活动水平 PAL▲							
轻 Light	9.62	7.94	2300	1900			
中 Moderate	10.87	8.36	2600	2000			
重 Heavy	13.00	9.20	3100	2200			
60~					75	65	20~30
体力活动水平 PAL▲							
轻 Light	7.94	7.53	1900	1800			
中 Moderate	9.20	8.36	2200	2000			
70~					75	65	20~30
体力活动水平 PAL▲							
轻 Light	7.94	7.10	1900	1700			
中 Moderate	8.80	7.94	2100	1900			
80~	7.94	7.10	1900	1700	75	65	20~30

注：# 各年龄组的能量的 RNI 与其 EAR 相同。# The RNIs of energy are the same as the EARs.
* 为 AI，非母乳喂养应增加 20%。* AI value, add 20% to non-breastfeeding infants.
PAL▲ physical activity level.
（凡表中数字缺如之处表示未制定参考值）

表 2. 常量和微量元素的 RNIs 或 AIs
Table 2 RNIs or AIs of some elements

年龄 Age (岁 Year)	钙 Ca AI mg	磷 P AI mg	钾 K AI mg	钠 Na AI mg	镁 Mg AI mg	铁 Fe AI mg	碘 I RNI μg	锌 Zn RNI mg	硒 Se RNI μg	铜 Cu AI mg	氟 F AI mg	铬 Cr AI μg	锰 Mn AI mg	钼 Mo AI μg
0 ~	300	150	500	200	30	0.3	50	1.5	15(AI)	0.4	0.1	10		
0.5 ~	400	300	700	500	70	10	50	8.0	20(AI)	0.6	0.4	15		
1 ~	600	450	1000	650	100	12	50	9.0	20	0.8	0.6	20		15
4 ~	800	500	1500	900	150	12	90	12.0	25	1.0	0.8	30		20
7 ~	800	700	1500	1000	250	12	90	13.5	35	1.2	1.0	30		30
						男 M 女 F		男 M 女 F						
11 ~	1000	1000	1500	1200	350	16 18	120	18.0 15.0	45	1.8	1.2	40		50
14 ~	1000	1000	2000	1800	350	20 25	150	19.0 15.5	50	2.0	1.4	40		50
18 ~	800	700	2000	2200	350	15 20	150	15.0 11.5	50	2.0	1.5	50	3.5	60
孕妇 Pregnant women														
早期 1st trimester	800	700	2500	2200	400	15	200	11.5	50					
中期 2nd trimester	1000	700	2500	2200	400	25	200	16.5	50					
晚期 3rd trimester	1200	700	2500	2200	400	35	200	16.5	50					
乳母 Lactating mothers	1200	700	2500	2200	400	25	200	21.5	65					
50 ~	1000	700	2000	2200	350	15	150	11.5	50	2.0	1.5	50	3.5	60

（凡表中数字缺如之处表示未制定该参考值）

表 3. 脂溶性维生素和水溶性维生素的 RNIs 或 AIs

Table 3 RNIs or AIs of some vitamins

年龄 Age (岁 Year)	维生素 A Vitamin A RNI μg RE[#]		维生素 D Vitamin D RNI μg	维生素 E Vitamin E AI mg α-TE[*]	维生素 B_1 Vitamin B_1 RNI mg		维生素 B_2 Vitamin B_2 RNI mg		维生素 B_6 Vitamin B_6 AI mg	维生素 B_{12} Vitamin B_{12} AI μg	维生素 C Vitamin C RNI mg	泛酸 Pantothenic acid AI mg	叶酸 Folic acid RNI μg DFE[▲]	烟酸 Niacin RNI mg NE[△]		胆碱 Choline AI mg	生物素 Biotin AI μg
0 ~	400(AI)		10	3	0.2(AI)		0.4(AI)		0.1	0.4	40	1.7	65(AI)	2(AI)		100	5
0.5 ~	400(AI)		10	3	0.3(AI)		0.5(AI)		0.3	0.5	50	1.8	80(AI)	3(AI)		150	6
1 ~	500		10	4	0.6		0.6		0.5	0.9	60	2.0	150	6		200	8
4 ~	600		10	5	0.7		0.7		0.6	1.2	70	3.0	200	7		250	12
7 ~	700		10	7	0.9		1.0		0.7	1.2	80	4.0	200	9		300	16
11 ~	700		5	10	1.2		1.2		0.9	1.8	90	5.0	300	12		350	20
	男 M	女 F			男 M	女 F	男 M	女 F						男 M	女 F		
14 ~	800	700	5	14	1.5	1.2	1.5	1.2	1.1	2.4	100	5.0	400	15	12	450	25
18 ~	800	700	5	14	1.4	1.3	1.4	1.2	1.2	2.4	100	5.0	400	14	13	500	30
孕妇 Pregnant women																	
早期 1st trimester		800	5	14		1.5		1.7	1.9	2.6	100	6.0	600		15	500	30
中期 2nd trimester		900	10	14		1.5		1.7	1.9	2.6	130	6.0	600		15	500	30
晚期 3rd trimester		900	10	14		1.5		1.7	1.9	2.6	130	6.0	600		15	500	30
乳母 Lactating mothers		1200	10	14		1.8		1.7	1.9	2.8	130	7.0	500		18	500	35
50 ~	800	700	10	14	1.3		1.4		1.5	2.4	100	5.0	400	13		500	30

注：[#] RE 为视黄醇当量。 RE is retinol equivalent.

[*] α-TE 为 α-生育酚当量。 α-TE is tocopherol equivalent.

[▲] DFE 为膳食叶酸当量。 DFE is dietary folate equivalent.

[△] NE 为烟酸当量。 NE is niacin equivalent.

（凡表中数字缺如之处表示未制定该参考值）

表4. 某些微量营养素的 ULs
Table 4 ULs of some micronutrients

年龄 Age (岁 Year)	钙 Ca mg	磷 P mg	镁 Mg mg	铁 Fe mg	碘 I μg	锌 Zn mg	硒 Se μg	铜 Cu mg	氟 F mg	铬 Cr μg	锰 Mn mg	钼 Mo μg	维生素 A Vitamin A μg RE#	维生素 D Vitamin D μg	维生素 B_1 Vitamin B1 mg	维生素 C Vitamin C mg	叶酸 Folic acid μg DFE▲	烟酸 Niacin mg NE△	胆碱 Choline mg
0～				10			55		0.4							400			600
0.5～				30		13	80		0.8							500			800
1～	2000	3000	200	30		23	120	1.5	1.2	200		80			50	600	300	10	1000
4～	2000	3000	300	30		23	180	2.0	1.6	300		110	2000	20	50	700	400	15	1500
7～	2000	3000	500	30	800	28	240	3.5	2.0	300		160	2000	20	50	800	400	20	2000
						男 M 女 F													
11～	2000	3500	700	50	800	37 34	300	5.0	2.4	400		280	2000	20	50	900	600	30	2500
14～	2000	3500	700	50	800	42 35	360	7.0	2.8	400		280	2000	20	50	1000	800	30	3000
18～	2000	3500	700	50	1000	45 37	400	8.0	3.0	500	10	350	3000	20	50	1000	1000	35	3500
孕妇 Pregnant women	2000	3000	700	60	1000	35	400						2400	20		1000	1000		3500
乳母 Lactating mothers	2000	3500	700	50	1000	35	400							20		1000	1000		3500
50～	2000	3500*	700	50	1000	37 37	400	8.0	3.0	500	10	350	3000	20	50	1000	1000	35	3500

注：# RE 为视黄醇当量。 RE is retinol equivalent.

▲DFE 为膳食叶酸当量。 DFE is dietary folate equivalent.

△NE 为烟酸当量。 NE is niacin equivalent.

* 60 岁以上磷的 UL 为 3000mg。UL of phosphorus is 3000mg for people 60 years over.

（表中数字缺如之处表示未制定该参考值）

表 5. 蛋白质及某些微量营养素的 EARs

Table 5 EARs of protein and some micronutrients

年龄 Age (岁 Year)	蛋白质 Protein g/kg	锌 Zn mg		硒 Se μg	维生素 A Vitamin A μg RE#	维生素 D Vitamin D μg	维生素 B_1 Vitamin B_1 mg		维生素 B_2 Vitamin B_2 mg		维生素 C Vitamin C mg	叶酸 Folic acid μg DFE▲
0～	2.25～1.25	1.5			375	8.8*						
0.5～	1.25～1.15	6.7			400	13.8*						
1～		7.4		17	300		0.4		0.5		13	320
4～		8.7		20			0.5		0.6		22	320
7～		9.7		26	700		0.5		0.8		39	320
		男 M	女 F				男 M	女 F	男 M	女 F		
11～		13.1	10.8	36	700		0.7	0.7	1.0	1.0		320
14～		13.9	11.2	40			1.0	0.9	1.3	1.0	63	320
18～	0.92	13.2	8.3	41			1.4	1.3	1.2	1.0	75	320
孕妇 Pregnant women								1.3		1.45	66	520
早期 1st trimester			8.3	50								
中期 2nd trimester			+5	50								
晚期 3rd trimester			+5	50								
乳母 Lactating mothers	+0.18		+10	65				1.3		1.4	96	450
50～	0.92										75	320

注：# RE 为视黄醇当量。 RE is retinol equivalent.

▲DFE 为膳食叶酸当量。 DFE is dietary folate equivalent.

* 0～2.9 岁南方地区为 8.88μg，北方地区为 13.8μg。0～2.9years, 8.88μg for south China, 13.8μg for north China.

（凡表中数字缺如之处表示未制定该参考值）

食物名称中英文对照表
Chinese-English Food Names

编码 Code	食物名称 Food name	英文名称 English name
	谷类及制品	**CEREALS and CEREAL PRODUCTS**
小麦		**WHEAT**
01-1-206	小麦面粉 [标准粉]	Wheat flour, moderately refined, standard grade
01-1-207	小麦面粉 [富强粉、特一粉]	Wheat flour, refined, special grade 1
01-1-208	小麦面粉 (特制)	Wheat flour, specially refined
01-1-313	挂面 (富强粉)	Noodle, from refined wheat flour, dried, raw
01-1-314	龙须面 (素)	Vermicelli, from wheat flour, plain or vegetarian, dried, raw
01-1-315	龙须面 (鸡蛋)	Vermicelli, from wheat flour, egg powder added, dried, raw
01-1-316	面条 (富强粉, 切面)	Noodle, from refined wheat flour, fresh, raw
01-1-317	面条 (富强粉, 煮)	Noodle, from refined wheat flour, boiled, drained
01-1-410	花卷 (加牛奶)	Bun, twisted, from refined wheat flour, milk and salt added, leavened, steamed
01-1-411	馒头 (富强粉)	Bun, from refined wheat flour, leavened, steamed
01-1-503	面筋 (肉馅)	Wheat gluten, filled with mince pork
稻米		**RICE**
01-2-106	粳米 (极品精米)	Rice, round grain, refined, raw, from Jilin
01-2-107	粳米 (西域王米)	Rice, round grain, refined, raw, from Xinjing
01-2-108	粳米 (小站稻米)	Rice, round grain, refined, raw, from Tianjin
01-2-214	籼米	Rice, long grain, moderately refined, raw
01-2-215	香米	Rice, long grain, fragrant, refined, raw
01-2-408	籼米饭 (蒸)	Rice, long grain, moderately refined, steamed
01-2-409	籼米粥	Rice porridge, long grain, moderately refined, boiled
01-2-410	米粉	Rice noodle, dried, raw
01-2-411	河粉	Rice noodle, flattened, dried, raw
玉米		**CORN**
01-3-108	玉米粒 (黄, 干)	Corn grain, yellow, dried, raw
01-3-109	玉米面 (黄)	Corn flour, yellow, dried, raw
01-3-110	玉米糁 (黄)	Corn grits, yellow, raw
01-3-202	玉米面面条	Corn noodle, wheat flour added, dried, raw

编码 Code	食物名称 Food name	英文名称 English name
大麦		**BARLEY**
01-4-102	黑大麦	Barley grain, naked, black, raw
小米		**MILLET**
01-5-104	小米 (黄)	Foxtail millet, hulled, yellow, raw
其它		**OTHERS**
01-9-010	荞麦面	Buckwheat flour, refined
01-9-011	莜麦面	Naked oat flour, refined
01-9-201	高粱面面条	Sorghum noodle, wheat flour added, dried, raw
	薯类、淀粉及制品	**TUBERS, STARCHES and PRODUCTS**
薯类		**TUBERS**
02-1-104	马铃薯 [土豆、洋芋]	Potato, white flesh, raw
02-1-105	马铃薯 (烤)	Potato, baked, peeled
02-1-106	马铃薯 (蒸)	Potato, steamed, peeled
02-1-107	马铃薯 (煮)	Potato, boiled, peeled
02-1-108	马铃薯全粉	Potato flour
02-1-205	甘薯 (红心) [山芋、红薯]	Sweet potato, red flesh, raw
淀粉类		**STARCHES**
02-2-108	淀粉 (小麦)	Starch, wheat
02-2-109	淀粉 (大米)	Starch, rice
02-2-110	淀粉 (马铃薯)	Starch, potato
02-2-111	淀粉 (甘薯)	Starch, sweet potato
02-2-112	煎炸粉	Potato starch flour, for pan-frying
	干豆类及制品	**DRIED LEGUMES and LEGUME PRODUCTS**
大豆		**SOYBEAN**
03-1-104	黄豆	Soybean, yellow
03-1-206	豆奶粉 (维维牌)	Soybean milk powder, WEIWEI, cow's milk and sugar added
03-1-207	豆奶粉 (多力牌)	Soybean milk powder, MIGHTYI, cow's milk powder, egg powder and sugar added, calcium fortified
03-1-208	豆奶粉 (大磨牌)	Soybean milk powder, DAMO, cow's milk added, calcium and iron fortified, unsweetened
03-1-306	豆腐 (北豆腐)	Soybean curd, semisoft, northern style
03-1-307	豆腐 (南豆腐)	Soybean curd, soft, southern style
03-1-405	豆浆	Soybean milk, unsweetened

编码 Code	食物名称 Food name	英文名称 English name
03-1-406	豆浆(甜)	Soybean milk, sweetened
03-1-527	豆腐皮	Soybean sheet, dried, skimmed from soybean milk
03-1-528	腐竹	Soybean stick, dried, skimmed from soybean milk
03-1-529	豆腐干	Soybean curd slab, semisoft
赤豆		**ADZUKI BEAN**
03-3-204	红豆沙	Adzuki bean paste, skin removed, sweetened
03-3-205	红豆馅	Adzuki bean paste, with skin, sweetened
蚕豆		**BROAD BEAN**
03-5-203	蚕豆(煮)	Broad bean, immature seeds, cooked, boiled, drained, without salt
其它		**OTHERS**
03-9-204	豇豆(煮)	Cowpea, boiled
03-9-303	豌豆(煮)	Pea, boiled
03-9-401	鹰嘴豆[桃豆]	Chickpeas, dried, raw
	蔬菜类及制品	**VEGETABLES and VEGETABLE PRODUCTS**
根菜类		**ROOT VEGETABLES**
04-1-111	白萝卜[莱菔]	Radish, white skin and flesh, raw
04-1-112	白萝卜(圆)	Radish, white skin and flesh, round, raw
04-1-113	青萝卜	Radish, green skin and flesh, raw
04-1-114	变萝卜[红皮萝卜]	Radish, red skin and white flesh, round, raw
04-1-115	樱桃萝卜	Cherry radish, raw
04-1-204	胡萝卜	Carrot, yellow, raw
04-1-402	根芹[根洋芹、球根塘蒿]	Celeriac, raw
04-1-403	紫菜头	Garden beet, purple skin and flesh, raw
鲜豆菜和豆苗类		**LEGUMINOUS VEGETABLES, SPROUTS and SEEDLINGS**
04-2-118	扁豆	Hyacinth bean, green, with husk, raw
04-2-119	豇豆	Cowpea, common, with husk, raw
04-2-120	四季豆[菜豆、芸豆]	Kidney bean, green, with husk, raw
04-2-121	四棱豆[杨桃豆、翅豆]	Winged bean, with husk, raw
04-2-122	甜脆荷兰豆[甜豆]	Sugar pea, with husk, raw
04-2-205	黄豆芽	Sprout, soybean, raw
04-2-206	绿豆芽	Sprout, mung bean, raw
04-2-207	黑豆苗	Seedling, black bean, raw
04-2-208	豌豆苗	Seedling, pea, raw

编码 Code	食物名称 Food name	英文名称 English name
茄果、瓜菜类		**CUCURBITACEOUS and SOLANACEOUS VEGETABLES**
04-3-115	茄子（白皮，长）	Eggplant, long, white skin, raw
04-3-116	茄子（紫皮，长）	Eggplant, long, dark purple skin, raw
04-3-117	茄子（紫皮，圆）	Eggplant, round, dark purple skin, raw
04-3-118	香瓜茄	Pepino, raw
04-3-119	番茄 [西红柿]	Tomato, raw
04-3-120	樱桃番茄 [小西红柿]	Cherry tomato, raw
04-3-121	辣椒（小红尖辣椒）	Chilli or hot pepper, red, small, raw
04-3-122	辣椒（小红尖辣椒，干）	Chilli or hot pepper, red, small, dried, raw
04-3-123	辣椒（青，尖）	Chilli or hot pepper, green, pointed tip, raw
04-3-124	甜椒 [灯笼椒、柿子椒]	Pepper or capsicum, sweet, green, raw
04-3-125	彩椒	Pepper or capsicum, sweet, red, yellow or purple, etc., raw
04-3-126	秋葵 [黄秋葵、羊角豆]	Okra, raw
04-3-221	冬瓜	Chinese wax gourd or winter melon, raw
04-3-222	飞碟瓜	Scallop squash, raw
04-3-223	黄金西葫芦	Zucchini, golden, raw
04-3-224	黄茎瓜	Calabaza, raw
04-3-225	迷你黄瓜 [荷兰乳黄瓜]	Mini cucumber, raw
04-3-226	秋黄瓜 [旱黄瓜]	Cucumber, *Autumn*, raw
04-3-227	南瓜（栗面）	Pumpkin, raw
04-3-228	丝瓜	Sponge gourd, raw
葱蒜类		**ALLIUM VEGETABLES**
04-4-206	大葱	Scallion, raw
04-4-207	细香葱 [香葱、四季葱]	Chive, raw
04-4-404	韭菜	Chinese chive, raw
嫩茎、叶、花菜类		**STEM, LEAFY and FLOWERING VEGETABLES**
04-5-117	大白菜（白口）	Chinese cabbage, *Bok choi*, white leaves and stems, raw
04-5-118	大白菜（青口）	Chinese cabbage, *Bok choi*, green leaves and stems, raw
04-5-119	酸白菜 [酸菜]	Chinese cabbage, pickled
04-5-120	小白菜 [青菜]	Pak choi, petiole, raw
04-5-121	奶白菜	Pak choi, petiole, raw
04-5-122	鸡毛菜	Mini pak choi, leaf and stem, raw
04-5-123	娃娃菜	Mini Chinese cabbage, raw
04-5-124	乌塌菜 [塌菜、塌棵菜]	Flat cabbage
04-5-125	油菜	Rape, green, leaf and stem, raw

编码 Code	食物名称 Food name	英文名称 English name
04-5-126	油菜心	Rape, green, flowering stalk, raw
04-5-210	结球甘蓝 (绿) [圆白菜]	Cabbage, green, raw
04-5-211	结球甘蓝 (紫)	Cabbage, purple, raw
04-5-212	抱子甘蓝	Brussels sprouts, raw
04-5-213	羽衣甘蓝	Curled kale, raw
04-5-214	盖菜	Mustard greens, broad leaf, raw
04-5-215	芥蓝 [甘蓝菜、盖蓝菜]	Kale, raw
04-5-216	菜花 [花椰菜]	Cauliflower, white, raw
04-5-217	西兰花 [绿菜花]	Broccoli, raw
04-5-327	番杏 [新西兰菠菜、夏菠菜]	Common tetragonia, raw
04-5-328	樱桃萝卜缨	Cherry radish leaf and stem, raw
04-5-329	白凤菜	Green gynura, raw
04-5-330	紫背天葵 [红凤菜、血皮菜]	Gynura, raw
04-5-331	芹菜 (茎)	Chinese celery stem, raw
04-5-332	西芹 [西洋芹菜、美芹]	Celery stem, raw
04-5-333	生菜	Endive lettuce, curl-leafed, raw
04-5-334	油麦菜	Romaine lettuce, raw
04-5-335	叶甜菜 (白梗)	Leaf beet, raw
04-5-336	莴笋叶 [莴苣菜]	Lettuce, leaf, raw
04-5-337	蕹菜 [空心菜、藤藤菜]	Water spinach, raw
04-5-338	观达菜 [根达菜、牛皮菜]	Swiss chard, leaf and stem, raw
04-5-339	球茎茴香 [甜茴香、意大利茴香]	Anise, raw
04-5-415	芦笋 (绿) [石刁柏、龙须菜]	Asparagus stem, raw
04-5-416	芦笋 (紫)	Asparagus stem, purple, raw
04-5-417	结球菊苣	Chicory, red, raw
04-5-418	软化白菊苣	Chicory witloof, raw
水生蔬菜类		**AQUATIC VEGETABLES**
04-6-010	藕 [莲藕]	Lotus root, raw
薯芋类		**TUBERS**
04-7-203	芋头 [芋艿、毛芋]	Taro, raw
04-7-204	芋头 (煮)	Taro, boiled
野生蔬菜类		**WILD VEGETABLES**
04-8-081	苦苣菜 [苦菜、天精菜]	Common sow thistle, raw
04-8-082	苜蓿 [草头、金花菜]	Alfalfa, raw
04-8-083	鱼腥草 (叶) [蕺菜、臭菜]	Heartleaf houttuynia, leaf, raw
04-8-084	鱼腥草 (根)	Heartleaf houttuynia, root, raw

编码 Code	食物名称 Food name	英文名称 English name
	菌藻类	**FUNGI and ALGAE**
菌类		**FUNGI**
05-1-028	白蘑菇 [双孢蘑菇、洋蘑菇]	Button mushroom
05-1-029	北风菌 [荷叶离褶伞、一窝羊]	Fried-chicken mushroom
05-1-030	草菇 [大黑头细花草、稻菇]	Straw mushroom, soaked in salted water, canned
05-1-031	茶树菇 (干) [柱状田头菇、茶薪菇]	Agrocybe aegerila
05-1-032	干巴菌	Ganba fungus
05-1-033	红奶浆菌 [多汁乳菇、谷熟菌]	Weeping milk cap
05-1-034	黄蘑 (干)	Yellow mushroom, dried
05-1-035	黄伞菇 (干) [多脂鳞伞、黄丝菌]	Golden pholiota, dried
05-1-036	鸡腿菇 (干) [毛头鬼伞]	Shaggy mane, dried
05-1-037	鸡油菌 [黄丝菌、杏菌]	Chanterelle
05-1-038	鸡纵 [蚁纵、伞把菇、鸡纵菌]	Termite mushroom
05-1-039	鸡纵 (干)	Termite mushroom, dried
05-1-040	鸡纵 (油炸) [油鸡纵]	Termite mushroom, steamed, fried, salted, in oil
05-1-041	鸡纵花	—
05-1-042	白牛肝菌 [美味牛肝菌]	King bolete
05-1-043	白牛肝菌 (干) [美味牛肝菌]	King bolete, dried
05-1-044	黑牛肝菌 [铜色牛肝菌]	Queen bolete
05-1-045	黄皮牛肝菌 [黄皮疣柄牛肝菌、黄癞头]	—
05-1-046	乳牛肝菌 (干) [粘盖牛肝菌、松树菌]	Cow spunk, dried
05-1-047	牛眼睛菌 [马勃菌]	Puffball
05-1-048	平菇 [糙皮侧耳、青蘑]	Oyster mushroom
05-1-049	青头菌 [变绿红菇、绿菇]	Virescent russule
05-1-050	松蘑 (干) [松茸、松口蘑]	Matsutake, dried
05-1-051	杏鲍菇	King oyster mushroom
05-1-052	血红菇 (干)	Red mushroom, dried
05-1-053	元蘑 (干) [亚侧耳、冬蘑、黄蘑]	Late fall oyster, dried
05-1-054	竹荪 (干) [竹笙、竹参]	Long net stinkhorn
05-1-055	榛蘑 (干) [小蜜环菌]	Honey mushroom, wild, dried
藻类		**ALGAE**
05-2-009	螺旋藻 (干)	Spirulina, dried
05-2-010	裙带菜 (干) [海芥菜、海木耳]	Sea water fungus
05-2-011	海带菜	Kelp sliver, with sugar, sesame and salt

编码 Code	食物名称 Food name	英文名称 English name
	水果类及制品	**FRUITS and FRUIT PRODUCTS**
仁果类		**KERNEL FRUITS**
06-1-907	蛇果	Apple, red delicious
核果类		**DRUPE FRUITS**
06-2-115	蜜桃	Peach, *Honey* type
06-2-116	桃 (糖水罐头)	Peach, canned in syrup
06-2-207	布朗	American plum or hog plum
06-2-208	西梅	Prune or garden plum
06-2-312	冬枣	Winter jujube
06-2-313	小枣 (干)	Date, dried
浆果类		**BERRIES**
06-3-911	红提子葡萄	Grape or fox grape
06-3-912	无花果 (干)	Fig, dried
柑橘类		**CITRUS FRUITS**
06-4-303	葡萄柚 (台湾) [西柚]	Grapefruit, from Taiwan
06-4-304	葡萄柚 (以色列) [西柚]	Grapefruit, from Israel
热带、亚热带水果		**TROPICAL FRUITS**
06-5-021	桂圆 (干)	Longan, dried
06-5-022	红毛丹	Rambutan
06-5-023	火龙果 [仙蜜果、红龙果]	Pitaya or dragon fruit
06-5-024	荔枝 (干)	Litchi, dried
06-5-025	榴莲	Durian
06-5-026	芒果 (大头)	Mango, *Dato*
06-5-027	木瓜 [番木瓜]	Papaya
06-5-028	酸木瓜	—
06-5-029	蒲桃 [香果、水石榴]	Rose apple
06-5-030	山竹	Mangosteen
06-5-031	香蕉 (红皮, 海南)	Banana, red skin, from Hainan
06-5-032	香蕉 (红皮, 泰国)	Banana, red skin, from Thailand
瓜果类		**MELONS**
06-6-206	小西瓜 [地雷瓜]	Water melon, small

编码 Code	食物名称 Food name	英文名称 English name
	坚果、种子类	**NUTS and SEEDS**
树坚果		**NUTS**
07-1-026	山核桃 (熟)	Wild walnut or hickory nut, in shell, salted and roasted
07-1-027	栗子 (北京密云) [板栗]	Chestnut, in shell, raw, from Beijing
07-1-028	栗子 (河南) [板栗]	Chestnut, in shell, raw, from Henan
07-1-029	栗子 (山东) [板栗]	Chestnut, in shell, raw, from Shandong
07-1-030	栗子 (河北迁西) [板栗]	Chestnut, in shell, raw, from Qianxi, Hebei
07-1-031	栗子 (河北邢台) [板栗]	Chestnut, in shell, raw, from Xingtai, Hebei
07-1-032	栗子仁 (熟)	Chestnut, roasted, shell removed
07-1-033	松子 (熟)	Pine nut, in shell, salted and roasted
07-1-034	杏仁 (熟, 带壳)	Almond, in shell, salted and roasted
07-1-035	杏仁 (熟, 去壳)	Almond, shell removed, salted and roasted, large
07-1-036	腰果 (熟)	Cashew nut, salted and roasted
07-1-037	榛子 (熟)	Hazelnut, in shell, roasted
07-1-038	榛子仁 (熟)	Hazelnut, without shell, salted and roasted
07-1-039	开心果 (熟)	Pistachio, in shell, salted and roasted
07-1-040	香榧 (熟)	Chinese torreya, in shell, salted and roasted
种子		**SEEDS**
07-2-020	花生 (烤, 勤俭牌)	Peanut, in shell, salted and roasted, QINJIAN
07-2-021	花生 (烤, 密日兴牌)	Peanut, in shell, salted and roasted, MIRIXING
07-2-022	花生仁 (油炸)	Peanut, without shell, fried, salted
07-2-023	葵花子 (奶油香瓜子)	Sunflower seed, in shell, salted and roasted, butter flavor
07-2-024	葵花子 (熟)	Sunflower seed, in shell, salted and roasted
07-2-025	南瓜子 (熟) [白瓜子]	Pumpkin seed, in shell, salted and roasted
07-2-026	西瓜子 (熟) [黑瓜子]	Watermelon seed, in shell, salted and roasted
	畜肉类及制品	**MEAT and MEAT PRODUCTS**
猪		**PIG**
08-1-121	猪肉 (前臀尖, 杜长大猪)	Pork, picnic butt, *Duchangda*, raw, lean and fat
08-1-122	猪肉 (前臀尖, 良杂猪)	Pork, picnic butt, *Liangza*, raw, lean and fat
08-1-123	猪肉 (后臀尖, 杜长大猪)	Pork, rump, *Duchangda*, raw, lean and fat
08-1-124	猪肉 (后臀尖, 良杂猪)	Pork, rump, *Liangza*, raw, lean and fat
08-1-125	猪肉 (硬肋, 杜长大猪)	Pork, chop, without rib, *Duchangda*, raw, lean and fat
08-1-126	猪肉 (硬肋, 良杂猪)	Pork, chop, without rib, *Liangza*, raw, lean and fat
08-1-127	猪肉 (通脊, 杜长大猪)	Pork, eye muscle or loin, *Duchangda*, raw, lean

续表

编码 Code	食物名称 Food name	英文名称 English name
08-1-128	猪肉(通脊,良杂猪)	Pork, eye muscle or loin, *Liangza*, raw, lean
08-1-129	猪肉(里脊)	Pork, tenderloin, raw, lean and fat
08-1-130	猪皮	Hogskin, raw
08-1-131	猪小排(杜长大猪)	Pork, sparerib, *Duchangda*, raw, lean
08-1-132	猪小排(良杂猪)	Pork, sparerib, *Liangza*, raw, lean
08-1-213	猪肚	Pork, stomach, raw
08-1-214	猪肝	Pork, liver, raw
08-1-215	猪舌[口条]	Pork, tongue, raw
08-1-216	猪肾[猪腰子]	Pork, kidney, raw
08-1-318	火腿心全精肉	Pork, salted and flavoured, for ham, raw, lean
08-1-319	火腿心肉	Pork, salted and flavoured, for ham, with skin and bone, raw, lean and fat
08-1-320	腊肉	Pork, lean and fat, cured and salted, raw
08-1-321	叉烧肉	Pork, lean and fat, barbecued, cooked with salt and sugar
08-1-322	酱排骨	Pork, sparerib, cooked with salt, soy sauce and sugar
08-1-323	香糟块肉	Pork, lean and fat, stewed, flavored
08-1-324	熏烤小里脊	Pork, tenderloin, barbecued and smoked, cooked with salt and sugar
08-1-325	猪肉脯	Pork, jerky, lean, cooked with salt, soy sauce and sugar, dried
08-1-326	肉酥	Pork, crispy, cooked with salt and sugar
08-1-327	猪肉松	Pork, floss, cooked with salt and sugar, dried
08-1-328	扒猪脸	Pork, face, braised with salt, soy sauce and sugar
08-1-329	酱肘子	Pork, hock, stewed with salt, soy sauce and sugar
08-1-423	脆皮肠	Pork sausage, cooked, with crispy skin
08-1-424	热狗肠	Pork, *hotdog* sausage, cooked
08-1-425	火腿肠	Pork ham sausage, cooked
08-1-426	火腿	Pork ham, cooked
08-1-427	火腿(云南)	Pork ham, *Xuanwei* Ham, cooked, canned
08-1-428	三明治火腿	Pork ham, for sandwich, cooked
08-1-429	午餐肉	Pork ham, *luncheon meat*, cooked
牛		**CATTLE**
08-2-111	牛肉(背部肉)[上脑]	Beef, highrib, raw, lean and fat
08-2-112	牛肉(里脊肉)[牛柳]	Beef, fillet tenderloin, raw, lean
08-2-113	牛肉(臀部肉)[紫盖、白板]	Beef, rump, raw, lean
08-2-114	牛肉(肩部肉)[肩肉]	Beef, shoulder, raw, lean and fat
08-2-115	牛肉(胸部肉)[牛胸]	Beef, brisket, raw, lean and fat
08-2-116	牛肉(腹部肉)[牛腩]	Beef, belly steak, raw, lean and fat
08-2-117	牛肉(膝圆肉)[和尚头]	Beef, boneless knuckle or thick flank, raw, lean

编码 Code	食物名称 Food name	英文名称 English name
08-2-118	牛肉(股内肉)[针扒、米龙、黄瓜条]	Beef, boneless topside, raw, lean
08-2-119	牛肉(小腿肉)[牛展、牛腱子]	Beef, shank, raw, lean
08-2-210	牛百叶(黑)	Beef, tripe, black, raw
08-2-307	牛肉(酱,五香)	Beef, lean and fat, spiced, cooked with salt, soy sauce, etc.
08-2-308	牛肉(清香)	Beef, lean and fat, cooked with salt, etc.
08-2-309	牛腱子(香叶)	Beef, shank, cooked with salt, soy sauce, etc.
08-2-310	牛肉干(长富牌)	Beef, jerky, lean, processed with salt, sugar, etc., dried, CHANGFU
08-2-311	牛肉干(沙爹牌)	Beef, jerky, lean, processed with salt, sugar, etc., dried, SHADIE
羊		**MUTTON**
08-3-113	羊肉(上脑)	Mutton, highrib / meat of the back of the body, lean and fat, raw
08-3-114	羊肉(腰窝)	Mutton, shoulder, lean and fat, raw
08-3-115	羊肉(前腿)	Mutton, fore leg, lean, raw
08-3-116	羊肉(后腿)	Mutton, hind leg, lean, raw
08-3-117	羊肉片	Mutton, slice, raw
08-3-309	烧羊肉(五香)	Mutton, spiced, barbecued with salt, oil, etc.
08-3-310	羊肉串(生)	Mutton, hind leg, chunks of meat, pierced through a bamboo stick, salted and flavored, raw
驴		**ASS**
08-4-304	驴肉(五香)	Donkey meat, spiced, cooked with salt, sugar, etc.
其它		**OTHERS**
08-9-006	鹿肉(梅花鹿)	Venison, clubs deer, raw
	禽肉类及制品	**POULTRY and POULTRY PRODUCTS**
鸡		**CHICKEN**
09-1-112	鸡胸脯肉	Chicken, breast, without skin and bone, frozen, raw
09-1-113	鸡腿	Chicken, thigh, frozen, raw
09-1-114	鸡翅	Chicken, wing, frozen, raw
09-1-115	鸡块(带浆粉)	Chicken, mixed with starch and other spices, frozen in pieces, raw
09-1-116	野山鸡	Pheasant, frozen, raw, whole
09-1-308	扒鸡(五香脱骨)	Chicken, braised, seasoned, whole
09-1-309	烤鸡	Chicken, roasted, seasoned, whole
09-1-310	童子鸡(熟)	Chicken, spring, braised with salt, beer, etc., whole
鸭		**DUCK**
09-2-214	鸭豉片	Duck slice, cured with salt, sugar and wine, etc., raw

编码 Code	食物名称 Food name	英文名称 English name
09-2-307	烤鸭 (老唐牌)	Duck (Peking duck), roasted, whole, LAOTANG
09-2-308	烤鸭 (全聚德牌)	Duck (Peking duck), roasted, whole, QUANJUDE
鹅		**GOOSE**
09-3-302	腊鹅	Goose, cured, raw
火鸡		**TURKEY**
09-4-301	火鸡腿	Turkey, thigh, no skin, cooked
其它		**OTHERS**
09-9-003	乳鸽	Pigeon, young, cured, raw, whole
09-9-004	乳鸽 (红烧)	Pigeon, barbecued, whole
	乳类及制品	**MILK and MILK PRODUCTS**
液态乳		**LIQUID COW'S MILK**
10-1-105	牛乳 (光明牌)	Milk, whole, BRIGHT
10-1-106	牛乳 (乐百氏牌)	Milk, whole, ROBUST
10-1-107	牛乳 (帕玛拉特牌)	Milk, whole, PARMALAT
10-1-108	牛乳 (三元牌)	Milk, whole, SANYUAN
10-1-109	牛乳 (完达山牌)	Milk, whole, WONDERSUN
10-1-110	牛乳 (龙丹牌)	Milk, whole, LONGDAN
10-1-111	牛乳 (蒙牛牌)	Milk, whole, MENGNIU
10-1-112	牛乳 (新南洋牌)	Milk, whole, XINNANYANG
10-1-113	牛乳 (帕玛拉特)	Milk, whole, PARMALAT
10-1-114	牛乳 (伊利牌)	Milk, whole, YILI
10-1-115	牛乳 (部分脱脂, 帕玛拉特)	Milk, partly skimmed
10-1-116	牛乳 (脱脂, 帕玛拉特)	Milk, skimmed
10-1-117	牛乳 (强化锌、钙, 帕玛拉特)	Milk, recombined, enriched with zinc and calcium, PARMALAT
10-1-118	牛奶 (草莓味, 卡夫牌)	Milk, strawberry flavored, whole, sweetened
10-1-119	牛奶 (巧克力味, 卡夫牌)	Milk, chocolate flavored, whole, sweetened, KAFU
10-1-120	牛奶 (巧克力味, 三元牌)	Milk, chocolate flavored, whole, sweetened, SANYUAN
10-1-121	学生奶	Milk, whole, sweetened, for Chinese students
奶粉		**COW'S MILK POWDER**
10-2-105	全脂奶粉 (雀巢)	Whole milk powder, NESTLE
10-2-106	全脂奶粉 (三鹿牌)	Whole milk powder, SANLU
10-2-107	全脂奶粉 (伊利牌)	Whole milk powde, YILI, no sucrose, vitamins enriched
10-2-108	全脂甜奶粉 (三鹿牌)	Whole milk powder, sugar added, SANLU

编码 Code	食物名称 Food name	英文名称 English name
10-2-109	全脂甜奶粉 (伊利牌)	Whole milk powder, sugar added, instantly soluble, vitamins enriched, YILI
10-2-110	低脂奶粉 (高钙高铁, 雀巢)	Milk powder, semi-skimmed, enriched with calcium and iron, NESTLE
10-2-111	低脂奶粉 (高钙高铁, 伊利牌)	Milk powder, semi-skimmed, enriched with calcium and iron, YILI
10-2-112	高钙高铁奶粉 (可淇牌)	Milk powder, enriched with calcium and iron, KOCCI
10-2-113	儿童奶粉 (安儿健 A+, 美赞臣)	Formula milk powder, MEAD JOHNSON ENFAKID A+, for children 3~6 years old
10-2-114	儿童奶粉 (适体健, 美赞臣)	Formula milk powder, MEAD JOHNSON SUSTAGEN KID, vanilla flavor, for children more than 3 years old
10-2-115	儿童奶粉 (惠氏)	Formula milk powder, WYETH S-26 PROMISE GOLD, for children 3~7 years old
10-2-116	儿童奶粉 (可淇牌)	Formula milk powder, KOCCI, for children more than 3 years old
10-2-117	儿童奶粉 (三鹿牌)	Formula milk powder, SANLU, for children
10-2-118	儿童奶粉 (完达山牌)	Formula milk powder, WONDERSUN 3, for children 3~6 years old
10-2-119	孕妇乳母奶粉 (惠氏)	Formula milk powder, WYETH S-26 MAMA, for pregnant and lactating women, vanilla flavor
10-2-120	孕妇乳母奶粉 (美赞臣)	Formula milk powder, MEAD JOHNSON ENFAMAMA, for pregnant and lactating women
10-2-121	中老年奶粉 (可淇牌)	Formula milk powder, KOCCI, for middle-aged and elderly people
10-2-122	中老年奶粉 (雀巢)	Formula milk powder, NESTLE OMEGA, for middle-aged and elderly people
10-2-123	中老年奶粉 (三鹿牌)	Formula milk powder, SANLU, for middle-aged and elderly people
10-2-124	中老年奶粉 (森永牌)	Formula milk powder, MORINAGA, for middle-aged and elderly people
酸奶		**YOGURT**
10-3-007	酸奶 (调味)	Yogurt, whole milk, with sugar
10-3-008	酸奶 (果粒)	Yogurt, whole milk, with fruits
奶酪		**CHEESE**
10-4-012	奶酪 (光明牌)	Cheese, BRIGHT
10-4-013	奶酪 (骑士牌)	Cheese, CHIS
10-4-014	低脂奶酪	Cheese, semi-skimmed
10-4-015	硬质干酪	Cheese, hard, average
奶油		**CREAM**
10-5-008	奶油	Cream, full fat
其它		**OTHERS**
10-9-004	全脂甜炼乳 (雀巢)	Condensed whole milk, sweetened, NESTLE
10-9-005	全脂甜炼乳 (燕山牌)	Condensed whole milk, sweetened, YANSHAN
10-9-006	脱脂甜炼乳	Condensed milk, skimmed and sweetened

编码 Code	食物名称 Food name	英文名称 English name
	蛋类及制品	**EGGS and EGG PRODUCTS**
鸡蛋		**HEN EGG**
11-1-109	鸡蛋 (红皮)	Egg, hen, brown shell, whole, raw
11-1-110	藏鸡蛋	Egg, Tibetan hen, whole, raw
11-1-111	乌鸡蛋 (绿皮)	Egg, black-boned hen, whole, raw
11-1-204	鸡蛋 (煮)	Egg, hen, whole, boiled
11-1-205	毛蛋	Egg, hen, hatched, whole, raw
11-1-206	荷包蛋 (油煎)	Egg, hen, fried, shell removed
11-1-207	荷包蛋 (煮)	Egg, hen, poached, shell removed
鸭蛋		**DUCK EGG**
11-2-104	海鸭蛋	Egg, sea duck, whole, raw
11-2-203	咸鸭蛋 (煮)	Egg, duck, whole, salt preserved, boiled
鹅蛋		**GOOSE EGG**
11-3-104	鹅蛋 (煮)	Egg, goose, whole, boiled
	鱼虾蟹贝类	**FISH, SHELLFISH and MOLLUSC**
鱼		**FISH**
12-1-131	草鱼 [白鲩、草包鱼]	Grass carp, white, freshwater, raw
12-1-132	鲢鱼 [白鲢、胖子、连子鱼]	Silver carp, freshwater, raw
12-1-133	鲫鱼 [喜头鱼、海附鱼]	Goldfish carp, freshwater, raw
12-1-241	带鱼 (切段)	Hairtail or beltfish, marine, segmented, frozen, raw
12-1-242	黄鱼 (小黄花鱼)	Yellow croaker, red lip, small, marine, raw
12-1-243	金鳇鱼	—
12-1-244	鲭鱼	Mackerel, chub, marine, raw
12-1-245	双髻鲨	Shovel-nosed shark, marine, raw
12-1-303	金鲨鱼翅 (干)	Shark fin, dried
12-1-304	鱼排	White fish fillet, mixed with bread crumbs, starch and salt, frozen, raw
12-1-305	鱼丸	Fish ball, mashed with starch, salt and sugar, frozen, raw
12-1-306	鱼子酱	Caviar
12-1-401	草鱼 (熏)	Grass carp, smoked and cooked with oil, salt and wine, etc., canned
12-1-402	丁香鱼 (香辣味)	Anchovy, fried, savory, canned
12-1-403	凤尾鱼 (熟)	Estuarine tapertail anchovy, fried, canned
12-1-404	箭鱼 (炸)	Swordfish, fried, canned
12-1-405	金枪鱼 (盐水浸)	Tuna, canned in brine, drained

编码 Code	食物名称 Food name	英文名称 English name
12-1-406	金枪鱼（油浸）	Tuna, canned in oil, drained
12-1-407	鲮鱼（豆豉，熟）	Dace, fried, with salted black bean, canned
12-1-408	鳗鱼（红烧）	Ell, barbecued with oil, sugar and salt, etc.
12-1-409	鲭鱼（烤，150℃，10分）	Mackerel, baked, 150℃ for 10min, flesh only
12-1-410	鲭鱼（烤，150℃，20分）	Mackerel, baked, 150℃ for 20min, flesh only
12-1-411	鲭鱼（烤，150℃，30分）	Mackerel, baked, 150℃ for 30min, flesh only
12-1-412	鲭鱼（烤，180℃，10分）	Mackerel, baked, 180℃ for 10min, flesh only
12-1-413	鲭鱼（烤，210℃，10分）	Mackerel, baked, 210℃ for 10min, flesh only
12-1-414	鲭鱼（炸）	Mackerel, fried in salad oil, 180℃ for 3min, flesh only
12-1-415	鲭鱼（蒸）	Mackerel, steamed, 100℃ for 10min, flesh only
12-1-416	鲭鱼（煮）	Mackerel, boiled, 100℃ for 10min, flesh only
12-1-417	沙丁鱼（茄汁，熟）	Sardine, canned in tomato sauce
12-1-418	沙丁鱼（盐水浸）	Sardine, canned in brine, drained
12-1-419	沙丁鱼（油浸）	Sardine, canned in oil, drained
12-1-420	午餐鱼（香辣味）	*Luncheon fish*, round scad, cooked with salad oil, salt and sugar, etc., savory, canned
12-1-421	鳕鱼（烤）	Cod, spread with butter, baked
12-1-422	鳕鱼（炸）	Cod, in crumbs, frozen, pre-fried in oil
虾		**PRAWN and SHRIMP**
12-2-203	虾酱	Shrimp paste
12-2-204	虾仁（红）	Prawn, flesh, red, frozen, no shell, raw
12-2-301	虾仁肉丸	Pork and shrimp meat ball, mashed, cooked then frozen
蟹		**CRAB**
12-3-006	海蟹（小）	Sea crab, small, frozen, front shell removed, raw
12-3-301	蟹足棒	Crab stick, crab meat mixed with starch, salt and sugar, frozen, raw
贝		**SHELLFISH**
12-4-117	海蚌［西施舌］	Coelomactra antiquata, marine, raw
12-4-601	文蛤丸	*Wen*clam meat ball, mashed with starch, raw
其它		**OTHERS**
12-9-014	甲鱼蛋	Turtle egg, raw
12-9-301	墨鱼圈	Cuttlefish ring, mashed, frozen, raw
12-9-302	墨鱼丸	Cuttlefish meat ball, mashed, frozen, raw

编码 Code	食物名称 Food name	英文名称 English name
	婴幼儿食品	**INFANT FOODS**
婴幼儿配方粉		**INFANT FORMULAS**
13-1-101	婴儿配方奶粉(爱儿乐, 惠氏)	Infant formula milk powder, WYETH S-26 SMA, for infants 0~6 months old
13-1-102	婴儿配方奶粉(爱儿乐, 惠氏, 金装)	Infant formula milk powder, WYETH S-26 SMA GOLD, for infants 0~6 months old
13-1-103	婴儿配方奶粉(爱力大1, 美赞臣)	Infant formula milk powder, MEAD JOHNSON ALCTA 1, for infants 0~12 months old
13-1-104	婴儿配方奶粉(安婴儿, 美赞臣)	Infant formula milk powder, MEAD JOHNSON ENFAMIL, for infants 0~12 months old
13-1-105	婴儿配方奶粉(安婴儿A+, 美赞臣)	Infant formula milk powder, MEAD JOHNSON ENFAMIL A+, for infants 0~12 months old
13-1-106	婴儿配方奶粉(安婴乐, 美赞臣)	Infant formula milk powder, MEAD JOHNSON ENFOLAC, for infants 0~12 months old
13-1-107	婴儿配方奶粉(吉利蜜1, 森永牌)	Infant formula milk powder, MORINAGA, for infants 0~6 months old
13-1-108	婴儿配方奶粉(可淇牌)	Infant formula milk powder, KOCCI, for infants 0~6 months old
13-1-109	婴儿配方奶粉(力多精1, 雀巢)	Infant formula milk powder, NESTLE LACTOGEN 1, iron enriched, for infants 0~6 months old
13-1-110	婴儿配方奶粉(美素力1)	Infant formula milk powder, FRISOCARE FRISOLAC 1, for infants 0~6 months old
13-1-111	婴儿配方奶粉(美素力H)	Infant formula milk powder, FRISOCARE FRISOLAC H, for infants 0~6 months old
13-1-112	婴儿配方奶粉(美素力, 袋装)	Infant formula milk powder, FRISOCARE FRISOLAC, for infants 0~6 months old
13-1-113	婴儿配方奶粉(圣元牌)	Infant formula milk powder, SAINT U-SMART 1, for infants 0~6 months old
13-1-114	婴儿配方奶粉(完达山牌)	Infant formula milk powder, WONDERSUN 1, for infants 0~6 months old
13-1-115	婴儿奶粉(高钙, 圣元牌)	Infant formula milk powder, calcium enriched, SAINT, for infants 0~6 months old
13-1-116	婴儿配方豆粉(爱儿素, 惠氏)	Infant formula soybean milk powder, WYETH S-26 NURSOY
13-1-201	较大婴儿配方奶粉(爱力大2, 美赞臣)	Formula milk powder, MEAD JOHNSON ALCTA 2, for infants 6~12 months old
13-1-202	较大婴儿配方奶粉(安婴宝, 美赞臣)	Formula milk powder, MEAD JOHNSON ENFAPRO, for infants 6~12 months old
13-1-203	较大婴儿配方奶粉(安婴宝A+, 美赞臣)	Formula milk powder, MEAD JOHNSON ENFAPRO A+, for infants 6~12 months old
13-1-204	较大婴儿配方奶粉(健儿乐, 惠氏)	Infant formula milk powder, S-26 WYETH PROMIL, for infants 6~12 months old
13-1-205	较大婴儿配方奶粉(健儿乐, 惠氏, 金装)	Infant formula milk powder, S-26 WYETH PROMIL GOLD, for infants 6~12 months old
13-1-206	较大婴儿配方奶粉(可淇牌)	Formula milk powder, KOCCI, for infants 6~12 months old

编码 Code	食物名称 Food name	英文名称 English name
13-1-207	较大婴儿配方奶粉(美素乐2)	Infant formula milk powder, FRISOCARE FRISOMEL 2, for infants 6~12 months old
13-1-208	较大婴儿配方奶粉(美素乐，全能装)	Formula milk powder, FRISOCARE FRISOMEL, for infants 6~12 months old
13-1-209	较大婴儿配方奶粉(美素乐，袋装)	Infant formula milk powder, FRISOCARE FRISOMEL, for infants 6~12 months old
13-1-210	较大婴幼儿配方奶粉(吉利蜜2，森永牌)	Infant formula milk powder, MORINAGA , for infants 6~36 months old
13-1-211	较大婴幼儿配方奶粉(力多精2，雀巢)	Infant formula milk powder, NESTLE LACTOGEN 2, for infants more than 6 months old
13-1-212	较大婴儿配方奶粉(圣元牌)	Infant formula milk powder, SAINT U-SMART 2, for infants 6~12 months old
13-1-213	较大婴幼儿奶粉(高钙，圣元牌)	Infant formula milk powder, calcium enriched, SAINT, for infants 6~36 months old
13-1-214	较大婴幼儿配方奶粉(完达山牌)	Infant formula milk powder, WONDERSUN 2, for infants 6~36 months old
13-1-301	幼儿奶粉(爱力大3，美赞臣)	Infant formula milk powder, MEAD JOHNSON ALCTA 3, for infants more than 12 months old
13-1-302	幼儿奶粉(安儿宝，美赞臣)	Infant formula milk powder, protein enriched, MEAD JOHNSON ENFAGROW, for infants more than 12 months old
13-1-303	幼儿奶粉(安儿宝A+，美赞臣)	Infant formula milk powder, protein enriched, MEAD JOHNSON ENFAGROW A+, for infants more than 12 months old
13-1-304	幼儿奶粉(惠氏)	Infant formula milk powder, WYETH S-26 PROGRESS, for infants 12~36 months old
13-1-305	幼儿奶粉(惠氏，金装)	Infant formula milk powder, WYETH S-26 PROGRESS GOLD, for infants 12~36 months old
13-1-306	幼儿奶粉(可淇牌)	Infant formula milk powder, KOCCI, for infants 12~36 months old
13-1-307	幼儿奶粉(美素高)	Infant formula milk powder, FRISOCARE FRISOGROW, for infants 12~36 months old
13-1-308	幼儿奶粉(美素高，全能装)	Infant formula milk powder, FRISOCARE FRISOGROW, vanilla flavor, for infants 12~36 months old
13-1-309	幼儿奶粉(美素高，袋装)	Infant formula milk powder, FRISOCARE FRISOGROW, vanilla flavor, for infants 12~36 months old
13-1-310	幼儿奶粉(雀巢)	Infant formula milk powder, NESTLE NESLAC
13-1-311	幼儿奶粉(雀巢金牌)	Infant formula milk powder, NESTLE PREMIUM NESLAC
13-1-312	幼儿奶粉(森永牌)	Infant formula milk powder, MORINAGA, for infants more than 12 months old
13-1-313	幼儿奶粉(圣元牌)	Infant formula milk powder, SAINT U SMART 3, for infants 12~36 months old

编码 Code	食物名称 Food name	英文名称 English name
婴幼儿断乳期辅助食品		**FORMULATED WEANING FOODS**
13-2-001	胡萝卜苹果泥(亨氏)	Carrot and apple, mashed, HEINZ
13-2-002	鸡肝蔬菜泥(亨氏)	Potato, carrot and jackbean, mashed with chicken liver, HEINZ
13-2-003	香甜胡萝卜泥(亨氏)	Carrot, mashed, HEINZ
婴幼儿补充食品		**SUPPLEMENTARY FOODS**
13-3-009	米粉(雀巢)	Rice flour, NESTLE, for infants more than 6 months old
13-3-010	米粉(高蛋白, 雀巢)	Rice flour, protein enriched, NESTLE, for infants more than 6 months old
13-3-011	米粉(高蛋白, 亨氏)	Rice flour, enriched with protein, vitamin A and D, HEINZ
13-3-012	米粉(苹果, 雀巢)	Rice flour, apple added, NESTLE, for infants more than 6 months old
13-3-013	米粉(蔬菜, 亨氏)	Rice flour, milk powder, carrot and tomato, etc. added, HEINZ, for infants 6~24 months old
13-3-014	米粉(蔬菜, 雀巢)	Rice flour, tomato and spinach, etc. added, NESTLE, for infants more than 7 months old
13-3-015	米粉(胡萝卜, 亨氏)	Rice flour, carrot added, HEINZ, for infants 4~24 months old
13-3-016	米粉(胡萝卜, 雀巢)	Rice flour, carrot added, NESTLE, for infants more than 6 months old
13-3-017	米粉(番茄, 亨氏)	Rice flour, milk powder and tomato, etc. added, HEINZ, for infants 4~24 months old
13-3-018	米粉(猪肝蔬菜, 亨氏)	Rice flour, milk powder, pork liver, carrot and tomato, etc., added, HEINZ, for infants 6~24 months old
13-3-019	米粉(鱼肉蔬菜, 亨氏)	Rice flour, cod, carrot and tomato, etc. added, HEINZ, for infants 8~24 months old
13-3-020	麦粉(蜂蜜, 雀巢)	Wheat flour, honey and sugar added, NESTLE, for infants more than 6 months old
	小吃、甜饼	**ETHNIC FOODS and CAKES**
小吃		**ETHNIC FOODS**
14-1-038	春卷(素馅)	*Spring roll*, vegetarian, wheat flour skin, filled with cabbage, carrot and mushroom, etc., frozen, raw
14-1-039	黑芝麻汤圆	Dumpling, glutinous-rice flour case, filled with black sesame, peanut and sugar, etc., frozen, raw
14-1-040	醪糟	Glutinous rice steamed, mixed with water and sugar, fermented
14-1-041	煎饼	Foxtail millet pancake, made from wheat, corn and soybean flours, unleavened
14-1-042	过桥米线	Rice noodle, boiled, salt and other spices added, from YUNNAN

编码 Code	食物名称 Food name	英文名称 English name
蛋糕、甜点		**CAKES**
14-2-108	蛋糕(巧克力)	Cake, with chocolate flavored
14-2-109	蛋糕(水果)	Cake, with fruit
14-2-209	月饼(蛋黄)	*Mooncake*, filled with salted egg yolk and lotus seed paste
14-2-210	月饼(豆沙)	*Mooncake*, filled with adzuki bean paste
14-2-211	月饼(桂花板栗)	*Mooncake*, filled with chestnut and osmanthus flower
14-2-212	月饼(奶油莲芸)	*Mooncake*, filled with cream and lotus seed paste
14-2-332	沙琪玛蛋酥	Egg crisp, sachima
14-2-333	香橙水果馅饼	Fruit pie, orange flavour
	速食食品	**FAST FOODS**
快餐食品		**HANDY FOODS**
15-1-001	鸡柳汉堡(肯德基)	Hamburger, chicken, KENTUCKY
15-1-002	香芋甜心(肯德基)	Taro, in starch, sweetened and fried, KENTUCKY
15-1-003	鸡肉汉堡(肯德基)	Hamburger, chicken and vegetables, KENTUCKY
15-1-004	鸡肉卷(肯德基)	Chicken roll, steamed, KENTUCKY
15-1-005	上校鸡块(肯德基)	Chicken, fried, KENTUCKY
15-1-006	辣鸡翅(肯德基)	Chicken wing, fried, hot, KENTUCKY
15-1-007	新奥尔良鸡翅(肯德基)	Chicken wing, fried, KENTUCKY
15-1-008	劲爆鸡米花(肯德基)	Chicken dollop, fried, KENTUCKY
15-1-009	甜玉米籽粒(肯德基)	Corn grain, sweetened, baked, KENTUCKY
15-1-010	薯条(肯德基)	Potato bar, fried, KENTUCKY
15-1-011	比萨饼(夹奶酪)	Pizza with cheese
15-1-012	比萨饼(夹奶酪、肉和蔬菜)	Pizza with cheese, meat and vegetables
15-1-013	三明治(夹火腿、干酪)	Sandwich, with ham and cheese
15-1-014	三明治(夹鸡蛋、干酪)	Sandwich, with egg and cheese
15-1-015	三明治(夹鸡肉片, 无调料酱)	Sandwich, with chicken fillet, plain
15-1-016	三明治(夹烤牛肉片)	Sandwich, with roast beef fillet, plain
15-1-017	三明治(夹鱼肉片)	Sandwich, with fish fillet
15-1-018	干酪汉堡包(夹熏肉, 加调料酱)	Cheeseburger, large, single meat patty, with bacon and condiments
15-1-019	干酪汉堡包(普通型, 夹单层肉饼, 无调料酱)	Cheeseburger, regular, single meat patty, plain
15-1-020	干酪汉堡包(普通型, 夹奶酪、单层肉饼, 加调料酱)	Cheeseburger, regular, single meat patty, with condiments
15-1-021	干酪汉堡包(普通型, 夹奶酪、单层肉饼, 加调料酱和蔬菜)	Cheeseburger, regular, single meat patty, with condiments and vegetables

编码 Code	食物名称 Food name	英文名称 English name
15-1-022	干酪汉堡包(普通型，夹奶酪、双层肉饼、双层面包，加调料酱和蔬菜)	Cheeseburger, regular, double meat patty, double-decker bun, with condiments and vegetables
15-1-023	汉堡包(普通型，夹肉饼，加调料酱和蔬菜)	Hamburger, regular, single meat patty, with condiments and vegetables
15-1-024	热狗(原味)	Hotdog, plain
方便食品		**CONVENIENCE FOODS**
15-2-105	早餐奶	Milk, for breakfast, wheat flakes and hen egg added
15-2-106	八宝粥(康师傅牌)	*Eight treasure* congee, canned, with glutinous rice, adlay, wheat, adzuki bean, peanut, longan and silver ear fungus, etc., sweetened, MR. KON
15-2-107	八宝粥(亲亲牌)	*Eight treasure* congee, canned, with glutinous rice, adlay, wheat, adzuki bean, mung bean, peanut and longan, etc., sweetened, QINQIN
15-2-108	八宝粥(同茂牌)	*Eight treasure* congee, canned, with glutinous rice, wheat, adzuki bean, mung bean, peanut and longan, etc., sweetened, TONGMAO
15-2-109	八宝粥(娃哈哈牌)	*Eight treasure* congee, canned, with glutinous rice, adlay, adzuki bean, silver ear fungus, lotus seed and longan, etc., sweetened, WAHAHA
15-2-110	八宝粥(无糖，娃哈哈牌)	*Eight treasure* congee, canned, with glutinous rice, adlay, adzuki bean, peanut, silver ear fungus, lotus seed and arum, etc., unsweetened, WAHAHA
15-2-111	八宝粥(椰树牌)	*Eight treasure* congee, canned, with glutinous rice, adlay, adzuki bean, mung bean, peanut, longan and date, etc., sweetened, YESHU
15-2-112	黑芝麻糊粉	Black sesame powder, mixed with black rice, peanut and walnut powder, etc.
15-2-113	麦片	Wheat flake, with millet, corn, etc.
15-2-114	麦片(原味香奶)	Wheat flake, with milk powder
15-2-115	燕麦片	Oatmeal flake
15-2-116	燕麦片(果仁，甜)	Oatmeal flake, nuts added, sweetened
15-2-117	苦荞麦片(无糖)	Buckwheat flake, no sugar
15-2-118	玉米片	Corn flake
15-2-119	玉米片(低钠)	Corn flake, low sodium
15-2-202	鸡汁味干脆面(面饼+调味料)	Instant crisp noodle, with chicken soup flavor, condiments added
15-2-203	海鲜味方便面(面饼+调味料+油料)	Instant wheat noodle, with sea food flavor, condiments and oil added
15-2-204	海鲜味方便面(面饼+调味料)	Instant wheat noodle, with sea food flavor, condiments added
15-2-205	油料(海鲜味方便面)	Oil packet, for instant wheat noodle with sea food flavor
15-2-206	红烧牛肉方便面(面饼+调味料+蔬菜+肉酱)	Instant wheat noodle, with braised beef flavor, condiments, vegetable and beef paste added
15-2-207	红烧牛肉方便面(面饼+调味料+蔬菜)	Instant wheat noodle, with braised beef flavor, condiments and vegetable added
15-2-208	肉酱(红烧牛肉方便面)	Beef paste, for instant wheat noodle with braised beef flavor

编码 Code	食物名称 Food name	英文名称 English name
15-2-209	鳕鱼方便面 (面饼 + 调味料 + 珍料 + 调味油 + 蔬菜)	Instant wheat noodle, with cod fish flavor, condiments, cod paste, vegetable and oil
15-2-210	鳕鱼方便面 (面饼 + 调味料 + 蔬菜)	Instant wheat noodle, with cod fish flavor, condiments and vegetable added
15-2-211	油酱料 (珍料 + 调味油料，鳕鱼方便面)	Oil and cod paste, for instant wheat noodle with cod fish flavor
15-2-212	铁板牛肉炒面 (面饼 + 汤料 + 蔬菜 + 调味酱)	Instant stir-fried wheat noodle, with baked beef flavour, condiments, vegetable and beef paste added
15-2-213	铁板牛肉炒面 (面饼 + 汤料 + 蔬菜)	Instant stir-fried wheat noodle, with baked beef flavour, condiments and vegetable added
15-2-214	调味酱 (铁板牛肉炒面)	Beef paste, for instant stir-fried wheat noodle with baked beef flavor
15-2-215	玉米红烧牛肉味方便面 (面饼 + 调味料 + 蔬菜 + 肉酱)	Instant corn noodle, with braised beef flavor, condiments, vegetable and beef paste added
15-2-216	玉米红烧牛肉味方便面 (面饼 + 调味料 + 蔬菜)	Instant corn noodle, with braised beef flavor, condiments and vegetable added
15-2-217	肉酱 (玉米红烧牛肉味方便面)	Beef paste, for instant corn noodle with braised beef flavor
15-2-218	海鲜鸡汁味米线 (米线 + 调味料 + 蔬菜 + 肉酱)	Instant rice noodle, with seafood and chicken soup flavor, condiments, vegetable, and chicken and shrimp paste added
15-2-219	海鲜鸡汁味米线 (米线 + 调味料 + 蔬菜)	Instant rice noodle, with seafood and chicken soup flavor, condiments and vegetable added
15-2-220	肉酱 (海鲜鸡汁味米线)	Chicken and shrimp paste, for instant rice noodle with seafood and chicken soup flavor
15-2-221	冬菜虾仁馄饨	Dumpling, wheat flour dough, filled with shrimp, fish, vegetables and salt, boiled then frozen
15-2-222	韭菜合子	Dumpling, wheat flour dough, filled with chinese chives, salt, etc., fried
15-2-223	糯米饭团	Glutinous rice lumps, steamed, filled with pork floss and vegetables
15-2-224	什锦炒饭	Long grained rice steamed, mixed with ham, vegetables, frozen, for frying
15-2-225	虾仁炒饭	Long grained rice steamed, mixed with shrimp flesh and vegetables, frozen, for frying
15-2-314	面包条 (白)	Bread loaf, white
15-2-315	面包屑	Bread crumbs
15-2-316	葡萄干面包	Bread, raisin added
15-2-415	饼干 (三明治)	Biscuit, sandwich, custard filled, LEZHI
15-2-416	饼干 (夹心)	Biscuit, sandwich, custard filled, DANONE
15-2-417	饼干 (甜酥夹心)	Cracker, sandwich, lemon custard filled
15-2-418	饼干 (苏打夹心)	Soda cracker
15-2-419	饼干 (咸)	Biscuit, salted
15-2-420	曲奇饼 (加奶油)	Cookies, cream added
15-2-421	早茶饼	*Morning tea* biscuit, wheat flour, oil, sugar, milk powder, salt added
15-2-501	饺子 (素馅)	Dumpling, wheat flour, filled with vegetables, wood ear fungus, egg, oil and salt added, frozen, raw

编码 Code	食物名称 Food name	英文名称 English name
15-2-502	饺子(三鲜馅)	Dumpling, wheat flour, filled with shrimp, wood ear fungus, egg or pork, oil and salt added, frozen, raw
15-2-503	饺子(猪肉白菜馅)	Dumpling, wheat flour, filled with pork, Chinese cabbage, oil and salt added, frozen, raw
15-2-504	饺子(猪肉韭菜馅)	Dumpling, wheat flour, filled with pork, Chinese chive, oil and salt added, frozen, raw
15-2-505	饺子(猪肉芹菜馅)	Dumpling, wheat flour, filled with pork, celery, oil and salt added, frozen, raw
15-2-506	饺子(猪肉茴香馅)	Dumpling, wheat flour, filled with pork, fennel, oil and salt added, frozen, raw
15-2-507	饺子(猪肉香菇馅)	Dumpling, wheat flour, filled with pork, shiitake mushroom, cod, frozen, raw
15-2-508	饺子(猪肉虾仁馅)	Dumpling, wheat flour, filled with pork, shrimp, stiitake mushroom, frozen, raw
15-2-509	饺子(鸡肉蘑菇馅)	Dumpling, wheat flour, filled with chicken, pork, mushroom, frozen, raw
15-2-510	饺子(海鳗猪肉馅)	Dumpling, wheat flour, filled with eel, pork, frozen, raw
15-2-511	饺子(海鳗虾仁馅)	Dumpling, wheat flour, filled with eel, shrimp, pork, frozen, raw
15-2-512	包子(三鲜馅)	Steamed bun, filled with shrimp, wood ear fungus, egg or pork, oil and salt added, frozen, raw
15-2-513	包子(猪肉馅)	Steamed bun, filled with pork, oil and salt added, frozen, raw
休闲食品		**SNACKS**
15-3-101	米饼(鸡蛋牛奶味)	Rice cake, oil, sugar and salt added, egg and milk flavored
15-3-102	雪米饼	Rice cracker
15-3-103	蛋酥卷	Egg roll, crispy
15-3-104	巧克力派	Chocolate pie
15-3-105	法式卷饼	Roll pie, French style
15-3-106	立体脆	Corn crispy ball
15-3-107	粟米脆	Corn chip crispy, with oil and salt
15-3-108	通心脆	Crispy chip, potato slab, with oil and potato flour
15-3-109	洋葱圈	Crispy roll, wheat flour, onion flavored
15-3-201	虾片	Cracker, shrimp
15-3-202	锅巴(豆香)	Rice chips, soybean flour added
15-3-203	锅巴(小米)	Millet crisps
15-3-204	海苔	Seaweed, flavored
15-3-205	香菇片	Oak mushroom chips
15-3-206	薯片(烧烤味)	Potato chips, barbecued flavor
15-3-207	薯片(香辣味)	Potato chips, hot and spicy
15-3-208	薯圈	Potato ring, crispy
15-3-301	怪味胡豆	Broad bean, roasted with sugar, oil and salt
15-3-302	奶油五香豆	Broad bean, roasted with sugar and salt, cream flavor
15-3-303	夹心米果	Rice pie, custard filled
15-3-304	乐芙球	Mini puff ball, wheat flour mixed with milk and egg powder, oil and sugar

编码 Code	食物名称 Food name	英文名称 English name
15-3-305	玉米花	Popcorn, mixed with oil and salt, edible upon heating
15-3-306	果仁脆枣	Crispy dates, with nuts
15-3-307	空心脆枣	Crispy dates, core removed
15-3-308	鱼肉粒	Salmon grain, mixed with wheat flour, soybean powder and sugar
15-3-401	果冻 (草莓水果冻)	Jelly, strawberry flavor
15-3-402	果冻 (蒟蒻冻)	Jelly, coconut flavor, PO-LI
15-3-403	果冻 (蒟蒻椰果冻)	Jelly, coconut flavor, LIUCHUAN
15-3-404	果冻 (AD 钙果冻)	Jelly, calcium, vitamin A and D fortified
	饮料类	**BEVERAGES**
碳酸饮料		**CARBONATED DRINKS**
16-1-009	可口可乐	Cola, carbonated, contains caffeine
果汁及果汁饮料		**FRUIT JUICES and FRUIT FLAVOURED DRINKS**
16-2-012	菠萝汁饮料 (百果洲牌)	Pineapple juice, BAIGUOZHOU
16-2-013	菠萝汁饮料 (大湖牌)	Pineapple juice, GREAT LAKE
16-2-014	苹果汁饮料 (光明牌)	Apple juice, BRIGHT
16-2-015	苹果汁饮料 (亨氏)	Apple juice, HEINZ
16-2-016	苹果果肉饮料	Apple juice, with flesh
16-2-017	橙汁饮料 (光明牌)	Orange juice, BRIGHT
16-2-018	橙汁饮料 (茹梦牌)	Orange juice, ZIPU
16-2-019	橙汁饮料 (汇源牌)	Orange juice, HUIYUAN
16-2-020	橙汁饮料 (三得利牌)	Orange juice, SANDELI
16-2-021	芒果汁饮料	Mango juice
16-2-022	沙棘果浆	Sea buckthorn berry juice, with flesh
16-2-023	山楂果肉饮料	Hawthorn juice, with flesh
16-2-024	酸枣果汁饮料	Wild spine date juice
16-2-025	西番莲汁饮料	Passionflower juice
16-2-026	西柚汁饮料	Grapefruit juice
16-2-027	椰子汁饮料	Coconut juice
16-2-028	杏仁椰汁饮料	Coconut juice, almond juice added
蔬菜汁饮料		**VEGETABLE JUCES and DRINKS**
16 3 002	胡萝卜汁饮料	Carrot juice
含乳饮料		**MILK DRINKS**
16-4-003	AD 钙奶	Milk drink, vitamin A, D enriched, YESHU
16-4-004	健康快车奶饮料	Milk drink, vitamin A, D enriched

编码 Code	食物名称 Food name	英文名称 English name
16-4-005	粒粒果奶饮料	Milk drink, vitamin A, D enriched
16-4-006	酸乳饮料	Yogurt drink, sweetened
16-4-007	酸乳饮料 (发酵)	Yogurt drink, with actobacillus, sweetened
植物蛋白饮料		**VEGETABLE PROTEIN DRINKS**
16-5-003	核桃乳 (儿童型)	Walnut juice, for children
16-5-004	核桃乳 (女性型)	Walnut juice, for women
16-5-005	核桃乳 (中老年型)	Walnut juice, for middle-aged and elderly people
16-5-006	核桃乳 (佐餐调和型)	Walnut juice, for cooking
16-5-007	杏仁露	Almond juice
茶叶及茶饮料		**TEA and TEA BEVERAGES**
16-6-111	大麦茶	Tea, green, mixed with roasted broom rice
16-6-202	大麦茶水	Green tea and roasted broom rice mixed, infusion
固体饮料		**POWDERED BEVERAGES**
16-7-011	高乐高营养饮品	Beverage, Cola Cao, in powder
16-7-012	菓珍	Beverage, Tang, in powder
16-7-013	桂花酸梅晶	Bayberry beverage, in crystal, with osmanthus flower powder and hawthorn berry crystal
16-7-014	柠檬茶	Lemon tea, instant powder, sweetened, lemon flavor
16-7-015	巧克力麦芽营养饮品	Cocoa malted beverage, in powder, milk and cocoa added
16-7-016	咖啡豆	Coffee bean
16-7-017	咖啡粉	Coffee, instant, regular, powder
16-7-018	咖啡伴侣	Coffee mate
冰激凌、棒冰类		**ICE CREAM and POPSICLES**
16-8-009	冰激凌 (草莓味)	Ice cream, strawberry flavor
16-8-010	冰激凌 (苦咖啡味)	Ice cream, coffee flavor
16-8-011	冰激凌 (加奶油)	Ice cream, butter added
16-8-012	冰激凌 (草莓圣代)	Ice cream, strawberry sauce added
16-8-013	冰激凌 (巧克力圣代)	Ice cream, chocolate sauce added
16-8-014	冰激凌 (脆皮甜筒)	Ice cream, crispy cone
16-8-015	冰激凌 (花心筒)	Ice cream, cone
16-8-016	冰激凌 (金百合)	Ice cream, *Jinbaihe*
16-8-017	雪糕 (百乐宝)	Ice cream bar, *Bailebao*
16-8-018	雪糕 (红豆缘)	Ice cream bar, *Hongdouyuan*, adzuki bean powder added
16-8-019	棒冰 (可乐冰)	Popsicle, *Cola*
16-8-020	棒冰 (奇彩旋)	Popsicle, *Qicaixuan*

编码 Code	食物名称 Food name	英文名称 English name
其它		**OTHERS**
16-9-002	纯净水 (康师傅牌)	Bottled water, distilled, MR. KON
16-9-003	纯净水 (乐百氏牌)	Bottled water, distilled, ROBUST
16-9-004	纯净水 (娃哈哈牌)	Bottled water, distilled, WAHAHA
16-9-005	纯净水 (椰树牌)	Bottled water, distilled, YESHU
16-9-006	饮用水 (农夫山泉牌)	Natrual water, NONGFUSPRING
16-9-007	饮用水 (雀巢)	Bottled water, NESTLE
16-9-008	矿泉水 (获特满牌)	Natural mineral water, WATERMAN
16-9-009	矿泉水 (康师傅牌)	Natural mineralized water, MR. KON
16-9-010	矿泉水 (蓝涧牌)	Natural mineral water, LANJIAN
16-9-011	矿泉水 (乐百氏牌)	Natural mineral water, ROBUST
16-9-012	矿泉水 (雀巢)	Natural mineral water, NESTLE
16-9-013	矿泉水 (椰树牌)	Natural mineral water, YESHU
	含酒精饮料	**LIQOUR and ALCOHOLIC BEVERAGES**
发酵酒		**FERMENTED ALCOHOLIC BEVERAGES**
17-1-115	啤酒 (4.3%, 青岛牌)	Beer, QINGDAO, alcohol 4.3%
17-1-116	啤酒 (4%, 燕京牌)	Beer, YANJING, alcohol 4%
17-1-117	啤酒 (5.1%, 生力牌)	Beer, SHENGLI, alcohol 5.1%
17-1-205	葡萄酒 (干白, 11%, 长城牌)	Wine, white, dry, grape, GREAT WALL, alcohol 11%
17-1-206	葡萄酒 (干白, 12%, 张裕牌)	Wine, white, dry, grape, ZHANGYU, alcohol 12%
17-1-207	葡萄酒 (半干白, 11.5%, 王朝牌)	Wine, white semi-dry, grape, alcohol 11.5%
17-1-208	葡萄酒 (干红, 11.5%, 长城牌)	Wine, red, dry, grape, GREAT WALL, alcohol 11.5%
17-1-209	葡萄酒 (干红, 11.5%, 王朝牌)	Wine, red, dry, grape, WANGCHAO, alcohol 11.5%
17-1-210	葡萄酒 (干红, 12%, 张裕牌)	Wine, red, dry, grape, ZHANGYU, alcohol 12%
17-1-211	黑加仑酒 (8%)	Wine, black currant, alcohol 8%
17-1-212	雪利酒	Sherry, medium
17-1-309	花雕酒 (16.5%)	Rice wine, HUADIAO, alcohol 16.5%
蒸馏酒		**LIQUORS**
17-2-127	董酒 (浓香型, 46%)	Liquor, DONGJIU, alcohol 46%
17-2-128	二锅头 (56%)	Liquor, twice distilled, ERGUOTOU, alcohol 56%
17-2-129	汾酒 (清香型, 53%)	Liquor, FENJIU, alcohol 53%
17-2-130	古井贡酒 (浓香型, 38%)	Liquor, GUJINGGONG, alcohol 38%
17-2-131	剑南春 (52%)	Liquor, JIANNANCHUN, alcohol 52%
17-2-132	剑南春 (浓香型, 38%)	Liquor, JIANNANCHUN, alcohol 38%
17-2-133	京酒 (浓香型, 38%)	Liquor, JINGJIU, alcohol 38%

编码 Code	食物名称 Food name	英文名称 English name
17-2-134	茅台酒 (53%)	Liquor, MAOTAI, alcohol 53%
17-2-135	五粮液 (52%)	Liquor, WULIANGYE, alcohol 52%
17-2-136	竹叶青酒 (45%)	Liquor, ZHUYEQING, alcohol 45%
17-2-137	金奖白兰地 (38%)	Brandy, alcohol 38%
17-2-138	伏特加	Vodka, distilled, 80 proof
17-2-139	威士忌	Whiskey, distilled, 86 proof
露酒		**CORDIALS**
17-3-105	苹果酒 (干型)	Apple cider, dry
17-3-106	苹果酒 (甜)	Apple cider, sweet
17-3-107	果汁朗姆酒 (9.9%)	Cocktail, pina colada, alcohol 9.9%
17-3-108	鸡尾酒	Cocktail, bourbon and soda
17-3-109	马提尼酒 (32%)	Martini, prepared from recipe, alcohol 32%
17-3-110	曼哈顿酒 (30.6%)	Cocktail, manhattan, alcohol 30.6%
17-3-111	酸味威士忌 (16.8%)	Whiskey sour, canned, alcohol 16.8%
	糖、果脯和蜜饯、蜂蜜	**SUGARS, PRESERVES and HONEYS**
糖果		**CONFECTIONERY**
18-2-101	夹心糖	Fruit flavored candy
18-2-102	水果味软糖	Jelly candy
18-2-201	牛奶糖	Milk candy
18-2-202	酸奶软糖	Jelly candy, yogurt flavor
18-2-203	太妃糖	Toffee candy
18-2-301	花生牛轧糖	Candy, coated with peanuts
18-2-302	花生芝麻糖	Candy, coated with sesames and peanuts
18-2-303	四味粽子糖	Candy, with nuts
18-2-401	巧克力 (充气)	Chocolate, filled with air
18-2-402	巧克力 (果仁)	Chocolate, with nuts
18-2-403	巧克力 (黑)	Dark chocolate
18-2-404	巧克力 (牛奶)	Milk chocolate
果脯和蜜饯		**PRESERVES**
18-3-012	冰糖酸角	Tamarind pulp, preserved with rock sugar
18-3-013	甘草杏	Apricot, preserved with sugar, salt and licorice
18-3-014	清凉杏肉	Apricot, preserved with sugar, only flesh
18-3-015	雪梅	Apricot, yellow, preserved with salt and licorice
18-3-016	九制梅肉	Plum, preserved with sugar and salt, only flesh
18-3-017	九制西梅	Plum, preserved with sugar, salt and licorice

编码 Code	食物名称 Food name	英文名称 English name
18-3-018	九制应子	Plum, preserved with sugar, salt and licorice
18-3-019	梅脯	Plum, preserved with sugar, only flesh
18-3-020	阿胶枣	*Ajiao* jujube
18-3-021	黑贡枣	Dateplum persimmon, core removed, preserved with sugar and honey
18-3-022	野酸枣	Wild spine date, preserved with sugar
18-3-023	多味山楂	Hawthorn slices, spiced
18-3-024	山楂脯	Hawthorn, preserved with sugar
18-3-025	地瓜干	Sweet potato, boiled and sliced, seasoned
蜂蜜		**HONEYS**
18-4-001	蜂蜜	Honey
18-4-002	蜂蜜 (槐花)	Honey, from Chinese scholar tree flower
18-4-003	蜂蜜 (天麻)	Honey, from tall gastrodia tuber
18-4-004	蜂蜜 (硬蜜)	Honey, from rugulose elsholtzia flower
18-4-005	蜂蜜 (油菜花)	Honey, from rape flower
	油脂类	**FATS and OILS**
植物油		**PLANTS OILS**
19-2-020	核桃油	Walnut oil
19-2-021	花生油	Peanut oil
19-2-022	葵花子油	Sunflower seed oil
19-2-023	粟米油 [玉米胚芽油]	Corn oil
19-2-024	米糠油	Chaff oil
19-2-025	油茶籽油	Camellia oil
19-2-026	芝麻油 [香油]	Sesame oil
19-2-027	大豆色拉油	Soybean oil
19-2-028	色拉油	Salad oil
	调味品类	**CONDIMENTS**
酱油		**SAUCES**
20-1-011	黄豆酱油	Soy sauce
20-1-012	老抽	Soy sauce, dark
20-1-013	生抽	Soy sauce, light
酱		**SAUCES and PASTES**
20-3-116	海鲜酱 (阿香婆)	Seafood sauce, savory
20-3-117	牛肉酱 (阿香婆)	Beef sauce, savory
20-3-118	花生酱	Peanut butter

编码 Code	食物名称 Food name	英文名称 English name
20-3-119	花生酱 (加巧克力)	Peanut butter, chocolate added
20-3-120	芝麻酱	Sesame paste
20-3-121	千岛沙拉酱	Thousand island salad dressing, HELLMANN'S
20-3-122	沙拉酱	Salad dressing or mayonnaise, KEWPIE
20-3-123	奶油攀司	Cream paste
20-3-207	草莓酱	Strawberry jam
20-3-208	番茄沙司	Tomato sauce
腐乳		**FERMENTED SOYBEAN CURD**
20-4-006	腐乳 (香辣味)	Fermented soybean curd, salted, pungent, white
20-4-007	腐乳 (白, 石宝寨牌) [酱豆腐]	Fermented soybean curd, salted, white, SHIBAOZAI
20-4-008	腐乳 (白, 王致和牌) [酱豆腐]	Fermented soybean curd, salted, white, WANGZHIHE
咸菜类		**PICKLES**
20-5-036	剁辣椒	Pepper pieces, salt added
20-5-037	酱八宝菜	Mixed vegetables and kernels in soy sauce
20-5-038	酱甘露	Artichoke, in soy sauce
20-5-039	酱花生米	Peanut, in soy sauce
20-5-040	酱籽萝	Radish, preserved in soy sauce
20-5-041	麻仁金丝	Turnip sliver, mixed with kernels, sugar and ginger in soy sauce
20-5-042	雪菜	Crispifolia mustard greens, preserved with chillies and salt in vegetable oil
20-5-043	腌大头菜	Turnip, preserved in soy sauce
20-5-044	腌芥菜头	Radish, preserved in soy sauce and salted
20-5-045	腌韭菜花	Chinese chives flower, salted, seasoned
20-5-046	腌萝卜条	Radish, slabbed, preserved in soy sauce
20-5-047	榨菜 (鱼泉牌)	Mustard root, preserved with salt and chili powder in vegetable oil, YUQUAN
20-5-048	榨菜 (正林牌)	Mustard root, preserved with salt and chili powder in sesame oil, ZHENGLIN
香辛料		**SPICES**
20-6-011	咖喱粉	Curry powder
盐、味精及其它		**SALT and OTHERS**
20-7-202	鸡粉	Chicken bouillon, granulated, JIALE
20-7-203	鸡精	Chicken bouillon, granulated, MAGGII
20-7-401	料酒	Cooking wine
	其它	**OTHERS**
21-9-014	蜂蛹 [蜂胚、蜂仔]	—

续表

编码 Code	食物名称 Food name	英文名称 English name
21-9-015	蜂蛹 (油蜂)	—
21-9-016	蜂蛹 (大黄蜂)	—
21-9-017	葛根	Kudzu root
21-9-018	花椒叶 (干)	Chinese prickly ash, leaf, dried
21-9-019	花粉 (油菜)	Pollen, rape
21-9-020	花粉 (油松) [松花粉]	Pollen, pine
21-9-021	花粉 (荞麦)	Pollen, buckwheat
21-9-022	牛蛙	Bull frog, raw
21-9-023	仙人掌 (食用)	Cactus
21-9-024	仙人掌果 [仙桃]	—
21-9-025	仙人掌籽	—

食物名称中拉文对照表
Chinese-Latin Food Names

编码 Code	食物名称 Food name	拉丁文名称 Latin name
谷类及制品		
01-2-106	粳米	Oryza sativa subsp jing
01-2-214	籼米	Oryza sativa subsp hsien
01-3-108	玉米	Zea mays
01-4-102	黑大麦	Hordeum vulgare
01-5-104	小米	Setaria italica
薯类、淀粉及制品		
02-1-104	马铃薯 [土豆、洋芋]	Solanum tuberosum
02-1-205	甘薯 [山芋、红薯]	Ipomoea batatas
干豆类及制品		
03-1-104	黄豆	Glycine max
03-5-203	蚕豆	Vicia faba
03-9-204	豇豆	Vigna sinensis
03-9-303	豌豆	Pisum sativum var. macrocarpon
03-9-401	鹰嘴豆 [桃豆]	Cicer arietinum L.
蔬菜类及制品		
04-1-111	白萝卜 [莱菔]	Raphanus sativus
04-1-112	圆白萝卜	Raphanus sativus
04-1-113	青萝卜	Raphanus sativus var. longipinnatus
04-1-114	变萝卜 [红皮萝卜]	Raphanus sativus
04-1-115	樱桃萝卜	Raphanus sativus
04-1-204	胡萝卜	Daucus carota var. sativa
04-1-402	根芹 [根洋芹、球根塘蒿]	Apium graveolens var. rapaceum
04-1-403	紫菜头	Beta vulgaris L. var. rapacea Koch
04-2-118	扁豆	Dolichos lablab L.
04-2-119	豇豆	Vigna sinensis
04-2-120	四季豆 [菜豆、芸豆]	Phaseolus vulgaris
04-2-121	四棱豆 [杨桃豆、翅豆]	Psophocarpus tetragonolobus
04-2-122	甜脆荷兰豆 [甜豆]	Pisum sativum var. macrocarpon

编码 Code	食物名称 Food name	拉丁文名称 Latin name
04-3-115	茄子	Solanum melongena
04-3-118	香瓜茄	Solanum muricatum
04-3-119	番茄 [西红柿]	Lycopersicon esculentum
04-3-120	樱桃番茄 [小西红柿]	Lycopersicon esculentum var. cerasiforme
04-3-121	辣椒	Capsicum frutescens L.
04-3-124	甜椒 [灯笼椒、柿子椒]	Capsicum frutescens var. grossum
04-3-125	彩椒	Capsicum frutescens var. grossum
04-3-126	秋葵 [黄秋葵、羊角豆]	Abelmoschus esculentus
04-3-221	冬瓜	Benincasa hispida
04-3-222	飞碟瓜	Cucurbita pepo
04-3-223	黄金西葫芦	Cucurbita pepo
04-3-224	黄茎瓜	Cucurbita moschata Duch
04-3-225	迷你黄瓜 [荷兰乳黄瓜]	Cucumis sativus L.
04-3-226	秋黄瓜 [旱黄瓜]	Cucumis sativus L.
04-3-227	南瓜	Cucurbita moschata
04-3-228	丝瓜	Luffa cylindrica
04-4-206	大葱	Allium fistulosum
04-4-207	细香葱 [香葱、四季葱]	Allium schoenoprasum
04-4-404	韭菜	Allium tuberosum Rottl.
04-5-117	大白菜 (白口)	Brassica pekinensis Rupr.
04-5-118	大白菜 (青口)	Brassica pekinensis Rupr.
04-5-120	小白菜 [青菜]	Brassica chinensis L.
04-5-121	奶白菜	Brassica chinensis L.
04-5-122	鸡毛菜	Brassica campestris L.
04-5-123	娃娃菜	Brassica campestris
04-5-124	乌塌菜 [塌菜、塌棵菜]	Brassica narinosa
04-5-125	油菜	Brassica campestris
04-5-126	油菜心	Brassica campestris
04-5-210	结球甘蓝 [圆白菜]	Brassica oleracea var. capitata
04-5-212	抱子甘蓝	Brassica oleracea var. gemmifera
04-5-213	羽衣甘蓝	Brassica oleracea var. acephala
04-5-214	盖菜	Brassica juncea
04-5-215	芥蓝 [甘蓝菜、盖蓝菜]	Brassica alboglabra
04-5-216	菜花 [花椰菜]	Brassica oleracea var. botrytis
04-5-217	西兰花 [绿菜花]	Brassica oleracea var. italica
04-5-327	番杏 [新西兰菠菜、夏菠菜]	Tetragonia expansa
04-5-328	樱桃萝卜缨	Raphanus sativus

编码 Code	食物名称 Food name	拉丁文名称 Latin name
04-5-329	白凤菜	Gynura divaricata
04-5-330	紫背天葵 [红凤菜、血皮菜]	Gynura bicolor
04-5-331	芹菜	Apium graveolens
04-5-332	西芹 [西洋芹菜、美芹]	Apium graveolens
04-5-333	生菜	Lactuca sativa var. capitata
04-5-334	油麦菜	Lactuca sativa var. longifolia
04-5-335	叶甜菜 (白梗)	Beta vulgaris
04-5-336	莴笋叶 [莴苣菜]	Lactuca sativa var. longifolia
04-5-337	蕹菜 [空心菜、藤藤菜]	Ipomoea aquatica Forsk.
04-5-338	观达菜 [根达菜、牛皮菜]	Beta vulgaris var. cicla
04-5-339	球茎茴香 [甜茴香、意大利茴香]	Foeniculum vulgare Mill.
04-5-415	芦笋 [石刁柏、龙须菜]	Asparagus schoberioidies Kunth
04-5-416	芦笋	Asparagus schoberioidies Kunth
04-5-417	结球菊苣	Cichorium intubus
04-5-418	软化白菊苣	Cichorium intubus
04-6-010	藕 [莲藕]	Nelumbo nucifera Gaertn
04-7-203	芋头 [芋艿、毛芋]	Colocasia esculenta
04-7-204	芋头	Colocasia esculenta
04-8-081	苦苣菜 [苦菜、天精菜]	Sonchus oleraceus
04-8-082	苜蓿 [草头、金花菜]	Medicago hispida Gaertn
04-8-083	鱼腥草 [蕺菜、臭菜]	Houttuynia cordata Thunb
菌藻类		
05-1-028	白蘑菇 [双孢蘑菇、洋蘑菇]	Agaricus bisporus
05-1-029	北风菌 [荷叶离褶伞、一窝羊]	Lyophyllum decastses
05-1-030	草菇 [大黑头细花草、稻菇]	Volvariella volvacea
05-1-031	茶树菇 [柱状田头菇、茶薪菇]	Agrocybe chaxingu Huang Sp.nor
05-1-032	干巴菌	Thelephora ganbajum
05-1-033	红奶浆菌 [多汁乳菇、谷熟菌]	Lactarius volemus
05-1-035	黄伞菇 [多脂鳞伞、黄丝菌]	Pholiota adiposa
05-1-036	鸡腿菇 [毛头鬼伞]	Coprinus comatus
05-1-037	鸡油菌 [黄丝菌、杏菌]	Cantharellus cibarius
05-1-038	鸡纵 [蚁纵、伞把菇、鸡纵菌]	Termitomyces albuminosus
05-1-041	鸡纵花	Mycena micyocarpa
05-1-042	白牛肝菌 [美味牛肝菌]	Boletus edulis
05-1-044	黑牛肝菌 [铜色牛肝菌]	Boleteus aereus
05-1-045	黄皮牛肝菌 [黄皮疣柄牛肝菌、黄癞头]	Leccinum crocipodium

编码 Code	食物名称 Food name	拉丁文名称 Latin name
05-1-046	乳牛肝菌 [粘盖牛肝菌、松树菌]	Suillus bovinus
05-1-047	牛眼睛菌 [马勃菌]	Calvatia
05-1-048	平菇 [糙皮侧耳、青蘑]	Pleurotus ostreatus
05-1-049	青头菌 [变绿红菇、绿菇]	Russula virescens
05-1-050	松蘑 [松茸、松口蘑]	Tricholoma matsutake
05-1-051	杏鲍菇	Pleurotus eryngii
05-1-052	血红菇	Russula sanguinea
05-1-053	元蘑 [亚侧耳、冬蘑、黄蘑]	Hohenbuehelia serotina
05-1-054	竹荪 [竹笙、竹参]	Dictyophora indusiata
05-1-055	榛蘑 [小蜜环菌]	Armillariella mellea
05-2-010	裙带菜 [海芥菜、海木耳]	Undaria pinnatifida
05-2-011	海带	Laminaria japonica
水果类及制品		
06-1-907	蛇果	Malus sylvestris
06-2-115	蜜桃	Prunus persica spp.
06-2-207	布朗	Prunus americana
06-2-208	西梅	Prunus domestica
06-2-313	小枣	Diaspyros lotus
06-3-911	红提子葡萄	Vitis labrusca
06-3-912	无花果	Ficus carica
06-4-303	葡萄柚 [西柚]	Citrus paradisi
06-5-021	桂圆	Dimocarpus longan
06-5-022	红毛丹	Nephelium lappaceum
06-5-023	火龙果 [仙蜜果、红龙果]	Hylocereus undatus Britt & Rose
06-5-024	荔枝	Litchi chinensis
06-5-025	榴莲	Durio zibethinus
06-5-026	芒果	Mangifera indica
06-5-027	木瓜 [番木瓜]	Carica papaya
06-5-029	蒲桃 [香果、水石榴]	Syzygium jambos Alston
06-5-030	山竹	Garcinia mangostana
06-5-031	香蕉	Musa nana Lour.
06-6-206	小西瓜 [地雷瓜]	Citrullus vulgaris
坚果、种子类		
07-1-026	山核桃	Carya cathayensis
07-1-027	栗子 [板栗]	Castanea mollissima Blume
07-1-033	松子	Pinus koraiensis

编码 Code	食物名称 Food name	拉丁文名称 Latin name
07-1-034	杏仁	Prunus armeniaca
07-1-036	腰果	Anacardium occidentale
07-1-037	榛子	Corylus heterophylla
07-1-038	榛子仁	Corylus chinesis
07-1-039	开心果	Pistacia vera
07-1-040	香榧	Torreya grandis
07-2-020	花生	Arachis hypogaea
07-2-023	葵花子	Helianthus annuus
07-2-025	南瓜子 [白瓜子]	Cucurbita moschuta
07-2-026	西瓜子 [黑瓜子]	Citrullus lanatus spp.
鱼虾蟹贝类		
12-1-131	草鱼 [白鲩、草包鱼]	Ctenopharyngoden idellus
12-1-132	鲢鱼 [白鲢、胖子、连子鱼]	Hypophthalmichthys molitrix
12-1-133	鲫鱼 [喜头鱼、海附鱼]	Carassius auratus
12-1-241	带鱼	Trichiurus haumela
12-1-242	黄鱼 (小黄花鱼)	Pseudosciaena polyactis
12-1-243	金鳇鱼	Gymnocypris przewalskii
12-1-244	鲭鱼	Pneumatophorus japonicus
12-1-245	双髻鲨	Sphyrna zygaena
12-1-403	凤尾鱼	Coilia ectenes
12-1-404	箭鱼	Xiphias gladius
12-1-407	鲮鱼	Cirrhina molitorella
12-1-408	鳗鱼	Muraenesox cinereus
12-1-417	沙丁鱼	Sardinops melanosticta
12-4-117	海蚌 [西施舌]	Mactra antiquata Spengler
其它		
21-9-017	葛根	Pueraria thomsonii Benth
21-9-022	牛蛙	Rana catesbeiana
21-9-023	仙人掌	Opuntia dillenii

注：与“食物描述”相比，此处的食物名称只保留了主词，不包括描述性用语。

Compared with the ones in the Table of Food Description, the food names in Chinese here just contain the main words. The words on food description were removed.

附录 5　Appendix 5

中国食物与营养发展纲要（2001 ～ 2010）

National Developing Plan on Food and Nutrition in China (2001 ～ 2010)

国务院办公厅

从新世纪开始，我国人民生活在总体达到小康水平的基础上继续改善，向全面建设小康社会迈进。今后十年，将是我国居民食物结构迅速变化和营养水平不断提高的重要时期。加快食物发展，改善食物结构，提高全民营养水平，增进人民身体健康，是国民整体素质提高的迫切需要，也是我国社会主义现代化建设的重大任务。为指导我国食物与营养持续，协调发展，特制定本纲要。

一、食物与营养发展的基本状况

（一）我国食物与营养发展的成就

《九十年代中国食物结构改革与发展纲要》颁布以来，我国国民经济持续发展，农业和农村经济发展进入了新阶段，实现了农产品供给由长期短缺到总量基本平衡，丰年有余的历史性转变，人民生活水平不断提高，推动了食物需求持续增长。全民营养状况得到全面改善。社会主义市场经济体制的逐步建立，为食物发展创造了良好的外部环境。科技进步已经渗透到食物发展的各个环节，加速了传统食物的改造，拓宽了食物发展的空间。我国食物与营养进入了一个新的发展阶段。

1. 食物综合生产能力显著增强。我国粮食的年均生产能力已达到5亿吨的水平，人均粮食占有量达到400公斤左右。在粮食生产稳步增长的同时，肉、蛋、水产品以及水果、蔬菜生产都有了快速的增长，为提高人民生活水平奠定了坚实的物质基础。

2. 食物消费质量明显提高。1990 年到 2000 年，全国居民人均收入从 904 元增加到 1625 元（1990 年不变价）。人均食物消费支出占生活消费总支出的比重逐步降低，恩格尔系数从 60.3% 下降到 46.0%。食物消费结果得到了显著改善。2000 年人均消费口粮 206 公斤，蔬菜 110 公斤，食用植物油 8.2 公斤，食糖 7.0 公斤，肉类 25.3 公斤，蛋类 11.8 公斤，奶类 5.5 公斤，水产品 11.7 公斤。与 1990 年相比，蛋、奶、水产品人均消费量有较大幅度提高。

3. 居民营养结构有较大改善。20 世纪 90 年代以来，全国居民摄入能量比较稳定，摄入的蛋白质总量中动物性蛋白质所占的比重有一定增长，膳食质量显著改善。通过 90 年代后期部分地区典型监测表明，居民人均每日摄入能量 2387 千卡，蛋白质 70.5 克，脂肪 54.7 克。其中城镇居民人均摄入能量 2253 千卡，蛋白质 69.2 克，脂肪 72 克；农村居民人均摄入能量 2449 千卡，蛋白质 71.1 克，脂肪 46.7 克，基本达到了营养素供给量标准。

（二）当前食物与营养发展中存在的问题

4. 食物生产、消费、营养不协调，生产结构不能满足营养结构改善需要。从目前情况看，一是我国优质农产品比重偏低，奶类、大豆等优质食物消费明显不足。二是城乡居民营养不平衡，地区差异较大，城市居民因膳食不平衡或营养过剩导致的疾病迅速增多，农村地区特别是贫困地区营养不良现象存在。三是食品工业发展滞后，产品结构不合理，技术装备总体水平偏低，食品工业值不足农业产值的40%，加工食品消费量仅占食品消费量的30%，与世界先进国家的差距较大。

5. 食物质量、安全和卫生存在隐患。部分地区食物生产的环境恶化，受到工业和城市的污染，生产过程中化肥、农药、兽药、饲料添加剂使用不当，加工中食品添加剂和技术使用不尽合理，导致部分食物有害物质残留超标，严重影响人民健康。

（三）食物与营养发展面临的新形式

6. 食物与营养面临新的形式：一是居民生活水平的不断提高，对事物多样化，优质化需求明显增加；对食物安全卫生要求不断提高。二是居民食物消费正处于由小康向更加富裕转型的时期，急需加强对居民食物与营养的指导工作，促进居民形成良好的饮食习惯。否则，既会造成资源浪费，也可能会影响一代甚至几代人身体素质的提高。三是世界经济和现代科技的发展，使国际食物与营养产业呈加速发展趋势，必须加快我国食物与营养工作，以跟上世界发展步伐。

因此，今后十年，我国食物与营养工作面临着十分艰巨的任务，必须调整战略，转变观念，明确发展重点，制定有效的政策措施，促进食物与营养取得新的发展。

二、食物与营养发展的指导思想、基本原则和目标

（一）食物与营养发展的指导思想和基本原则

7. 食物与营养发展的指导思想。适应我国人民生活水平提高和营养改善的要求，为提高中华民族素质，实现中华民族伟大复兴，动员和号召全社会力量，加快我国食物与营养的发展。紧紧围绕食物发展的重点领域，重点地区，重点人群，分类指导，全面推进，建设现代食物生产、加工和市场体系，调整引导我国食物结构向营养、卫生、科学、合理的方向发展，经过不懈努力，使我国居民的食物消费与营养整体水平有较大幅度提高。

8. 食物与营养发展的基本原则。坚持食物生产与消费协调发展的原则，适应居民营养改善的需要，建立以农业为基础，以食品工业为龙头的现代食物产业体系；坚持食物资源利用与保护相结合的原则，合理开发利用各种食物资源，实现可持续发展；坚持食物质量与安全卫生管理质量和安全卫生水平；坚持优化结构与预防疾病相结合的原则，调整优化食物与营养结构，预防营养性疾病，提高全民营养和健康水平；坚持继承与创新相结合的原则，发扬中华饮食文化的优良传统，全面提高食物发展的科技水平，走有中国特色的食物与营养发展道路。

（二）食物与营养发展的目标

9. 2010年食物与营养发展总体目标。保障合理的营养素摄入量。人均每日摄入能量为2300千卡（供给能量为 2600 千卡），其中 80% 来自植物性食物，20% 来自动物性食物；蛋白质 77 克，其中 30% 来自动物性食物；脂肪 70 克，提供的能量占总能量的 25%；钙 580 毫克，铁 23 毫克，锌 12 毫克；维生素B_1 1.2 毫克，维生素B_2 1.4 毫克，维生素A 775 毫克。

保障合理的食物摄入量。人均每年主要食物摄入量为：口粮 155 公斤，豆类 13 公斤，蔬菜 147 公斤，水果 38 公斤，食用植物油 10 公斤，食糖 9 公斤，肉类 28 公斤，蛋类 15 公斤，奶类 16 公斤，水产品 16 公斤。

保障充足的事物供给。2010 年全国主要食物生产总量的安全保障目标为：粮食 5.7 亿吨，豆类 2300 万吨，蔬菜 3.7 亿吨，水果 7300 万吨，油料 3400 万吨，糖料 1.3 亿吨，肉类 7600 万吨，蛋类 2700 万吨，奶类 2600 万吨，水产品 5000 万吨。

降低营养不良性疾病发病率。5 岁以下儿童低体重发病率降至 5%，生长迟缓发病率降至 15%。孕妇和儿童贫血患病率分别降至 20% 和 15%。4 个月以内婴儿的母乳喂养达到普及，4 个月以上的婴儿，应逐步补充各种辅助食品。

10. 2010 年城乡居民食物与营养发展目标。城市居民：人均每日摄入能量 2250 千卡，其中 75% 来自植物性食物，25%来自动物性食物；蛋白质80克，其中35%来自动物性食物；脂肪80克，提供的能量占总能量的28%。人均每年主要食物摄入量为：口粮 135 公斤，豆类 12 公斤，蔬菜 160 公斤，水果 52 公斤，食用植物油 10 公斤，食糖 10 公斤，肉类 32 公斤，蛋类 18 公斤，奶类 32 公斤，水产品 22 公斤。

农村居民：人均每日摄入能量 2320 千卡，其中 84% 来自植物性食物，16% 来自动物性食物；蛋白质 75 克，其中 27% 来自动物性食物；脂肪 65 克，提供的能量占总能量的 24%。人均每年主要事物摄入量为：口粮 165 公斤，豆类 13 公斤，蔬菜 140 公斤，水果 30 公斤，食用植物油 10 公斤，食糖 8 公斤，肉类 26 公斤，蛋类 13 公斤，奶类 7 公斤，水产品 13 公斤。

三、食物与营养发展的重点领域、地区与群体

今后十年，针对我国食物与营养发展现状和存在的问题，要优先发展奶类产业、大豆产业和食品加工业三个重点食物领域，努力解决好农村和西部两个重点地区以及少年儿童、妇幼、老年三个重点人群的食物与营养发展问题。

（一）食物与营养发展的重点领域

我国食物与营养发展的内容多，任务重，领域广，要在整体推进的基础上，把涉及食物与营养发展的难点和薄弱环节作为今后十年的重点内容，优先发展。

11. 奶类产业。加快发展奶业，提高居民奶类消费水平。扶持奶源基地建设，调整奶畜群结构，改善奶业基础薄弱的状况。加快发展乳制品加工业，支持开发新的奶产品，促进奶产品的升级换代。大力加强奶业科学研究，提高奶业发展的科技含量。支持并形成若干个对全国具有带动作用的大型乳品加工企业集团。加大对奶业发展的支持力度，尽快提高我国居民的奶类食品消费水平，到 2010 年居民的乳制品人均消费量比 2000 年要有大幅度增加。

12. 大豆产业。大力发展大豆产业，促进大豆及其产品的生产和消费，提高大豆食品的供给水平。支持开展大豆资源、生产、精深加工等方面的科学研究。大力开拓大豆及其制品的消费市场，优先支持开发新型的大豆食品，用现代高新技术改造传统豆制品；到 2010 年，以大豆为基础的优质蛋白质消费量以及深加工产品消费量要有明显增加，质量要有明显改进。

13. 食品加工业。优先支持对主食的加工，加快居民主要制成品食物的发展步伐，重点发展符合营养科学要求的方便食品，速冻食品。加快发展食物营养强化工作，重点推进主食品营养强化，减轻食物营养素缺乏的状况。优先支持我国传统食品的工业化技术改造，选择并支持若干种具有市场前景和示范作用的传统食品，提高其科技含量，加快其工业化步伐。优先支持大宗农产品深度开发与加工利用，逐步提高农产品加工转化程度。

（二）食物与营养发展的重点地区

食物与营养发展需要全民参与，协调发展。要把相对落后的地区作为重点，加大力度，努力推进。

14. 农村地区。广大农村地区，食物发展不平衡，营养状况相对落后。要加快农村经济发展，大力推进农业和农村经济结构的调整，切实增加农民收入，提高食物消费能力。重视农村营养改善，加强农村食物与营养发展的基础设施建设，改善食物购买与消费环境，开拓农村食物市场。力争到 2010 年广大农村地区营养状况有较大改善，农村居民生活质量不断提高。

15. 西部农村地区。西部农村地区食物发展基础较差，食物资源丰富但未能充分开发利用。要加强食物发展基础设施建设，建立西部食物发展主导产业，保护生态环境，促进西部地区食物消费，降低西部地区农民营养不良的发生率。采取综合措施，促进西部地区农民食物与营养状况的不断改善。

（三）营养改善的重点人群

营养改善是长期的任务，在注重各类人群营养改善的同时，要切实抓好弱势人群的营养改善工作。

16. 少年儿童群体。提高民族整体素质，基础在少年儿童。积极组织实施有关少年儿童营养改善的国家计划。优先保证这一群体的营养供给，提高身体素质。定期对少年儿童营养健康状况进行监测，实行有针对性的营养指导，使少年儿童从小形成良好的饮食习惯。建立贫困地区少年儿童营养保障制度，切实解决少年儿童营养失调问题，使农村营养不良儿童所占的比例比 2000 年减少一半，城市营养失调儿童所占的比例减少 1/3。

17. 妇幼群体。妇女具有特殊营养需要，婴幼儿正处于生命的早期，他们的营养状况关系到人体一生的健康。要加大妇幼群体营养改善的力度，逐步建立孕妇，婴儿营养保障制度，防止妇女尤其是孕妇、产妇、哺乳期妇女的营养失衡。在全面普及母乳喂养的基础上，针对妇幼群体的特殊需要，大力开发适合妇幼群体消费的系列食品，加强对妇幼食品的市场管理。重点搞好 3 岁以下幼儿的营养改善，为提高中华民族新一代的身体素质打下良好基础。

18. 老年人群体。我国60岁以上老年人比例逐渐增大，老年人的营养与健康越来越成为一个非常重要的社会问题。要建立老年人营养保障制度，关心老年人膳食营养，做好孤寡老人的膳食供给，加强对老年人的营养保障工作。研究开发适合老年人消费的系列食物，重点发展营养强化食品和低盐，低脂，低能量食品。减少老年人营养性疾病的发生率，提高老年人的生活质量和健康水平。

四、促进食物与营养发展的政策措施

（一）调整结构，提高食物综合供给能力

19. 调整农业结构，提高食物质量。在稳定提高粮食生产能力的基础上，着力优化食品品种，优化食物品质，优化食物布局，促进食物生产效益大幅度增长。种植业要由传统的粮食作物－经济作物“二元结构”向粮食作物－经济作物－饲料作物“三元结构”转变，大力发展名、特、优农产品，形成各具特色的优质农产品及其加工专用生产区，建立优质食品加工专用原料生产基地，大力发展适合食品加工业需要的标准化农产品生产。合理和充分利用草地，农作物秸秆等资源，建立规模养殖场，加快牛羊，禽特别是奶畜发展，生产优质畜禽食品。在合理保护渔业资源和水域生态环境的前提下，加快发展水产养殖业，积极开发大洋性渔业资源。

20. 加强管理，加快食品工业发展。转变政府职能，加强行业规划和协调，加强监管和服务，实行食品工业产供销一体化。调整食品工业结构，加速传统食品工业的优化升级，促进传统食品工业向现代食品工业的转化，建立现代食品工业体系。开展食品加工机械、包装、贮运技术创新，大力发展现代食品科技，提高我国食品工业科技水平。加强食品工业基础设施建设，做好产品标准化包装、运输。加强对大宗食物的加工，提高综合利用率。采取措施，严格控制对人们身心健康危害较大的烟草业、烈性酒的发展。

21. 加强食物市场体系建设，提高食物国际竞争力。逐步建立和完善食物产地批发市场，城乡集贸市场，连锁超市等零售市场，进行合理布局，形成规范的生产－批发－零售一体化的市场网络。建立食物快捷运输通道，建设发达的食物流通体系。参照世界贸易规则，制定我国食物进出口贸易政策，采用国际标准进行食物生产、加工，发展外向型食品产业。以市场为导向，加强优势食物出口的生产，提高水果、蔬菜、畜产品、水产品等劳动密集型产品的质量，增强国际市场竞争能力。加强对食物进出口的检验检疫。

（二）加强法制建设，保护食物资源环境

22. 加强对食物与营养法制建设，完善食物与营养标准体系。加快食物与营养立法步伐，制定食品管理法规，保证食品安全卫生与人民身体健康。抓紧制定关于营养师、营养标识、儿童营养等方面的法规，把居民营养改善工作纳入法制化轨道。加强食物生产、加工、流通过程的标准化建设，加快食物质量、安全、卫生的标准体系建设，制定不同类别食物与营养标准，科学的指导食物生产和消费。在大中城市和有条件的地区逐步实行农产品认证制度，规范直接上市农产品的质量要求。加快食物流通体系的法制建设，规范企业行为，保护生产者与消费者的权益。

23. 保护食物资源环境，保障食物质量、安全与卫生。加大耕地、草地、水资源等生态建设和环境保护的力度的，逐步改善食物资源环境，保证食物资源可持续利用。大力推广节地、节水、节能型等食物生产技术，缓解耕地、水资源紧缺的压力。强化食物生产过程的环境保护，加大食品生产经营企业的治污力度。大力发展无污染、安全优质、营养丰富的食物生产，加快发展绿色食品和有机食品，逐步增加名牌精品食物的市场供给。积极稳妥地发展高质量、高效能的保健食品，满足城乡居民多层次、多样化的需要。加强对食物种植、养殖阶段农药、兽药的管理，完善有关农药、兽药安全使用管理规定。建立健全食物质量、安全与卫生检验检测体系，加强对食物生产全过程的监督管理，提高食物质量，确保食物安全与卫生。

（三）依靠科技进步，提高全民营养意识

24. 加强科技研究，提高食物与营养发展的科技水平。增加食物生产、食品工业、食物营养卫生及相关领域前瞻性、战略性、公益性科研投入，加强食物发展各领域的基础研究和技术开发工作，促进产、学、研相结合，使相关学科相互渗透和交融，不断增强开发新产品、新技术、新工艺的能力。加强生物技术、信息技术等高新技

术在食物与营养领域的应用研究，显著提高食物产量、质量、安全和卫生水平。开展食物、营养与健康的相关研究，培养和造就食品与营养科学研究领域的高层次人才。吸收发达国家的先进经验，注重引进、消化、吸收国外有关食物与营养的先进技术。

25. 全面普及营养知识，提高全民营养意识。加强对居民食物与营养的指导，建立用科学的营养知识引导消费和用消费带动生产的新机制，使生产机构、消费机构和营养机构合理协调。开展多种形式、多种类型的营养知识教育，充分发挥各新闻媒体的作用，加强营养知识宣传，提高城乡居民的营养科学知识和自我保健意识，引导居民的食物消费方向，提高全民科学，合理膳食的自觉性。加强对中小学生和家长的营养知识教育，把营养健康教育纳入中小学教育的内容。提高营养师的社会地位，逐步在医院、幼儿园、学校、企事业单位的公共食堂及餐饮服务业推行营养师制度。

（四）改善居民营养结构，保障我国食物安全

26. 实施有关营养改善行动计划。继续和规范实施国家营养改善行动计划、国家大豆行动计划、国家学生饮用奶计划等。积极推广学生营养餐，作为国家营养改善的一项重要工作，成立相应协调机构，制定相关法规，依法加强管理。力争到 2010 年，全国大中城市要有一半以上的中小学生吃上学生营养餐。在经济落后地区，采取不同形式，保证居民营养供给。对发生严重营养不良的地区，当地政府要及时采取营养改善措施。

27. 加强营养监测，建立食物安全保障系统。建立和完善食物与营养监测系统，坚持重点监控与系统监测结合，监测不同地区、不同人群的营养状况。加强全民食物供给和消费安全。要从国内外两种资源、两个市场来考虑我国食物的安全，密切关注和研究市场变化、重大自然灾害对食物供给带来的影响，提前做好各种应对准备，确保我国食物安全。

（五）加强对食物与营养工作的领导

28. 分级管理，部门分工配合，建立现代食物管理体制。《中国食物与营养发展刚要（2001 ~ 2010）的实施由农业部牵头协调，国务院各有关部门要紧密协作，积极配合，加强对食物与营养发展工作的指导，进一步发挥国家食物与营养咨询委员会的重要作用。地方各级人民政府要高度重视和加强食物与营养发展工作，结合本地实际，充分考虑不同地区、不同人群的差别和习惯，研究制定本地区的国民经济和社会发展计划。加快我国食物与营养管理体制改革，建立现代食物发展管理体系，保证食物与营养发展目标的顺利实现。

参考文献
References

1. 杨月欣, 王光亚编著. 中国食物成分表 2002. 北京：北京大学医学出版社, 2002
2. 杨月欣, 王光亚主编. 实用食物营养成分分析手册. 北京：中国轻工业出版社, 2002
3. 中国营养学会编著. 中国居民膳食营养素参考摄入量. 北京：中国轻工业出版社, 2000
4. 中国营养学会编著. 中国居民膳食营养指南. 拉萨：西藏人民出版社, 2008
5. 全国食品工业标准化技术委员会秘书处编. 食品标签通用标准实施指南续编. 北京：中国标准出版社, 1999
6. 《中国传统蔬菜图谱》编委会编. 中国传统蔬菜图谱. 杭州：浙江科学技术出版社, 2001
7. 张光亚编著. 中国常见食用菌图鉴. 昆明：云南科技出版社, 1999
8. 沈同, 王镜岩主编. 生物化学. 北京：高等教育出版社, 2000
9. 沈亢川, 林升清主编. 福建省食物营养成分表. 福州：福建科学技术出版社, 1991
10. 赵玉堂, 周玲仙主编. 云南食物成分表. 昆明：云南科技出版社, 2003
11. Deutache Forschungsanstalt fur Lebensmittelchemie, Garching b. Munchen. Food Composition and Nutrition Tables. Sixth Revised and completed edition. German：Scientific Publisher Stuttgart, 2000
12. Food Composition Table. Sixth Revision. Korea：National Rural Living Science Institute, 2001
13. 科学技术厅资料调查会. 日本食物标准成分表. 五订. 东京：大藏省印刷局, 2000
14. Food Standards Agency. McCance and Widdowson's The Composition of Foods. Sixth Summary Edition. Cambridge：The Royal Society of Chemistry, 2002
15. Greenfield H, Southgate DAT. Food Composition Data: production, management and use. FAO Publishing Management Service, 2003
16. Rand WM, Windham CT, Young VR. Food Composition Data: a user's perspective. Tokyo：The United National University, 1987
17. Rand WM, Pennington JAT. Compiling Data for Food Composition Databases. Tokyo：The United Nations University, 1991
18. Royal Society. Metric units, conversion factors and nomenclature in nutritional and food sciences. Report of the subcommittee on metrication of the British National Committee for Nutritional Sciences, 1972
19. FAO/WHO. Energy and protein requirement. Report of a Joint FAO/WHO Ad Hoc Expert Committee. FAO Nutrition Meetings Report Series, No. 52; WHO Technical Report Series, No. 522, 1973
20. Foster-Powell K, Miller JB. International tables of glycemic index. Am J Clin Nutr, 1995 Oct; 62(4): 871S-890S
21. Ahuja JKC, Gebhardt Se. New challenges for the national survey nutrient databases. FASEB Journal, 2002 Mar; 16(40), A656
22. Klensin JC. INFOODS Food Composition Data Interchange Handbook. Tokyo：The United Nations University, 1992
23. http://www.fao.org/infoods/
24. http://www.nal.usda.gov/fnic.foodcomp/

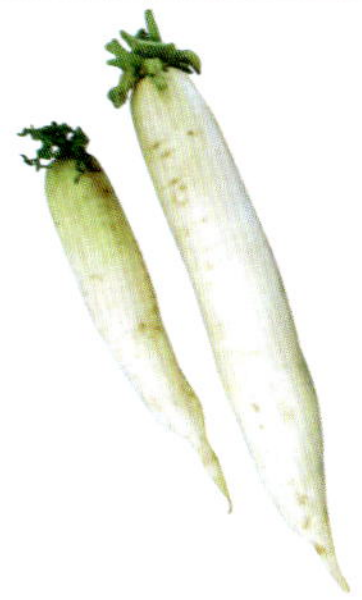
白萝卜

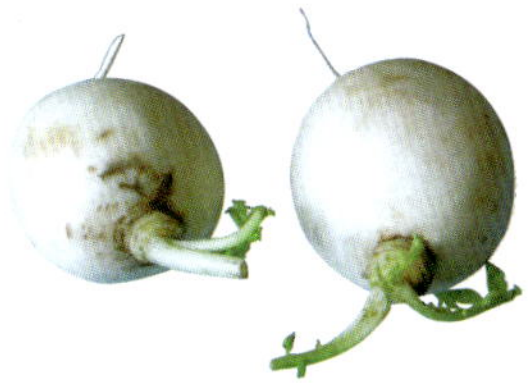
小圆白萝卜

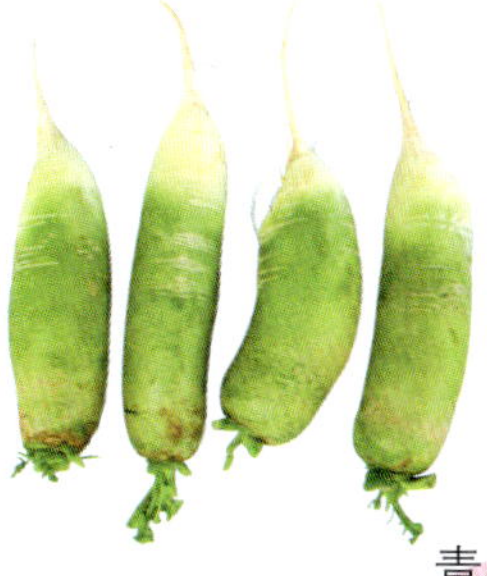
青萝卜

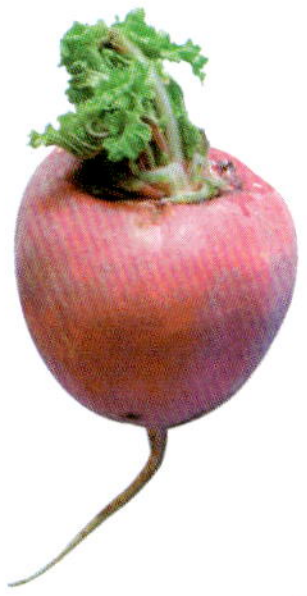
变萝卜

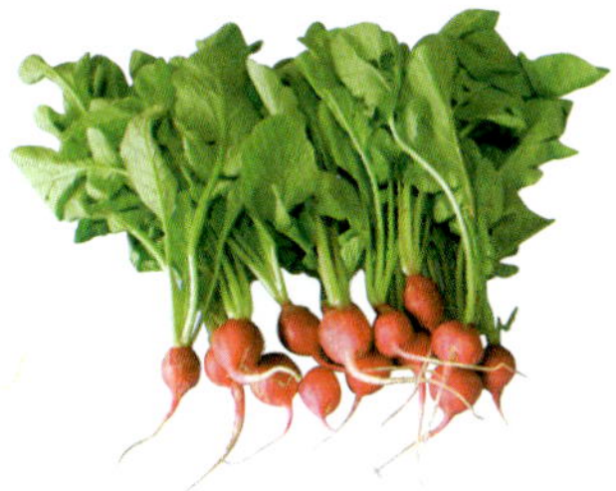
樱桃萝卜

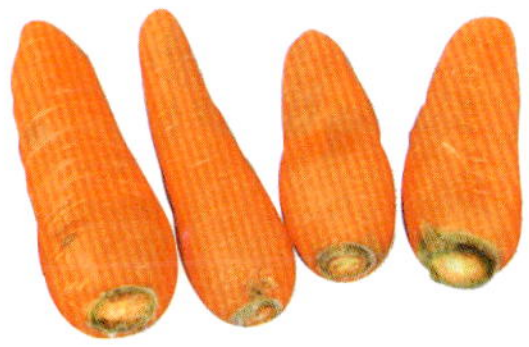
胡萝卜

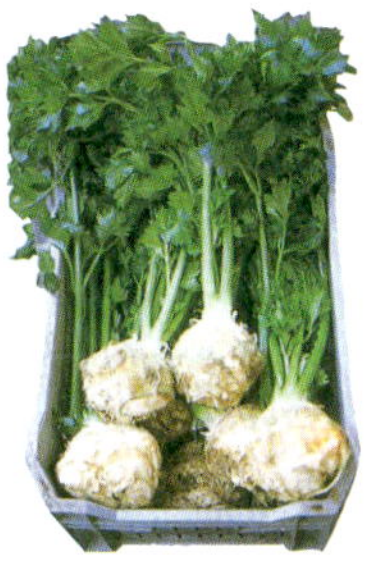
根芹

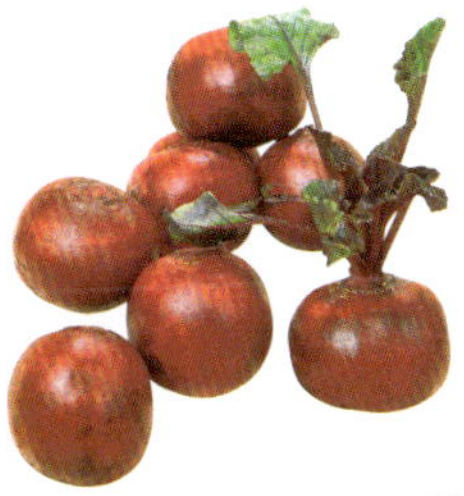
紫菜头

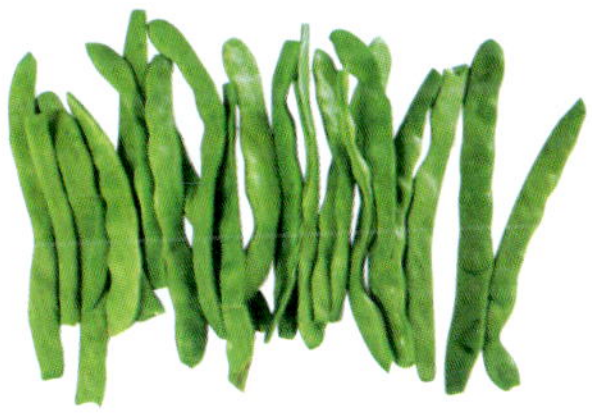
扁豆

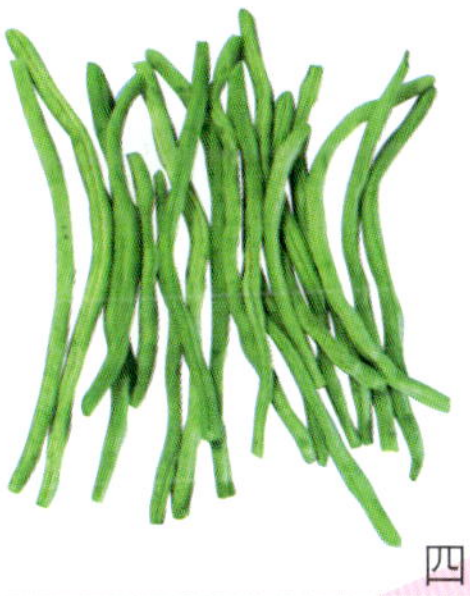
四季豆

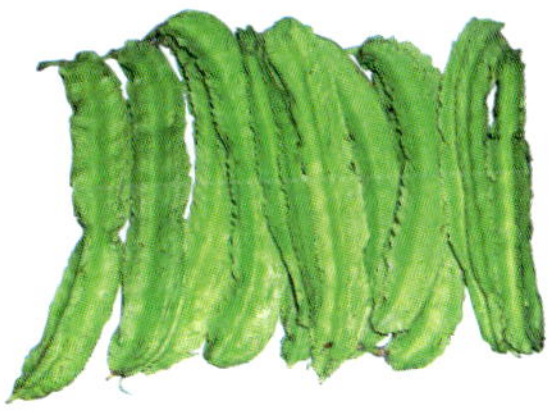
四棱豆

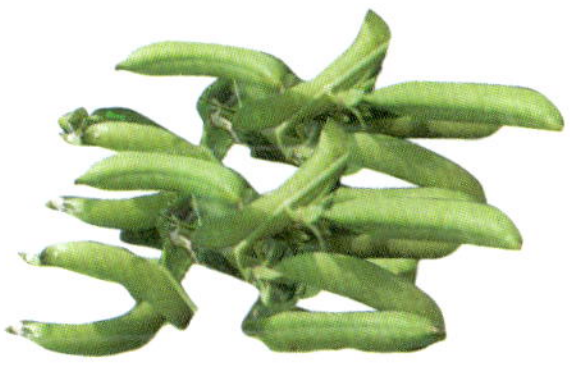
甜脆荷兰豆

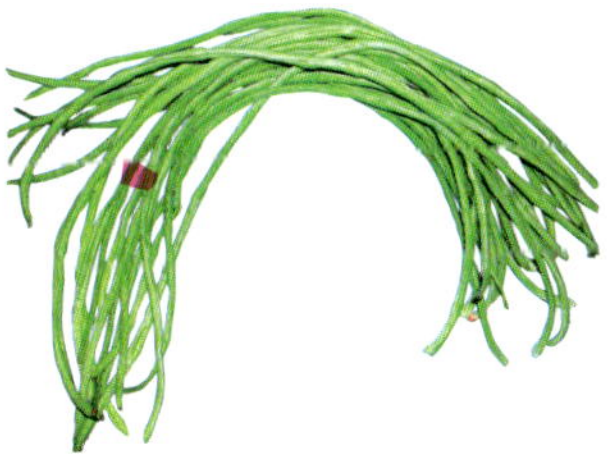
豇豆

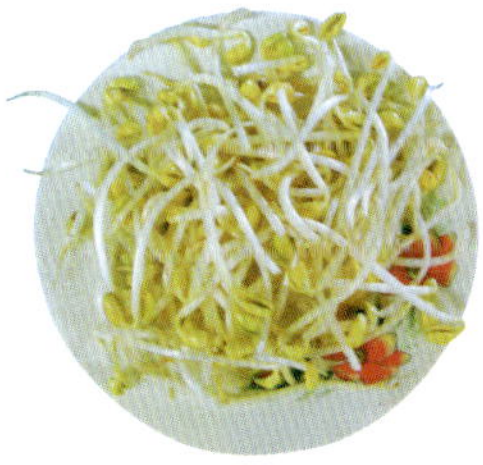
黄豆芽

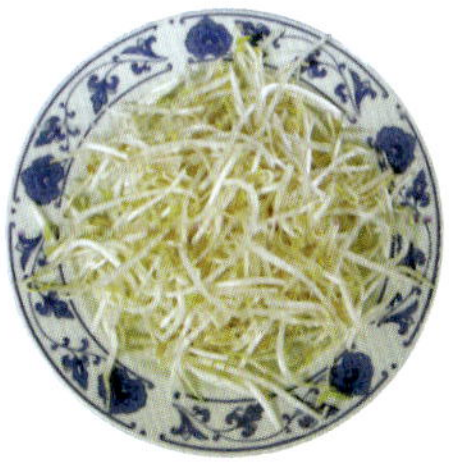
绿豆芽

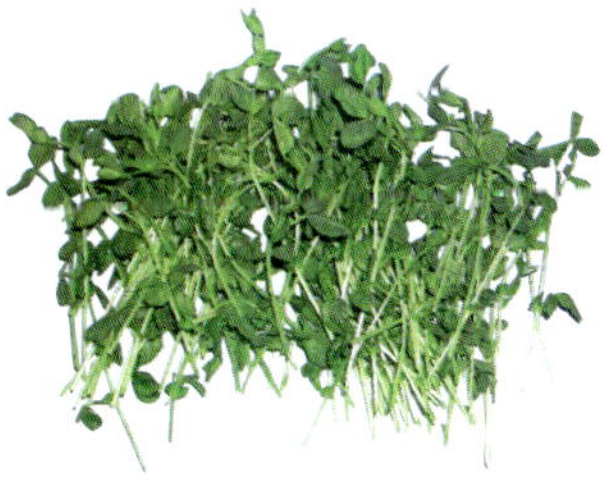
豌豆苗

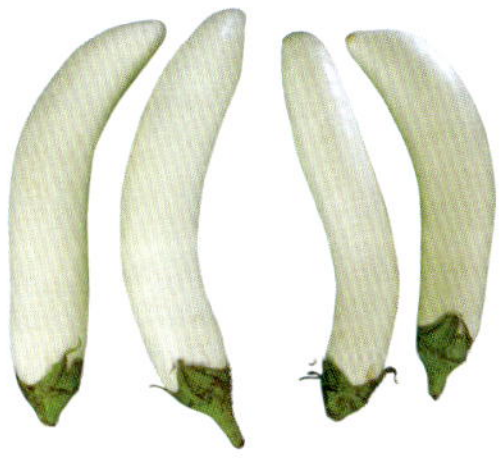
茄子（白皮，长）

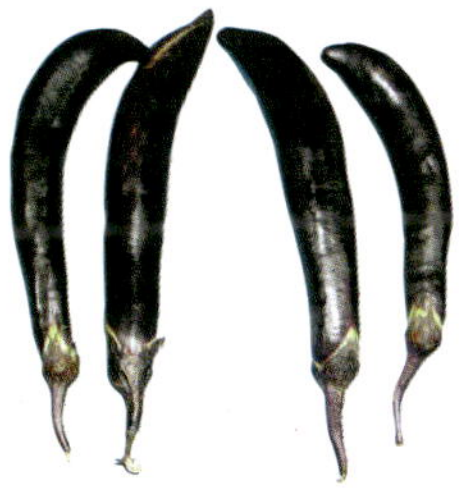
茄子（紫皮，长）

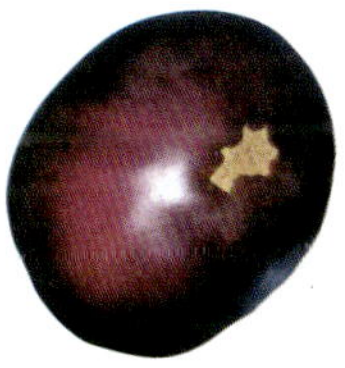
茄子（紫皮，圆）

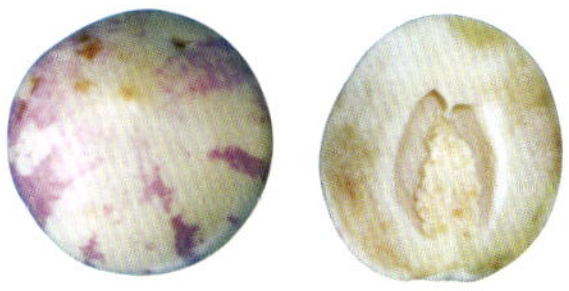
香瓜茄

蔬菜

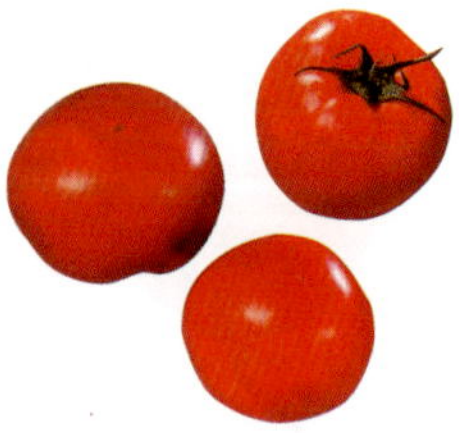
番茄

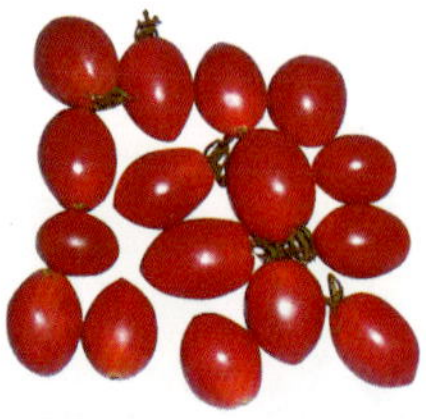
樱桃番茄（紫樱柿）

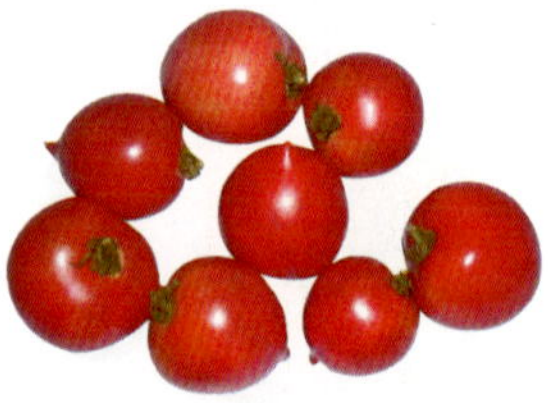
樱桃番茄（春桃圣女）

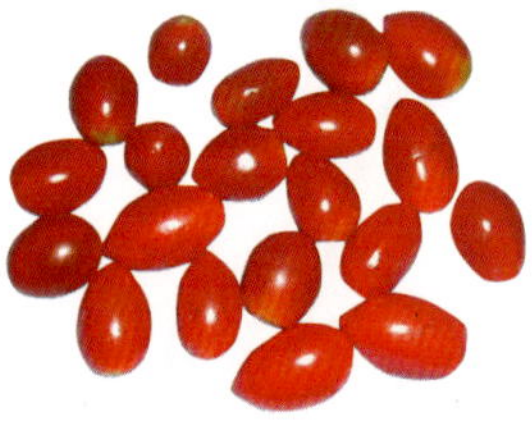
樱桃番茄（圣女果）

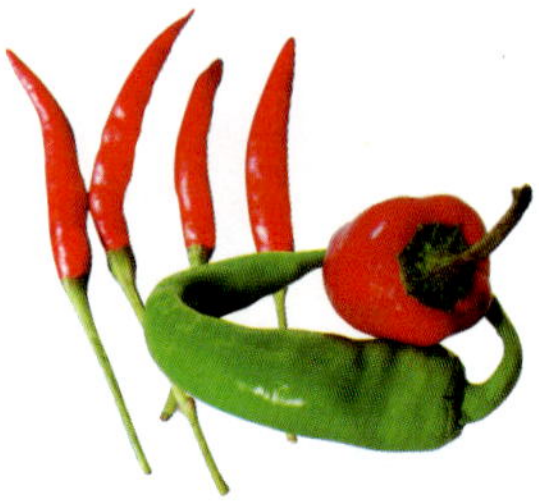
辣椒

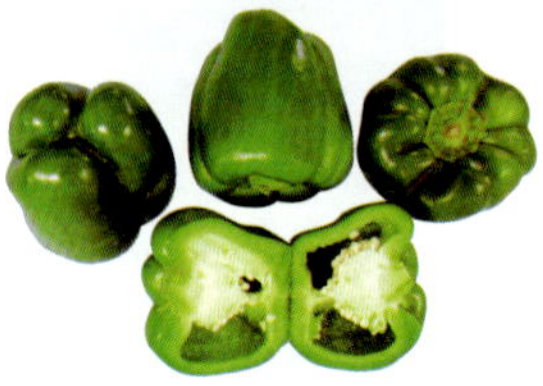
甜椒

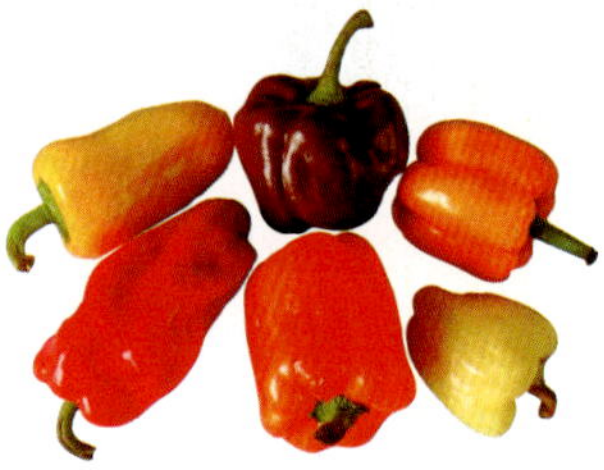
彩椒

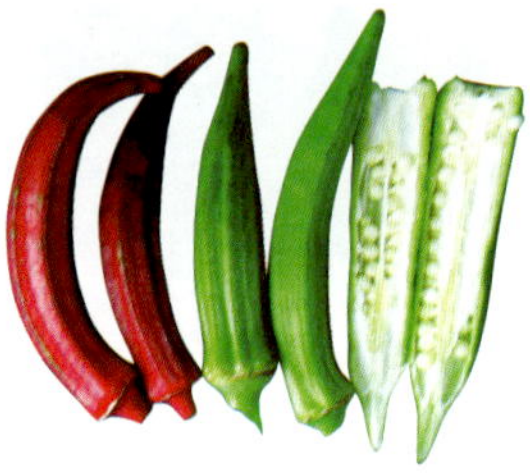
秋葵

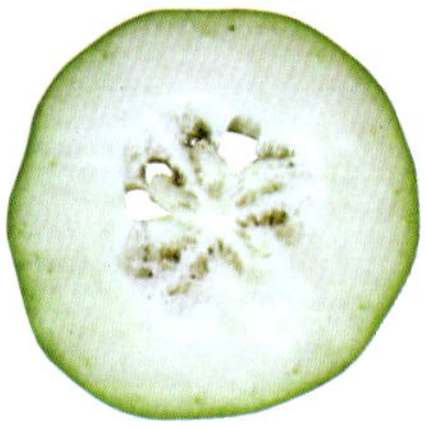
冬瓜

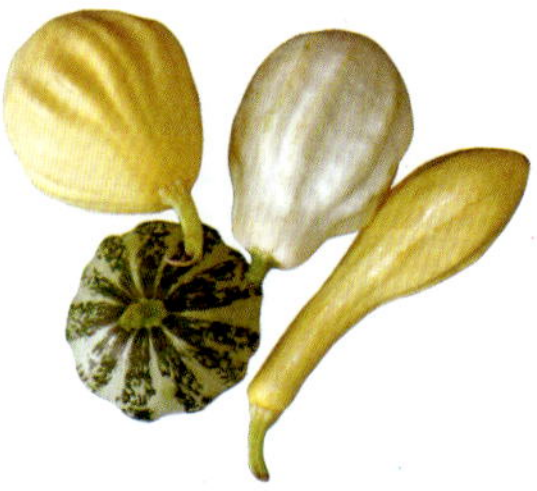
飞碟瓜

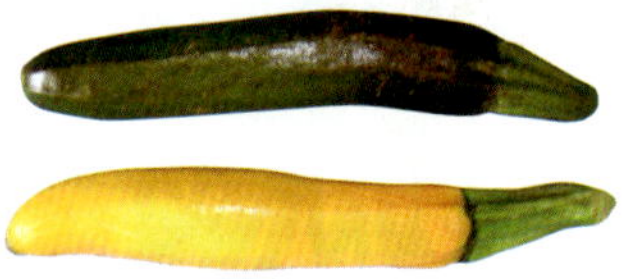
黄金西胡芦

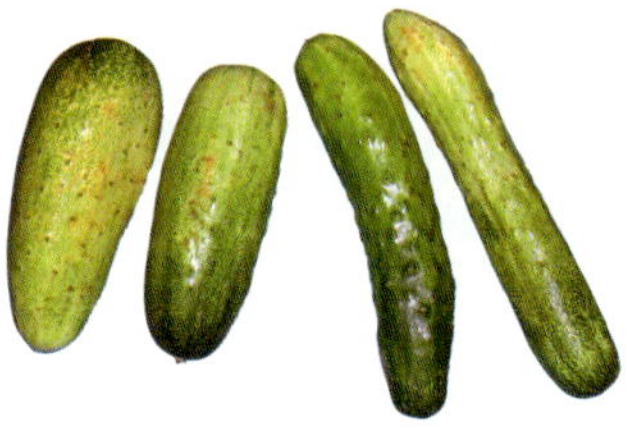
秋黄瓜

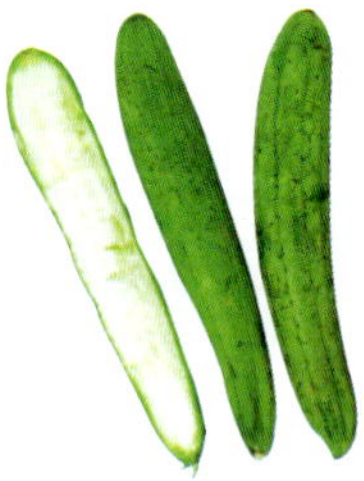
丝瓜

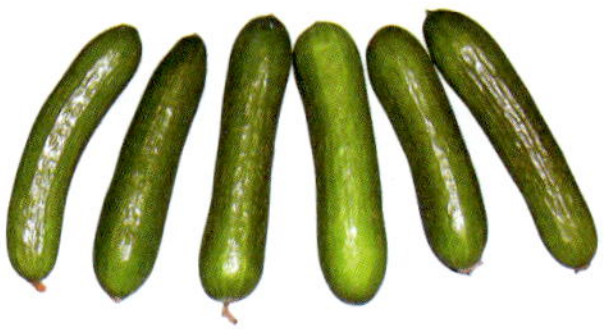
迷你黄瓜

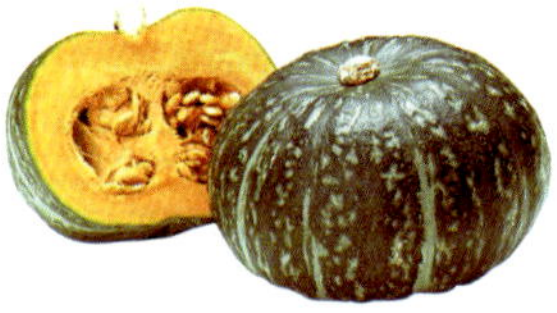
栗面南瓜

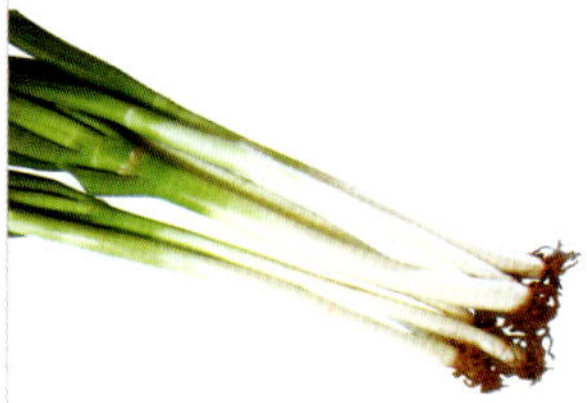
大葱

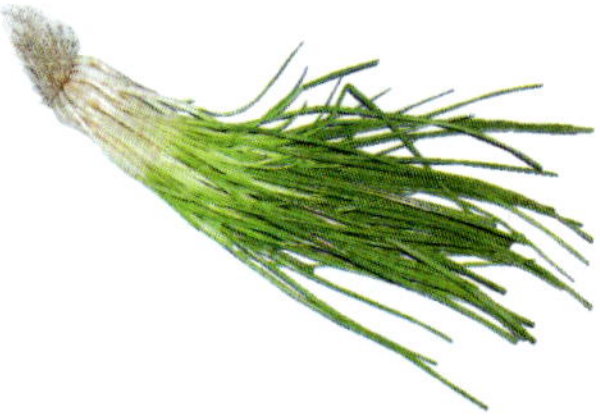
细香葱

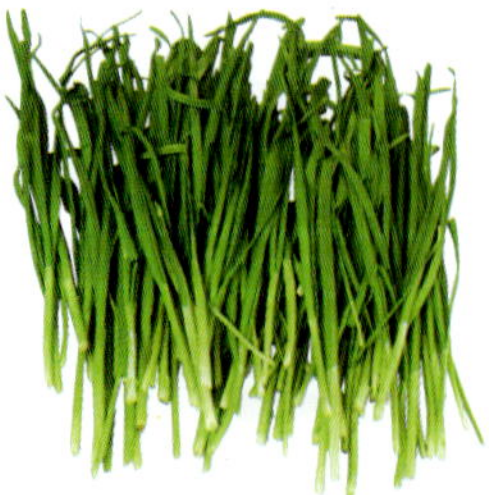
韭菜

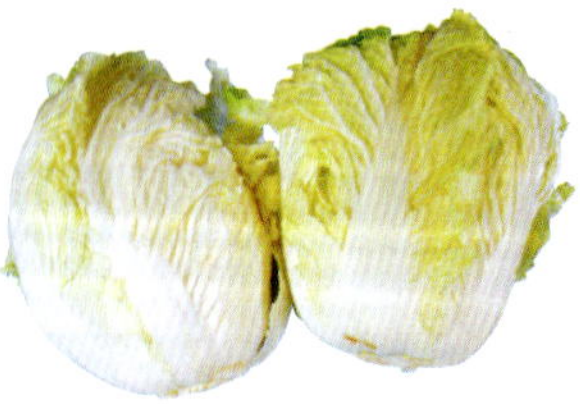
大白菜(白口)

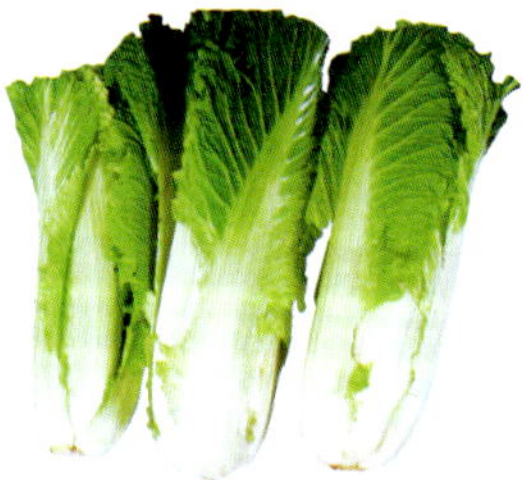
大白菜(青口)

蔬菜

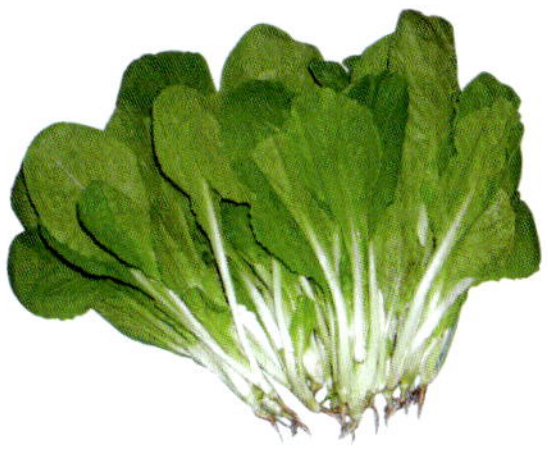
小白菜

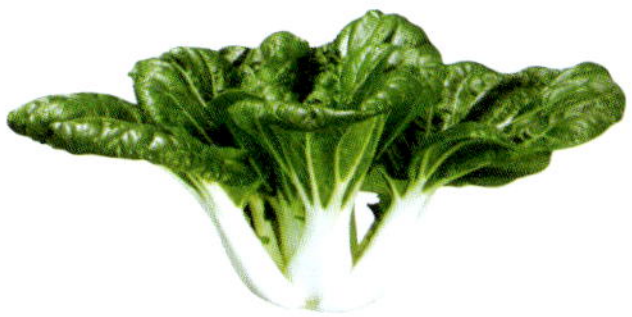
奶白菜

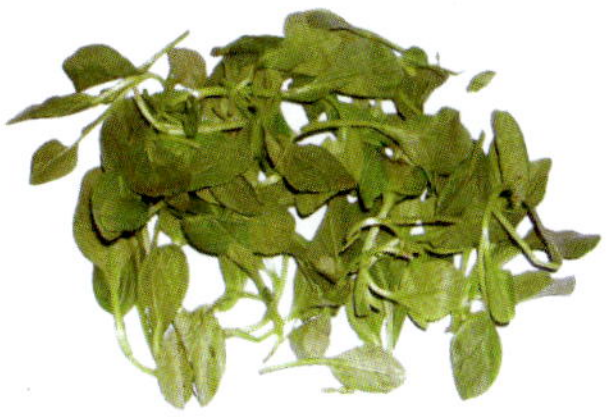
鸡毛菜

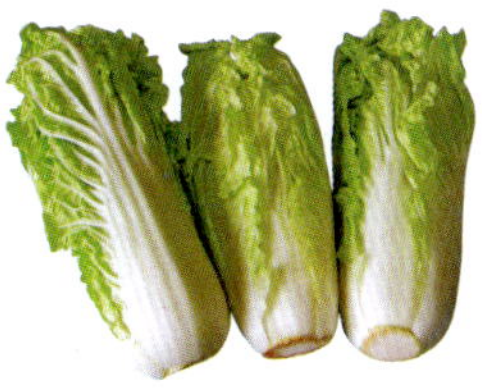
娃娃菜

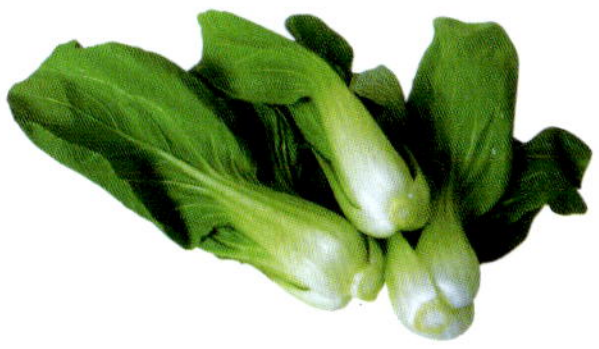
油菜

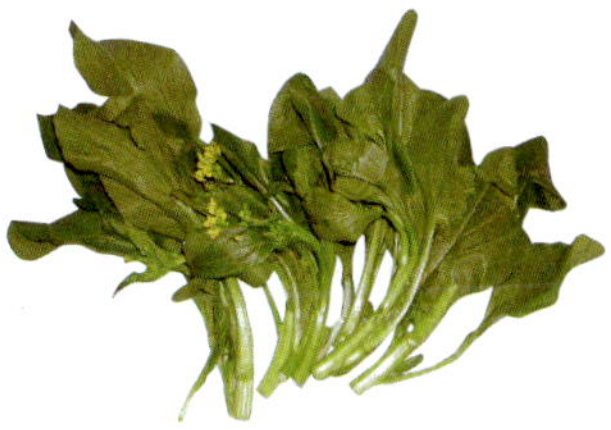
油菜心

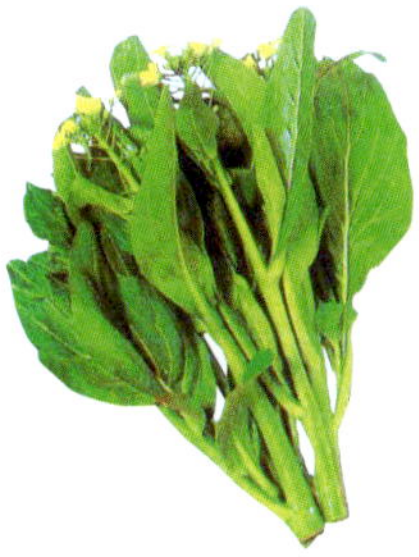
菜苔

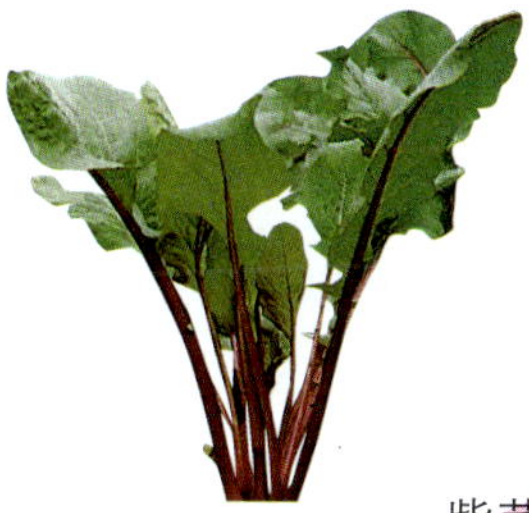
紫菜苔

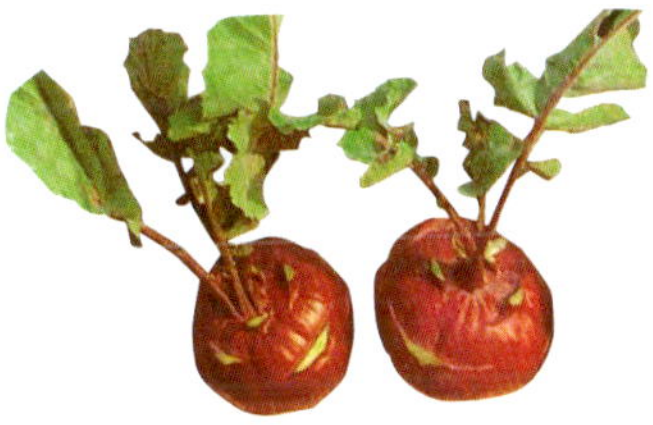
球茎甘蓝

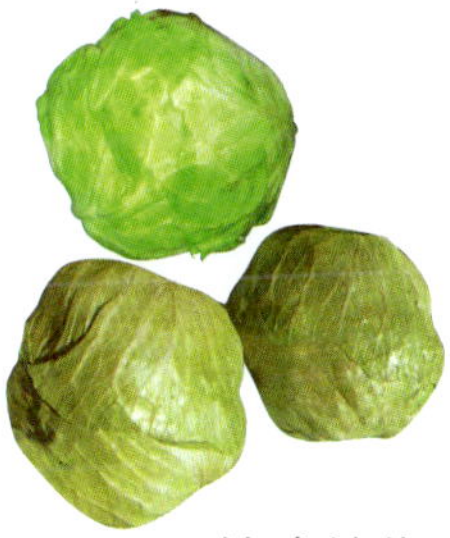
结球甘蓝（绿）

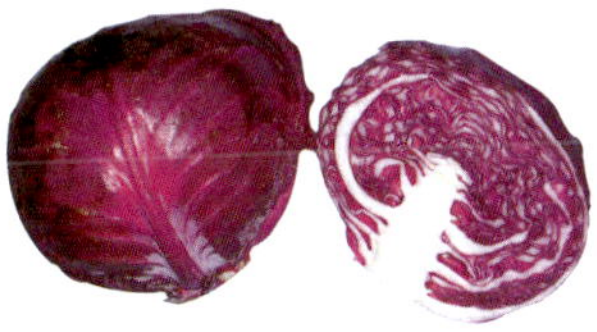
结球甘蓝（紫）

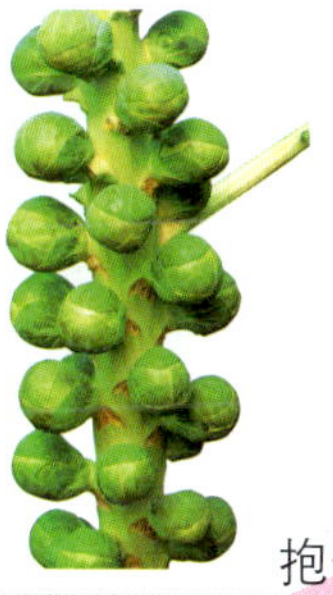
抱子甘蓝

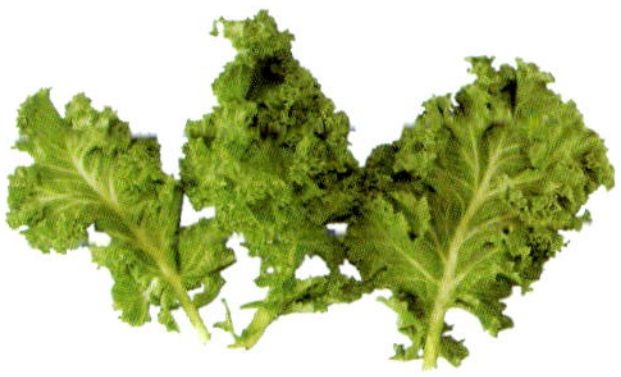
羽衣甘蓝

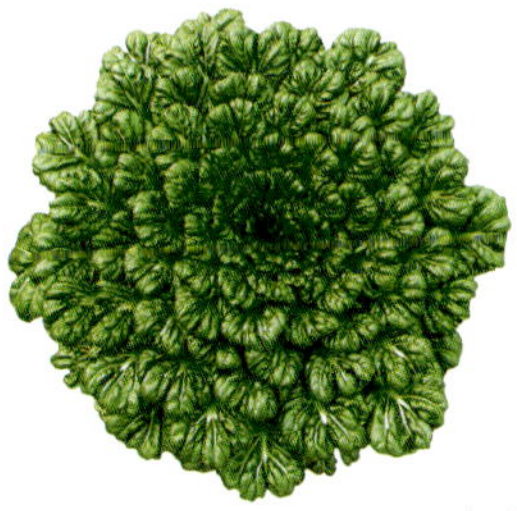
乌塌菜

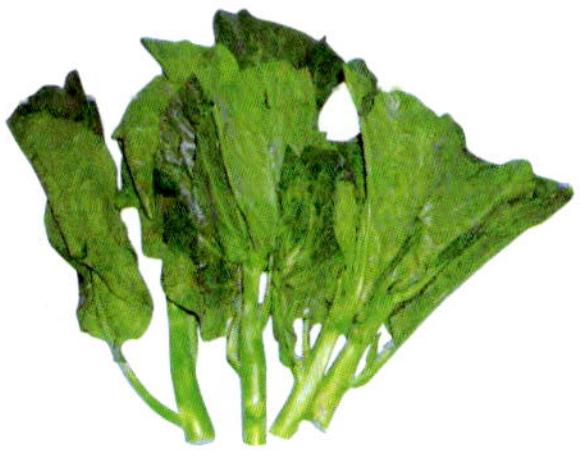
芥蓝

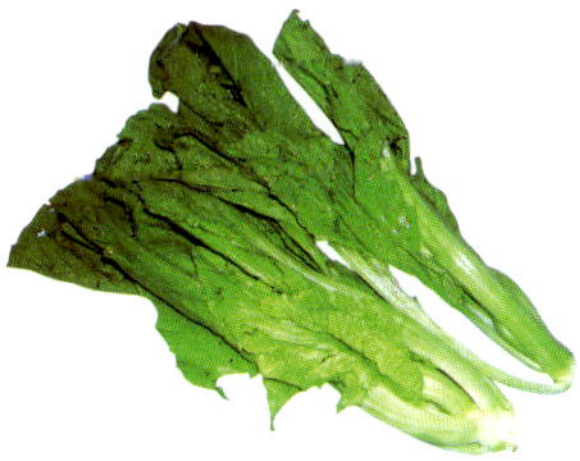
盖菜

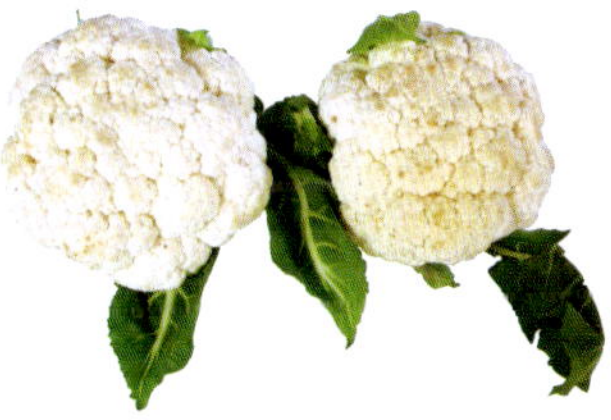
菜花

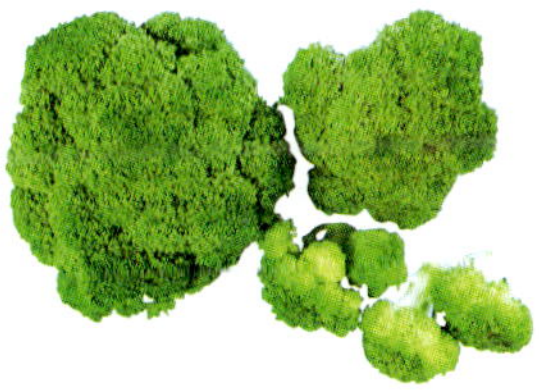
西兰花

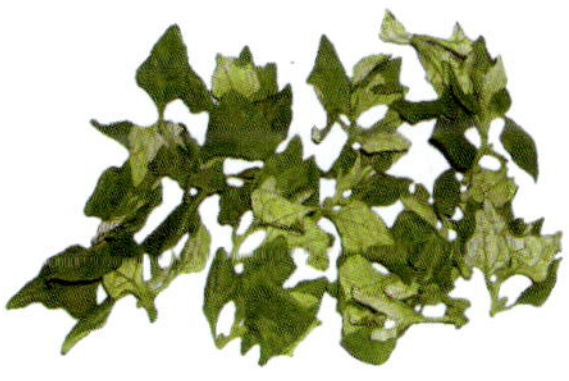
番杏

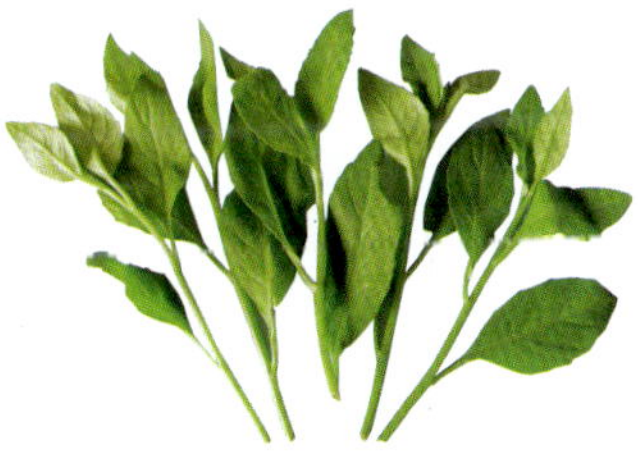
白凤菜

蔬菜

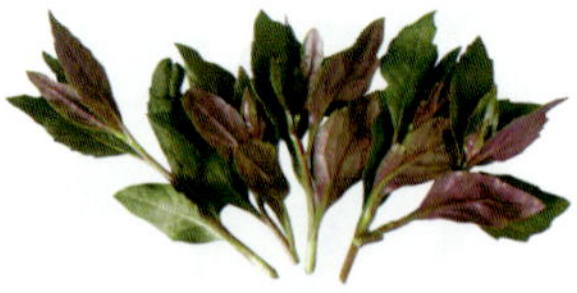
紫背天葵

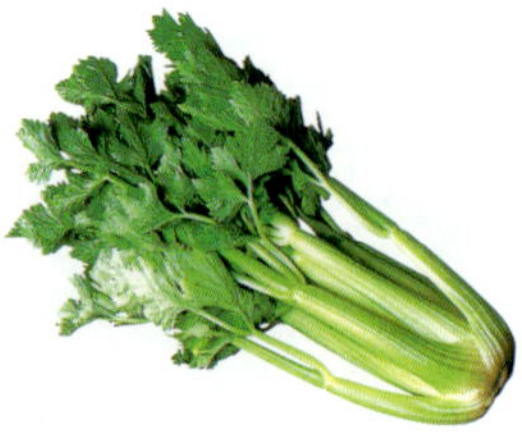
西芹

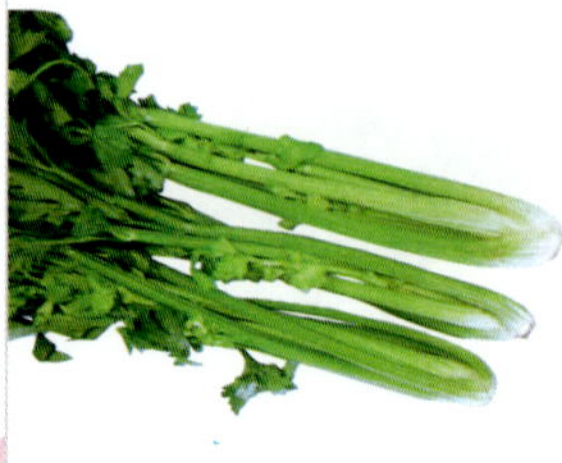
芹菜

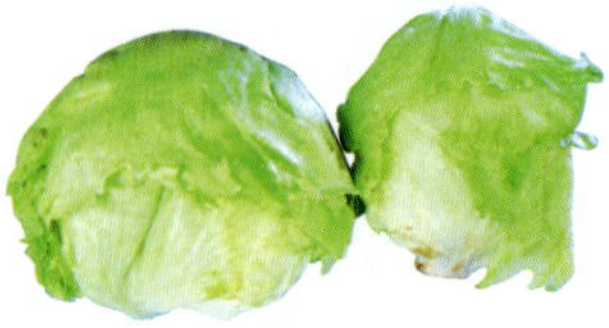
生菜

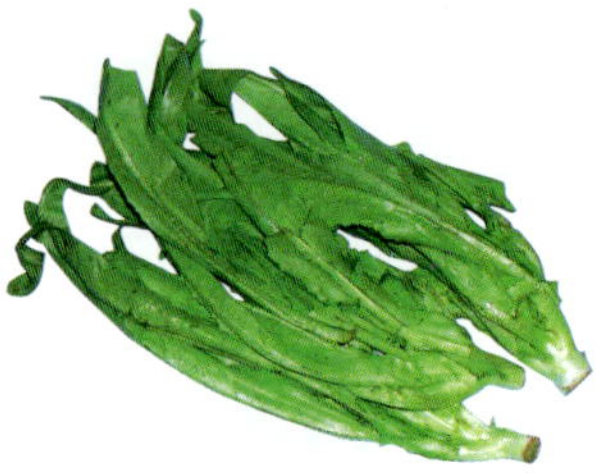
油麦菜

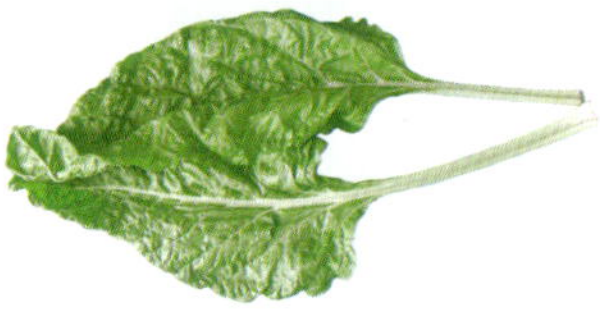
甜菜叶（白梗）

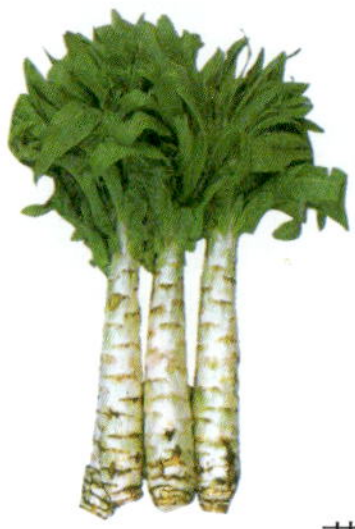
茎用莴苣

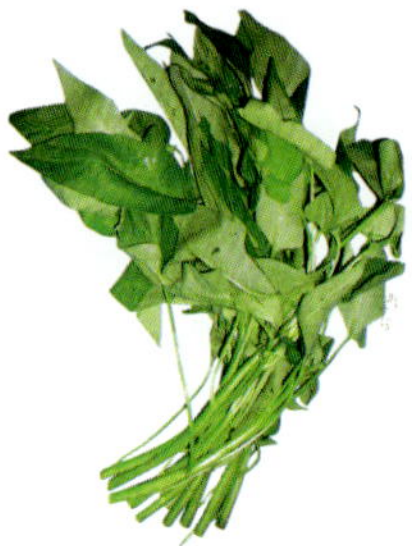
蕹菜

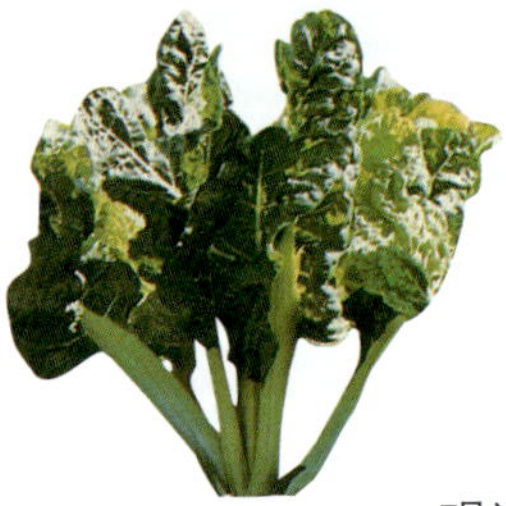
观达菜

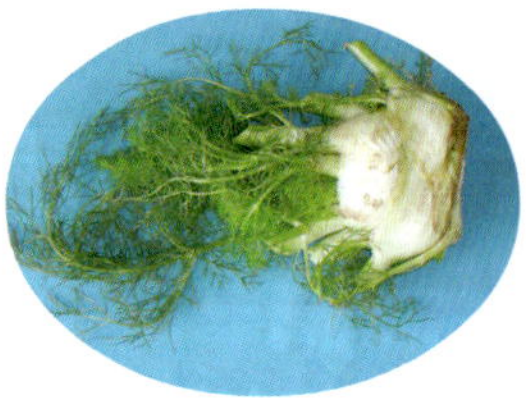
球茎茴香

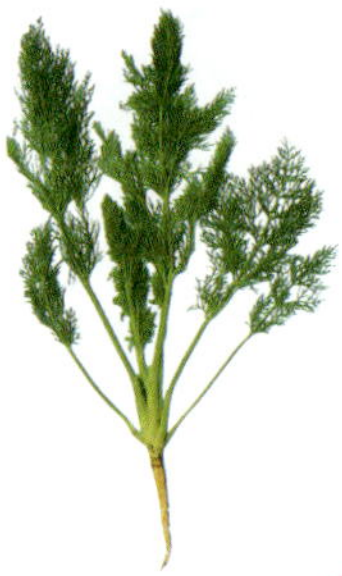
茴香

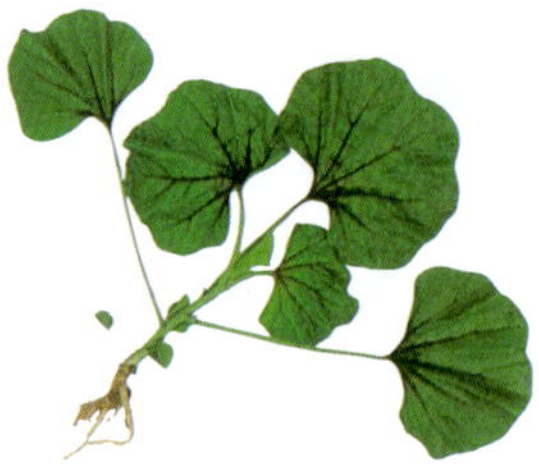
冬寒菜

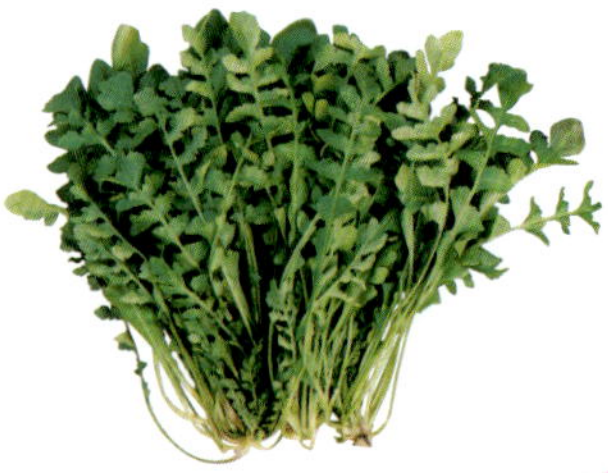
荠菜

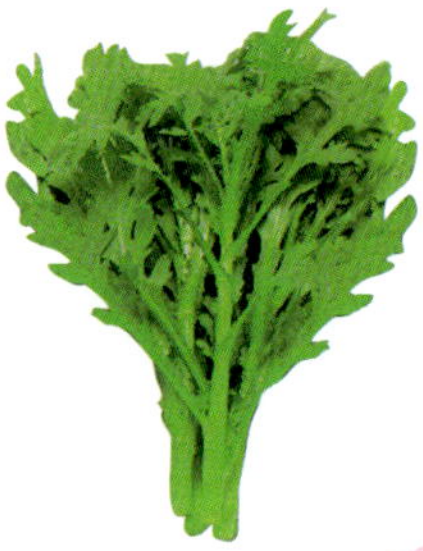
茼蒿

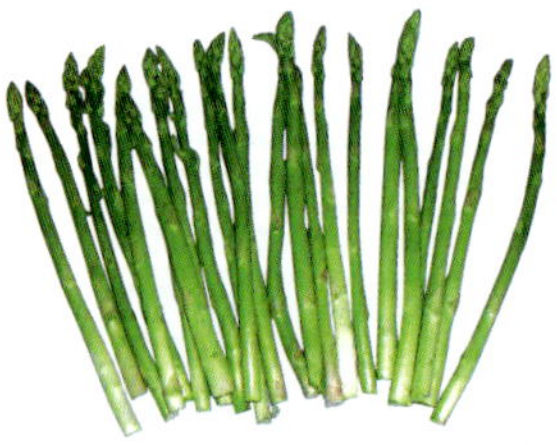
芦笋（绿）

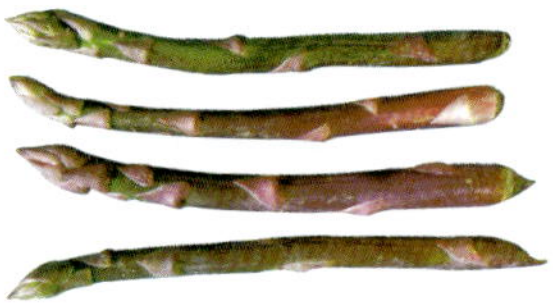
芦笋（紫）

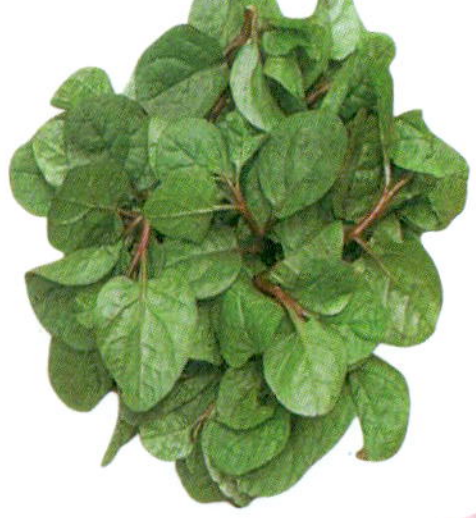
落葵

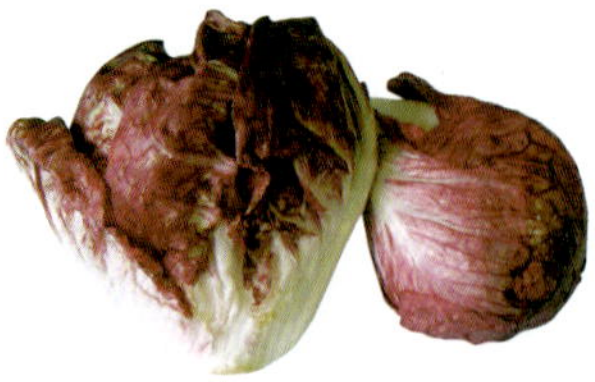
结球红菊苣

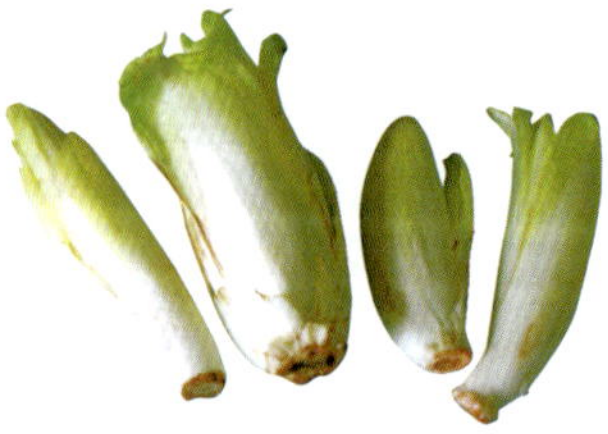
软化白菊苣

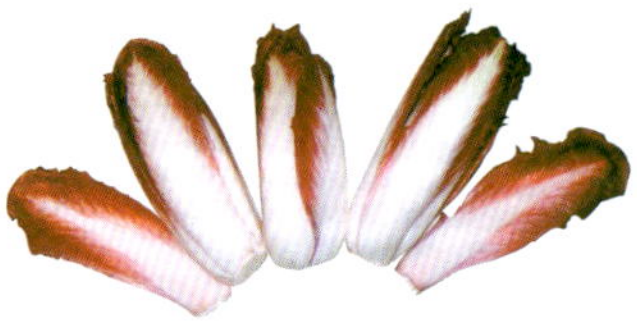
软化红菊苣

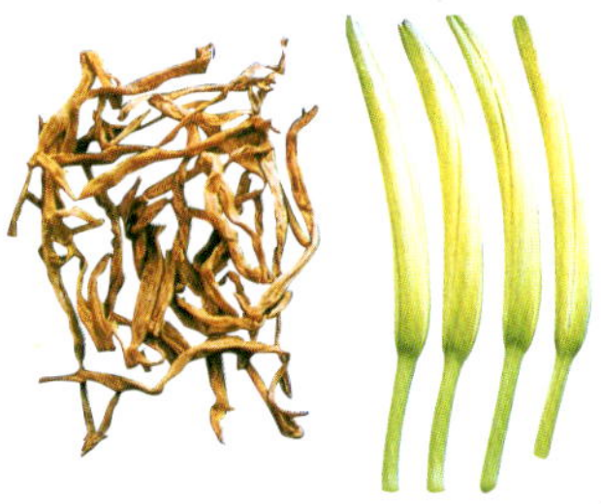
金针菜

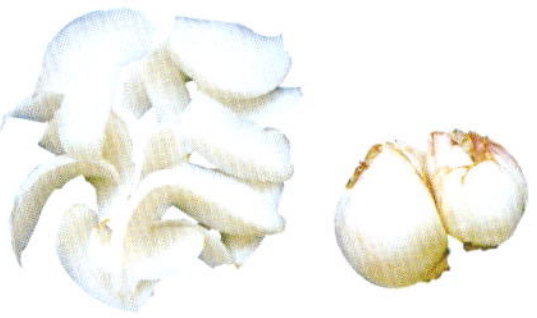
百合

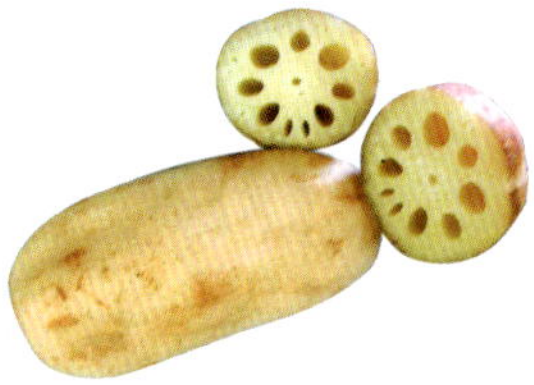
藕

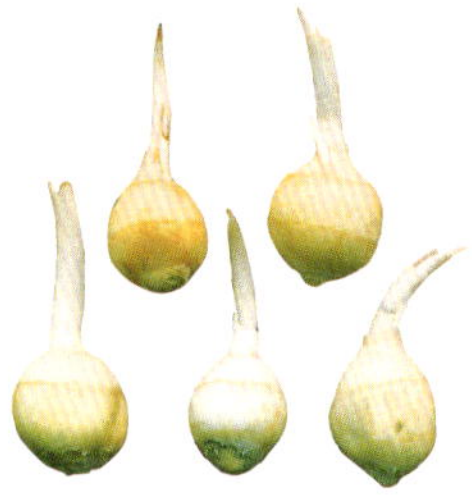
慈姑

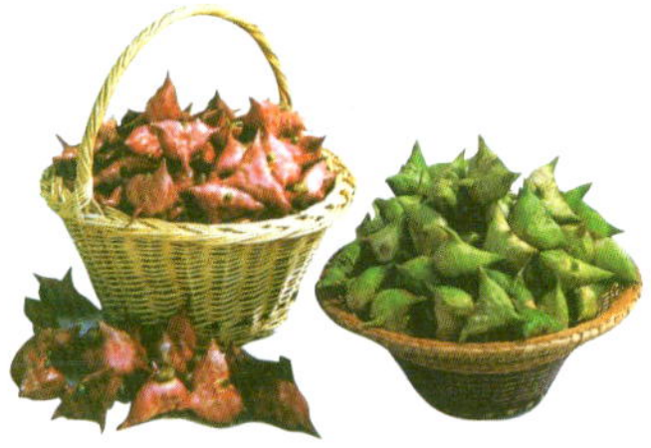
菱角

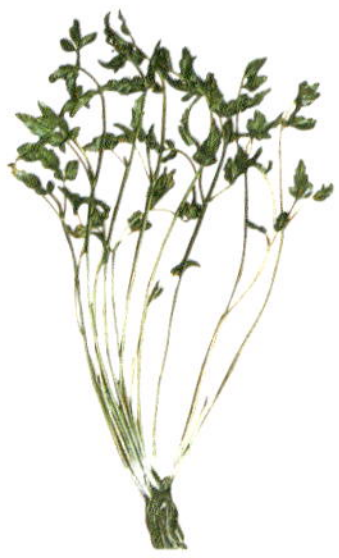
水芹菜

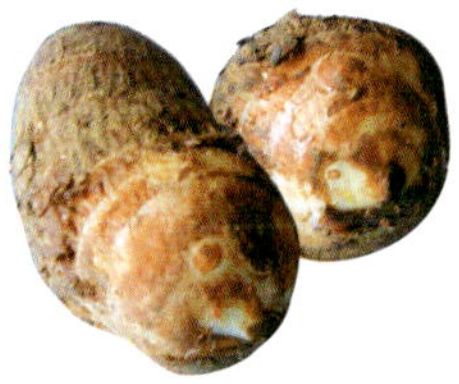
芋头

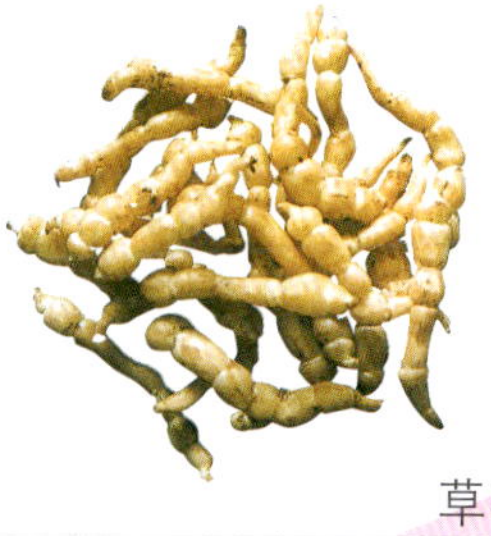
草石蚕

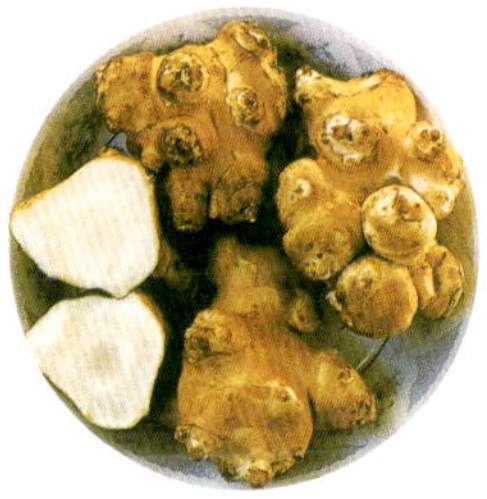
菊芋

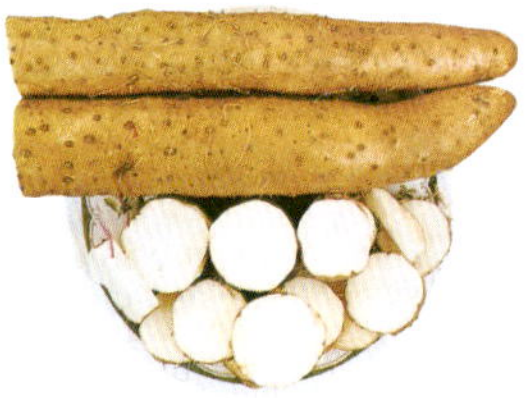
山药

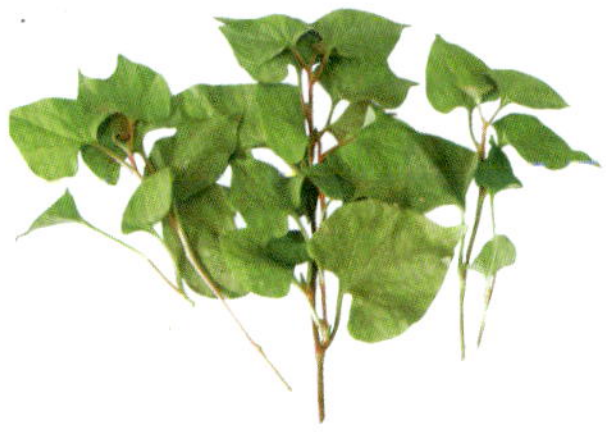
鱼腥草叶

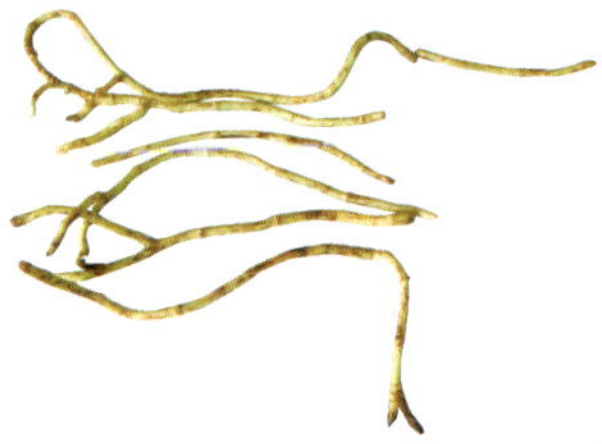
鱼腥草根

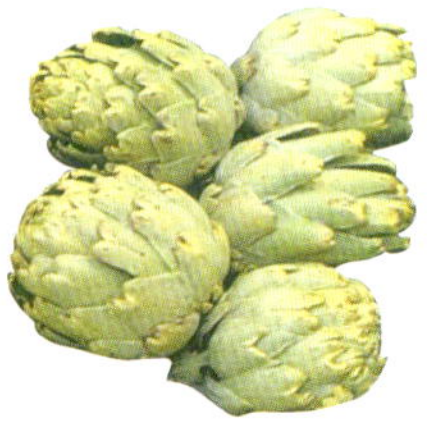
朝鲜蓟

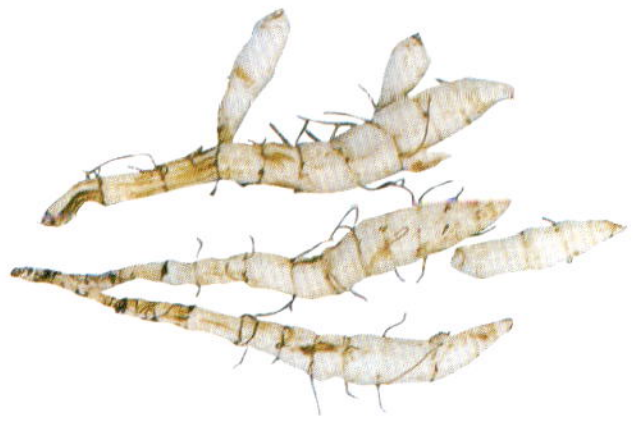
地笋

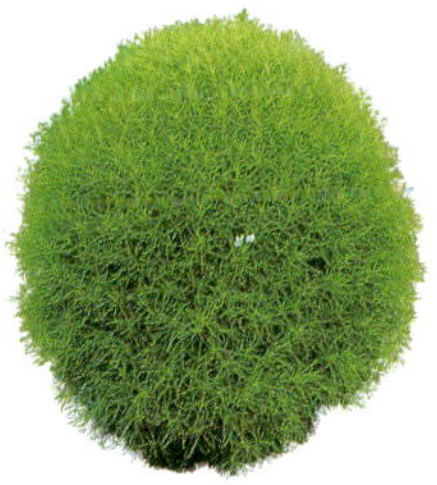
地肤

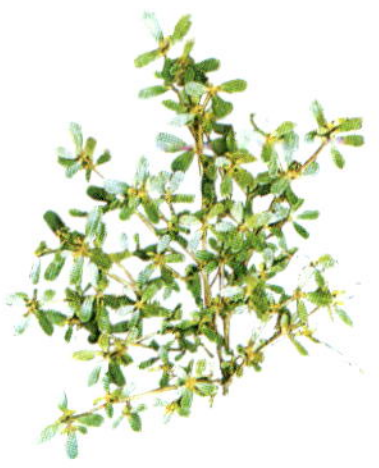
马齿苋

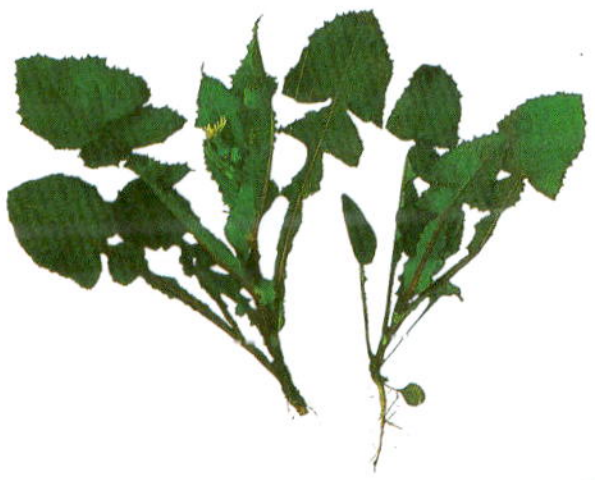
苣荬菜（苦苣菜）

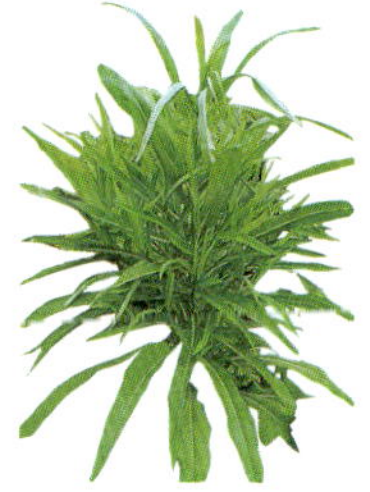
苣荬菜

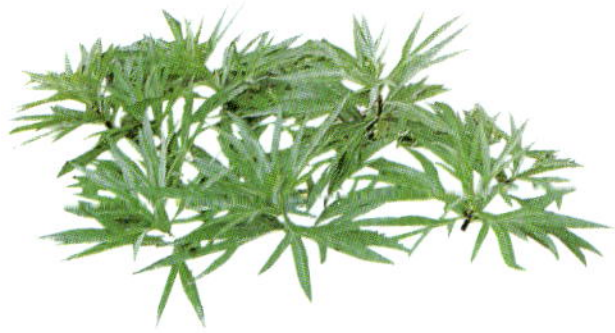
蒌蒿

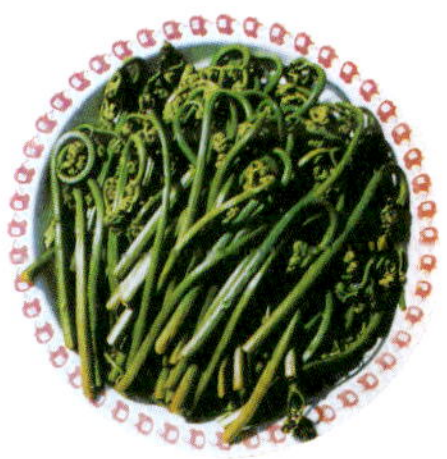
蕨菜

菌类

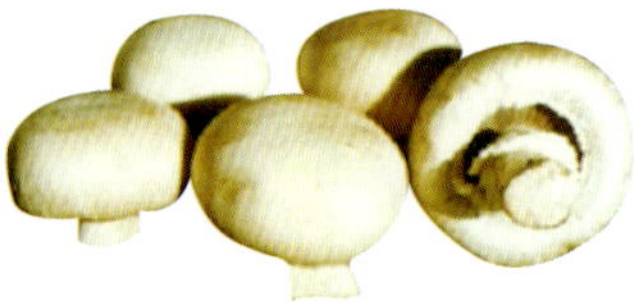
白蘑菇

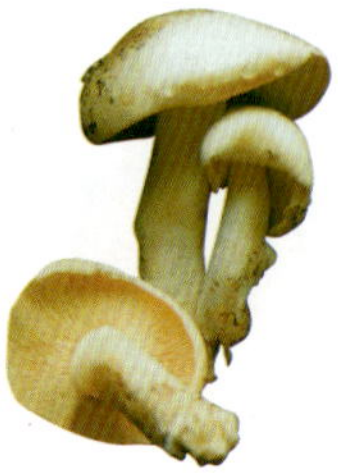
北风菌

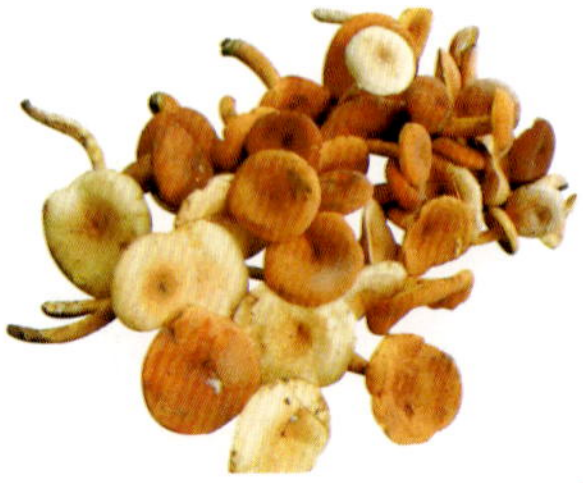
奶浆菌

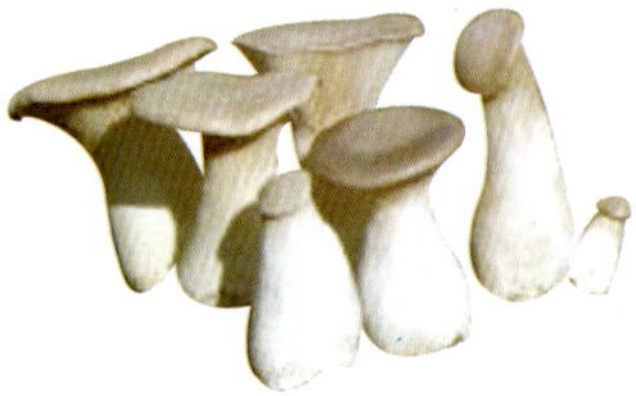
杏鲍菇

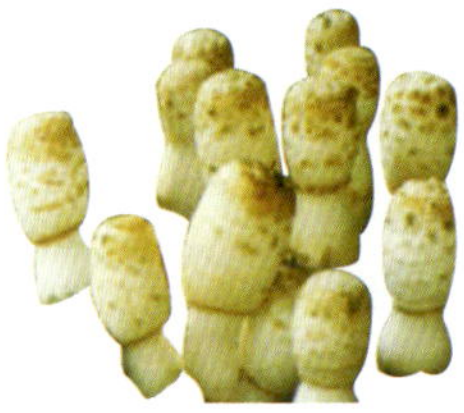
鸡腿菇

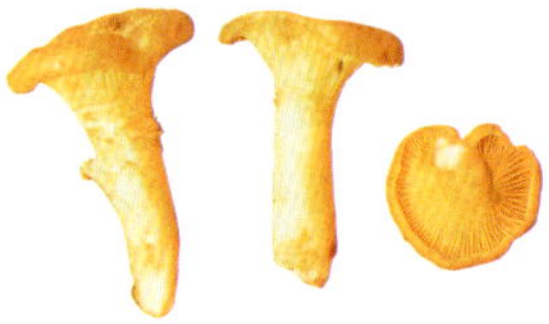
鸡油菌

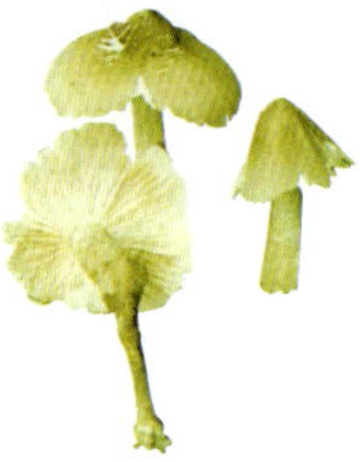
鸡纵

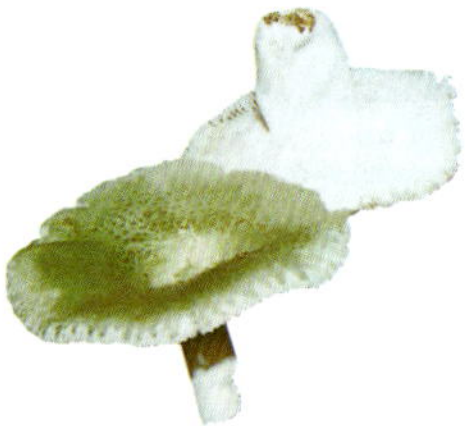
青头菌

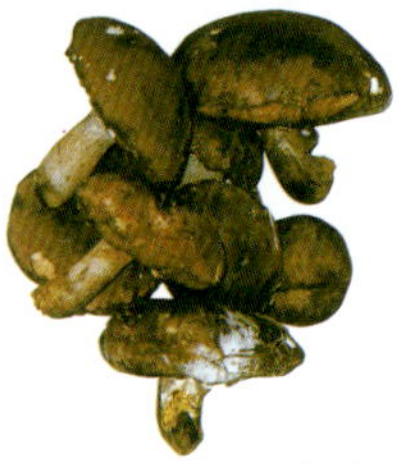
铜色牛肝菌

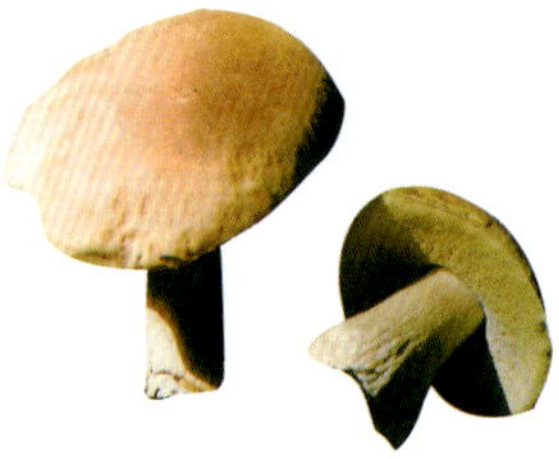
美味牛肝菌

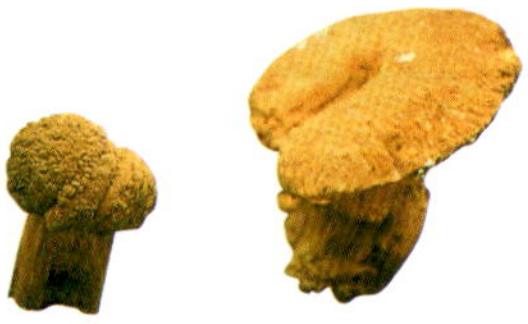
黄皮疣柄牛肝菌

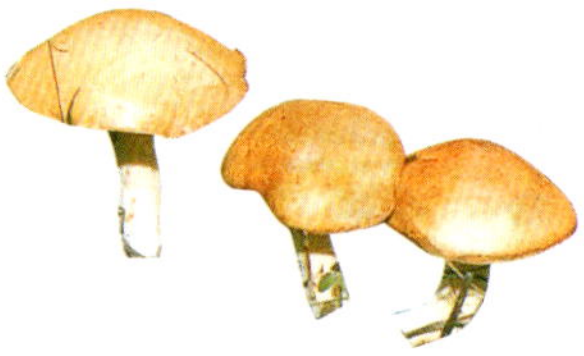
乳牛肝菌

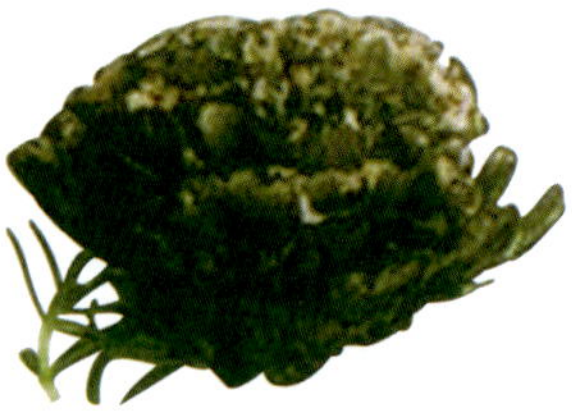
干巴菌

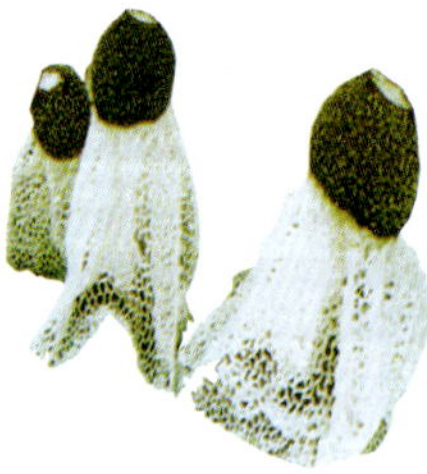
竹荪

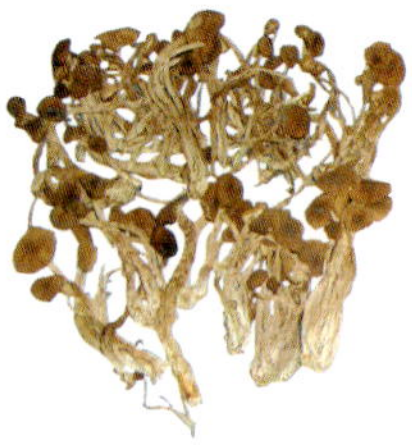
茶树菇（干）

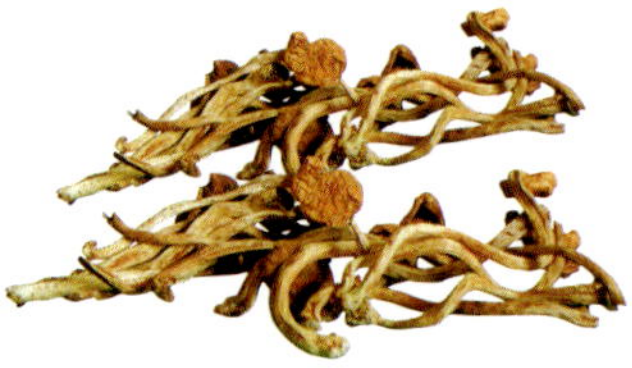
黄伞菇（干）

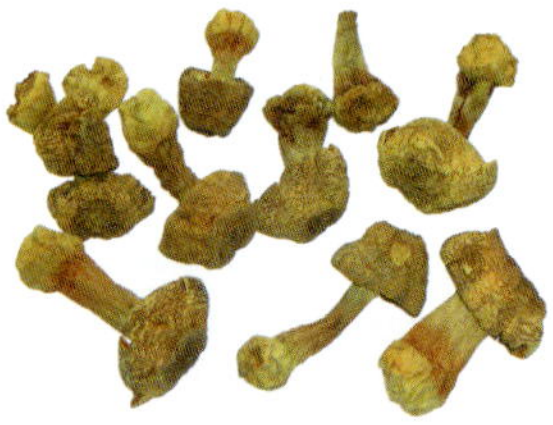
松茸（干）

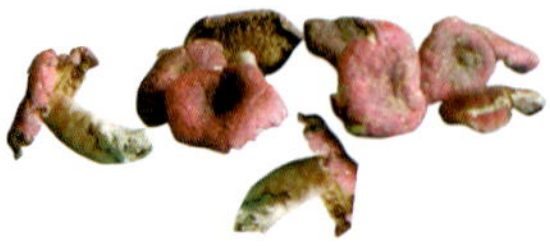
血红菇（干）

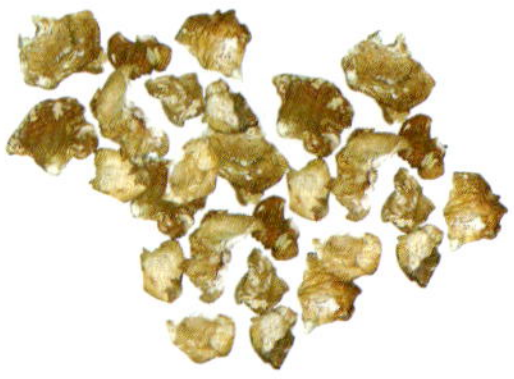
元蘑（干）

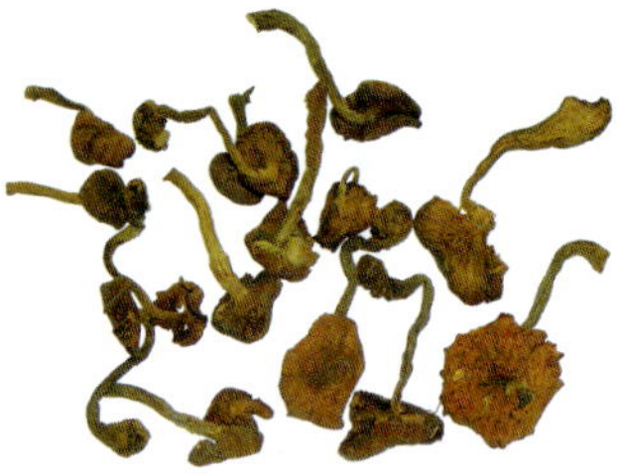
榛蘑（干）

水果

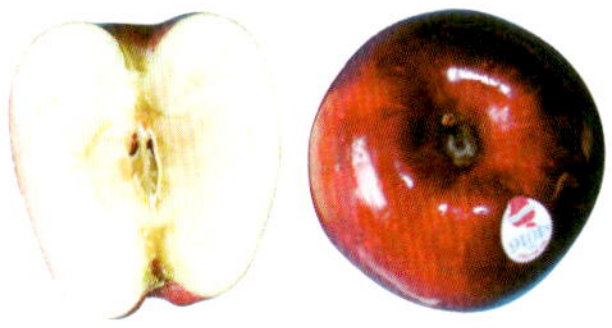
蛇果

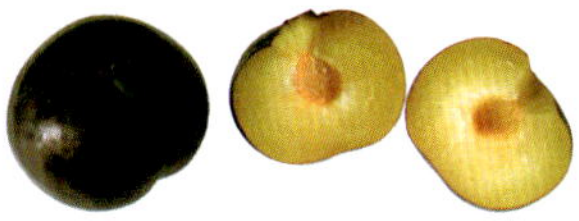
布朗

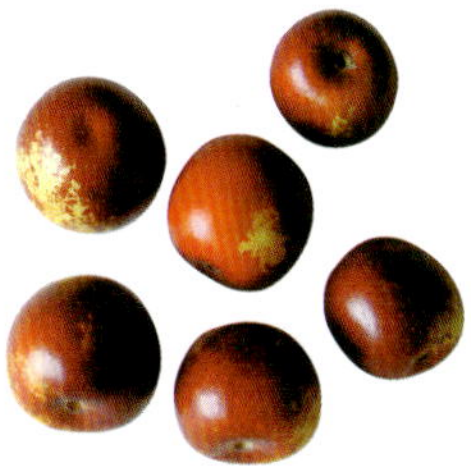
冬枣

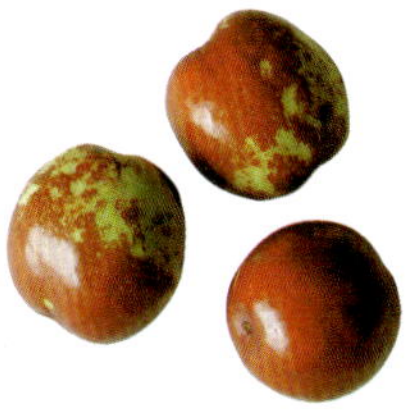
梨枣

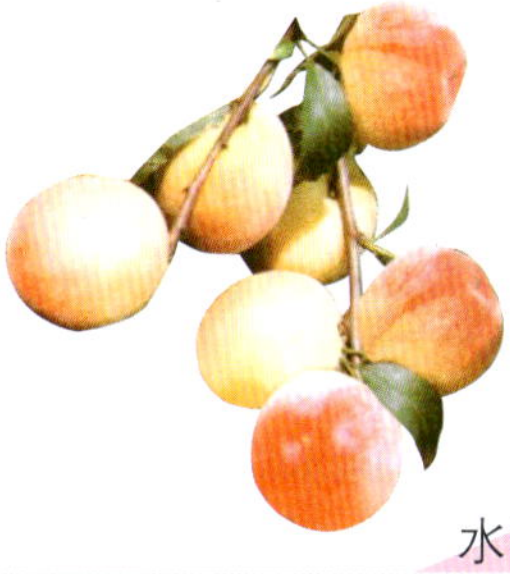
水蜜桃

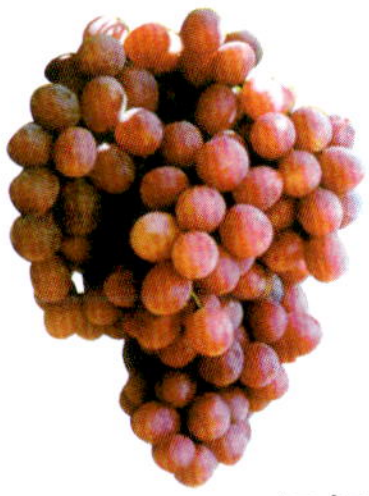
红提子葡萄

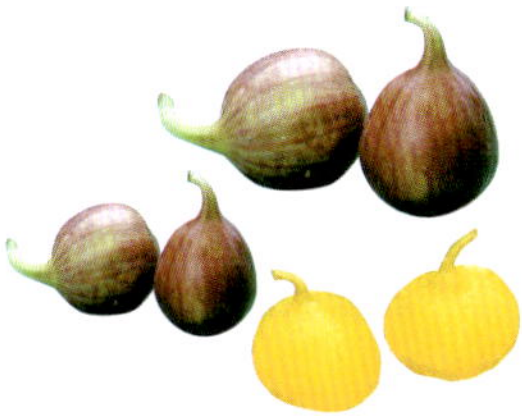
无花果

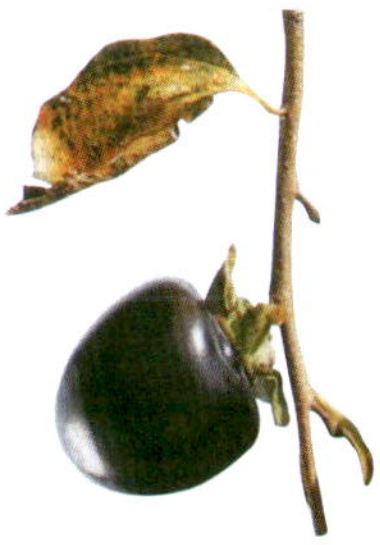
黑柿

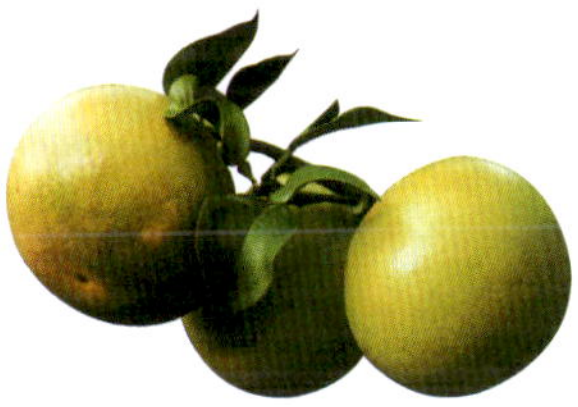
葡萄柚

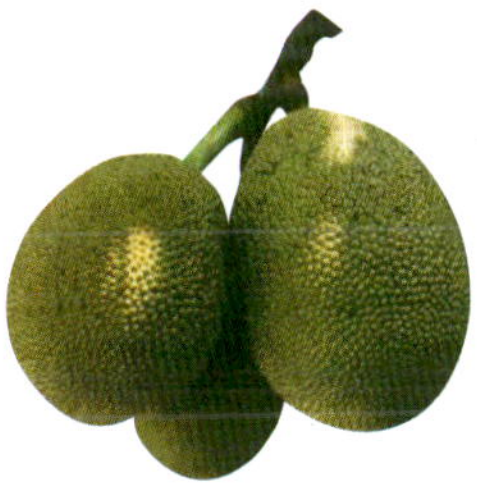
菠萝蜜

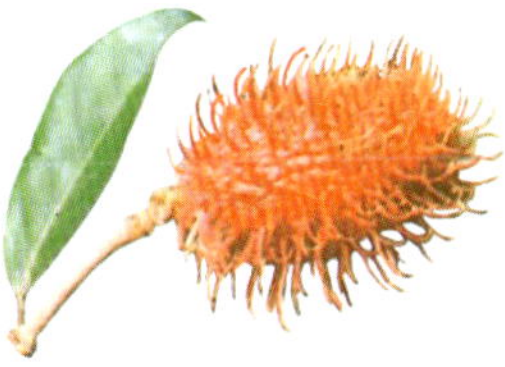
红毛丹

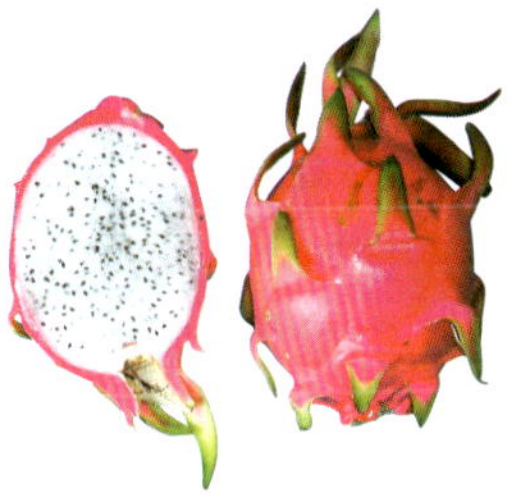
火龙果

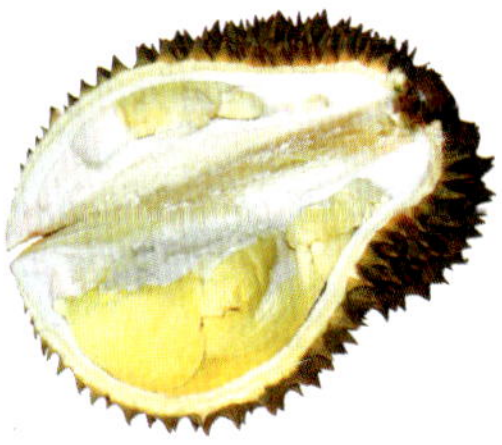
榴莲

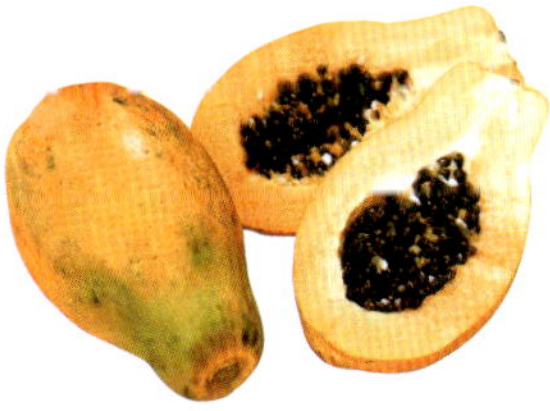
木瓜（番木瓜）

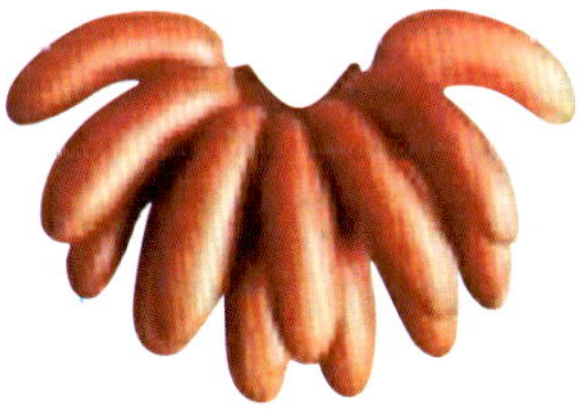
香蕉（红皮）

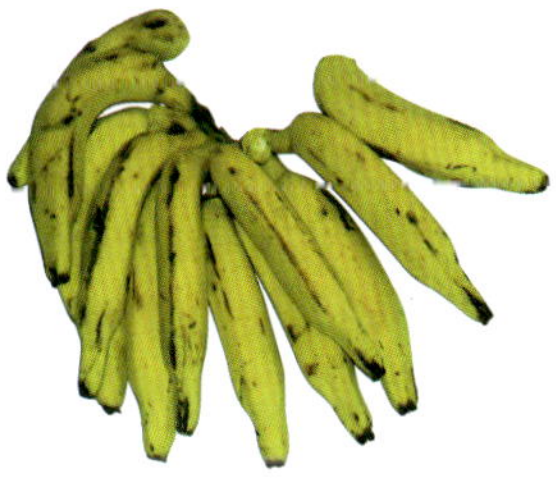
芝麻香蕉

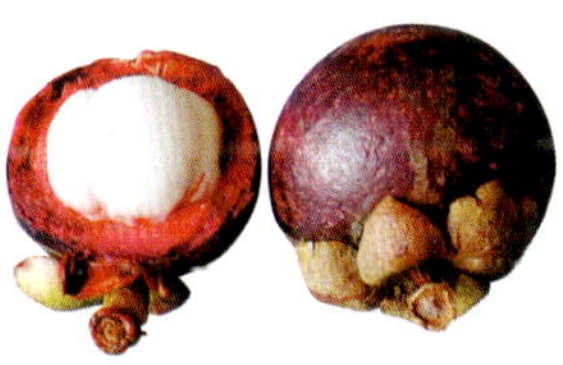
山竹

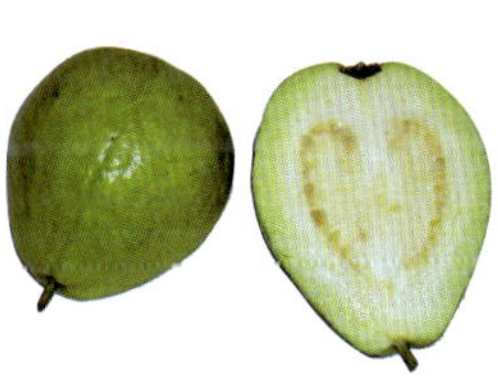
番石榴

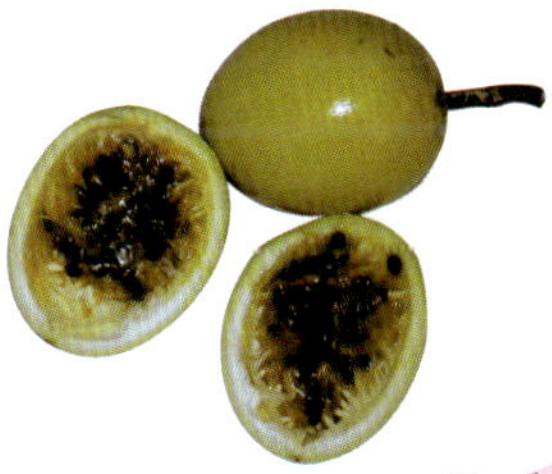
西番莲

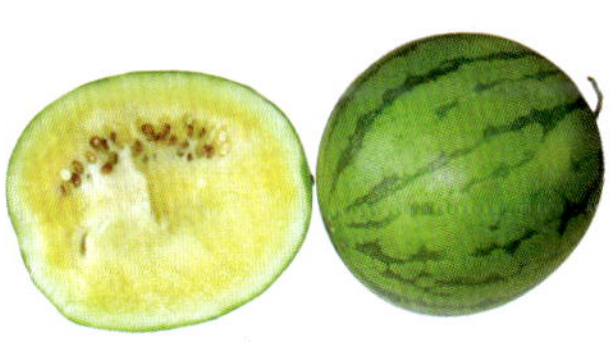
小西瓜

速食食品

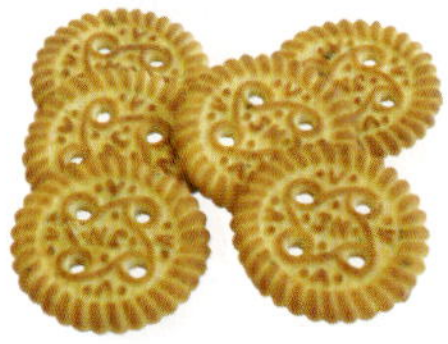
9g/片 饼干

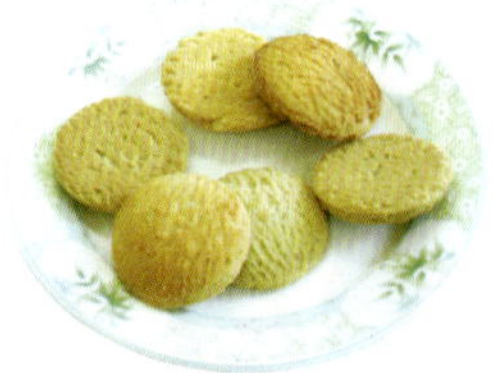
9g/片 曲奇饼干

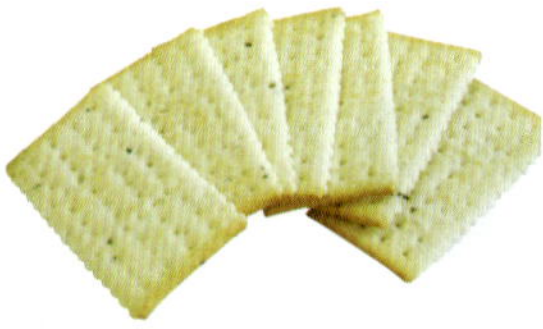
7g/片 苏打饼干

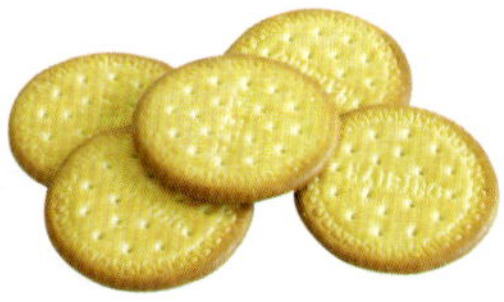
6g/片 早餐饼

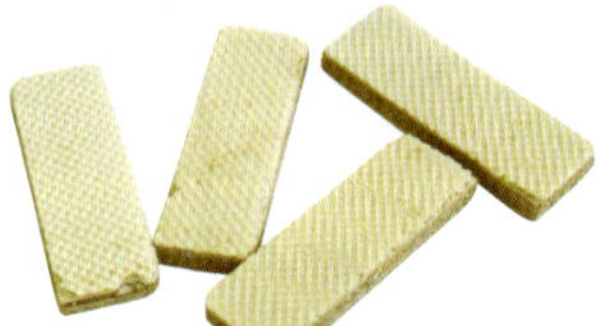
12g/片 白华夫饼干

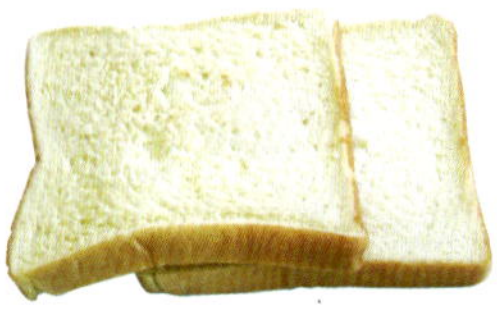
36g/片 面包片

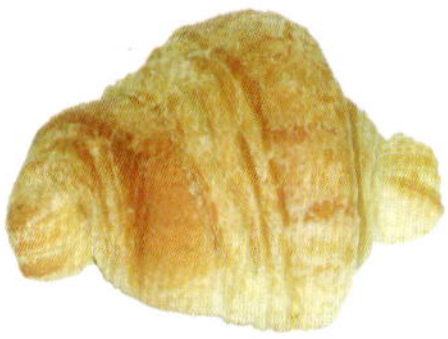
33g/个 牛角面包

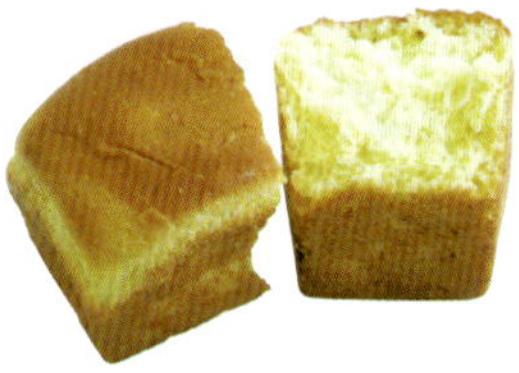
135g/个 维生素面包

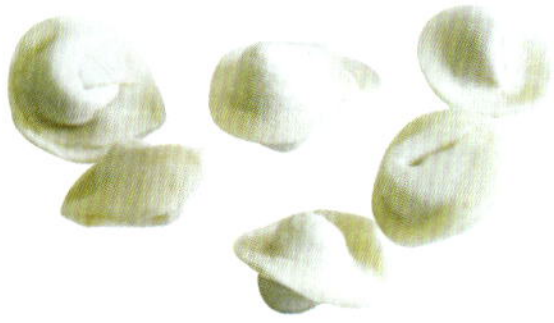
4g/个 混饨(猪肉大葱馅,生)

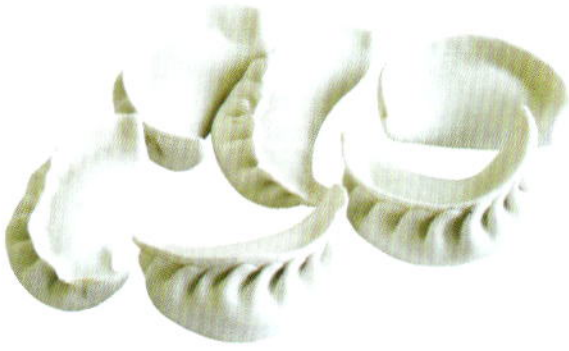
17g/个 饺子(猪肉大葱馅,生)

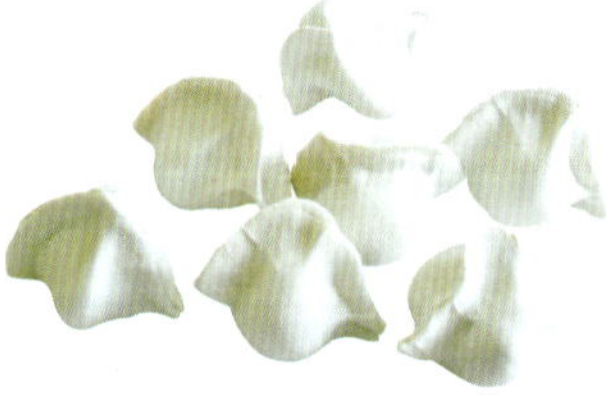
18g/个 饺子(猪肉茴香馅,生)

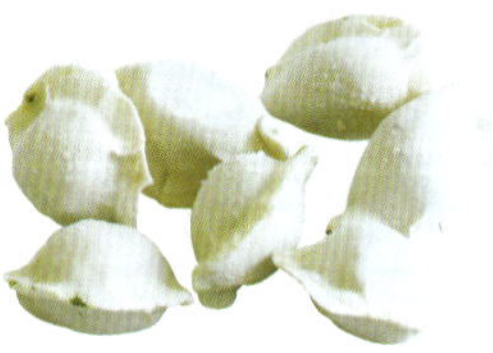
19g/个 饺子(韭菜鸡蛋馅,生)

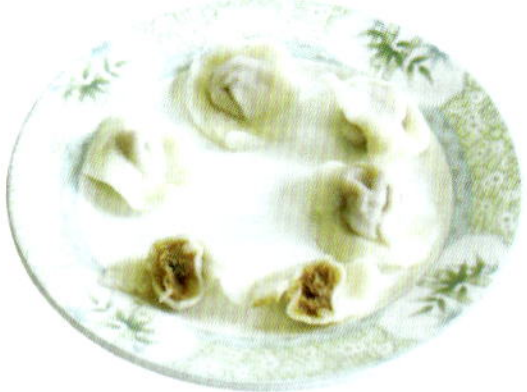
6g/个 混饨(猪肉大葱馅,熟)

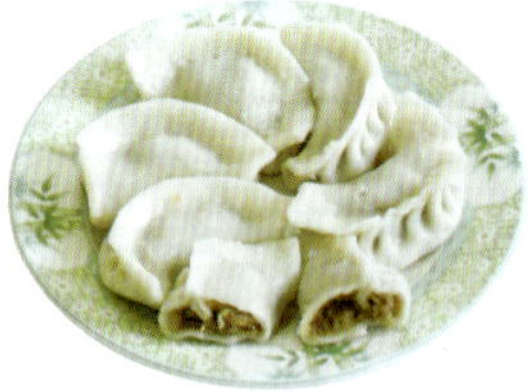
20g/个 饺子(猪肉大葱馅,熟)

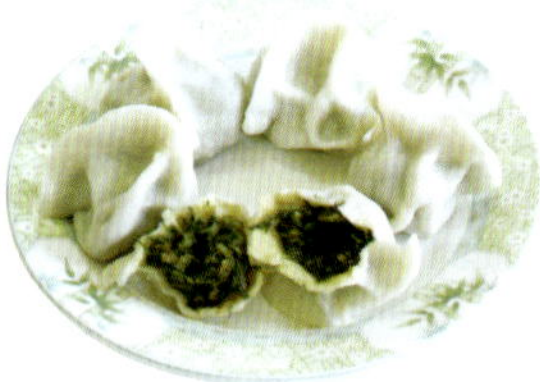
22g/个 饺子(猪肉茴香馅,熟)

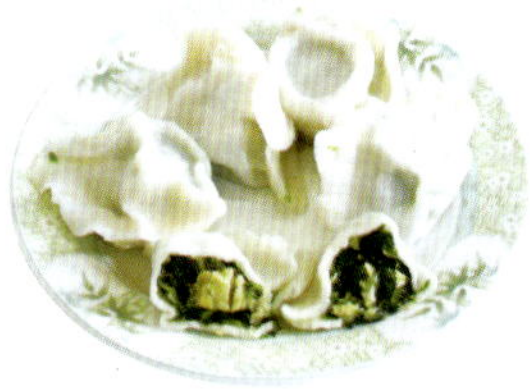
23g/个 饺子(韭菜鸡蛋馅,熟)

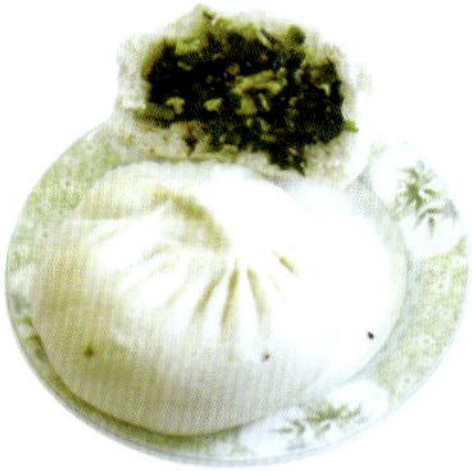
120g/个 大包子(韭菜鸡蛋馅)

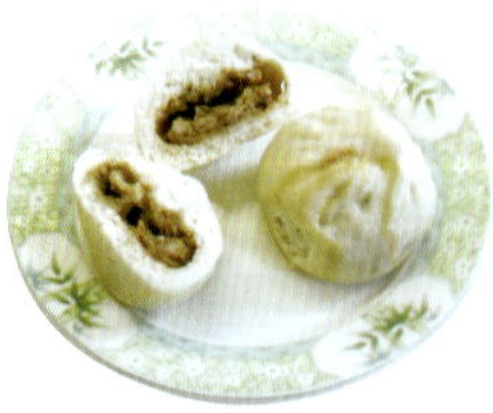
43g/个 小包子(猪肉白菜馅)

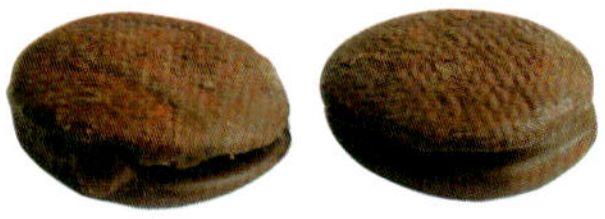
40g/个 巧克力派

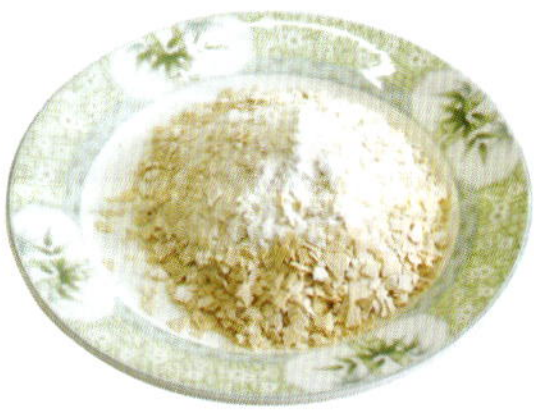
35g 奶香麦片

速食食品

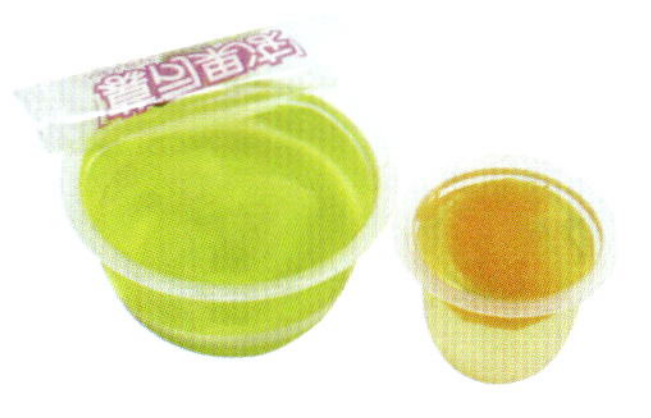

80g/个, 30g/个 果冻

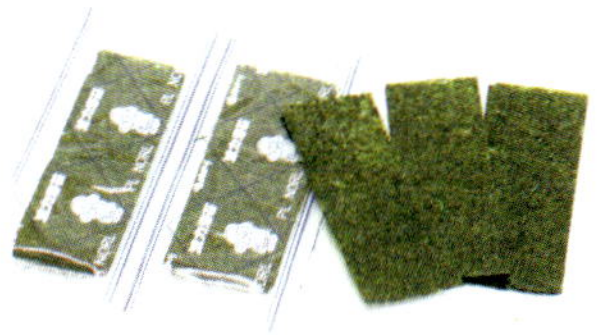

1g/片 海苔

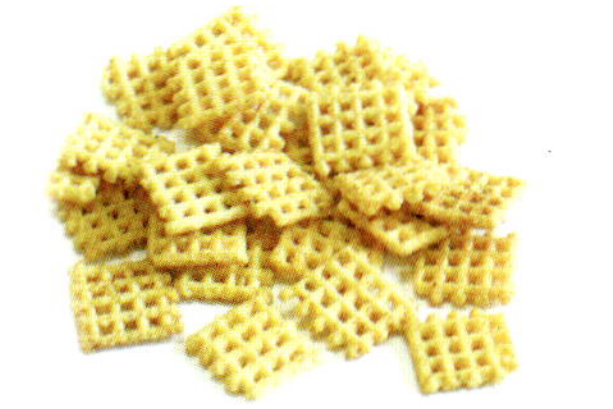

25g 锅巴

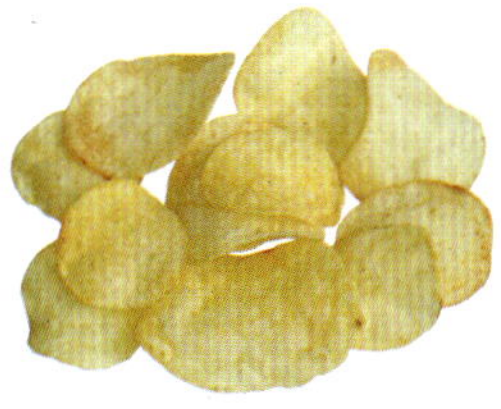

10g 薯片

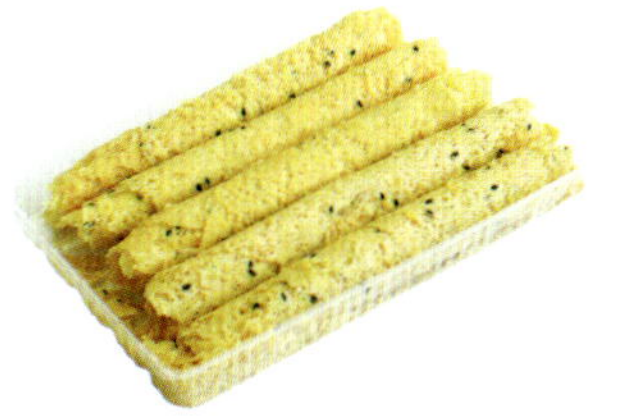

18g/根 蛋酥卷

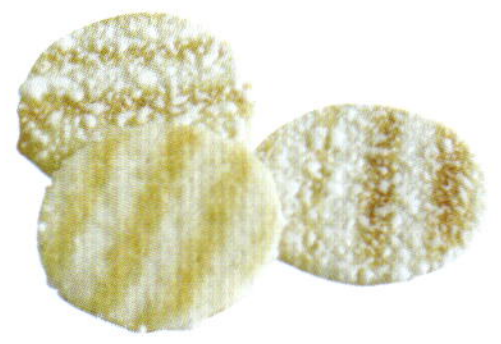

6g/片 雪米饼

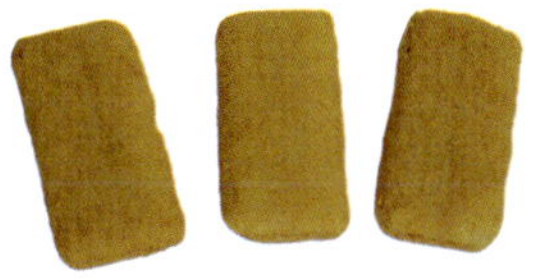

6g/块 夹心米果

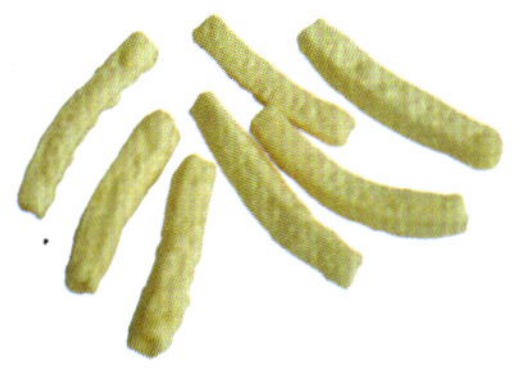

5g 通心脆

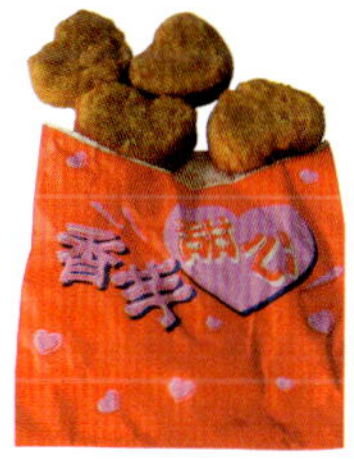

65g/份 香芋甜心

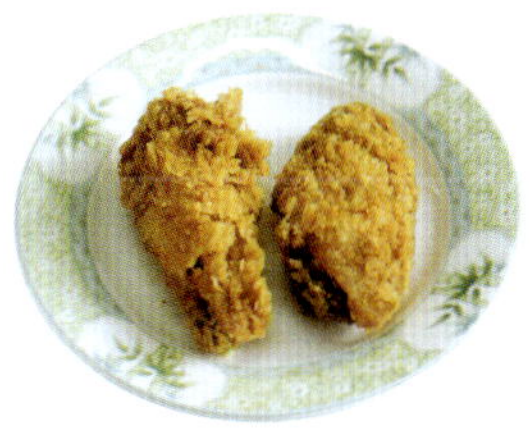

80g/对 香辣鸡翅

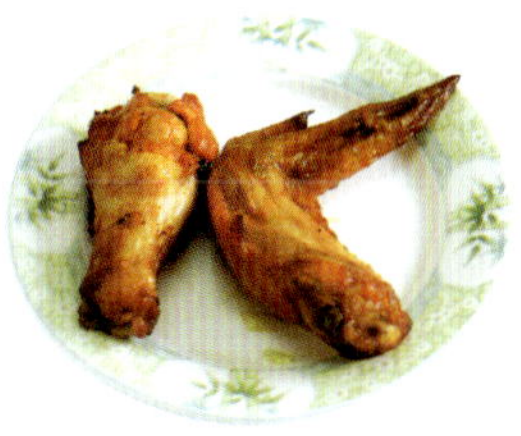

90g/对 鸡翅(炸)

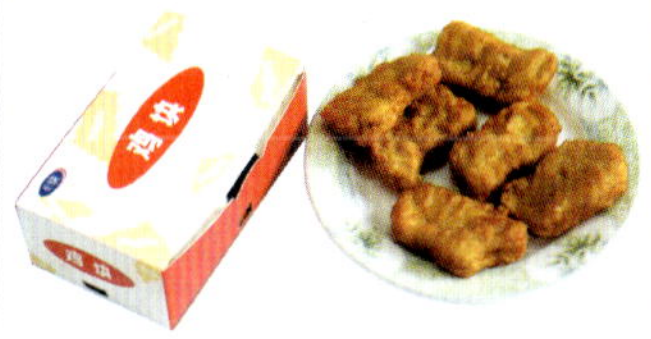

30g/块 鸡块(炸)

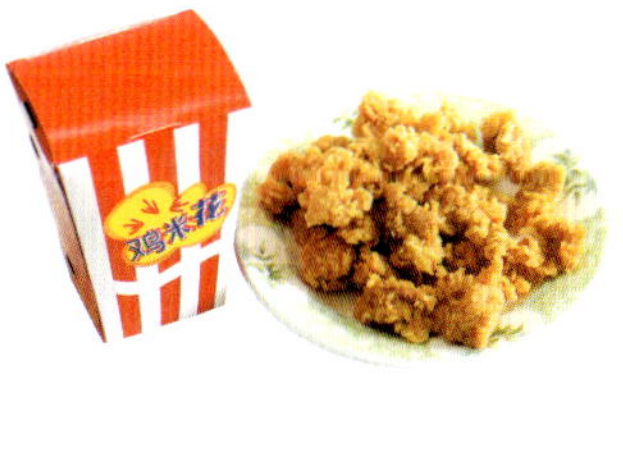

120g/盒 劲爆鸡米花

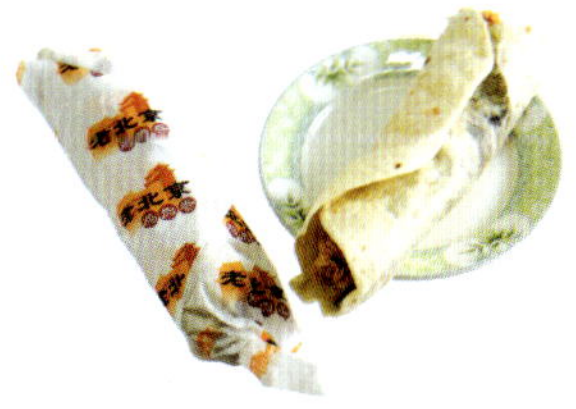

180g/个 老北京鸡肉卷

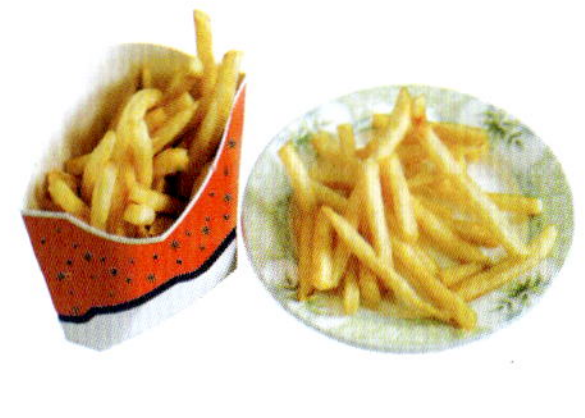

100g/盒 薯条（中号）

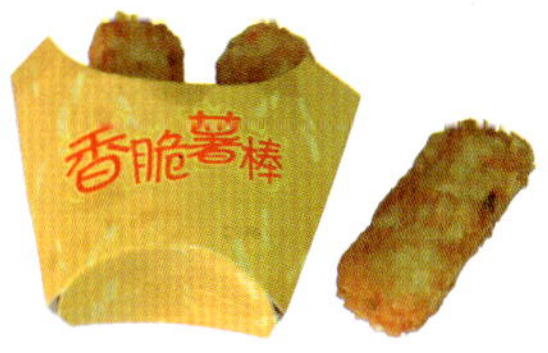

10g/个 香脆薯棒

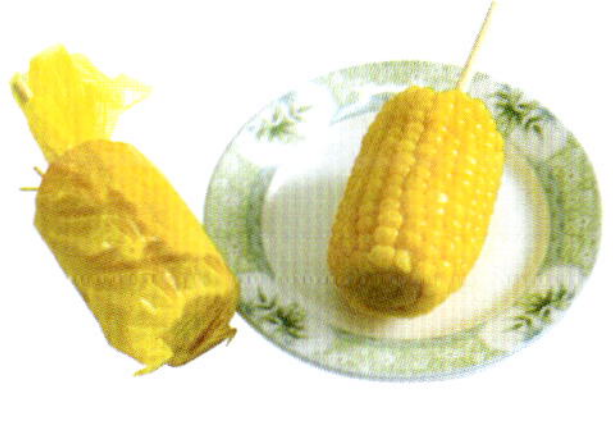

150g/个 甜玉米籽粒

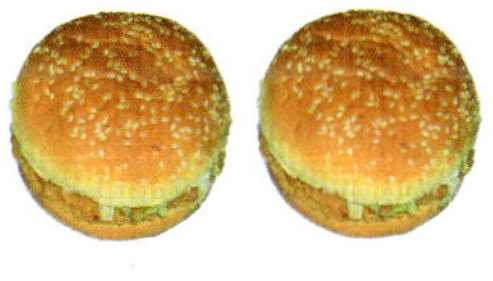

137g/个 田园脆鸡堡

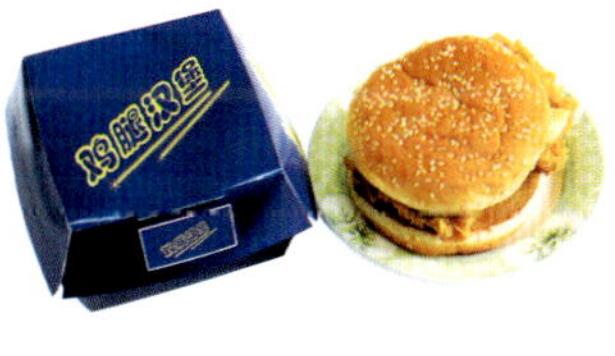

200g/盒 劲脆鸡腿堡

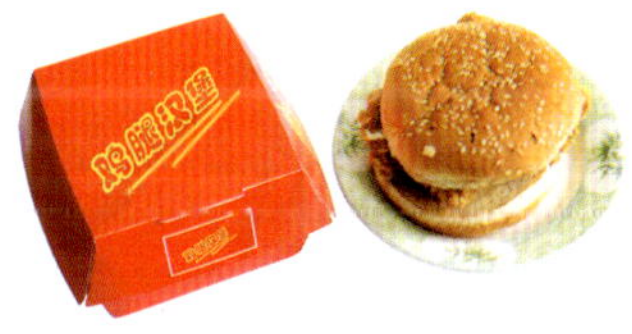

200g/盒 香辣鸡腿堡

速食食品及其它

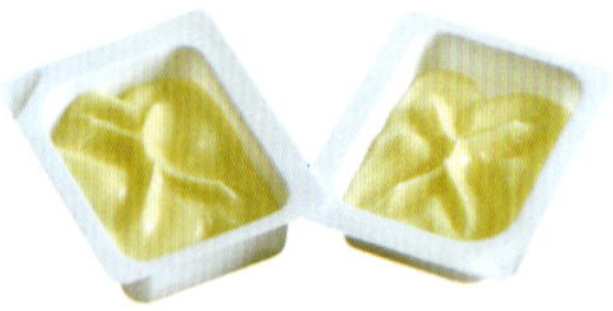
10g/盒 黄油

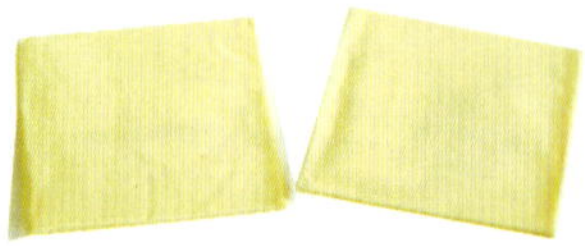
19g/片 鲜奶酪

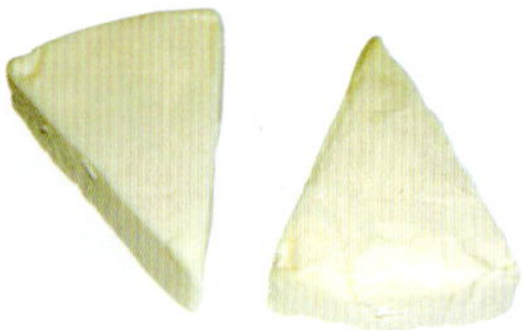
18g/块 原味奶酪

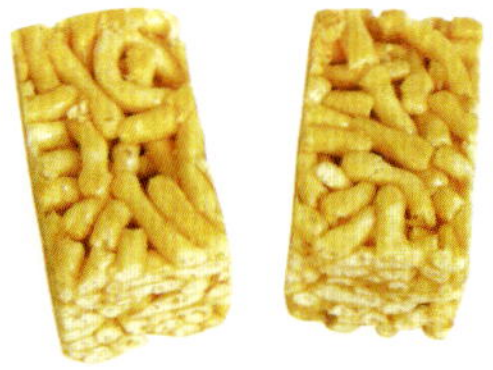
20g/块 沙琪玛

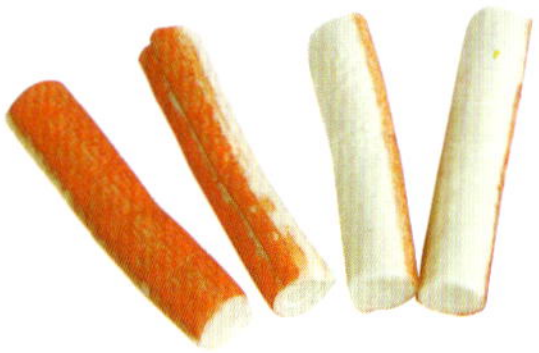
22g/根 蟹足棒(生)

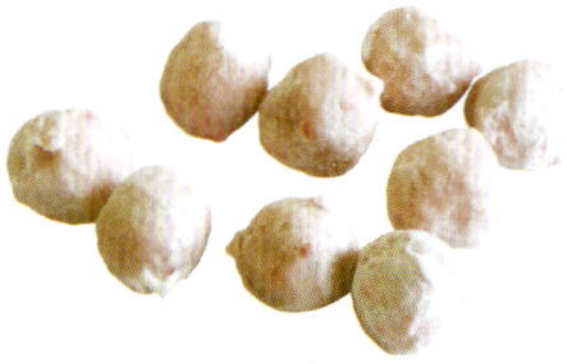
7g/个 虾丸(生)

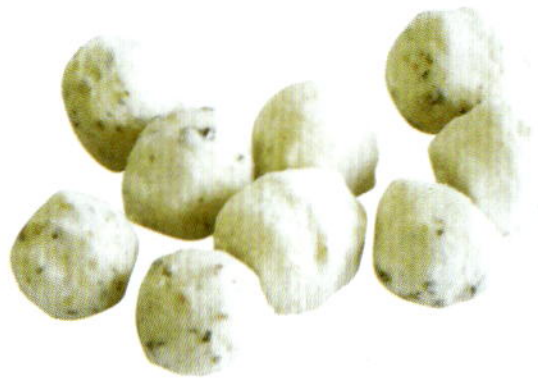
7g/个 鱼丸(生)

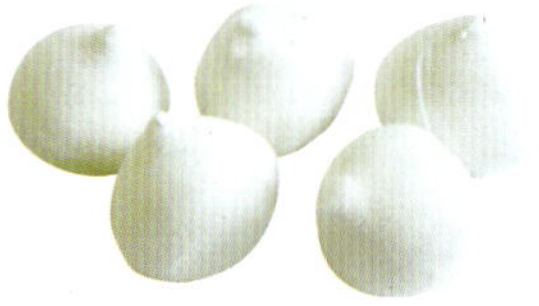
21g/个 芝麻汤圆(生)

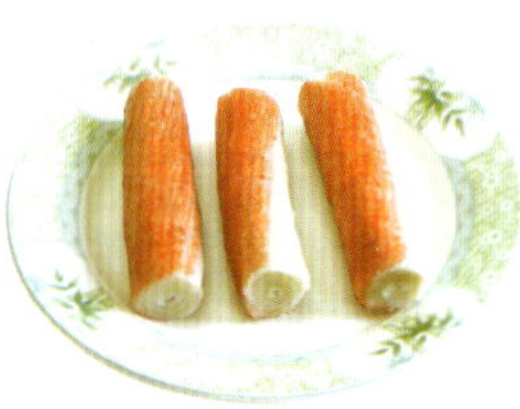
24g/根 蟹足棒(熟)

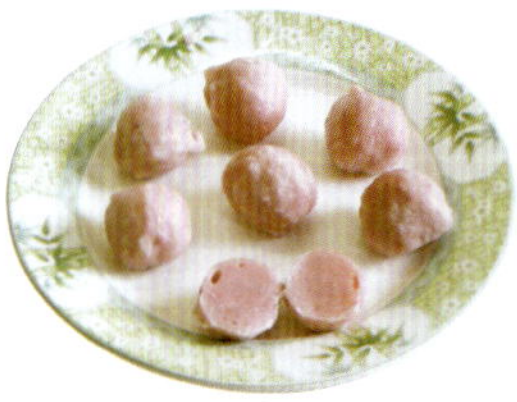
8g/个 虾丸(熟)

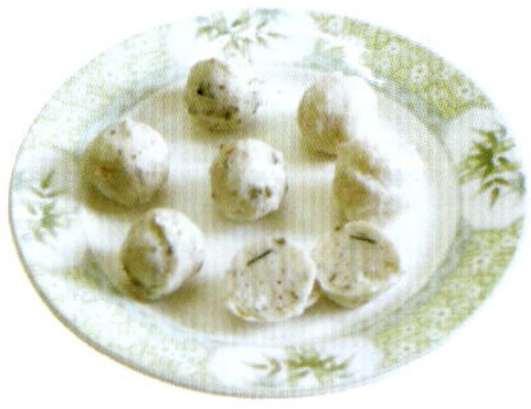
8g/个 鱼丸(熟)

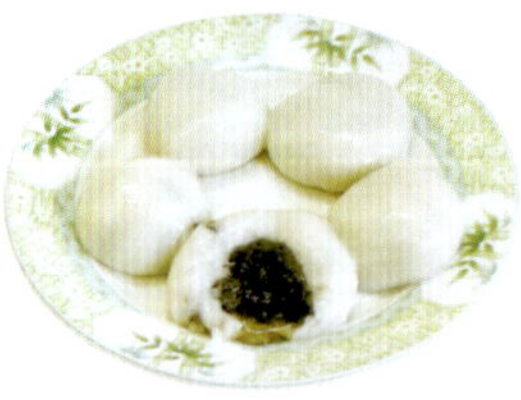
23g/个 芝麻汤圆(熟)

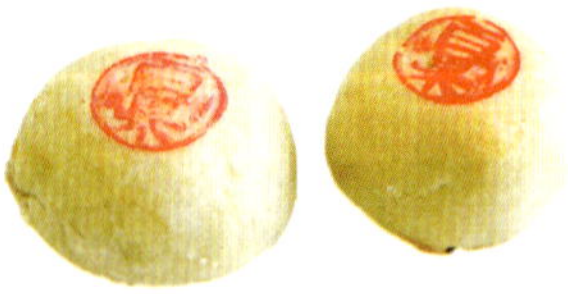
70g/个 月饼(自来白)

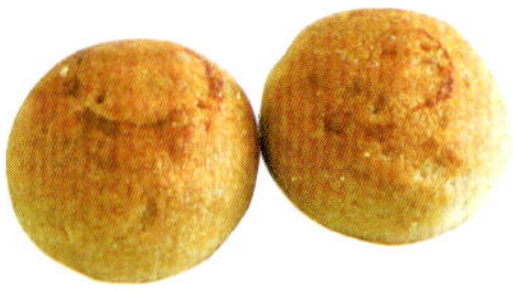
60g/个 月饼(自来红)

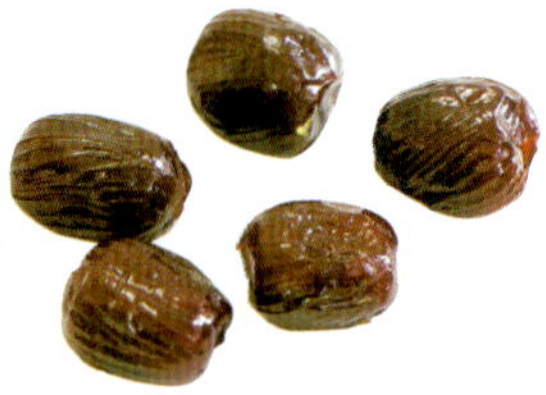
14g/粒 蜜枣(无核)

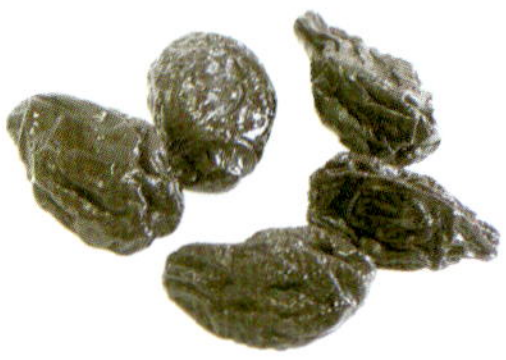
6g/粒 西梅

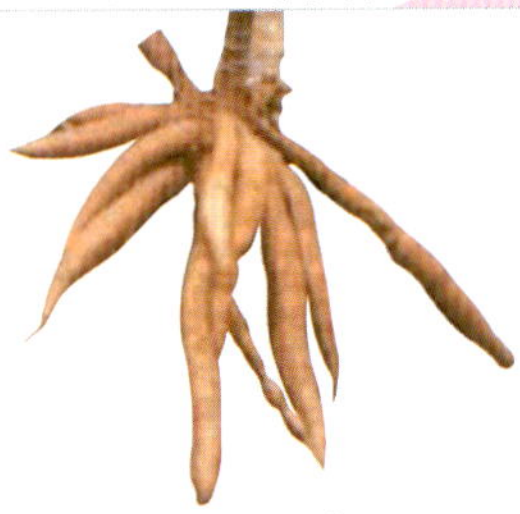
木薯

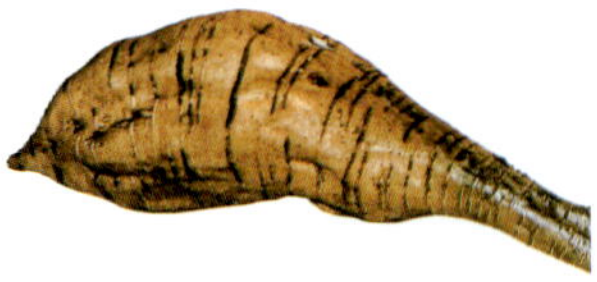
葛根

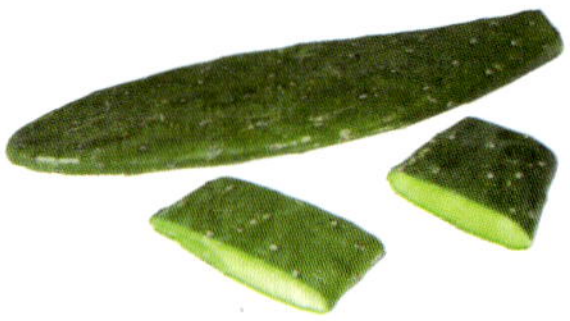
仙人掌

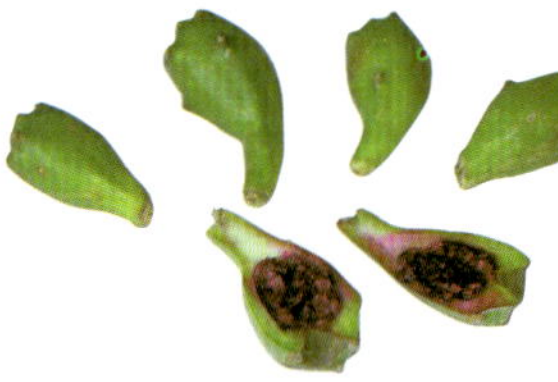
仙人掌果

牛解剖部位图

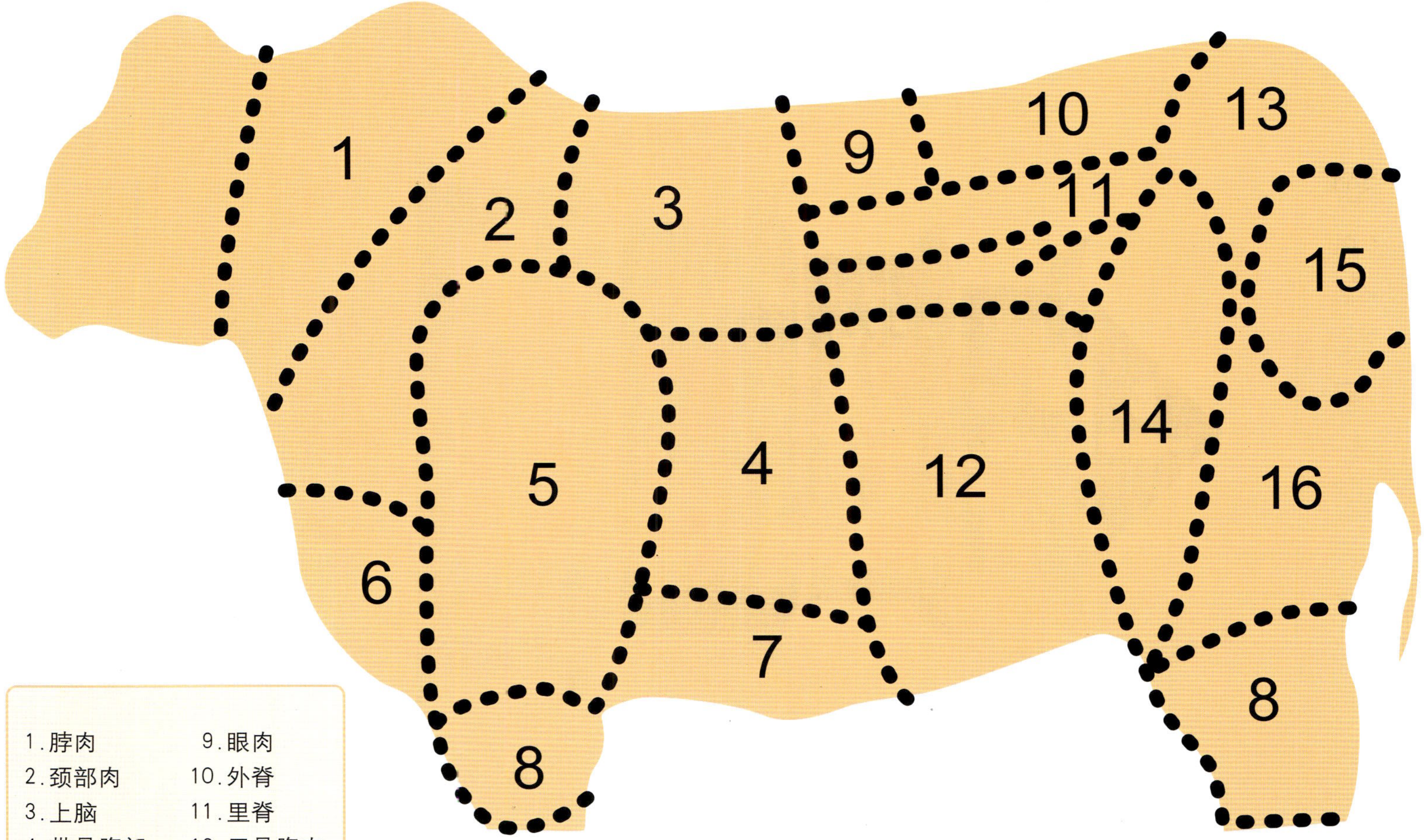

1.脖肉
2.颈部肉
3.上脑
4.带骨腹部
5.肩肉
6.前胸肉
7.后胸肉
8.腱子肉
9.眼肉
10.外脊
11.里脊
12.无骨腹肉
13.臀肉
14.和尚头
15.米龙
16.黄瓜条

中国居民平衡膳食宝塔

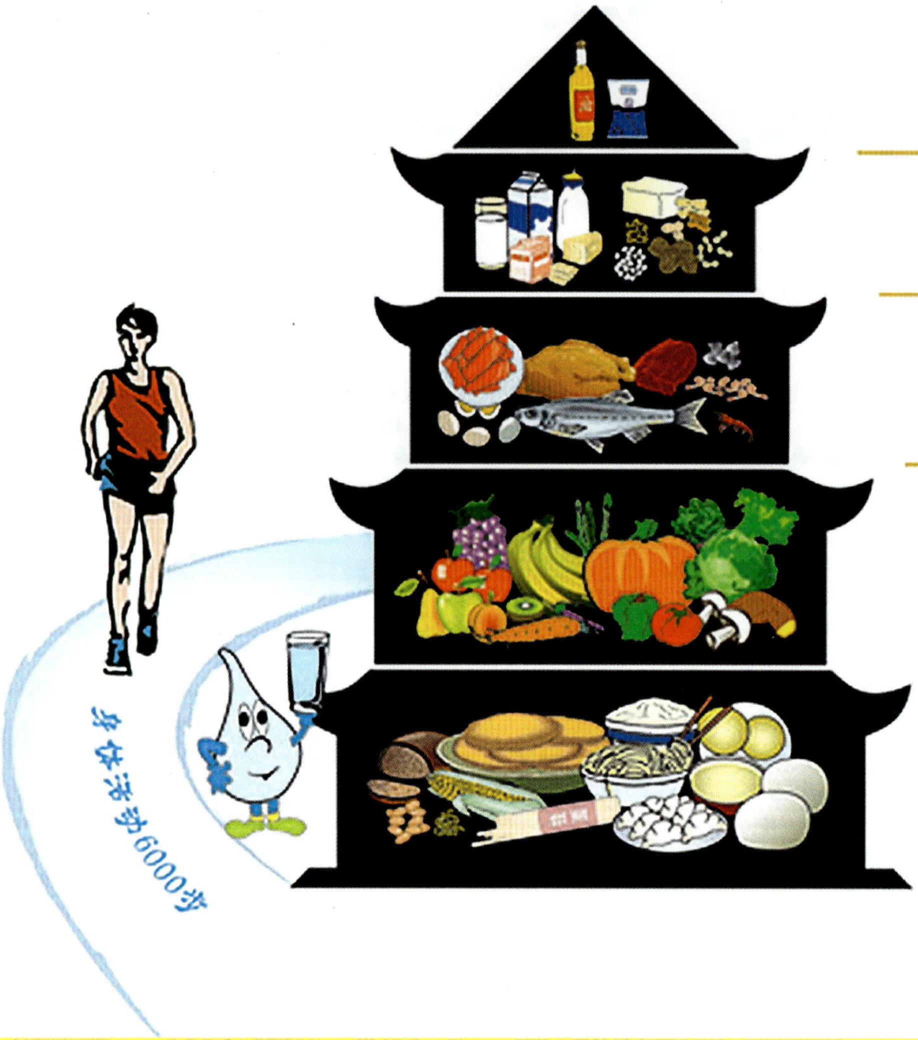

中国营养学会